Third Edition

Handbook of Medical Laboratory Technology

Foreword by

Dr Atul Goel
Director General of Health Services
Ministry of Health & Family Welfare
Government of India

Third Edition

Handbook of Medical Laboratory Technology

Chief Editor

VH Talib
MBBS, MD, PhD, FIC (Path), FIMSA, FCAIC Delhi (India), FIMSA, FRSH (London)

Ex-Head, Department of Pathology and Laboratory Medicine
Safdarjung Hospital, New Delhi
Course Director, Medical Laboratory Technology
(Under Directorate General of Health Services,
Ministry of Health and Family Welfare, Government of India)
VMMC and Safdarjung Hospital, New Delhi

Co-editors

SR Khurana MBBS, DCP
Ex-Senior Medical Officer, Department of Clinical Pathology
Safdarjung Hospital, New Delhi

Saba Talib Groves MBBS, MSc (Micro)
Ex-Resident, Safdarjung Hospital
New Delhi

Sunil Ranga MBBS, MD
Ex-Head, Department of Pathology and Laboratory Medicine
Vardhman Mahavir Medical College and Safdarjung Hospital
New Delhi

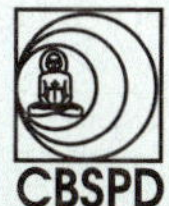

CBS Publishers & Distributors Pvt Ltd
New Delhi • Bengaluru • Chennai • Kochi • Kolkata • Lucknow • Mumbai
Hyderabad • Jharkhand • Nagpur • Patna • Pune • Uttarakhand

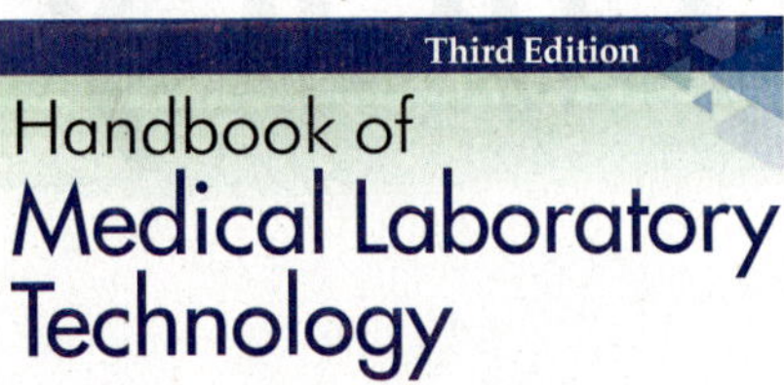

ISBN: 978-93-5466-760-2

Third Edition: 2025
First Edition: 1998
Reprint: 1991, 1993, 1995, 1996, 1998
Second Edition: 1999
Reprint: 2000, 2002, 2003, 2004, 2006, 2007, 2008, 2009, 2011, 2012, 2013, 2014, 2015, 2017, 2019, 2022, 2023

Published by Satish Kumar Jain and produced by Varun Jain for

CBS Publishers & Distributors Pvt Ltd
4819/XI Prahlad Street, 24 Ansari Road, Daryaganj, New Delhi 110 002, India
Ph: 011-23289259, 23266838 Website: www.cbspd.com
e-mail: delhi@cbspd.com

Corporate Office: 204 FIE, Industrial Area, Patparganj, Delhi 110 092, India
Ph: 011-4934 4934 Fax: 011-4934 4935 e-mail: publishing@cbspd.com; publicity@cbspd.com

Branches

- **Bengaluru:** Seema House 2975, 17th Cross, K.R. Road, Banasankari 2nd Stage, Bengaluru 560 070, Karnataka, India
  Ph: +91-80-26771678/79 Fax: +91-80-26771680 e-mail: bangalore@cbspd.com
- **Chennai:** 18/8B, Subbarayan Street, Shenoy Nagar, Chennai 600 030, Tamil Nadu, India
  Ph: +91-44-42032115, 26681266 e-mail: chennai@cbspd.com
- **Kochi:** 42/1325, 1326, Power House Road, Opposite KSEB, Power House, Ernakulum 682018, Kochi, Kerala, India
  Ph: +91-484-4059061–65, 67 Fax: +91-484-4059065 e-mail: kochi@cbspd.com
- **Kolkata:** 147, Hind Ceramics Compound, 1st Floor, Nilgunj Road, Belghoria, Kolkata 700056, West Bengal, India
  Ph: +91-33-25633055/56 e-mail: kolkata@cbspd.com
- **Lucknow:** Basement, Khushnuma Complex, 7 Meerabai Marg (behind Jawahar Bhawan), Lucknow 226001, UP, India
  Ph: +91-522-4000032 e-mail: tiwari.lucknow@cbspd.com
- **Mumbai:** PWD Shed, Gala No. 25/26, Ramchandra Bhatt Marg, Next JJ Hospital Gate No. 2, Opp. Union Bank of India, Noorbaug, Mumbai 400009, Maharashtra, India
  Ph: +91-22-66661880/89 e-mail: mumbai@cbspd.com

Representatives

- **Hyderabad** 0-9885175004
- **Patna** 0-9334159340
- **Jharkhand** 0-9811541605
- **Pune** 0-9664372571
- **Nagpur** 0-8692091830
- **Uttarakhand** 0-9716462459

Printed at: Gokul offset Pvt. Ltd., Okhla Industrial Area, New Delhi, India

Contributors

VH Talib MBBS, MD, PhD, FIC (Path), FIMSA, FCAIC Delhi (India), FIMSA, FRSH (London)
Ex-Head, Department of Pathology and Laboratory Medicine
Safdarjung Hospital, New Delhi

Sunil Ranga MBBS, MD
Ex-Head, Department of Pathology and Laboratory Medicine
Vardhman Mahavir Medical College and Safdarjung Hospital
New Delhi

SR Khurana MBBS, DCP
Ex-Chief Medical Officer, Safdarjung Hospital
New Delhi
CGHS, Delhi

Geeta Ashok Raj MBBS, MD, MNAMS (Morbid Anatomy)
Ex-Professor, Department of Pathology (CIO)
and Professor of Pathology
Dharan, Nepal

Late SN Haldar MBBS
Ex-Head, Blood Bank and Transfusion Services
Safdarjung Hospital, New Delhi, and
Ex-Director, CGHS
Nirman Bhawan, New Delhi

Shashi Gupta MBBS, MD
Ex-Senior Resident
(Clinical Pathology)
Consultant Pathologist, New Delhi

Neha Trivedi MD
Ex-Senior Resident
Laboratory Medicine
Safdarjung Hospital
New Delhi

SH Talib MBBS, MD (Medicine)
Ex-Professor and Head, Department of Medicine
Govt. Medical College and
MGM Medical College
Aurangabad (MS)

Atul Goel MBBS, MD
Director General of Health Services
New Delhi

Kaiser Saleem MBBS, MD
Ex-Senior Resident (Medicine) and
Consultant Medicine
Raipur (MP)

Saba Talib Groves MBBS, MSc (Micro)
Ex-Resident, Safdarjung Hospital
New Delhi

Farah Talib DMD, USA
University of Illinois, College of Dentistry
Angleton Family Dental
Texas 77515

Foreword to the Third Edition

प्रो.(डॉ.) अतुल गोयल
Prof. (Dr.) Atul Goel
MD (Med.)
स्वास्थ्य सेवा महानिदेशक
DIRECTOR GENERAL OF HEALTH SERVICES

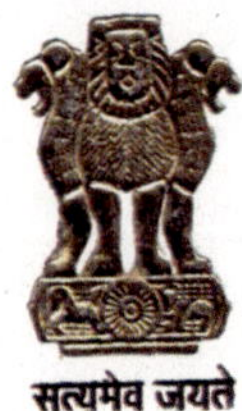

भारत सरकार
स्वास्थ्य एवं परिवार कल्याण मंत्रालय
स्वास्थ्य सेवा महानिदेशालय
Government of India
Ministry of Health & Family Welfare
Directorate General of Health Services

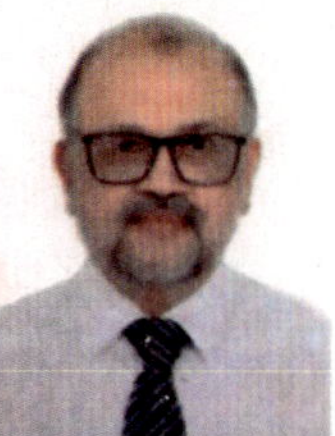

I am pleased to write the Foreword to this book. I was closely associated as one of the contributors (as a house surgeon in Clinical Pathology at Safdarjung Hospital) to its first edition, which was published for the Directorate General of Health Services, Ministry of Health and Family Welfare, in the year 1987. That edition was sponsored by the World Health Organization. It was the first organized source of information for those who underwent training as 'Medical Laboratory Technologists'. While I appreciate the fact that I was acknowledged as a contributor, despite being the junior most staff member of the Department of Clinical Pathology, Safdarjung Hospital, I would have been happier if it had remained a Government Publication as it was to begin with. I would urge the Editors to approach the Ministry of Health and Family Welfare, so that the publication can once again become a Government of India publication, despite being published by CBS Publishers & Distributors.

I am sure it will continue to be of immense usefulness to personnel being trained as Medical Laboratory Technicians. My sincere compliments to all contributors and editors. I end this Foreword with quite a bit of nostalgia fondly remembering people like Mr. Bahuguna (Sr Technician), Dr Shashi Gupta (Senior Resident), Dr SR Khurana (Chief Medical Officer and I/c Blood Bank) and Dr VH Talib (Head, Department of Pathology and Laboratory Medicine) from the Department in 1986–87.

Atul Goel

14th October 2024
New Delhi

Foreword to the Second Edition

This book is a cumulation of the cooperative efforts of the staff of department of clinical pathology, Blood Bank, histopathology and microbiology, Safdarjung Hospital, New Delhi. Although there are many authoritative and exhaustive books on medical laboratory technology yet there is dearth of a handbook in the subject. I appreciate the great pains, hard labour and dedication of the Course Director, Medical Laboratory Technology, in writing and editing of this handbook for the benefit of medical undergraduate and postgraduate students as well as practitioners.

There was a need for such a comprehensive handbook which deals at the same time with subjects of haematology, clinical pathology, biochemistry, microbiology and histopathology, immunology and blood banking with standard methods and their interpretations.

Editors and contributors deserve credit for the excellent hard work and presentation of this handbook which is first of its kind from this country for inservice training course of medical laboratory technology as well as to all medical undergraduate and postgraduate students. I hope the handbook will receive a warm welcome not merely because no Indian book exists in this field but also because comprehensive contents presented in each field of laboratory technology.

Late Dr GK Vishwakarma
Ex-Director General of Health Services

Nirman Bhawan
New Delhi
December 22nd 1987

Preface to the Third Edition

The present edition of the book is the third revision. It was a long pending demand to revise the edition of this book, from all areas of the country which has acquired an outstanding reputation. To keep the revision updated and to incorporate recent advances, we could not keep this book handy and comprehensive yet is most beneficial to medical laboratory technologist, medical undergraduates and postgraduate students. The book is also suitable for all undergraduate and postgraduate students of all allied health sciences.

The revision has been done mostly in sections of haematology, body fluids, immunology and microbiology. Addition and deletion have been done in most of these chapters. A few diagrams and tables have been deleted and more illustrative diagrams and tables have been added. The second edition had 46 chapters and the third edition has 59 comprehensive chapters. Recent advances in automation, quality control, laboratory safety and waste disposal have been much stressed earlier in these chapters. All above mentioned chapters have been revised and updated up to July 2024. Rest of the other chapters will be updated in the next incoming editions.

I keep this opportunity to thank all my students and readers who suggested for revision and updating of this book. I have tried my level best to bring the third edition up-to-date and confirmatory with the demands of all the readers. In spite of this there is still chances of some omission. I shall be grateful if any such is brought to the notice for consultation and corrections in future revision and edition. I am confident this book will be of immense value and help to one and all.

I will remain grateful for the help rendered by the co-author Dr Saba Talib Groves and I owe special thanks to Dr Ambreen Salena Hussain and Dr Farah for the guidance given for the upgradation and revision of the book.

VH Talib

Preface to the First Edition

There is a great need and demand of the comprehensive book in the field of medical laboratory technology. Medical diagnostic laboratory is a backbone not only to clinician but also to the patient. Better diagnosis does mean better patient care.

In preparing this handbook on technology, I have fully utilized the opportunity to include all branches of medical laboratory technology including haematology, clinical pathology, histopathology, biochemistry, microbiology, blood banking and immunology. Most of the important and common tests are now included to make this book as much useful and complete as possible.

All students, technical staff, practitioners and individuals related to diagnostic and/or therapeutic medicine would find this book very useful.

I have tried my level best to bring this first edition up-to-date in confirmatory with limitations of a common laboratory in both urban and rural areas of our country. Being a handbook of laboratory technology, quite a few theoretical aspects have not been dealt due to limitations of space.

In spite of this, there is still a chance of some omissions. I shall be grateful, if any such is brought to notice for consideration in the next edition.

I take this opportunity to thank my friends and colleagues who have contributed various chapters of this handbook, to whom I remain grateful.

VH Talib
Department of Clinical Pathology
Safdarjung Hospital

New Delhi
July 30, 1988

Contents

Section 3A: Microbiology

Section 3B: Virology

Section 3C: Mycology

Section 3D: Parasitology

Section 4: Immunology

Section 1

Haematology

1. Phlebotomy: Peripheral Blood Examination
2. Anticoagulants
3. Haemopoiesis (Haematopoiesis)
4. Anaemias in General and Iron Deficiency Anaemias
5. Megaloblastic Anaemia and Pernicious Anaemia
6. Haemolytic Anaemia and Other Anaemias
7. Normal and Abnormal Haemoglobin—Haemoglobinopathies
8. Aplastic Anaemia
9. Bone Marrow Examination (BME) and Diagnostic Significance of Peripheral Blood Examination
10. Leukaemias, Myelodysplastic Syndromes, and Myeloproliferative Disorders
11. Normal Haemostasis and Haemostatic Disorders
12. LE Cell Phenomenon and Systemic Lupus Erythematosus

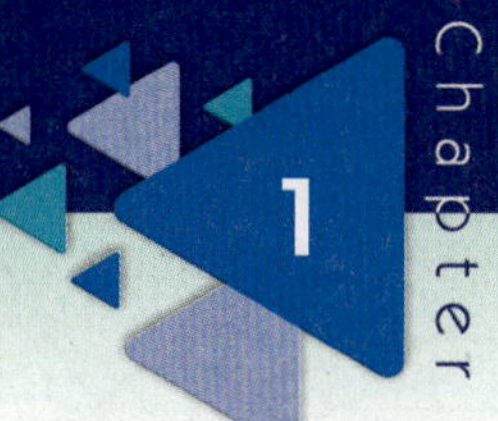

Phlebotomy: Peripheral Blood Examination

Chapter Outline

- Collection of Blood
- Relevant Anatomy
- Equipment
- Venous Blood
- Contraindications
- Hospitalised Patients
- Capillary Blood
- Artery Blood
- Arterial and Venous Anatomy
- Complications Related to Arterial Blood Sampling
- Vacutainer System
- Vacutainer Needle Parts

All staff should be trained in, phlebotomy, to prevent unnecessary risk of exposure to blood and to reduce adverse events for patients.

- Groups of health workers who historically are not formally trained in phlebotomy should be encouraged to take up such training; lax infection prevention and control practices result in poor safety for staff and risk to patients.

COLLECTION OF BLOOD

There are three ways of obtaining the samples

i. From the vein
ii. From the capillary
iii. Arterial blood.

Venous blood is preferred because a number of investigations can be done and repeated on the same sample and because the examination can be done at leisure.

Relevant Anatomy

- The median cubital and cephalic veins are preferred for blood sampling, but other arm and hand veins may be used.
- The cephalic vein is located on the lateral (radial) side of the arm, and the basilic vein is located on the medial (ulnar) side. These veins extend through and branch within the antecubital fossa, creating the large antecubital and proximal forearm veins.

Equipment

- Skin-cleansing materials: Alcohol, chlorhexidine, or povidone-iodine swabs or wipes.
- Nonsterile gloves (sterile gloves if blood cultures are being obtained)
- Tourniquet, single-use
- Needle system, e.g. needle and syringe, or needle and vaccum tube, typically 21-gauge needles for adults; 22- or 23-gauge for neonates, small children, and sometimes older.
- Butterfly needles attached to a syringe may be preferred for difficult venipuncture (e.g. small veins in neonates, fragile veins in older people).
- If a suitable vein is difficult to locate, try lowering the extremity and/or applying warm compresses or nitroglycerin ointment to help dilate veins.
- Well-fitting gloves make palpation of the vein easier.

Venous Blood

Venous blood is obtained by venepuncture. Good light and a comfortable position for both the patient and the operator are necessary. Ideally, the patient should be lying down. In the adult, one of the veins in the antecubital fossa is chosen. Make the veins prominent by applying a tourniquet or a blood pressure cuff kept at the diastotlic pressure; further, the patient is asked to open and close his hand several times vigorously and then keep the first clinched on a roll of bandage. Select the vein that is both visible and palpable and well fixed to the surrounding tissue (Fig. 1.1). Check all the pieces of equipment, the needle should be sharp (19–20 swg) patent and tight fitting. The syringe should be dry and with all the air expelled from it; and the bottle or the tube to receive the sample must be ready at hand. The patient is reassured and the part-cleaned with clean gauge or cotton moistened with rectified spirit. The patient's forearm is grasped with left hand and to steady the vein, the thumb retracts downwards soft tissues below the site of the

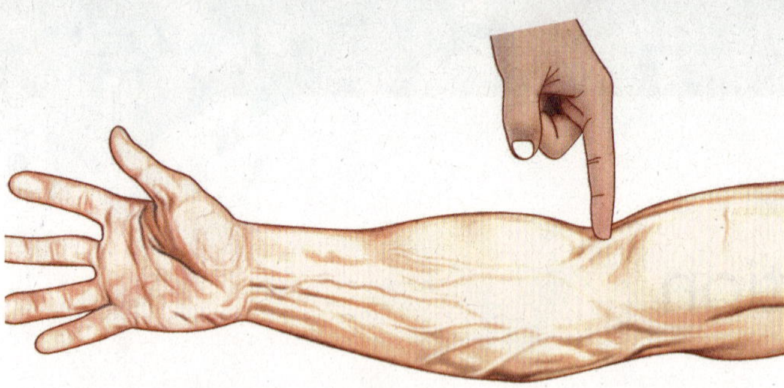

Fig. 1.1: Visible, palpable veins in antecubital fossa

puncture. The needle is brought to the skin over the vein, the bevel of the needle turned up. If the vein is large and well fixed, the skin and the vein may be punctured with a single short thrust. If the vein is small or slippery, the skin is punctured first and the vein next, the plunger is pulled back gently. When the blood starts flowing into the syringe, the tourniquet is released and after sufficient blood has been collected the needle is withdrawn. The punctured site is gently pressed with a swab of cotton or gauge moistened with spirit for two minutes, the patient elevates the arm and is asked maintain the pressure for a few minutes more to prevent a haematoma. Before emptying the syringe into the bottle, the needle must be removed. The contents are delivered slowly and mixed with anticoagulant by gentle shaking for 1 minute.

Warnings and Common Errors

- If the vein is not entered, do not try to reposition the needle by moving the tip to one side or another; this can push the vein out of the way and also damage tissue. Instead, withdraw the needle partway before changing the angle and direction of insertion.
- It is no longer recommended to flex the elbow after antecubital venipuncture.

Contraindications

Relative Contraindications

- Infection or haematoma at a prospective venipuncture site.
- Injured or massively edematous extremity
- Thrombotic or phlebitic vein
- Intravenous catheter distal to a prospective venipuncture site (may affect laboratory results if IV fluids or drugs are infusing distal to the venipuncture site)
- Arteriovenous graft or fistula
- Ipsilateral mastectomy

In the above situations, use another site (e.g. the opposite arm) for venipuncture.

Coagulopathy is not a contraindication, but sites must be compressed for a longer time after venipuncture.

Complications

Complications are uncommon and include

- Local infection
- Arterial puncture
- Haematoma or bleeding
- Damage to the vein
- Nerve damage
- Vasovagal syncope

Aftercare

- Recheck the site after a few minutes to verify the absence of haemorrhage/haematoma.

Hospitalised Patients

- In hospitalised patients, do not take blood from an existing peripheral venous access site because this may give false results. Haemolysis, contamination and presence of intravenous fluid and medication all can alter the results. Nursing staff and physicians may access central venous lines for specimens following protocols. However, specimens from central lines carry a risk of contamination or erroneous laboratory test results.

Additional Considerations

- Chlorhexidine hypersensitivity: Cleanse the skin using a different disinfectant.
- Latex hypersensitivity: Use latex-free gloves and tourniquet.
- Efficient, expeditious performance of the procedure is required to avoid prolonged tourniquet placement and blood stasis.
- If povidone-iodine is used to cleanse the skin, allow it to dry and then remove it with isopropyl alcohol, to avoid erroneous blood test resutls (e.g. hyperkalemia, hyperphosphatemia, or hyperuricemia) and also to avoid skin irritation.

Tips and Tricks

- If a suitable vein is difficult to locate, try lowering the extremity and/or applying warm compresses or nitroglycerin ointment to help dilate veins.
- Well-fitting gloves make palpation of the vein easier.
- Instruct patients to look away from the equipment and the procedure to help prevent a vasovagal episode.

Capillary Blood

Capillary blood is obtained by pricking the skin. Only a few drops of blood can be collected in this manner. Blood is collected directly in appropriate pipettes and has to be manipulated it immediately. Haemoglobin estimation, red cell count, leucocyte count, platelet count and reticulocyte count can be done with capillary blood.

For preparing smears for a differential count, capillary blood without an anticoagulant is perferred.

In adult, capillary blood is obtained from the ball of the fingers and the lobes of the ear; in infants, the sites are the ball of the thumb, great toe or the heel.

Technique

Examine the site of the puncture to make sure that there is no oedema or congestion or that the site is not too cold or blood less. In the last, place the part in warm water for prompt congestion. Both the patient and the operator should be seated comfortably and in good light. All the apparatus must be ready to hand before the site is punctured. The site chosen is cleaned with spirit and the part must be allowed to dry completely before puncture is made. The point of the needle is touched to the skin and a bold quick prick is made. The prick must be deep enough (2–4 mm) to ensure a free flow of blood. The needle must be sharp and sterilized. Blood must flow spontaneously from the stab. The first drop is wiped off and the second one used for filling pipette. Squeezing of the finger is not permissible as this will dilute the blood with the tissue fluid.

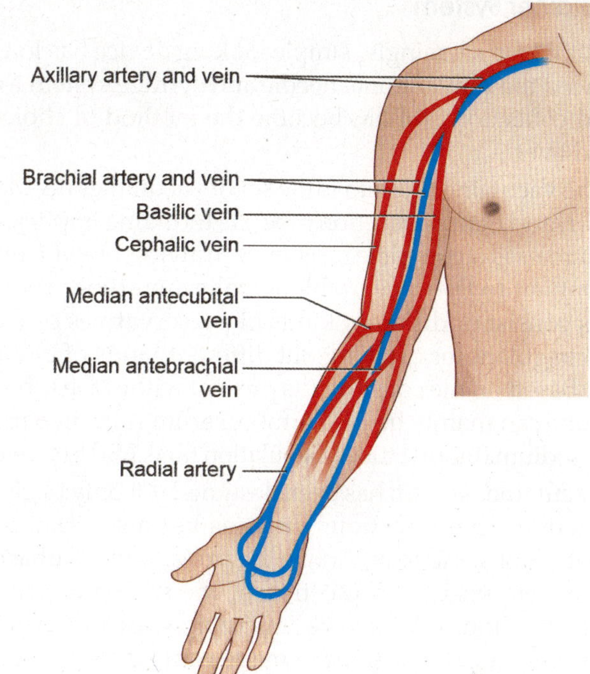

Fig. 1.2: Anatomy of arterial and venous system

Artery Blood

Choice of Site

Several different arteries can be used for blood collection. The first choice is the radial artery, which is located on the thumb side of the wrist; because of its small size, use of this artery requires extensive skill in arterial blood sampling.

Arterial and Venous Anatomy

- The radial artery lies close to the skin over the ventrolateral distal wrist, just medial to the radial styloid process and lateral to the flexor carpi radialis tendon. The artery runs deeper in the more proximal wrist and the forearm (Fig. 1.2).
- Avoid pushing too hard on the artery while palpating the pulse during needle insertion; doing so may compress the artery and make it harder to cannulate.
- Some arterial lines are sensitive to wrist position; be alert to changes in the pressure and/or waveform with patient movement. The wrist may need to be immobilized in the most satisfactory position.

Alternative sites for access are brachial or femoral arteries, but these have several disadvantages.

An arterial blood sample is collected from an artery, primarily to determine arterial blood gases. Arterial blood sampling should only be performed by health workers for whom the procedure is in the legal scope of practice for their position in their country and who have demonstated proficiency after formal training.

The sample can be obtained either through a catheter placed in an artery, or by using a needle and syringe to puncture an artery. These syringes are pre-heparinized and handled to minimize air exposure that will alter the blood gas values.

Complications Related to Arterial Blood Sampling

There are several potential complications related to arterial blood sampling. The points below list some of the complications related to the procedure, and how they can be prevented.

- *Arteriospasm* or involuntary contraction of the artery may be prevented simply by helping the patient relax; this can be achieved, for example, by explaining the procedure and positioning the person comfortably.
- *Haematoma* or excessive bleeding can be prevented by inserting the needle without puncturing the far side of the vessel and by applying pressure immediately after blood is drawn. Due to the higher pressure present in arteries, pressure should be applied for a longer time than when sampling from a vein, and should be supervised more closely, to check for cessation of bleeding.
- *Fainting* or a *vasovagal response* can be prevented by ensuring that the patient is supine (lying down on their back) with feet elevated before beginning the blood draw. Patients requiring arterial blood sampling are usually inpatients or in the emergency ward, so will generally already be lying in a hospital bed. Children may feel a loss of control and fight more if placed in a supine position; in such cases, it may be preferable to have the child sitting on the parent's lap.

Vacutainer System

Vacutainer, a seemingly, simple looking device has long replaced the conventional needle and syringe system for blood collection and has become the method of choice world over.

The vacutainer system is the set of vacutainer needle, holder, and blood collection tube. As the name implies, a vacutainer is a complete system of drawing blood from the patient to the vaccum blood collection tube. These tubes consist of different kinds of preservatives or the anti-coagulant for carrying out different kinds of blood tests. Based on the constituents present within the tubes, the tube can mainly be EDTA tube, serum tube, heparin tube, sodium fluoride tube, coagulation tube, ESR tube, etc.

Vacutainer system has been designed not only to give protection from infectious diseases but also ensure a high level of standardisation in the pre-analytical phase. The system ensures protection of the specimen from contamination, haemolysis, microclots, evaporation, etc. The system has also been made compatible to most modern automated analytical machines of laboratory, eliminating many of the manual steps, further improving the handling of test procedures.

Vacutainer Needle Parts

A vacutainer needle is a type of needle, that is used to draw blood from the patient.

As shown in Figs 1.3 to 1.5, the major components of the vacutainer needles are the bevel, shaft, threaded tub, and rubber sleeves covering the needle.

The sizes of the needle generally range from 1 to 1.5 inches with the gauge value ranging from 19 to 22.

The procedure of blood drawn is shown in Fig. 1.6 (1–3).

Vacutainer collection tube is like a self-aspirating syringe and is evacuated to draw certain volume of blood (Fig. 1.7). Vacuum is retained by a special hemogard stopper, which makes it leakproof and eliminates any chance of blood exposure due to spillage. In addition, these collection tubes come with precise and accurate amount of high quality additive and preservatives, identifiable by international colour codes. The precise vacuum in the tube ensures a right mix of additive and blood ratio, very vital for correct analysis of specimen in the laboratory in order to achieve accurate and true result for analyte.

Various types of colour coded vacutainer collection tubes available in the market, mostly by and large BD company in use (Fig. 1.8).

Various types of collecting tubes with type of colour indicated in their respective caps and label on tubes with their uses information given in Table 1.1.

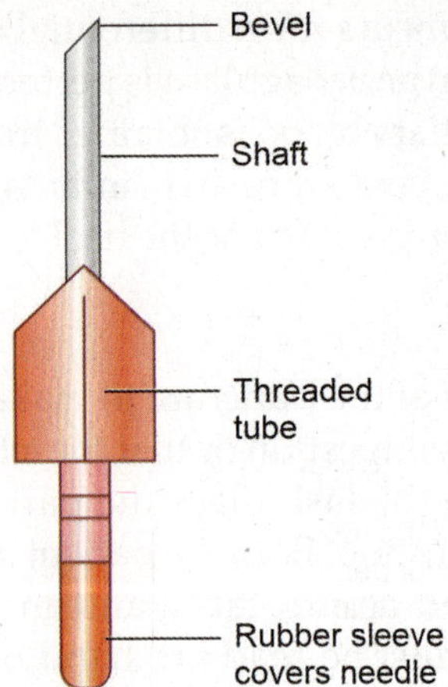

Fig. 1.3: Vacutainer multi-sample needle

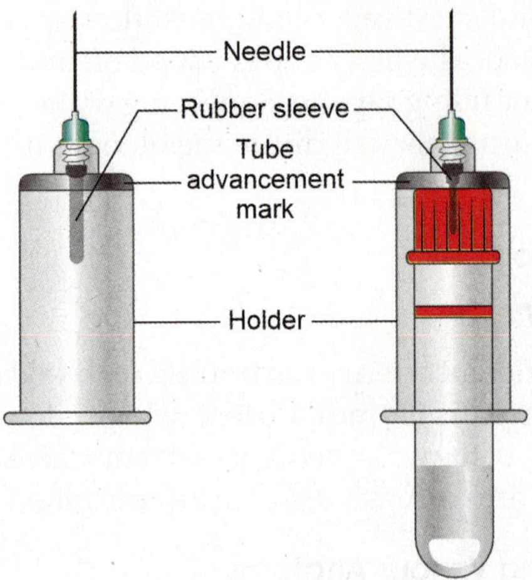

Fig. 1.4: Vacutainer label diagram

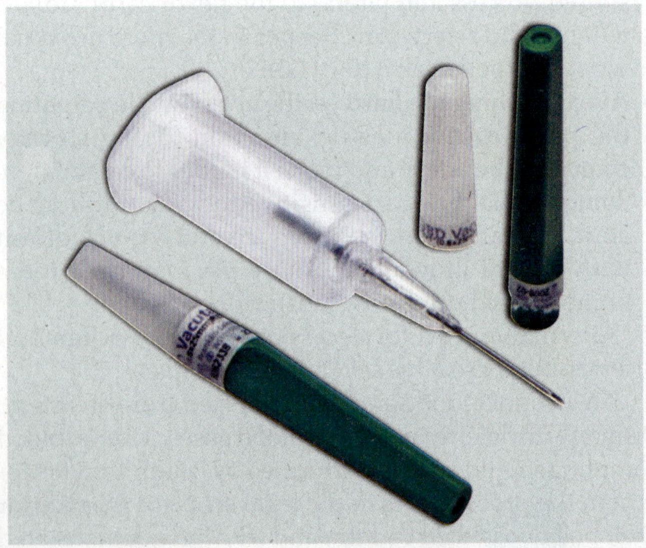

Fig. 1.5: Parts of vacutainer needle covers

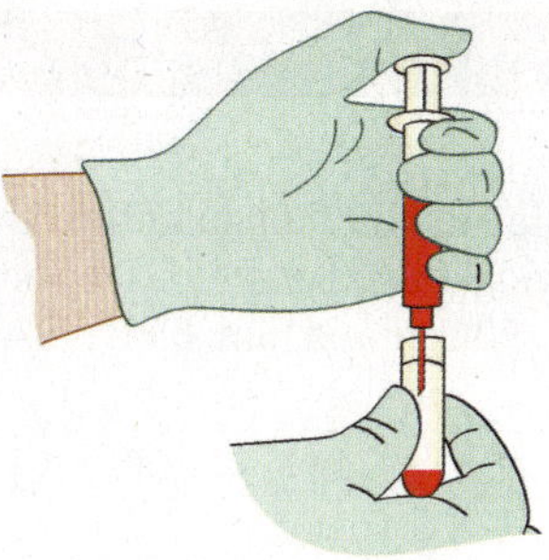

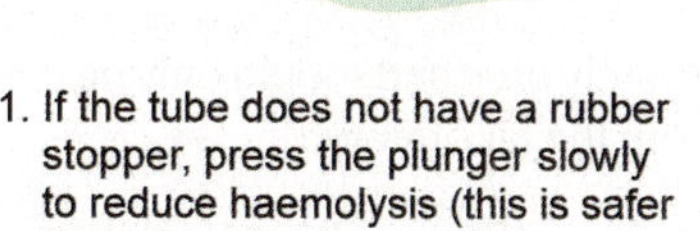

1. If the tube does not have a rubber stopper, press the plunger slowly to reduce haemolysis (this is safer than removing the needle)

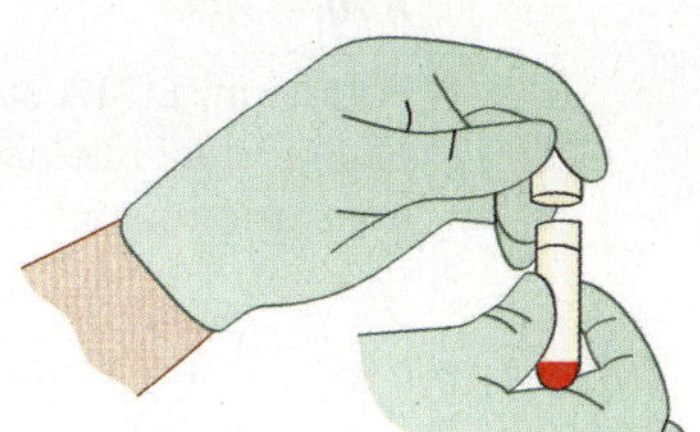

2. Place the stopper in the tube

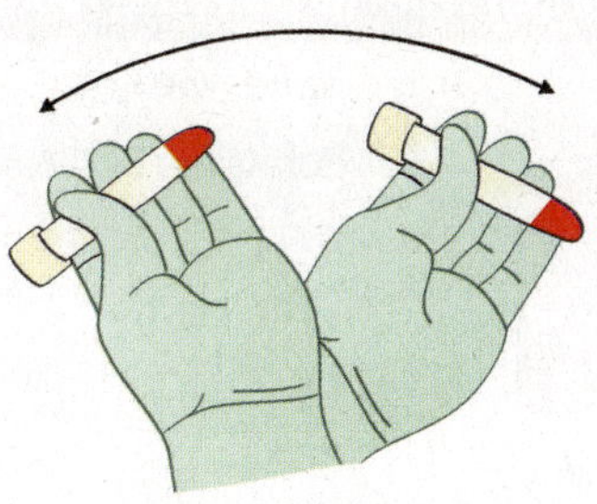

3. Following laboratory instructions invert the sample gently to mix the additives with the blood before dispatch

Fig. 1.6: Procedure of blood for further processing

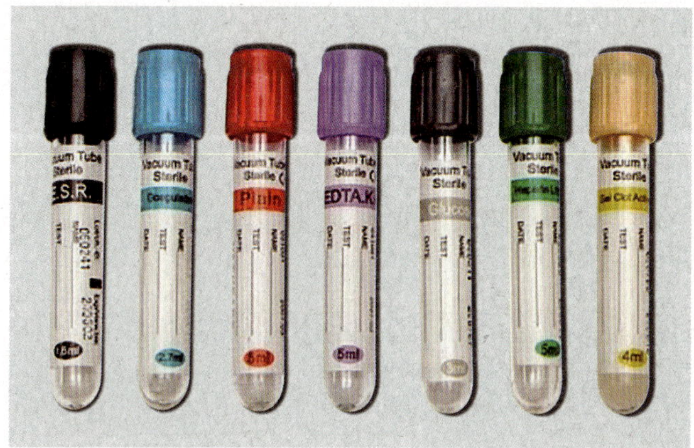

Fig. 1.7: Vacutainer collecting tubes (Chinese) in different standard colours in use

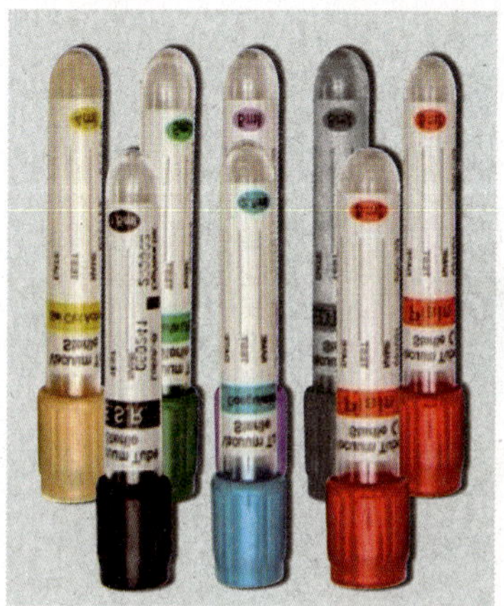

Fig. 1.8: Collecting tubes (BD company)

Table 1.1: Various types of collecting tubes

Tube colour	*Tube type*	*Information*
Gold	Serum separating tube (SST)	This tube type is used for the vast majority of biochemistry immunology and serology tests. Please check the website if unsure of the correct sample type.
Green	Lithium heparin/plasma separating tube	A few of the tests that use this tube type require the plasma to be frozen within half an hour of the sample being take. Please check the test information on the website
Royal Blue	Sodium heparin tube	These samples are used to check the levels of trace metals—lead and mercury in the blood.

Contd.

Table 1.1: Various types of collecting tubes (Contd.)

Tube colour	*Tube type*	*Information*
Lavender	Potassium EDTA tube	Potassium EDTA serves as the anticoagulant for the performance of almost all haematological tests. Larger EDTA bottles are used for transfusion samples only. FBC, blood film, ESR, HBA1c
Red	Plain tube	These tubes are very rarely used and should only be used for a specimen under instruction from the laboratory.
Grey	Fluoride oxalate tube	Anticoagulant and fluoride salt act as a glycolysis inhibitor to stabilise the glucose concentration in the sample. Main tests analysed on the sample: Glucose, lactate and alcohol
	Coagulation screen INR D-dimer	
	U+E, CRP, LFTs, amylase, calcium, phosphate, magnesium TFTs, lipid profile, troponins	

The supply of tubes comes in package of 100 tubes as in case of EDTA tubes as shown in Fig. 1.9.

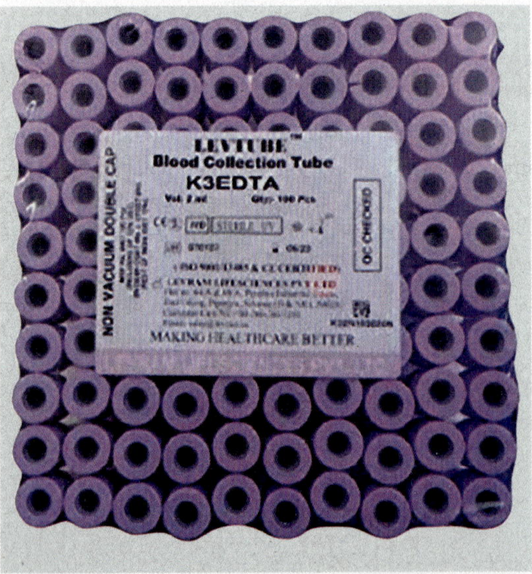

Fig. 1.9: Collection tube of EDTA tube package in 100 tubes supply

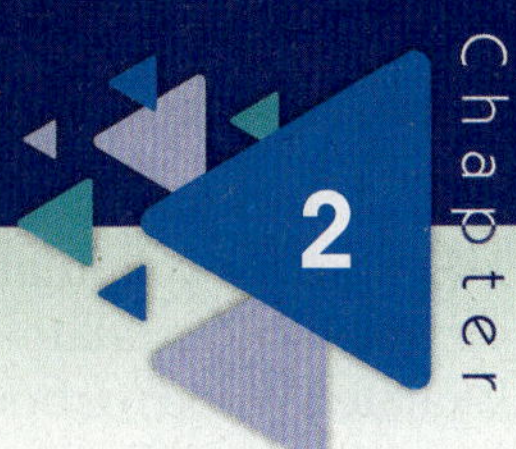

Anticoagulants

Chapter Outline

ANTICOAGULANTS

For various purposes a number of different anticoagulants available. The anticoagulants in use are:

1. Disodium or dipotassium ethylenediaminetetraacetic acid (EDTA; Sequestrene).
2. Ammonium and potassium oxalate mixture
3. Tri-sodium citrate
4. Heparin and
5. Acid-citrate-dextrose (ACD) solution

1. Ethylenediaminetetraacetic acid (EDTA)

The sodium and potassium salts of EDTA are powerful anticoagulants and they are the anticoagulants of choice for routine haematological work. EDTA acts by its chelating effect on the calcium molecules in blood. To achieve this requires a concentration of 1.2 mg (approximately 4 μmol) of the anhydrous salt per ml of blood. The recommended concentration of the dipotassium salt is 1.50 ± 0.25 mg/ml of blood.

The dilithium salt of EDTA is equally effective as an anticoagulant, and its use has the advantage that the same sample of blood can be used for chemical investigations. However, it is less soluble than the dipotassium salt (160 g/L).

EDTA is not suitable for use in the investigation of coagulation problems and should not be used in the estimation of prothrombin time.

2. Ammonium and potassium oxalate mixture

This consists of a mixture of 2 parts of potassium oxalate and 3 parts of ammonium oxalate. Take 1% solution of potassium oxalate 0.4 ml and 1% solution of ammonium oxalate 0.6 ml in a test tube. Evaporate to dryness in the incubator. This amount of oxalates is sufficient to prevent coagulation of 5 ml blood.

3. Trisodium citrate

0.109 mol/L trisodium citrate (32 g/L $Na_3C_6H_5O_7 2H_2O$) is the anticoagulant of choice in coagulation studies. Nine volumes of blood are added to 1 volume of the sodium citrate solution and immediately well mixed with it. Sodium citrate is also the anticoagulant most widely used in the estimation of the sedimentation rate (ESR); for 4 volumes of venous blood are diluted with 1 volume of the sodium citrate solution.

4. Heparin

This may be used at a concentration of 15 ± 2.5 IU per ml of blood. Heparin is an effective anticoagulant and does not alter the size of the red cells and a good dry anticoagulant when it is important to reduce to a minimum the chance of lysis occurring after blood, has been withdrawn. However, heparinized blood should not be used for making blood films as it gives a faint blue colouration to the background when the films are stained by Romanowsky dyes. This is especially marked in the presence of abnormal proteins. Heparin is the best anticoagulant to use for osmotic fragility tests; otherwise it is inferior to EDTA for general use and should not be used for leucocyte count as it tends to cause the leucocytes to clump.

5. Acid-citrate-dextrose (ACD) solution

This is preferred for blood transfusions, for preserving red cells, for enzyme studies, and for the study of haemolytic processes. A standard preparation consists of sodium citrate 1.32 gm, citric acid 0.48 gm, dextrose 1.40 gm, and distilled water to 100 ml. One ml of ACD solution is sufficient to prevent coagulation of 4 ml of blood.

Mode of Action of Anticoagulants

EDTA and sodium citrate remove calcium which is essential for coagulation. Calcium is either precipitated as insoluble oxalate (crystals of which may be seen in oxalated blood) or bound in a non-ionized form. Heparin works in a different way; it neutralizes thrombin by inhibiting the interaction of several clotting factors in the presence of a plasma co-factor, antithrombih Ill. Sodium citrate or heparin can be used to render blood incoagulable before transfusion.

For better long-term preservation of red cell for certain tests and for transfusion purposes citrate is used in combination with dextrose in the form of acid-citrate-dextrose (ACD), citrate-phosphate-dextrose (CPD) or Alsever's solution.

Effects of Anticoagulants of Blood Cell Morphology

If blood is allowed to stand in the laboratory before films are made, degenerative changes occur. The'changes are not solely due to the presence of an anticoagulant for they also occur in defibrinated blood.

Irrespective of anticoagulant, films made from blood which has been standing for not more than 1 hr at room temperature (18–25°C), are not easily distinguished from films made immediately after collection of the blood. By 3 hours changes may be discernible and by 12–18 hours these become striking. Some but not all neutrophils are affected: their nuclei may stain more homogeneously than in fresh blood, the nuclear lobes may become separated and the cytoplasmic margin may appear ragged or less well defined; small vacuoles appear in the cytoplasm. Some or many of the large mononuclears develop marked changes; small vacuoles appear in the cytoplasm and the nucleus undergoes irregular lobulation which may almost amount to disintegration. Some of the lymphocytes, too, undergo a similar type of change; a few vacuoles may be seen in the cytoplasm and the nucleus may undergo major budding so as to give rise to nuclei with two or three lobes. Other lymphocyte nuclei may stain more homogeneously than usual.

The red cells (of normal blood at least) are little affected by standing for up to 6 hours at room temperature (18–25°C). Longer periods lead to progressive crenation and sphering.

The cells in defibrinated blood undergo degenerative changes at about the same rate as those in EDTA blood.

All the above changes are retarded but not abolished in blood kept at 4°C. Their occurrence underlines the importance of making films as soon as possible after withdrawal. But delay of up to 1–3 hours or so is certainly permissible.

The practice of making films of blood before it is added to the antfcoagulant (e.g. at the bedside) is to be commended, especially when screening for lead toxicity, as the granules of punctate basophilia may not stain in anticoagulated blood. In fresh blood films, however, the platelets usually clump and it is less easy to estimate the platelet count from inspection of the film. Such films are nevertheless of particular value in investigating patients suspected of suffering from purpura, as in certain rare conditions, the absence of platelet clumping is a useful pointer to the diagnosis.

PREPARATION AND STAINING OF PERIPHERAL BLOOD SMEARS

Peripheral smear provides information about red cells—their number, shape, size and variation in morphology to diagnose different types of anaemia and other haematologic disorders. It also provides information for differential leucocyte count, platelets, abnormal cells and haemoparasites.

Procedure

1. Take a drop of blood from a finger prick and put it on a clean slide 1 cm from the end.
2. Take another slide with a smooth edgespreader and place the edge over the drop so that blood spreads along the edge.
3. Keep the spreader slide at approximately 30–40° angle and make a smear with a forward movement of the spreader. Smear should be 2.5–3.5 cm in length and spreader should preferably have smaller edge than the slide on which smear is being made.
4. Air dry the smear.
5. Make at least 2 smears of each sample.

Fixation of the Smear

Smears should be fixed within 4 hours to get good staining of cells and avoid background staining of plasma.

Take methanol in a Coplin jar. Give 4–6 dips to the smear in methanol. Let it get air dry.

Staining of the Smear

Staining of the smears is carried out using Romanowsky's stains which stain red cells, white cells, platelets and parasites. Romanowsky's stains consist of mixture of methylene blue, eosin and methylene blue oxidation products—azures which are formed by interaction and chemical treatment of the stain.These products are responsible for different shades of staining, e.g. red cells—pink, eosinophilic granules—red—orange; basophilic granules—bluish black; neutrophilic granules—lilac (azurophilic granules combine with azures of the stain); nuclear chromatin—purple black; white cell cytoplasm—faint purple.

Following are the commonly used stains:

- Leishman stain
- Giemsa stain
- Wright's stain

- Jenner's stain
- Jenner-Giemsa stain

Most of the routine laboratories use

- Giemsa stain
- Leishman stain

The details are given as follows.

Leishman stain

Leishman stain powder	1 gm
Methanol (acetone free)	500 ml

Mix the two. Warm the mixture to 50°C for 15 minutes in a conical flask. Filter the stain and the stain is ready for use after 2 days.

Giemsa stain

Giemsa stain powder	1 gm
Glycerol	66 ml
Methanol	66 ml

Dissolve Giemsa stain in glycerol at 60°C for 2 hours. Cool it. Add 66 ml of methanol (acetone free) and mix. Keep it at 37°C for 1 week to ripen. Stain is filtered before use.

Buffer water (Sorensen's phosphate buffer)

Solution A

Potassium dihydrogen phosphate	9.08 gm/L

Solution B

Dibasic sodium phosphate	9.47 gm/L
For pH 6.8	
Solution A	50.8 ml
Solution B	49.2 ml

Mix the two solutions to get 100 ml of buffer water.

Leishman's Staining

- Place the PS (peripheral smear) on the staining rack.
- Pour the stain on the slide with a dropper and count the drops and cover the whole slide with the stain.
- After 2 minutes, pour double the number of drops of buffer water or distilled water on the slide and mix buffer with stain using a dropper.
- Let the slide be stained by this mixture for 15–30 minutes. Exact time to be decided for each batch of stain.
- Pour running water from one side of the slide so that the stain scum is drained off the slide and no more stain is left on the slide.
- Pick up the slide and keep it slanting for it to dry up.
- The slide is ready for examination.

Sources of Error

- If the pH of the buffer is too acidic, then red cells stain pink, and WBCs stain very light.
- If the pH of the buffer is too basic, red cells stain blue and WBCs take a bluish black hue. Hence for proper staining buffer with correct pH 6.8 should be used.
- Sometimes red cells demonstrate holes in them. These are due to air bubbles because of air drying in humid weather. To overcome this, smear should be dried up quickly by waving it vigorously in air.

Giemsa Staining

- Fixation of the smears 8–10 dips in methanol in a Coplin jar.
- Dry the slides and then pour the diluted (1 in 10) stain for 20–30 minutes. Exact dilution and time of staining to be determined for each batch of stain.
- Wash the slide (as in Leishman staining) and dry it.

Evaluation of a Peripheral Smear

Apply very thin layer of oil all over the smear and examine it under low power. Area for DLC-tail and edges of the smear should be avoided while doing DLC, since monocytes and neutrophils predominate in these areas. This area is better suited for parasites like malarial parasite, microfilaria, since these are heavier than red cells carried to the tail by the spreader. DLC should be carried out in thin part of the smear next to the tail. For red cell morphology, the best area is between tail and body of the smear. Tail, head and edges should be avoided.

HAEMOGLOBIN ESTIMATION

The haemoglobin (Hb) content in a blood sample may be determined by measurement of its colour, its power of combining with oxygen or carbon monoxide or by its iron content. The clinical methods for routine purpose are all based on colour or light intensity matching techniques:

A. i. Sahli or acid-haematin method (Fig. 2.1)
   ii. Alkaline-haematin method
   iii. Haldanes carboxyhaemoglobin method
   iv. Oxyhaemoglobin method
   v. Cyanmethaemoglobin method

B. Copper sulphate specific gravity method

Haemoglobin is a chromoprotein consisting of the colourless globin molecule attached to four red coloured haem molecules. The globin molecule consists of two alpha polypeptide chains and two beta polypeptide chains. Haem is a metal complex containing an iron atom in the centre of a porphyrin structure. Haemoglobin is formed in developing erythrocytes (normoblasts) in the marrow.

The biosynthesis of haemoglobin involves the triad of manufacture of haem, manufacture of globin and iron metabolism. Methods for estimation of haemoglobin are as follows:

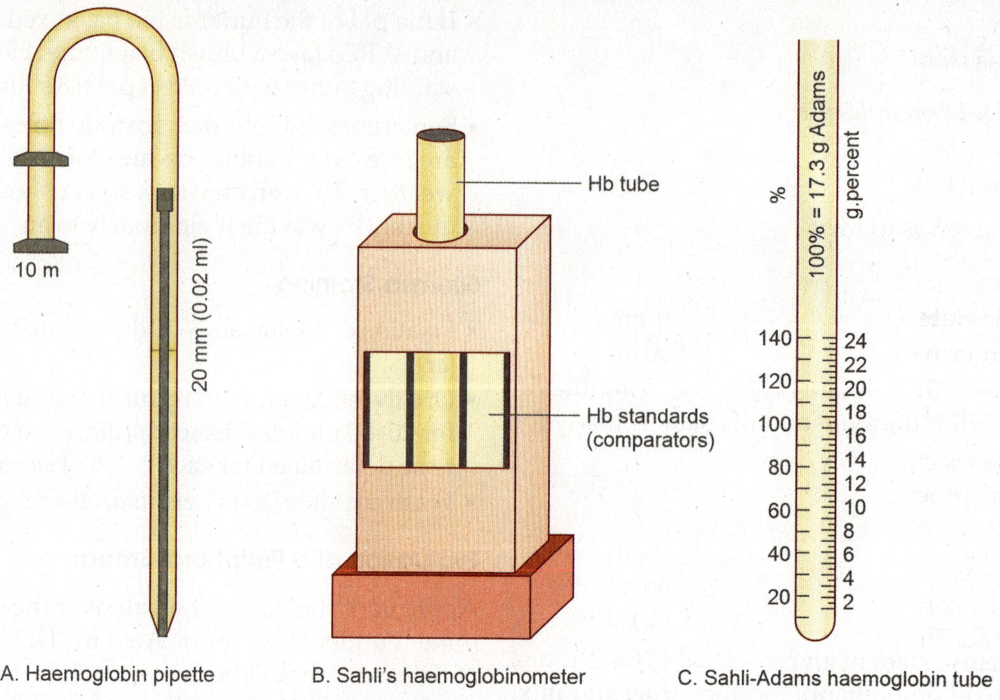

Fig. 2.1: Sahli's acid haematin method

A. i. Sahli's Acid Haematin Method

Principle: Hb is converted into acid haematin by hydrochloric acid. The brown colour of the compound is matched against a brown glass standard in a comparator.

Apparatus: Sahli-type haemoglobinometer consisting of the comparator with glass standards, a square Hb tube marked both grams and percentage figures and Hb pipette marked at 20 cu mm, 0.1 N HCl and distilled water.

Technique

1. Fill the Hb calibrated tube up to the mark 20 (not less) with 0.1 N HCl by means of a dropper.
2. Fill the Hb pipette exactly up to 20 cu mm mark by gently controlled sucking; the pipette is held horizontal while taking the blood. If a slight excess is drawn in, it may be removed by touching the point of the pipette with the finger or gauge. If a great excess has been drawn in, inaccuracy will result, in this case the pipette must be cleaned, dried and refilled. Wipe off with gauge the blood on the outside of the pipette.
3. Empty the pipette into acid in the tube by keeping the point of the pipette to the bottom of the tube and gently blowing off the blood without causing bubbles. Rinse the pipette at least three times by drawing in and discharging the blood acid mixture. Now withdraw the pipette half way up the tube and rinse the outside of pipette with a few drops of the acid.
4. Mix the acid haematin solution in the tube with the glass rod and allow the tube to stand for 10 minutes. In this interval at least 95% of the colour of acid haematin is developed.
5. Now dilute the solution of acid haematin by adding distilled water, drop by drop, stirring the mixture all the time wtih glass rod. The comparator is held against good daylight and the additon of water continued till the colour of solution matches perfectly with that of the standards. Take the reading in grams per cent. The bottom of the meniscus is read.

Normal Range

Males	13–18 gm
Females	11–16 gm
Newborns	14–19 gm%

Significance

Low Hb values are seen in various types of anaemias.

High Hb values are seen in polycythaemia rubra vera, secondary erythrocytosis.

ii. Alkaline-Haematin Method

Haemoglobin, methaemoglobin, carboxyhaemoglobin and sulphaemoglobin are converted to alkaline haematin by addition of sodium hydroxide, a strong alkali. It forms a true solution and the brown colour can be read against comparable standards or in a colourimeter. Foetal haemoglobin and Hb-Barts are alkali-resistant, but can be converted by heating in a boiling water bath for 4 minutes or by collecting the blood first into acid and then adding alkali (acid-alkali method).

iii. Haldane's Carboxyhaemoglobin Method

Haemoglobin is converted to carboxyhaemoglobin (which is bright red in colour), by exposing it to carbon monoxide (CO). It is a relatively accurate method but CO is dangerous.

iv. Oxyhaemoglobin Method

Haemoglobin is converted to oxyhaemoglobin by mixing blood with a dilute solution of sodium carbonate or ammonium hydroxide. The intensity of the colour obtained is measured colourimetrically. It is a fast and accurate method, but traces of copper can give errors.

v. Cyanmethaemoglobin Method

Principle: Potassium ferricyanide converts Hb from ferrous to ferric state to form meth-Hb. The resulting meth-Hb combines with potassium cyanide to produce the stable pigment cyanmeth-Hb. Cyanmeth-Hb represents the sum of oxy-Hb, carboxy-Hb and meth-Hb.

Apparatus: Photoelectric colourimeter with filter 540 nm, test tubes, 5 ml pipettes and 20 µl micropipette (an accurately calibrated Sahli's pipette may be used).

Precaution: Do not pipette reagent by mouth. This reagent is poisonous. The concentration of KCN in Hb diluting reagent is 50 mg/L. The lethal dose of Hb diluting reagent is about 4,000 mg/L.

Reagent Drabkin's solution: Dissolve 5 gm of sodium bicabonate in distilled water first. Add 0.250 gm of potassium cyanide KCN in the solution, add 1 litre of distilled water. Then add 1.0 gm of potassium ferricyanide $K_4Fe(CN)_6$ in the solution. Shake well, make final volume with distilled water to 5 litres.

Interfering substance: Gross lipemia may result in a positive error of up to 3 g/dl.

Calibration curve: Hb standard for the cyanmeth-Hb method is used for calibrating. Into three clean and dry test tubes add solutions as described below (Fig. 2.2):

1. Pipette 5 ml of Hb standard in the first tube (60 mg/100 ml)
2. Into the second test tube pipette exactly 2.5 ml of Hb standard and add in the same tube exactly 2.5 ml of Hb diluting reagent. Stopper the tube and mix by repeated inversion, this is 1:1 dilution of standards (30 mg cyanmeth-Hb per 100 ml).
3. In the third test tube add 5.0 ml of Hb diluting reagent which serves as a blank.

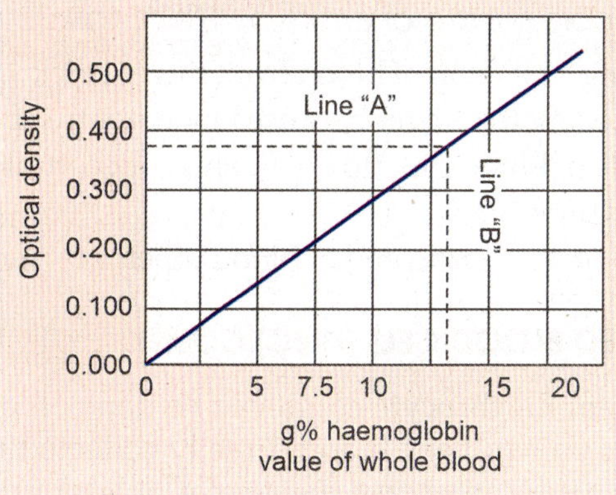

Fig. 2.2: Calibration curve

Measurement of Optical Density/Transmittance

1. Set the wavelength of photoelectric colourimeter at 540 nm, pour the blank (test tube no. 3) into the cuvette. Set the optical density to zero or transmission at 100%.
2. Pour the diluted Hb standard (test tube no. 2) into the cuvette and record the optical density or per cent transmission (cyanmeth-Hb standard).
3. Pour the undiluted Hb standard into the cuvette and record the optical density or per cent transmission.
4. If per cent transmission is determined, convert the reading to optical density.
5. Plot a graph Hb in mg/dl on horizontal axis and optical density on the vertical axis.
6. The value of cyanmeth-Hb in mg/dl is given on each vial. Half of this value will give the concentration of cyanmeth-Hb in the tube containing 1 : 1 dilution of Hb standard.
7. The equivalent g/dl Hb conc. in the undiluted and diluted standard can be calculated as shown below:
   Equivalent g/dl Hb value of undiluted standard.
   - g/dl Hb value of undiluted standard × dilution factor.
   - 0.06 × 251 (if the conc. of Hb standard is 60 mg/dl).
   - 15.06 equivalent g/dl Hb value of 1:1 diluted standard.
   - g/dl Hb value of diluted standard × dilution factor.
   - 0.03 × 251 (Half conc. of the Hb standard 60 mg/dl).
   - 7.53 = 7.5

> **Note:** The mg/dl Hb value (printed on the label divided by 1000 gives the g/dl Hb.

The procedure using 0.02 ml of whole blood in 5 ml Hb diluting reagent, the dilution factor is 251. Alternatively, the procedure using 0.02 ml of whole blood in 6 ml of Hb diluting reagent, the dilution factor is 301.

8. Draw a straight line connecting the two plotted points on the graph which should pass through origin. Reagents should be room temperature 25 ± 5°C.

Method

	Test	*Blar*
Hb diluting reagent	5.0 ml	5.0 ml
Fresh whole blood	0.02 ml	–

Mix well, allow to stand at room temperature for 3 minutes and measure optical density/transmittance of the test against blank 540 nm.

Record the readings: The colour is stable for more than 24 hours in well-stoppered tubes, kept in dark.

From the optical density reading of the test specimen determine the concentration of Hb in g/dl from the calibration curve.

If the optical density reading of test specimen is 0.385, then from the optical density reading of 0.385

draw a straight line parallel to the horizontal axis until it intersects the calibration curve. From this intersection draw a line parallel to the vertical axis down horizontal axis. Alternatively if a single standard reading is taken, the following calculation method may be used.

Calculation

$$\text{Hb} = \frac{\text{OD of unknown}}{\text{OD of standard}} \times \frac{\text{Conc. of standard in mg/dl} \times \text{dilution factor}}{1000} \text{ g/dl}$$

$$\text{Example: } \frac{0.385 \times 60 \times 251}{0.418 \times 1000} = 13.8 \text{ g/dl}$$

Normal range of Hb

Men	15.5 ± 2.5 g/dl
Women	14.0 ± 2.5 g/dl
Infants (full-term cord blood)	16.5 ± 3.0 g/dl
Children 3 months	11.0 ± 1.5 g/dl
Children 3–6 years	12.0 ± 1.0 g/dl
Children 10–12 years	13.0 ± 1.5 g/dl

B. Copper Sulphate Specific Gravity Method

The method is based on specific gravity and is a reasonably reliable method for determining the haemoglobin of the blood donor. It is indirect measure of the Hb value.

Preparation of Copper Sulphate Solution

1. Preparation of copper sulphate solution (sp. gravity 1100).

   Dissolve 159.63 g of pure air dried crystals of copper sulphate ($CuSO_4 \cdot 5H_2O$) in water and make up to exactly 1000 ml at 25°C. The specific gravity of the solution must be 1100.

2. Prepare standard copper sulphate solution of specific gravity 1052 to 1055 is given in Table 2.1.

The solution should be stored at room temperature in tightly capped containers to prevent evaporation.

Check specific gravity of $CuSO_4$ solution which must be within ±.0003 of required value. Specific gravity is determined using a 50 cc capacity specific gravity bottle and weighing in the 4th decimal place:

1. Weigh specific gravity bottle, clean and dry.
2. Weigh specific gravity bottle + distilled H_2O.
3. Weigh specific gravity bottle + $CuSO_4$ solution. Bottle is rinsed out three times with solution to be weighed before filling with that solution and weighing.

$$\frac{3\text{-}1}{2\text{-}1} = \frac{\text{Weight of } CuSO_4 \text{ solution}}{\text{Weight of water}} = \text{Sp. Gr. of } CuSO_4$$

Adjust specific gravity if necessary (a rough guide is 10 ml saturated $CuSO_4$ solution added to 1 litre of $CuSO_4$ solution increase that specific gravity by approx 0.001) and recheck specific gravity.

Table 2.1: Preparation of copper sulphate solution of 1052–1055 from stock solution

Sp. gravity	*Stock solution*	*Distilled water to make*	*Hb equivalent*
1052	51 ml	100 ml	12.0 g
1053	52 ml	100 ml	12.5 g
1054	53 ml	100 ml	13.0 g
1055	54 ml	100 ml	13.4 g

Method

A solution of specific gravity 1053 is used for determining haemoglobin level of 12.5 g/dl:

1. Dispense 30 ml of copper sulphate solution (specific gravity 1053) into appropriately labelled clean, dry, tubes or bottles. Change the solution daily of after 25 tests and be sure that the solution is properly mixed before performing tests daily.
2. The site of the skin puncture, i.e. fingertip is cleaned with antiseptic solution and allowed to dry.
3. Disposable lancet is used for puncture and there should be free flow of blood.
4. One drop of blood is collected either in capillary tube or pipette and allowed to fall generaly from a height of 1 cm above the surface of the copper sulphate solution.
5. The drop gets encased in a sac of copper proteinate, which prevents any change in specific gravity for about 12 seconds. If the drop of blood remains at the surface, or rises from the bottom of the solution, the drop is lighter than the $CuSO_4$ solution and the haemoglobin content of the blood is below normal levels. However, if the drop of blood has the specific gravity same or higher than the solution, it will sink within 15 seconds, i.e. haemoglobin will be equal to or higher than 12.5 ± 0.1 g%.

☞ **Note:** If plasma protein level of donors is on lower limit of normal, it is possible a donor may be rejected through he/she may be having required Hb.

Remediable source of errors in HB estimation

i. Taking first drop of blood from finger prick
ii. Squeezing the finger because blood not free flowing.
iii. Inside of blood pipette not flushed out completely.
iv. Dirty pipette.
v. Chip of delivering end of blood pipette.

TOTAL RED BLOOD CELL (TRBC) COUNT

Specimen: Erythrocyte count can be done on oxalated blood or on capillary blood directly collected into the pipette. In the former case, the sample, unless refrigerated must not be more than 6 hours old.

Apparatus

Red cell pipette	
Diluting fluid: 40% formaldehyde	10 ml
Trisodium citrate (3% w/v)	990 ml
or	
Trisodium citrate	3.8 gm
Formalin	1 ml
Distilled water	1 ml
Neubauer's chamber with coverslip	99 ml

Technique

1. If oxalated blood is to be used, first mix it thoroughly by gentle shaking.
2. Fill the red cell pipette exactly up to 0.5 mark by holding the pipette almost horizontally. The pipette must be clean and dry.
3. Now draw in the diluting fluid up to the mark 101 (dilution 1 in 200). While filling the bulb the pipette should be gently rotated to obtain good mixing (Fig. 2.3)

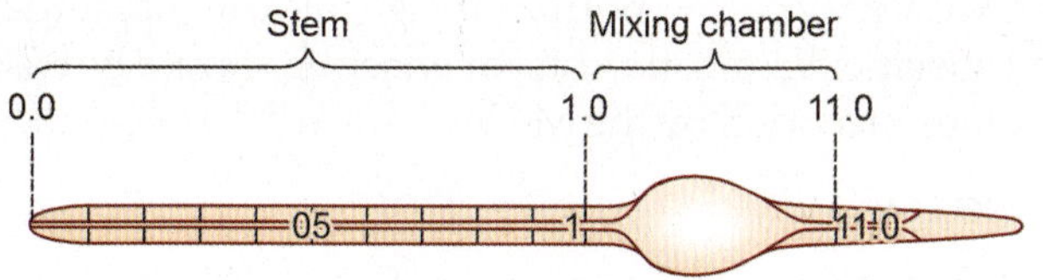

Fig. 2.3: RBC pipette

4. The coverslip is placed over the Neubauer's chamber so as to cover both the ruled platforms evenly.
5. Now load the chamber. This is done in three steps:
   a. Mix the contents of pipette for 3 minutes.
   b. Expel 6 drops from the pipette to remove the fluid in the stem which has not been mixed with blood.
   c. By holding the pipette at an angle of 45° and touching the space between the coverslip and the chamber by the point of the pipette, an appropriate drop of the mixture is allowed to run under the coverglass by capillary action. It must be large enough to cover the whole ruled area of platform of Neubauer chamber.
6. Allow two minutes for setting of the cells and then count.
7. The count is done as follows.

In the erythrocytic count, the central double ruled square is used. Red cells lying in 80 very small squares have to be counted. These 80 small squares comprise 5 medium-sized squares, each of which is bound by a triple line (Fig. 2.4). It is recommended that the five medium-sized squares chosen for counting cells should consist of four corners and one central; this is to secure an even distribution of cells. In counting, cells which touch the left hand lines or the upper lines of the square are taken to be within that square and those which touch the lower or right hand lines are omitted as outside the square.

To obtain accuracy at least 400 to 600 cells must be counted. If the count of the 80 small squares is less than this figure, more squares must be counted.

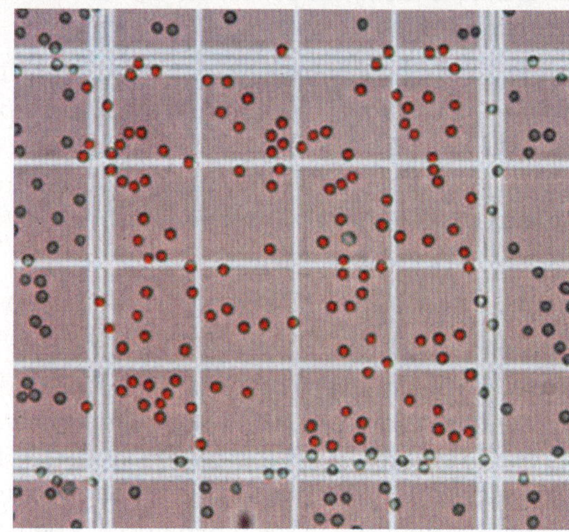

Fig. 2.4: Microphotograph showing RBC in Neubauer chamber

Calculation: The total area of the whole large central square is 1 sq mm. The smallest square has side of 1/20 mm so that its area is 1/400 sq mm and since the depth is 1/10 mm, its volume is 1/4000 cu mm. Total volume of 80 small squares is therefore 80/4,000 cu mm = 1/50 cu mm.

Dilution is 1 in 200

$$\text{Total RBC count} = \frac{\text{Dilution} \times \text{No. of cells counted}}{\text{Volume}}$$

$$= 200 \times N \times 50$$

$$= N \times 10{,}000 \text{ cells/cu mm}$$

Sources of Error

1. Sampling error in collection of blood.
2. Equipment error in the pipette and haemocytometer.
3. Technical errors involved in the exercise from the filling of the pipette to the final count.

Inherent or field errors of the distribution of cells in the counting chamber.

Normal Values

Men	$5.5 \pm 1.0 \times 10^{12}$/L
Women	$4.8 \pm 1.0 \times 10^{12}$/L
Infants (full term cord blood)	$5.0 \pm 1.0 \times 10^{12}$/L
Children 3 months	$4.0 \pm 1.0 \times 10^{12}$/L
Children 1 year	$4.4 \pm 0.8 \times 10^{12}$/L
Children 3–6 years	$4.8 \pm 0.7 \times 10^{12}$/L
Children 10–12 years	$4.7 \pm 0.7 \times 10^{12}$/L

DETERMINATION OF PACKED RED CELL VOLUME (PCV) AND ABSOLUTE INDICES

Principle: An oxalated sample of the blood is centrifuged to pack red cells to the maximum. The volume of packed red cells is determined. The procedure is reliable because of its reproducibility.

Specimen: Though haematocrit determination (PCV) can be done on capillary blood (with the use of special haematocrit) venous blood is preferred. The blood must be oxalated with the special mixture of potassium and ammonium oxalate. The sample must be processed within two hours of collection.

Apparatus: The Wintrobe haematocrit tubes, pasteur pipettes and a centrifuge with a speed of 3000 rpm.

Procedure: The haematocrit tube must be clean and dry. Mix the oxalated sample of blood thoroughly by gently shaking for 3 minutes. With the pasteur pipette fill the haematocrit tube to the 10 mark. This is done by passing the pipette to the bottom of the haematocrit. There must be no air bubbles.

Fill a second haematocrit with either another sample of blood or with water. This tube is to counterbalance the first one during centrifugation. Put the tubes in the centrifuge. Centrifuge at 3,000 rpm for 30 minutes, preferably for 60 minutes. Take the reading of packed red cells. Recentrifuge for 5 minutes more at the same speed and take the reading again. There should be no difference between the two readings if the packing has been complete. If there is a difference, further centrifugation is indicated.

At the uppermost portion of packed red cells, a narrow dark band (due to reduced haemoglobin) is seen. The reading is made at the uppermost level of the band. Above the band will be seen a reddish grey layer of white cells. The volume of packed red cells read is for 10 ml. Multiply by 10 to get the value for 100. This value is the PCV. Normal range for adult males 43 to 54 per 100 ml of blood for adult females 37 to 47 per 100 ml of blood.

Calculation of MCV, MCH and MCHC (absolute indices):

$$\underset{\text{(in cubic microns)}}{\text{MCV}} = \frac{\text{PCV}}{\text{RBCs in millions per cu mm}} \times 10$$

$$\underset{\text{(in percent)}}{\text{MCHC}} = \frac{\text{Hb in g per 100 ml}}{\text{PCV}} \times 100$$

$$\underset{\text{(in picograms)}}{\text{MCH}} = \frac{\text{Hb in gm per 100 ml}}{\text{RBCs in million per cu mm}} \times 10$$

Clinical Usefulness of Red Blood Cell Indices

Now with the Coulter counter type of automated equipment, a suspension of RBCs in a metered volume of electrolyte solution simply passes through a small orifice which is electrically charged. Since each RBC is a relative nonconductor, a change in the electrical charge occurs, which is then expressed as an RBC count. The magnitude of the charge change is proportional to the cell volume, and thus an MCV is derived as well. Finally, a haemoglobin is determined by an automated colourimetric method. Thus, only the Hb, MCV and RBC count are actually measured, while the Hct, MCH, and MCHC are computed internally using the above equations.

Normal Values for MCV, MCH, MCHC

The normal MCV in newborns is higher than at any other time of life, but beginning at a few months of age the MCV becomes lower than adult values. An MCV of 70, for example, may be normal for a 1-year-old infant. This development change in MCV is paralleled by changes in the MCH. The MCHC is fairly constant throughout the life.

The Significance of the MCV

The MCV may be low, normal or high in various disorders, and specific diagnostic tests for anaemia should be based on clues provided by the MCV.

A. The Low MCV

Iron deficiency: The earliest changes in iron deficiency are a fall in bone marrow iron and a concomitant fall in serum ferritin. This is followed by a decrease in serum iron and rise in the quantity of RBC free erythrocyte porphyrin (FEP). The MCV then falls and finally the Hb drops. Currently, the MCV and the FEP are the most widely used screening tests for iron deficiency, but the serum ferritin may soon be both then screening and the diagnostic test.

Lead (Pb) poisoning: Microcytosis may be seen in lead poisoning but is not uniformly present, while a rise in FEP is almost invariably found. The FEP is now the standard screening test for Pl poisoning. The FEP tends to be much higher in Pb poisoning than in iron deficiency, although some overlap may exist.

Thalassaemia minor: A low MCV is the hallmark of thalassaemia minor, and the MCV may be used as a screening test of high sensitivity in the detection of beta thalassaemia minor. In alpha thalassaemia, the MCV on the average is slightly higher than in beta thalassaemia. A Hb electrophoresis is best considered a confirmatory test for thalassaemia.

A very simple calculation may be used to distinguish iron deficiency and lead poisoning from thalassaemia minor based on the MCV and RBC count. The RBC count falls in iron deficiency in Pb poisoning but is normal in thalassaemia minor.

If the MCV divided by the RBC count, a discriminate index is obtained where

$$\frac{MCV}{RBC} < 12 = \text{Thalassemia minor}$$

$$\frac{MCV}{RBC} > 14 = \text{Iron deficiency or Pb poisoning}$$

Values between 12 and 14 are indiscriminate. Since these formulae are correct 95% of the time, a more rational selection of confirmatory tests is possible.

Miscellaneous: Other causes of microcytosis are much less common but include the anaemia of chronic disorders (this is usually normocytic, but 10% are microcytic), severe protein malnutrition, sideroblastic anaemia, and copper deficiency.

B. Normocytic Anaemia

Anaemia with a normal MCV is usually caused by bone marrow failure, recent blood loss, or haemolysis.

C. The High MCV

Unlike in adults, macrocytosis in a child should not call B_{12} deficiency to mind first. The causes of a high MCV include:

1. **Normal newborn:** All normal newborns are macrocytic. In fact, an MCV of 94 or less should suggest a diagnosis of alpha thalassaemia minor, the most common cause of microcytosis in newborns.
2. **Reticulocytosis:** Reticulocytes are very large and, when averaged with more mature RBCs, may produce a high MCV. A review of the peripheral blood smear will show that an elevated MCV is merely a reflection of young RBCs.
3. **Down's syndrome:** In Down's syndrome, the MCV averages 10 fl higher than normal.
4. **Liver disease:** This will deposit excessive lipids on the RBC, producing enlargement.
5. **Hypothyroidism:** A low T_4 commonly produces large speculated and targeted RBC.
6. **Drugs:** Any drug such as methotrexate which alters the DNA synthesis causes macrocytosis.
7. **Folate deficiency**
8. **B_{12} deficiency:** B_{12} and folate deficiency, in addition to producing macrocytosis, will cause hypersegmentation of neutrophils, distinguishing them from other causes of macrocytosis.
9. **Miscellaneous:** Other causes include preleukemic states and congenital pure RBC aplasia (Blackfan-Diamond syndrome).

Alterations of MCH and MCHC

Since the MCH falls as the Hb falls, relatively a little information is obtained from the MCH itself. The same is somewhat true of a low MCHC, which adds nothing to what is already known from the MCV. A high MCHC is important to recognize, since it indicates that the haemoglobin content of the RBC is being very tightly packed. A high MCHC almost invariably means spherocytes are present and suggests such diagnosis as hereditary spherocytosis, AHU incompatibility, autoimmune haemolytic anaemia, and occasionally microangiopathic haemolytic anaemias. Normal values of MCV, MCH and MCHC at different ages are given in Table 2.2.

Table 2.2: Normal values of MCV, MCH and MCHC at different ages

	MCV (fl)	*MCH (pg)*	*MCHC*
Normal adult	90 ± 10	31 ± 4	34 ± 3
Normal newborn	119 ± 9.0	36 ± 2	32 ± 2
Ages 10–17 months	77 ± 7	26.1 ± 2.8	34.2 ± 1.6
18–48 months	80 ± 6	27.0 ± 3.0	33.6 ± 1.4
4–7 years	81 ± 5	27.6 ± 2.4	33.6 ± 1.6

ERYTHROCYTE SEDIMENTATION RATE (ESR)

If an anticoagulant is added to the blood and the specimen allowed to stand in a tube, red cells slowly sediment to the bottom of the tube leaving clear plasma as the supernatant. The rate of sedimentation estimated under standard conditions is known as the erythrocyte sedimentation rate (ESR). Sedimentation takes place in three stages:

1. Formation of rouleaux.
2. Sinking of rouleaux.
3. Packing of the rouleaux.

Influencing Factors

1. Difference in specific gravity between red cells and plasma.
2. The extent to which the red cells form rouleaux, which sediment more rapidly than single cells.
3. The ratio of red cells to plasma, i.e. the PCV.
4. Plasma viscosity.
5. Verticality or otherwise of the sedimentation tube.
6. The bore of the tube .
7. Dilution, if any, of the blood.

Methods of Estimation

1. Wintrobe Method

Wintrobe Tube

Length	110 mm
Diameter	3. 0 mm

Graduation of lower 100 mm from 0–100

Anticoagulant used: Double oxalate

Method: The tube is filled up to the 100 mm mark, allowed to stand in a vertical position at the room temperature, read the fall of red cells at the end of one hour (Fig. 2.5).

Advantages: Can be used for

1. Packed cell volume.
2. Buffy coat preparation.

2. Westergren Method

Westergren tube

Length 300 mm

Diameter 2.5 mm

Graduation in mm from 0 to 200

Anticoagulant used: 3.13% sodium citrate solution (0.106 M). 0.5 ml of anticoagulant is used for 2 ml blood.

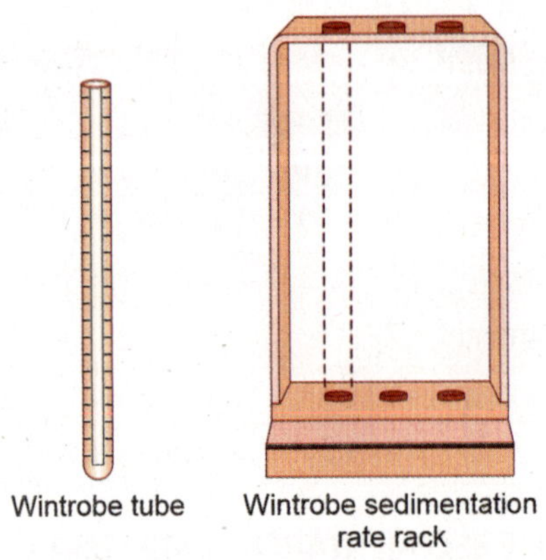

Fig. 2.5: Wintrobe tube and rack for ESR

Method: The mixture is drawn into a Westergren tube up to the zero mark and the tube set upright in a stand with a spring clip on top and rubber at bottom.

The level of the top of the red cell column is read at the end of 1 hour.

Precautions

1. The tubes must be scrupulously clean.
2. They must be filled properly without air bubbles.
3. They must be kept vertically.
4. Anaemia, if present, will raise the ESR, irrespective of the primary condition.

Normal Values

Wintrobe method: Men—0 to 9 mm in 1st hour
Women—0 to 20 mm in 1st hour

Westergren method: Men—0 to 5 mm in 1st hour
Women—0 to 7 mm in 1st hour

Corrected ESR

The corrected ESR is needed to eliminate the influence of anaemia on sedimentation rate. The rate is then corrected according to the volume of cells by referring to chart for correction (Fig. 2.6).

Find the horizontal line which represents the sedimentation in mm for 1st hour. Follow this across the chart until it intersects the vertical line which represents the blood cell volume per cent.

Follow the nearest curved line until it intersects the heavy line at 42% per 100 ml, if the patient is female, or

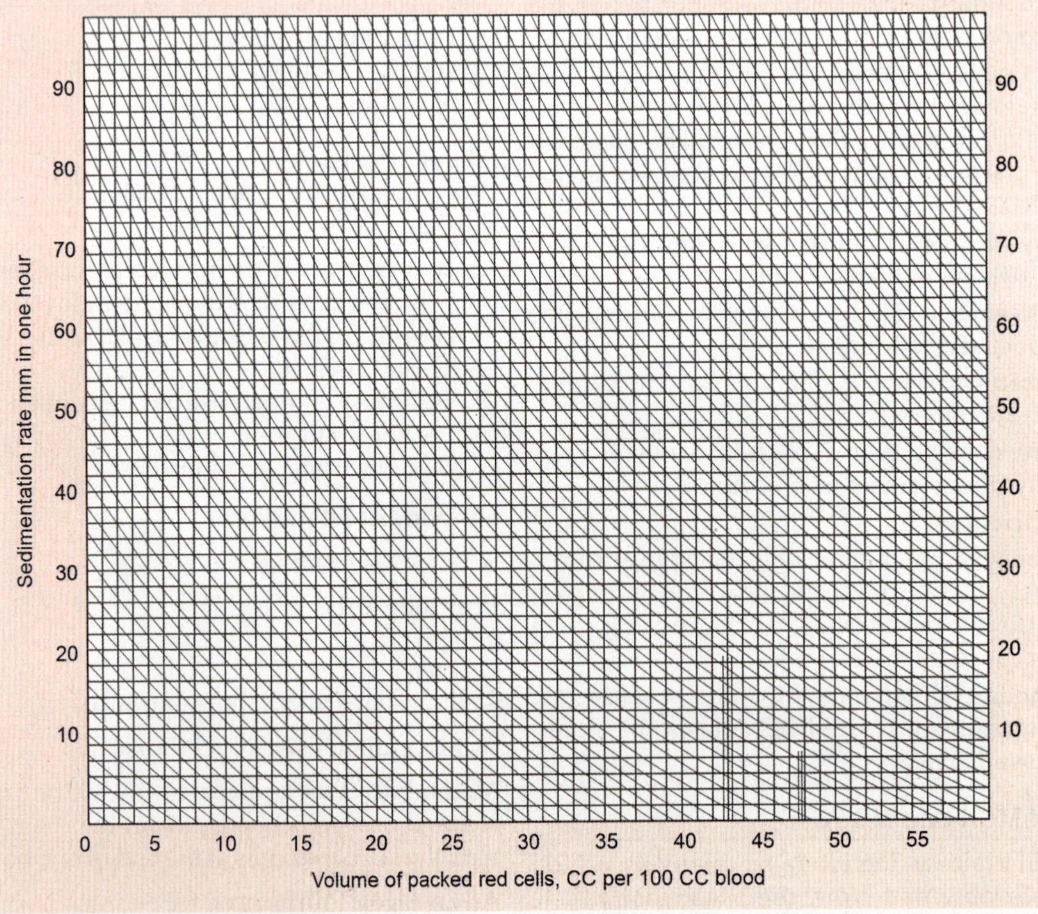

Fig. 2.6: Graph 1: Wintrobe and Landsberg chart for correcting the sedimentation rate for variations resulting from differences in the concentration of erythrocytes as measured by the volume of packed cells

the line at 47% if the patient is male. Then, at the point of intersection, read the value on the horizontal line for the corrected sedimentation rate. The normal average sedimentation in one hour by this method is 9.6 mm for healthy female (0–20 mm) and 0–9 mm for healthy male.

Total Leucocyte Count (TLC)

Specimen: The leucocyte count may be done on oxalated blood or capillary blood. In the former case the sample must be examined within 6 hours of collection.

Apparatus

- A white cell pipette (white lead).
- Diluting fluid—4% acetic acid with two drops of gentian violet per litre.
- Neubauer's chamber with coverslip.
- Microscope.

Procedure

1. Draw blood in a clean dry pipette up to the mark 0.5 (Fig. 2.7) with all possible accuracy. The oxalated sample must be thoroughly mixed before use.
2. Wipe off the outside of the pipette with gauge.
3. Now draw the diluting fluid up to mark 11 (dilution 1 in 20). While drawing the fluid rotate the pipette.
4. Mix the contents of the pipette for 3 minutes.
5. Dispel the first 4 drops of the contents.
6. Adjust the Neubauer's chamber. It must be clean and dry. By holding the coverglass between the fingers at the edges, place it in such a manner that both the ruled platforms are evenly covered by it. Load it with the mixture, by holding the pipette at angle of 45° and touching the space between the coverglass an the chamber by the point of the pipette, and appropriate drop of the mixture is allowed to run under the coverglass by capillary action. It must be sufficiently large to cover the whole ruled platform, yet not large enough to fill the moat. Also there must be no air bubbles.
7. Allow 2 minutes for setting of cells, then count.
8. The count is done as follows: The improved Neubauer chamber has two central platforms each of which is ruled. When the coverglass is in place, there is a space of 0.1 mm depth over the ruled area. The surface of the ruled area is 3 × 3 mm (9 sq mm) (Fig. 2.8). Nine large squares can be recognised in the ruled area; the four corner squares are single ruled and the five central squares are double ruled. Each of the corner single ruled square is divided into 16 smaller squares (Fig. 2.9). The central double ruled square is divided into 400 very small squares. Each of the four large corner squares (with 16 small squares) has an area of 1 sq mm; each of the very small squares (400 in all) in the central square has an area of 1/400 sq mm. The central square is meant for the erythrocyte count; the four large corner squares are used for the leucocytic count. Figure 2.10 shows pattern of good and poor distribution of white blood cells and Fig. 2.11 shows procedure and score of counting. In counting, cells which touch the left hand lines or the upper lines of the square are taken to be within that square and those which touch the lower and right lines are omitted as outside the square. WBC as viewed under low power magnification are shown in Fig. 2.12.
9. **Calculation:** The area of each large square is 1 sq mm, the depth of the chamber being 0.1 mm, the volume of the square is 0.1 cu mm.

   Volume of four corner squares = 0.1 × 4 = 0.4 cu mm

   No. of cells in four corner squares = N

   0.4 cu mm contains = N cells.

   $$1 \text{ cu mm contains} = \frac{N \times 20 \text{ (dilution factor)}}{0.4}$$

   $$= N \times 50$$

Sources of Error

1. Sampling error in collection of blood.
2. Equipment error in the pipette and chamber.
3. Technical errors involved in the exercise from the filling of the pipette to the final count.
4. Inherent or field errors of the distribution of cells in the counting chamber. This can be minimised by counting a large number of cells.

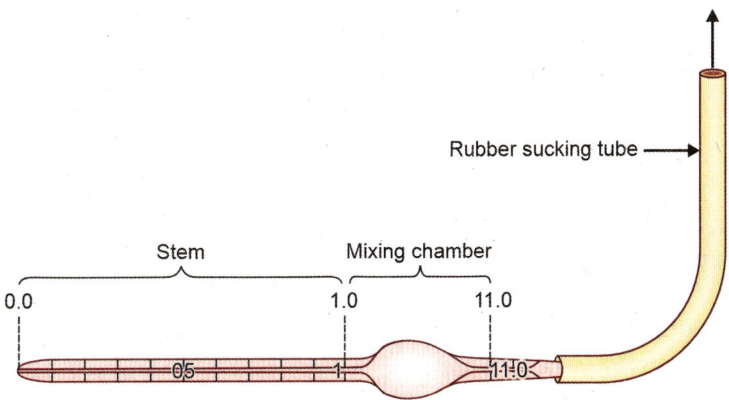

Fig. 2.7: White cell pipette with markings

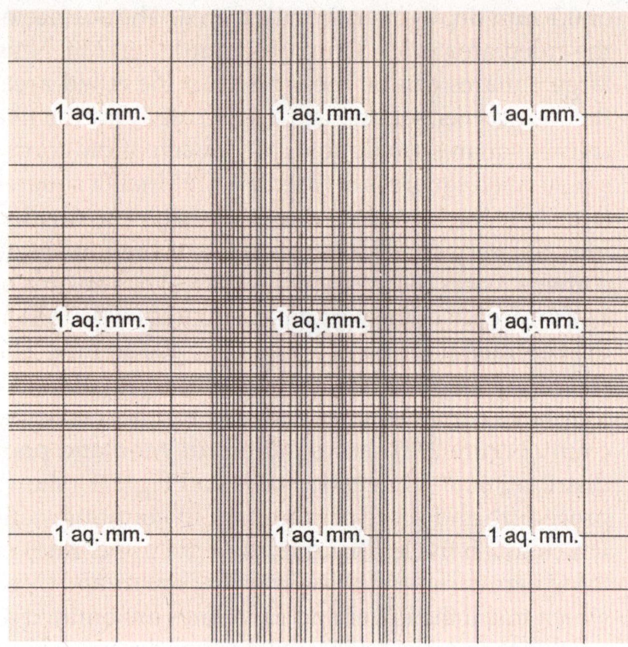

Fig. 2.8: Ruled area of Neubauer chamber

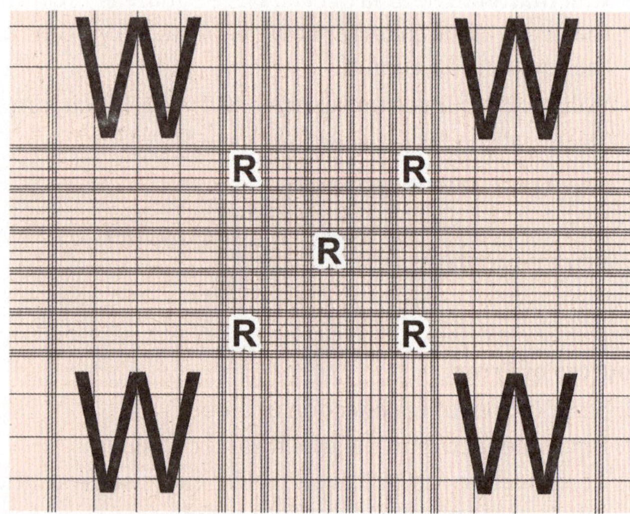

Fig. 2.9: 'W' areas for white cell count

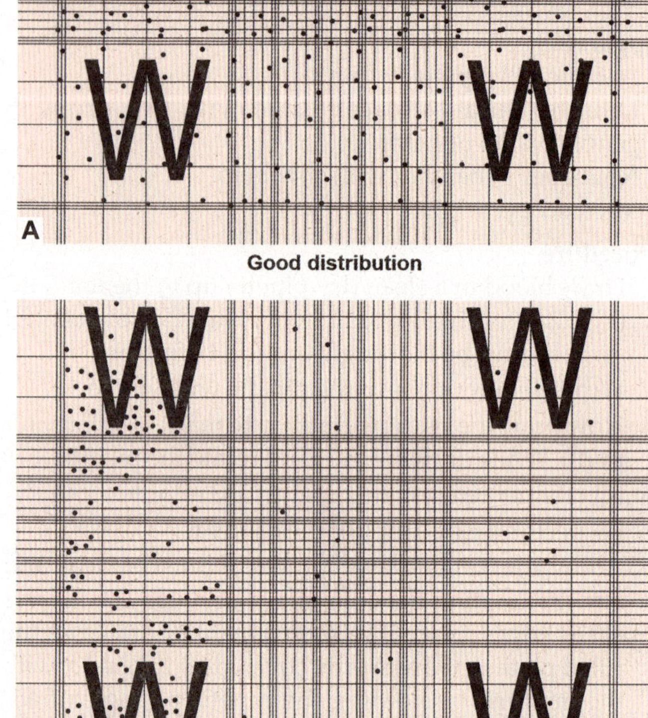

Fig. 2.10A and B: Pattern of good and poor distribution of WBC

Range of TLC

Adults	$7.5 \pm 3.5 \times 10^3$/cu mm
Infants (full term 1st day)	$18 \pm 8 \times 10^3$/cu mm
Infants, 1 year	$12 \pm 6 \times 10^3$ cumm
Children 4–7 years	$10 \pm 5 \times 10^3$/cu mm
Children 8–12 years	$9 \pm 4.5 \times 10^3$/cu mm

The spreader

1. Should have a smooth edge.
2. Should be narrower in breadth than the slide on which film is to be made so that the edges of the film may be readily examined.
3. Should not be used for making more than six slides in succession without being cleaned.
4. Should be washed in running water and dried immediately after being used.

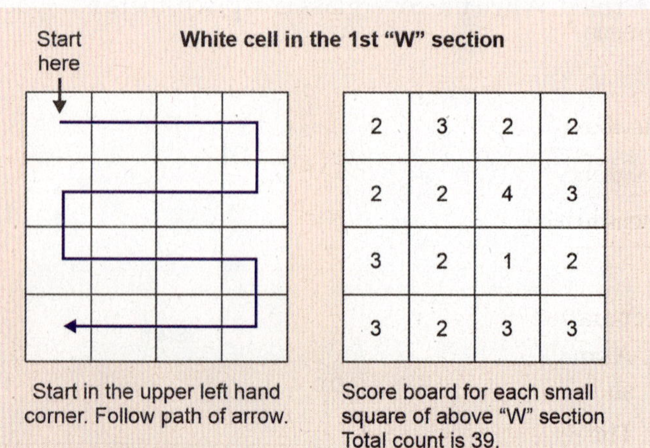

Fig. 2.11: Procedure and score of counting

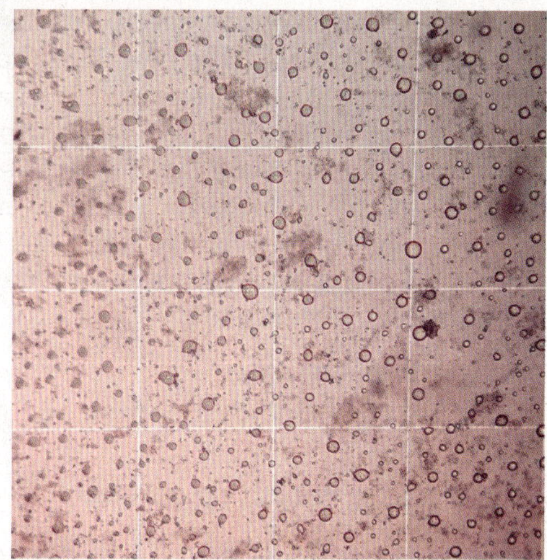

Fig. 2.12: WBC as viewed under low power magnification (× 10)

Table 2.3: Conditions accompanied by abnormal white cell counts

High white cell count (leucocytosis)	*Low white cell count (leucopenia)*
Appendicitis	Measles
Pneumonia	Influenza
Leukaemia	Brucellosis
Tonsillitis	Typhoid fever
Meningitis	Agranulocytosis
Abscesses	Infectious hepatitis
Rheumatic fever	Lupus erythematosus
Diphtheria	Cirrhosis of liver
Smallpox	Paratyphoid fever
Chickenpox	Protein therapy
Peritonitis	Radiation
Erythroblastosis fetalis	Myxedema
Uremia	Psittacosis
Ulcers	Sandfly fever
Newborn	Scrub typhus
Pregnancy	Dengue
Menstruation	Rheumatoid arthritis

Preparation of Film

1. A small drop of blood is placed in the central line of a slide about 1–2 cm. from one end.
2. The spreader is placed at an angle of 45° to the slide and then moved back to make contact with the drop.
3. The drop should spread out quickly alone the line of contact of the spreader with the slide (Fig. 2.13).

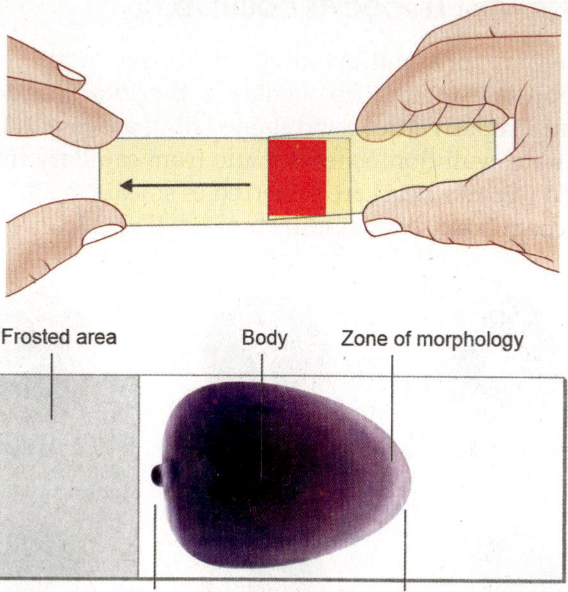

Fig. 2.13: Method of preparation of blood smear

4. The moment this occurs the film should be spread by a rapid smooth, forward movement of the spreader.
5. The drop should be of such size that the film is 3–4 cm in length.

Sources of error: If the film is made too thin or if a rough edged spreader is used, many of the leucocytes, perhaps even 50% of them, accumulate at the edges and in the tail. Moreover, a gross qualitative irregularity in distribution is the rule. Polymorphonuclear neutrophils and monocytes predominate at the margins and the tail and lymphocytes in the middle of the film. This separation probably depends upon differences in stickiness, size and specific gravity among the different classes of cells (Fig. 2.14).

Qualities of a Good Film

1. Should not be too thin and the tail of the film should be smooth (diagrammatic representation Fig. 2.14).
2. There should be some overlap of the red cells. diminishing to separate near the tail.
3. The leucocytes in the body of the film should not be badly shrunken.

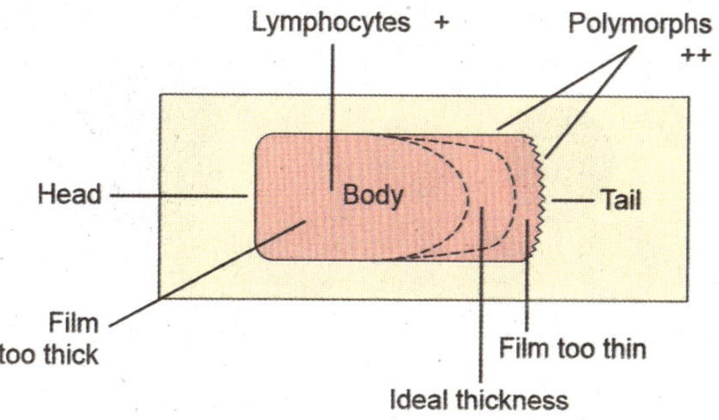

Fig. 2.14: Diagrammatic representation of distribution of cells and parts of the smear

DIFFERENTIAL LEUCOCYTE COUNT (DLC)

Gives an information about the type of the cells responsible for the rise or fall in the total leucocyte count. Properly spread and stained films are essential for accurate evalution. Smears made from capillary finger blood (direct smear) are preferred to smears made from anticoagulated blood (indirect smear) (Fig. 2.15).

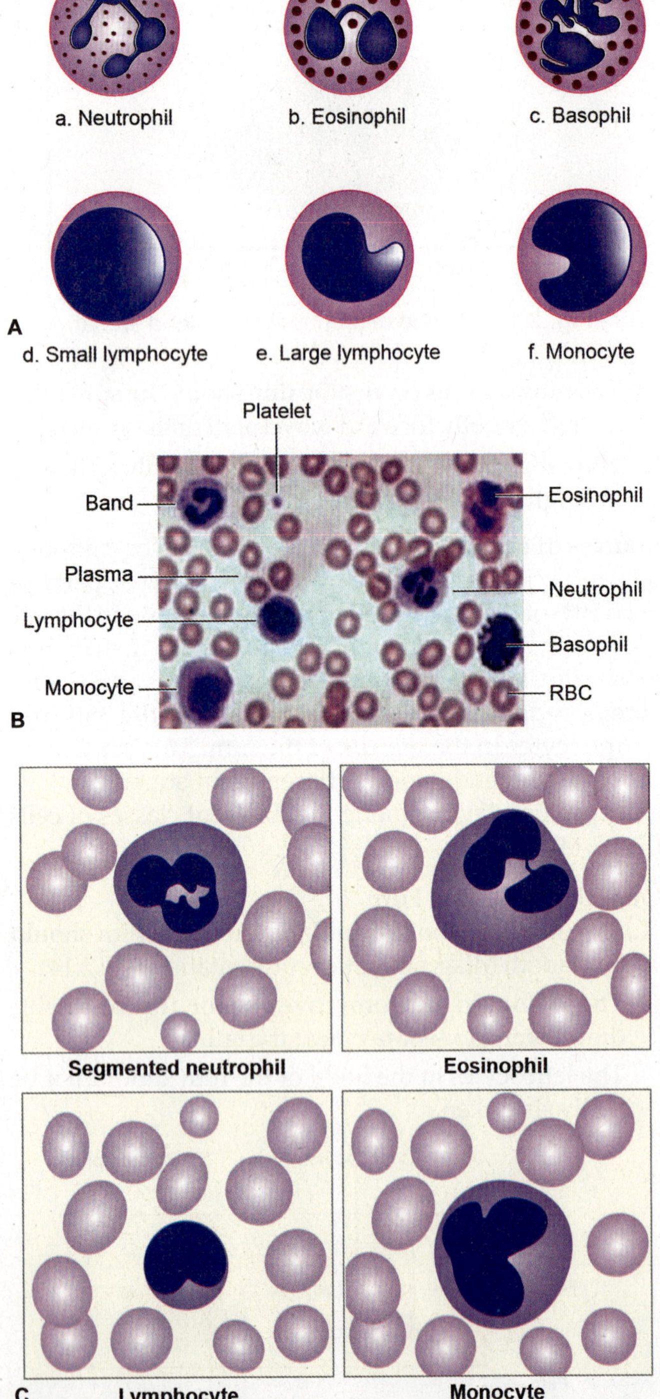

Fig. 2.15: (A) Labelled DIC (a–f) diagram; (B) Labelled photograph DLC; (C) Diagram labelled—segmented neutrophil, eosinophil, lymphocyte and monocyte

Method: A small drop of blood is placed on a clean glass slide, 1–2 cm from one end. The spreader (having a smooth edge, narrower breadth) is placed at an angle of 45° in front of the drop and moved backwards to touch the drop. The drop will spread along the line of contact. The smear is made by a rapid, smooth, forward movement of the spreader. The angle is important to avoid aggregation of leukocytes at the periphery. The smear should be dried rapidly in the air and never heated.

Characteristics of a good smear

- Good film has a thick and thin portion and gradual transition.
- The film should have smooth, even appearance and free from ridges, waves or holes.
- The edge of spreader must be smooth, if it is rough, the film has ragged tails containing many leukocytes.
- The film has some overlap of red cells in much of the film but even distribution and separation of red cells towards the thin tail.
- The faster the film is air dried, the better is the spreading of the individual cells and there is no shrinkage of cells. The slide is labeled by writing with a lead pencil on thick end of the film.

Fixation of smears: Most Romanowsky stains are dissolved in methyl alcohol and combine fixation with staining. Wright's and Leishman stains are alcoholic stains that fix the smears during staining. For Giemsa stain, a prior fixation in methyl alcohol (2–3 minutes) is necessary. If staining is delayed, all the smears must be fixed in methyl alcohol.

Staining of the smears: Romanowsky stains are used in routine practice. Romanowsky stains include Wright's stain, Leishman stain, Giemsa stain (common ones) May-Grunwald stain and Jenner stain.

Staining the smear with Wright's stain/Leishman stain

1. Cover the air dried smear with Wright's stain.
2. Add double the volume of buffered water or distilled water after 1 minute. The water should not run of the slide.
3. Mix the stain and the water by blowing gently on the surface. Keep the slide for 5–8 minutes, till a scum with metallic sheen is formed on the surface.
4. Wash the slide directly under running water (to avoid deposition of the scum on the stained film).
5. Clean the back of the slide, and air dry the smear. Examination of smear is done under oil immersion.

Procedure of Count

1. The cells should be counted using high power coil immersion lens in a strip running the whole length of the film.
2. The lateral edges of the film are avoided.
3. The film should be inspected from the head to the tail.

4. If less than 100 cells are encountered in a single narrow strip, one or more additional strips should be examined until at least 100 cells have been counted.
5. In patients with very high counts (as in leukaemia) the cells should be counted in any well spread area where the cell types are easy to identify.

Cell Identification

Leucocytes include segmented cell of myeloid series and mononuclear cells of lymphoid and monocytic cells. *Mature cells of myeloid series include*:

1. Neutrophil
2. Eosinophil
3. Basophil

These are segmented cells of 10–12 μ size. The nucleus shows lobes connected by filaments, cytoplasm contains granules.

- **Neutrophil or polymorph:** Nucleus may show 2–5 lobes. Cytoplasmic granules are fine and pale pink violet.
- **Eosinophil:** Nucleus usually bilobed like a spectacle. Cytoplasmic granules are coarse and orange.
- **Basophil obscure:** Cytoplasmic granules are large deep purple and nucleus.

Mature Cells of Lymphoid Series

Small Lymphocytes

- Size same as that of RBC
- Round, dark staining nucleus fills the cell
- Scanty pale blue cytoplasm.

Size 10–14 μm

- Pale nucleus large, rounded or indented
- Cytoplasm abundant, pale blue, may show a few reddish blue granules.

Monocytes

- Large cell, 14–20 μm
- Nucleus round, oval kidney-shaped, convoluted
- Cytoplasm abundant, grayish blue.

Normal Range of DLC

- Neutrophils, 40–60%
- Lymphocytes, 20–45%
- Monocyte, 2–10%
- Eosinophil, 1–6%
- Basophils, 0–1%.

Abnormalities of Leucocytes

Increase in neutrophils with toxic granules	Pyogenic infections
Increase in lymphocytes	Viral infections
Increase in eosinophils	Allergies parasitic infestation
Increase in monocytes	Chronic infections
Presence of immature leucocytes	Infections, leukaemia

ABSOLUTE EOSINOPHIL COUNT

Apparatus

- WBC pipette
- Eosinophil diluting fluid (Dunger's solution)

Stock Solution

- Eosin yellow: 0.5 gm
- Formaldehyde (40%): 0.5 ml
- Phenol (95%) (aqueous): 0.5 ml
- Distilled water up to: 100 ml

Working solution: 6 ml of stock solution diluted with distilled water up to 100 ml.

- Neubauer's chamber with coverslip
- Microscope.

Procedure: Suck blood up to 0.5 mark in a WBC pipette and dilute up to 11 mark with the diluting fluid. Gently rotate the pipette. Discard first 3 or 4 drops of fluid. Charge the Neubauer counting chamber and allow it to stand for 3 minutes, so that the cells settle down (Fig. 2.16).

Count all the eosinophils in the whole of the ruled area (i.e. 9 squares).

Calculation

$$\text{Absolute eosinophil count (AEC)} = \frac{N \times \text{Dilution}}{\text{Volume}}$$

Where N = No. of cells counted

$$\text{Volume} = \text{length} \times \text{breadth} \times \text{depth} = 3 \times 3 \times 0.1 = 0.9 \text{ cu mm}$$

$$\text{Dilution is 1 in 20} = \frac{N \times 20}{0.9}$$

$$\therefore \text{AEC} = N \times 22.2 \text{ cu mm}$$

Normal range of AEC = 40–440 cell/cu mm

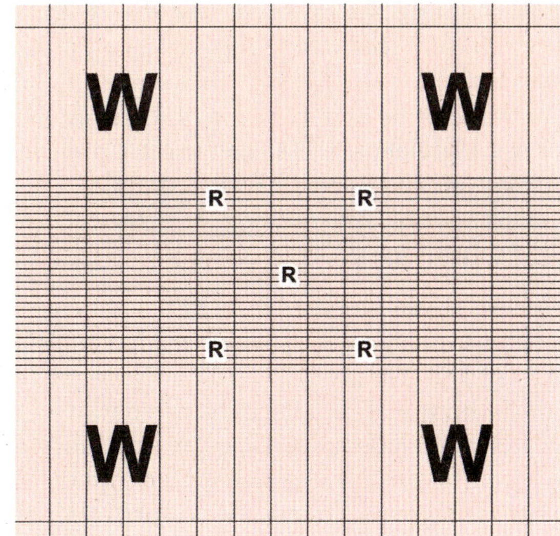

Fig. 2.16: Ruled area of Neubauer's chamber showing counting areas

Interpretation: An increase in eosinophil count or eosinophilia is seen in:

- Allergic diseases such as bronchial asthma.
- Skin disorders, e.g. eczema.
- Parasitic infestation.

PLATELET COUNT

Direct Method (1)

Specimen: Venous blood is collected by a clean puncture and delivered without frothing into a bottle or a tube containing the anticoagulant dipotassium EDTA. EDTA prevents the clumping of platelet or it may be collected finger prick. Venous blood is preferred.

Procedure

1. Draw the blood into a clean dry RBC pipette up to the mark 0.5. The accuracy in filling the pipette has to be of high order.
2. Wipe off the outside of the pipette.
3. Draw the diluting fluid up to the mark 101.

   The diluting fluid (Rees-Ecker) has the following formula:

Sodium citrate	3.8 g
Brilliant cresyl blue	0.05 g
Neutral formalin	0.65 ml
Distilled water	100 ml

   Filter and centrifuge at 2,800 rpm for 30 minutes. Stock the solution in a refrigerator in a well-stoppered bottle and filter before use every time.

   Another good diluent is the formol citrate solution used for red cell count.
4. Shake the pipette for 5 minutes.
5. Discard the first 4 drops. Load the chamber; both the haemocytometer and the coverslip must be scrupulously clean.
6. Allow the preparation to stand for 15 minutes in a moist chamber. An inverted Petri dish with a piece of wet filter paper in the top makes a good moist chamber.
7. Count under the high power with the light partially cut off. Platelets are lilac-coloured. Count at least 300 platelets and calculate by the formula.

Platelet counts can be made by visual counting or by electronic counters. Accuracy in visual counting (direct or indirect method) is only achieved by scrupulous cleanliness during blood preparation and by experience in differentiating platelets from extraneous matter. Phase contrast microscopy helps considerably in recognising and counting platelets. 1% ammonium oxalate can be used as a diluent in which red cells are lysed.

Count: Calculation

$$\frac{\text{No. of platelets counted} \times 10 \times \text{dilution}}{\text{No. of 1 mm squares counted}} = \text{Platelets per cu mm}$$

Normal values—1,50,000 to 4,00,000 cells/cu mm

Direct Method (2)

The blood is diluted in 1% ammonium oxalate stored refrigerated at 4°C which haemolyzes the red blood cells. (Prepared by dissolving 1 gm of ammonium oxalate in 100 ml of distilled water.)

Fill blood and diluent (in this case 1% ammonium oxalate) as described for the RBC count and using the RBC pipette. If platelet count is low, a WBC pipette can be used instead:

- Charge the chamber with the help of the pipette employed.
- Using 40 x objective with reduced condenser aperture count the platelets in the same squares as indicated for RBC counting.
- Calculate as (if RBC pipette used) =

$$\frac{\text{Cells counted} \times \text{blood dilution} \times \text{chamber depth factor}}{\text{Area of chamber counted}}$$

$= N \times 200 \times 5 \times 10$

$= N \times 10000$

(However, if a WBC pipette is employed the appropriate formula and method should be used. Platelet counts are made in the small 5 RBC squares only. Platelet count $= N \times 20 \times 5 \times 10$ or $N \times 1000$).

Indirect method

1. A drop of 14% magnesium sulfate is placed on the fingertip and the finger is pricked through it to dilute the blood at once in order to prevent the clumping or disintegration of platelets.
2. With a drop, a thin smear is prepared and stained with Leishman's or Wright's stain.
3. With another drop of blood, the RBC count is done simultaneously.
4. On the smear 1000 RBCs are counted and the number of platelets seen whilst counting is noted.

PLATELET COUNT (by visual impression)

A peripheral smear prepared from EDTA anticoagulated blood helps to judge roughly whether adequate platelets are present and usually if 2 to 10 platelets per 100 red cells or if clumps of platelets are present; it suggests that platelets are adequate. The size and morphology of the platelets can also be studied by peripheral smear examination. They are bluish, spherical or oval structures, 2–4 microns in diameter. With Romanowsky's stain azure granules are seen in the hyaline, light blue cytoplasm, no nucleus is present.

Platelet count (per litre).

$$\frac{\text{Number of platelets counted} \times \text{Red cell count}}{1000}$$

Normal platelet counts = 1.5–4.0 Lakhs/cu mm.
Raised platelet count (thrombocytosis).
Reduced platelet count (thrombocytopenia).

Causes of Thrombocytosis

1. During infections
2. Immediately after surgery and following bleeding
3. Iron deficiency anaemia
4. Chronic myeloid leukaemia
5. Polycythaemia vera
6. Myelofibrosis
7. Trauma
8. Acute haemolytic states
9. Hemorrhagic thrombocythaemia
10. Hereditary spherocytosis
11. Spleenectomy
12. Thalasemia

Causes of Thrombocytopenia

a. Causes of platelet production failure
  i. Selective megakaryocyte depression:
    - *Drugs:* Antazoline, benzene compounds and chemicals
      • Chloramphenicol
      • Chlorothiazide
      • Chlorpropamide
      • Digitoxin
      • Phenobarbitone
      • Phenylbutazone
      • Quinidine
      • Quinine
      • Salicylates
      • Sulphonamides
    - *Viral infections:* Measles, infectious mononucleosis, rubella, scarlet fever, septicemia, tuberculosis
  ii. Part of general bone marrow failure:
    - Aplastic anaemia
    - Leukaemia
    - Myelosclerosis
    - Marrow infiltration, e.g. in carcinoma, lymphoma
    - Multiple myeloma
    - Megaloblastic anaemia.
b. Increased destruction of platelets
  - Acute or chronic (ITP) idiopathic thrombocytopenic purpura
  - Secondary immune thrombocytopenia (post-infection, SLE, CLL, and lymphomas)
c. Abnormal distribution of platelets
  - Splenomegaly.
d. Dilutional loss
  - Massive transfusion of old blood to bleeding patients

RETICULOCYTE COUNT

Reticulocytes are young red cells which contain basophilic ribonucleoprotein but no nucleus. With Romanowsky stains they may shown in Fig. 2.17.

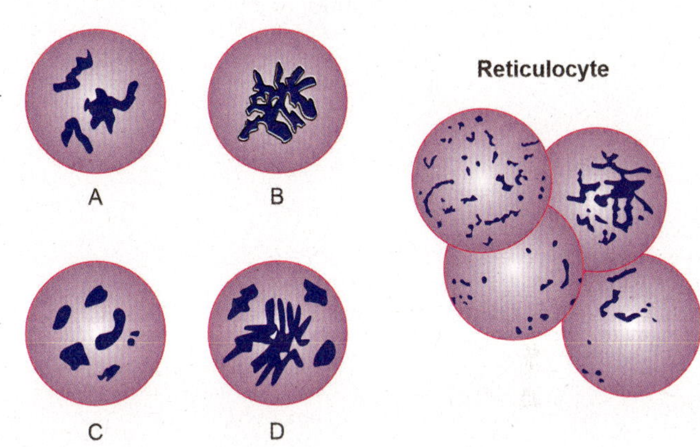

A. Basophilic multiple granules
B. Confluent basophilic granular, branching pattern
C. Confluent ganular rod type
D. Basophilic, branching bush appearance

Fig. 2.17: Reticulocytes stained with methylene blue

1. Diffuse basophilia (polychromasia)
2. Punctate basophilia
3. Filaments in the cells (Skein cells)

Basophilic ribonucleoprotein (RNP) reacts with brilliant cresyl blue to form blue precipitate of granules or filaments. They take 1–2 days to ripe to mature RBC in spleen or peripheral blood. In smear they may be confused with:

1. Papenheimer bodies which usually contain single dot like granular material and stain darker blue shade.
2. Heinz bodies stain lighter blue as compared to reticulocytes.

Staining Solution

Brilliant cresyl blue	1.0 gm
Sodium carbonate (anhydrous)	400 gm
Nomal saline	100 ml

First dissolve dye in normal saline, then add sodium carbonate. Mix and filter the stain and keep at room temperature.

Procedure: Put 3–4 drops of staining solution in a small test tube. Add equal amount of oxalated or EDTA blood. Mix and keep in incubator at 37°C for 15–20 minutes. After that, gently mix the solution and prepare smears. If patient is anaemic, add more blood. If patient is polycythaemic, add less blood. Films are examined without fixing or counter staining, under oil immersion.

Calculation

Count 100 reticulocytes

For example: No. of reticulocyte in 150 fields = 100

Total no. of red cells in 150 fields = 3,000

Therefore,

$$\text{Reticulocyte\%} = \frac{100}{3000} \times 100 = 3.3\%$$

Normal Range

Adults and children	0.2–2.0%
Newborn infants	2.0–6.0%

Decreased Reticulocyte Count

In aplastic anaemia and in conditions where the bone marrow is not producing red blood cells.

Increased Reticulocyte Count

In haemolytic anaemias, iron deficiency anaemias receiving iron therapy, thalassaemia, sideroblastic anaemias, and acute and chronic blood loss.

Chapter 3

Haemopoiesis (Haematopoiesis)

Chapter Outline

- Haematopoiesis
- Normal Erythropoiesis
- Abnormalities of Erythrocytes

HAEMATOPOIESIS

Haematopoiesis is the formation of blood cells. The site for blood formation varies with age (Fig. 3.1).

Haematopoiesis first begins in the yolk sac around third week of foetal life. These are clusters of large nucleated erythrocytes called 'blood islands'. These cells contain embryonic haemoglobin. By 6 weeks some of these cells migrate to liver where small non-nucleated erythrocytes are produced. The haemoglobin now changes to foetal haemoglobin. After 3 months of foetal life, spleen becomes an additional site of haematopoiesis. Bone marrow haematopoiesis which starts at fourth month becomes fully established by the time of birth. From birth till 4 years of age the medullary cavities of all the bones are densely packed with blood forming cells. However, by adulthood the medullary cavities in peripheral bones become fatty and haemapoietically inactive. Only the axial skeleton remains active. However, in a number of diseases the liver and spleen can again become an active site of haematopoiesis even in adults. This is referred to as extra medullary haematopoiesis.

Haemopoiesis starts in the bone marrow at the 4th month of fetal life. At birth, the marrow is the main site of haemopoiesis. Until puberty all marrow throughout the skeleton is red. By 18–20 years, only the vertebrae, sternum, skull, pelvis and proximal humerus and femur contain red marrow, the rest is yellow and inactive.

At times of increase demand when RBC production must increase, the yellow marrow turns red and RBC production can increase 7–8 times. Also areas like liver, spleen can take over haemopoisis (extramedullary haemopoiesis).

Origin of blood cells: All blood cells (RBC, granulocytes, monocytes, platelets and lymphocytes) arise from a totipotent stem cell (Fig. 3.2).

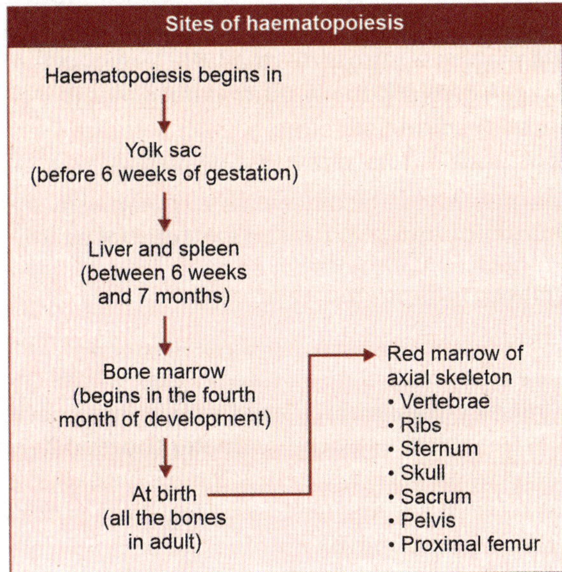

Fig. 3.1: Sites of blood formation during foetal development

NORMAL ERYTHROPOIESIS (Figs 3.2 and 3.3)

In the adult normal erythropoiesis is described as 'normoblastic'. According to the monophyletic theory, the various cells concerned in normoblastic erythropoiesis are the haemocytoblast, the pro-erythroblast, three types of normoblasts, the reticulocyte and the mature erythrocyte

1. **Haemocytoblast:** A large cell, 18 to 24 microns in diameter, a larger nucleus fills almost the whole cell; two or more nucleoli; cytoplasm agranular and stained dark blue. The cell is not readily identifiable, either by morphologcial or histochemical criteria.
2. **Pro-erythroblast (Pro-normoblast):** Formed by differentiation from the haemocytoblast; measures 14 to 19 microns (2 to 3 times the mature erythrocyte); a large round nucleus fills three-fourths of the cell; nuclear chromatin delicate with a reticulated pattern; nucleoli present; cytoplasm agranular and deep

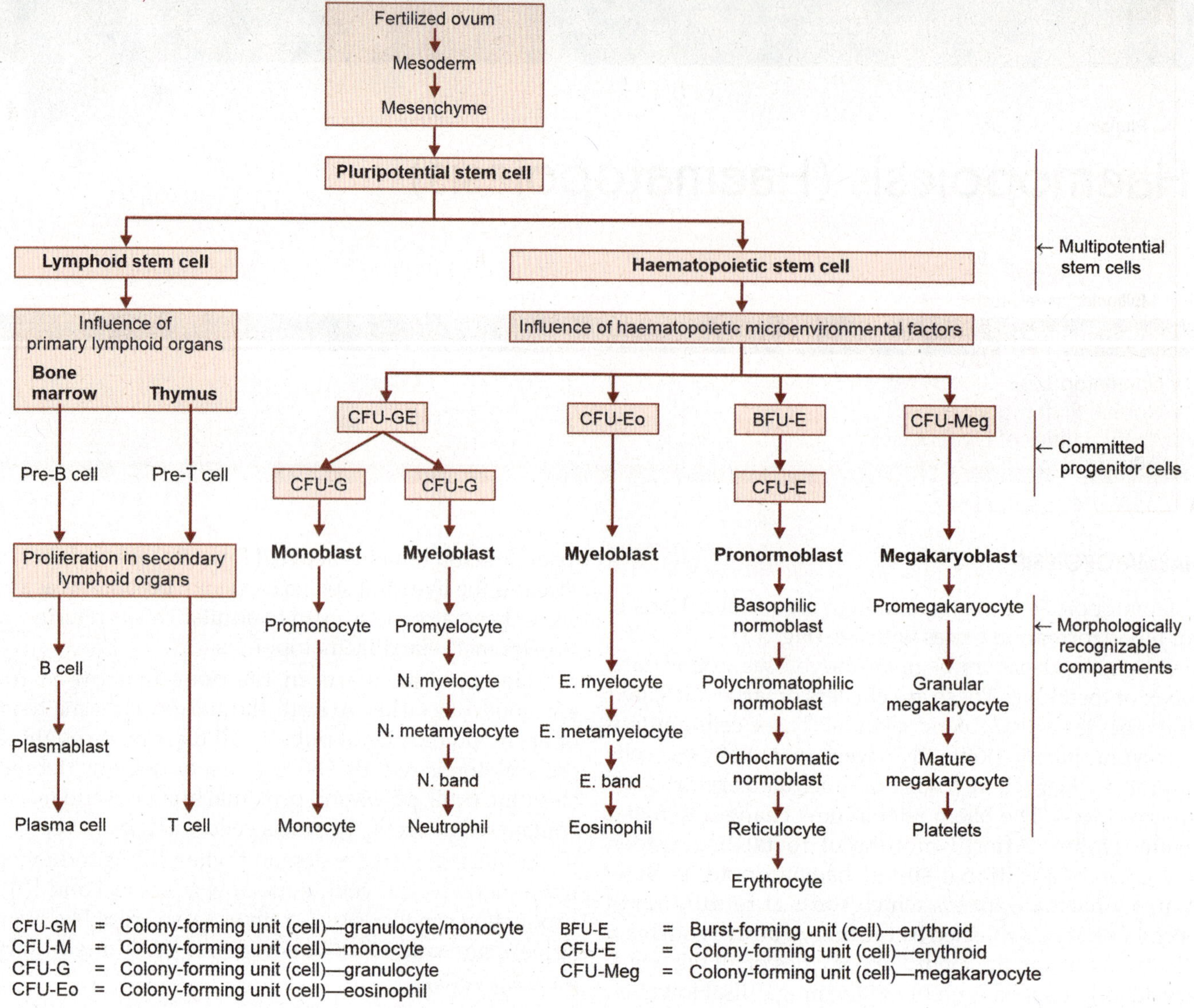

Fig. 3.2: Normal haemopoiesis

blue (non-haemoglobinised with a high content of ribonucleoprotein).

3. **Early normoblast (basophilic normoblast type I):** Formed from the pro-erythroblst by division; measures 11 to 17 microns: nucleus large but without neucleoli; nuclear chromatin coarse and shows some lumps due to condensation; cytoplasm agranular and blue (non-haemoglobinised).
4. **Intermediate normoblast (polychromatophilic normoblast type II) (Fig. 3.4):** Formed by division from the early normoblast; measures 10 to 14 microns; nucleus smaller than that of the precursor and nuclear chromatin coarser with many lumps; cytoplasm bluish red (partial haemoglobinisation).
5. **Late normoblast (orthochromatic normoblast type III):** Formed by ripening of the intermediate normoblast measures 7 to 10 microns (a little larger than the mature erythrocyte); nuclear chromatin very coarse, almost lumpy, cytoplasm red (fully haemoglobinised).
6. **Reticulocyte:** The smear has been stained supravitally by brilliant cresylblue. A non-nucleated cell of the size of a mature erythrocyte or a little larger, cytoplasm shows a network of reticulum stained blue (basophilic ribonucleoprotein).
7. **Mature erythrocyte:** Measure 7.2 microns in diameter, non-nucleated, biconcave disc, cytoplasm stained almost uniformly red with a faint central pallor.

ABNORMALITIES OF ERYTHROCYTES

Size: With some experience it is possible to say if the red cells are of normal size (normocytosis), diminished in size (microcytosis) or increased in size (macrocytosis). One judges the size by the diameter (normal average: 7.2 microns). In severe anaemia there is variation in the size of cells; this is anisocytosis. Megalocytes are large oval cells found in megaloblastic anaemias.

Shape: Red cells with an irregular shape are called poikilocytes. The commonest irregularity is a pear-shaped

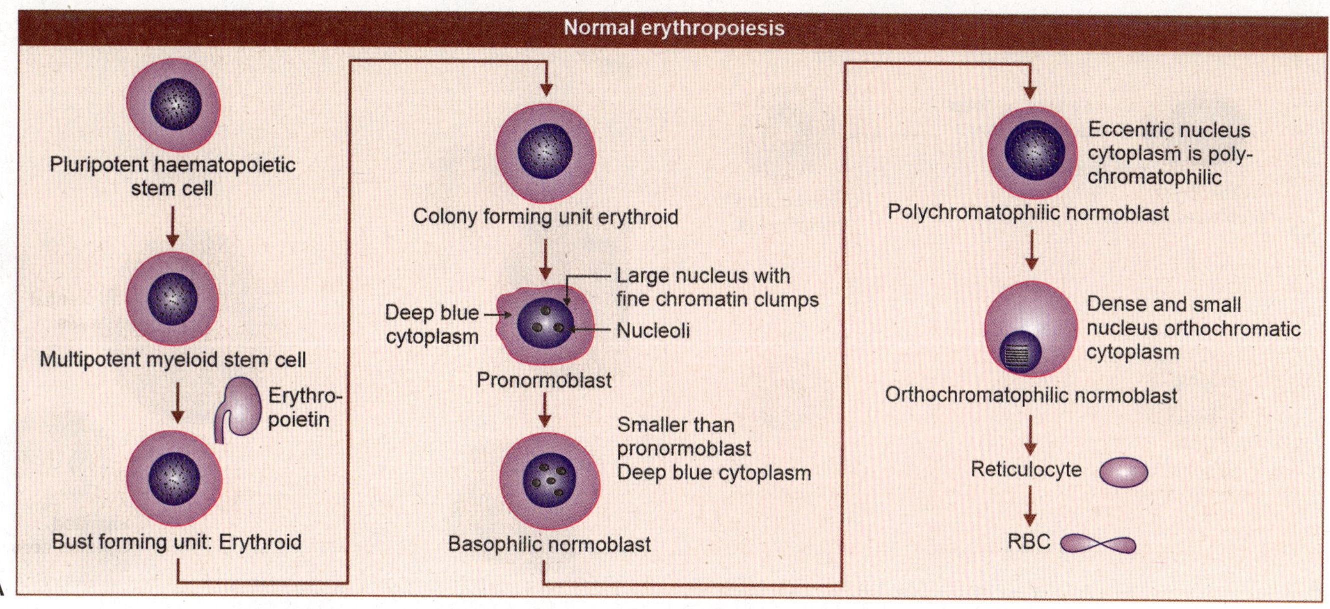

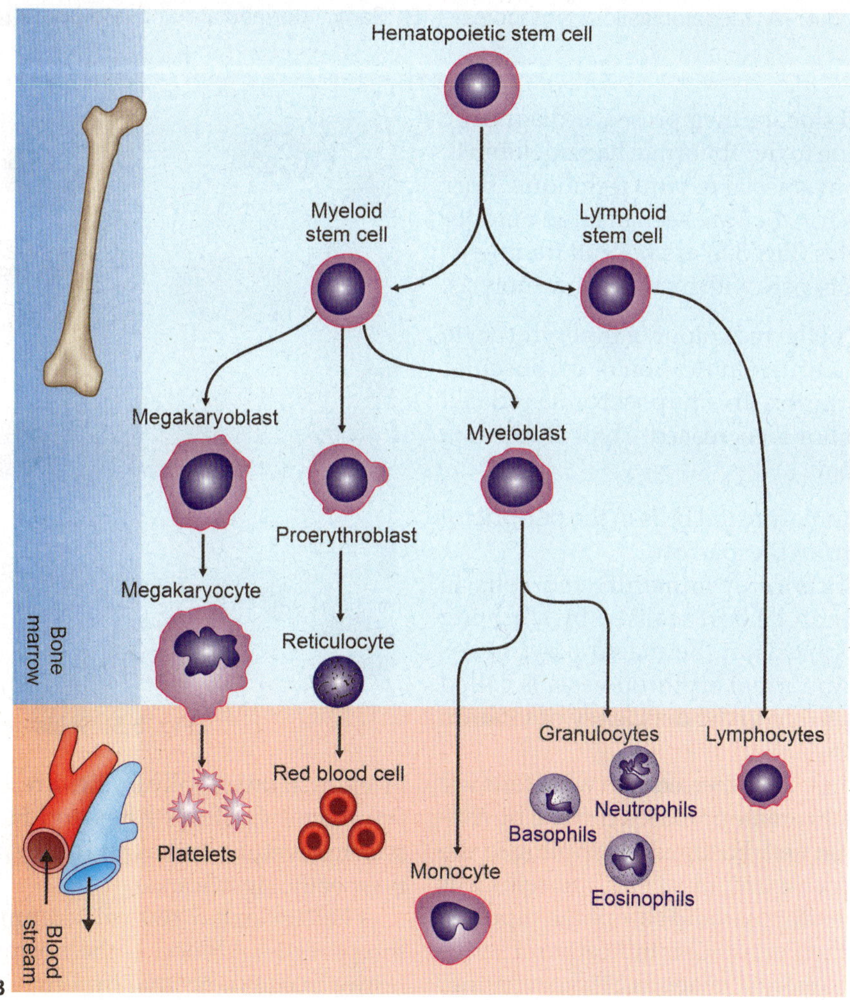

Fig. 3.3: (A) Normal erythropoiesis; (B) Normal haemopoiesis

cell. Poikilocytosis, like anisocytosis, is a non-specific phenomenon found in all severe anaemias. In haemolytic anaemias the red cells are abnormally thick; they look like densely stained microcytes: the abnormality is known as micropherocytosis. Target cells are thin red cells with a relatively large diameter and resemble the concentric circles of a rifle target; they are seen in various anaemias, in obstructive jaundice and after splenectomy. Sickle cells

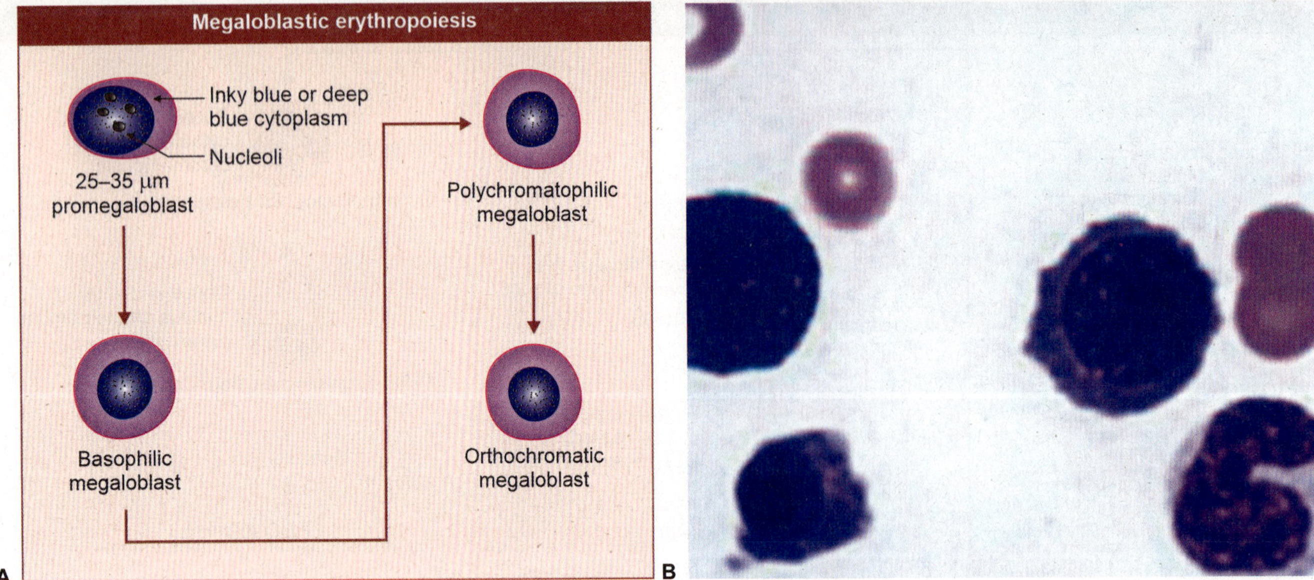

Fig. 3.4: (A) Megaloblastic erythropoiesis; (B) Early, intermediate and late normoblast

may be seen in stained smears; their presence, diagnostic of sickle cell disease due to the abnormal haemoglobin S, is best demonstrated by special *in vitro* technique. Burr cell with spiny periphery; they are seen in large number in uraemia. Schistocytes (Fig. 3.5) are red cell fragments found in many blood diseases with increased haemolysis.

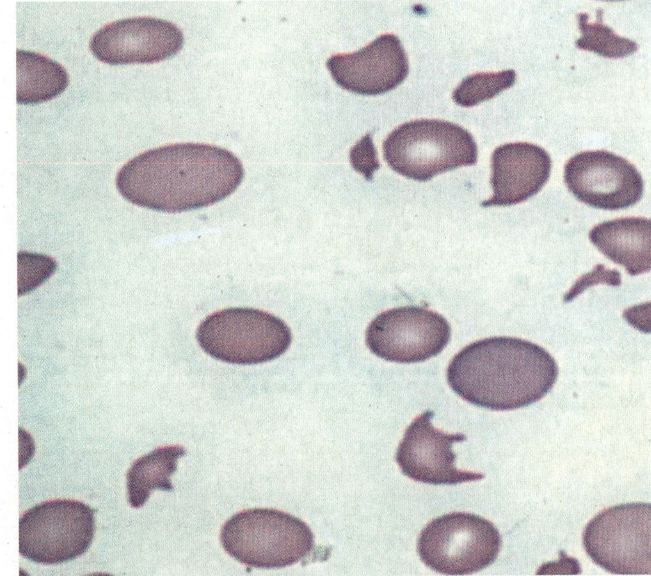

Fig. 3.5: Schistocytes

Colour: The intensity of the red colour of the erythrocyte in a stained smear is a rough indication of corpuscular haemoglobin concentration. In a hypochromic red cell the normal central pallor is increased. Hypochromasia indicates iron deficiency.

Immature red cells: Immature red cells in the peripheral blood can only come from the marrow.

The correct significance of immature red cells in the peripheral blood can be best realised by studying their source, erythropoiesis in the marrow by means of marrow, biposy. Abnormal erythropoiesis is called 'Meagaloblastic' and is due to the deficiency of vitamin B_{12} or folic acid, or both.

Only common findings are referred to in what follows: Polychromasia (polychromatophilia) is diffuse bluish-grey staining of the red cell. Basophilic stippling is the presence of multiple coarse granules in the red cell. Cells which show polychromatophilia and basophilic stippling are reticulocytes and their presence is indicative of active erythropoiesis, as in heamolytic anaemias; Pappenheimer bodies are small scanty basophilic granules in the red cell; unlike the granules of basophilic stippling, these bodies give a positive prussian blue reaction; they are siderophilic granules. Pappenheimer bodies are characteristically present after splenectomy. Cells with pappenheimer bodies or siderophil granules are known as siderocytes. Cabbot's rings are reddish purple rings or like the figure of eight. Howell-Jolly bodies are reddish blue nucleated fragments. Cabbot's rings and Howell-Jolly bodies are seen in severe anaemias and after splenectomy. They have no specific significance.

The nucleated red cell commonly encountered in the peripheral blood is the normoblast. An occasional normoblast is a normal findings in the newborn. A few normoblasts 2 to 5 per 100 leucocytes may be present in any severe anaemia. If present in large numbers, a haemolytic anaemia with an actively regenerating marrow is suspected. The presence of a megaloblast in the peripheral blood means that erythropoiesis must be megablastic and that the patient must be suffering from a megaloblastic anaemia.

Normal Leucopoiesis

1. Cells of the myeloid or the granular series are produced normally only in the marrow.
2. Cells of the lymphoid series arise in the marrow to a small extent; their chief source is the lymphoid tissue small extent; lymph nodes and lymphoid tissue of the tonsils, the pharynx, the gastrointestinal tract, the spleen and the thymus.
3. Cells of the monocytic series are probably derived from the reticulum cells of the marrow and the spleen. However, some consider myeloblasts and even lymphocytes as their ancestors.

Myeloid Cells

Myeloid cells develop from pluripotent stem cells in the marrow. The earliest cell which can be recognised with certainty as belonging to the myeloid series is myeloblast. Myeloblast constitutes less than 1 to 5% of normal marrow cells. They are never present in normal peripheral blood.

Myeloblast (Fig. 3.6)

- Large, round nucleus
- Two or more pale blue nucleoli
- Scanty blue cytoplasm

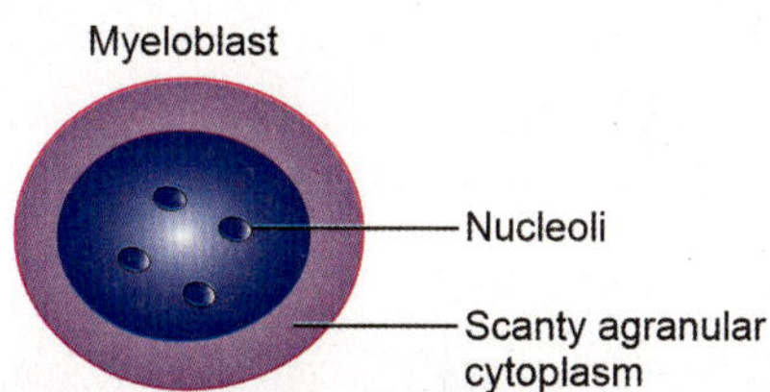

Fig. 3.6: Myeloblast

Myeloblast differentiates into promyelocyte. During this differentiation the lysosomal granules (azurophil granules) are produced.

Promyelocyte (Fig. 3.7)

- Cytoplasm contains coarse blue or violet, dense granules.
- Granules are located in the periphery of the cell.
- Histochemically, the granules are positive for myeloperoxidase.
- Nucleus is eccentric and has nucleoli like the myeloblast.
- Promyelocyte differentiates to produce the myelocyte.

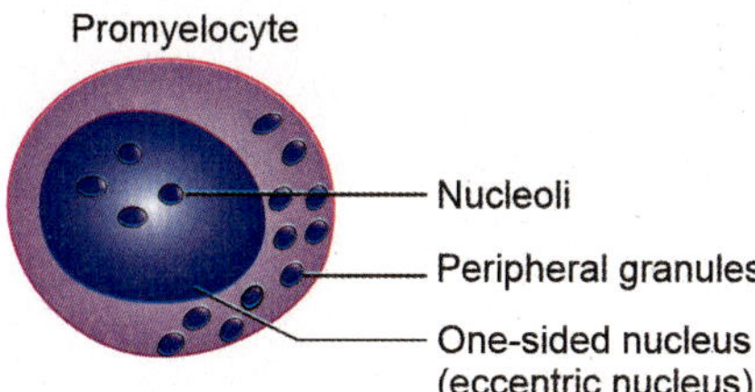

Fig. 3.7: Promyelocyte

Myelocyte (Fig. 3.8)

- Clumping of nuclear chromatin begins
- Nucleoli are less distinct compared to previous cells

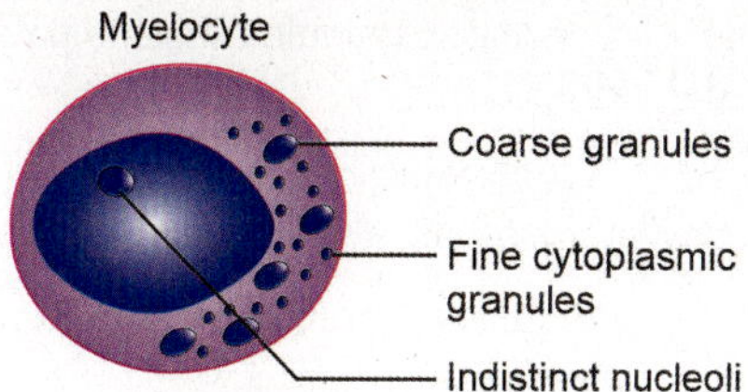

Fig. 3.8: Myelocyte

- Nucleus is eccentric.
- Cytoplasm starts becoming pinkish.

Towards the final stage of maturation, cells loose the ability to divide. They just differentiate into metamyelocytes and then to band neutrophils before finally maturing into neutrophils.

Metamyelocyte (Fig. 3.9)

- Cytoplasm matures to uniform pink colour
- Cytoplasmic granules are fine pinkish blue in colour and scattered throughout cytoplasm.
- Nuclear chromatin is coarse, clumped and condensed in the periphery.
- The nucleus is bean shaped (indented). This is the beginning of nuclear segmentation.

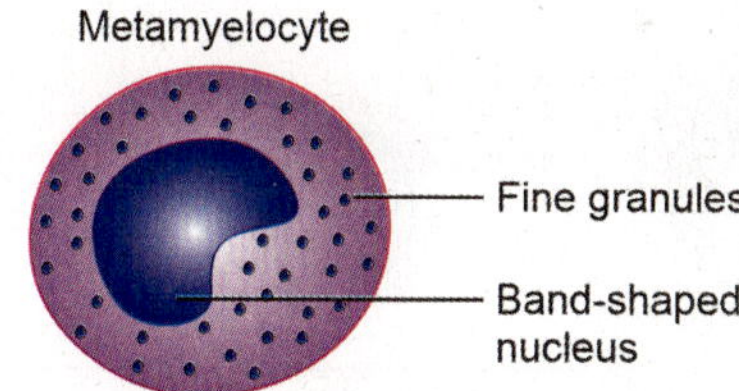

Fig. 3.9: Metamyelocyte

Band Form (Stab Form) (Fig. 3.10)

- Band form are the first cells to appear in normal peripheral blood (3–5%).
- Mature pink cytoplasm
- Fine bluish or azure cytoplasmic granules
- Elongated, sausage or band-shaped nucleus
- Coarse and clumped nuclear chromatin

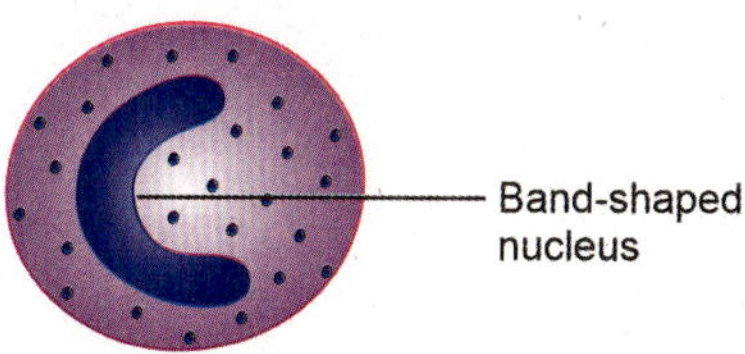

Fig. 3.10: Band form

Segmented cell (polymorphonuclear cells). Size 10 to 12 microns; nucleus shows lobes connected by filaments; cytoplasm contains granules.

(a) Neutrophil segmented	Cytoplastic granules fine and pale pink violet
(b) Basophil segmented	Cytoplasmic granules coarse and pink; nucleus like a spectacle (bilobed)
(c) Basophil segmented	Cytoplasmic granules large, deep purple and obscure the nucleus.

Summary of stages in the formation of polymorphs is shown in Fig. 3.11.

Abnormalities of Leucocytes (Fig. 3.12)

These mainly consist of the presence of immature leucocytes and of granulocytes with toxic granulations. Normally an occasional metamyelocytes or juvenile cells (about 1%) are present. In pyogenic infections (with leucocytosis) their count goes up. A few myelocytes are common in the blood of infants and children. In adults a few myelocytes and an occasional myeloblast (without leucocytosis) may be found in severe anaemias and when the marrow is the seat of metastatic deposits of a carcinoma. However, in chronic myeloid leukaemia, the blood shows a large number of myelocytes (10 to 50%) and fewer myeloblast (2 to 5%). In acute myeloid leukaemia, the myeloblast is the predominant cell in the blood (up to 90%). In chronic lymphatic leukaemia, the predominant cell in the blood is the small lymphocyte, forming 85–99% of leucocytes; lymphoblasts are rare. In acute lymphatic leukaemia, the lymphoblast is the predominant cell. In monocytic leukaemia, 50 to 90% of leucocytes are monocytes and precursors (monoblasts), a few myelocytes and myeloblasts are also encountered. In infectious Mononucleosis (glandular fever), 40 to 80% of leucocytes are ordinary lymphocytes, lymphocytoid monocytes 'abnormal cells'. The last are primitive monocytes. Morphologically infectious mononucleosis can be confused with monocytic leukaemia; in the former the patient's serum contains agglutinins for sheep's red cells (Paul-Bunnel's test).

In severe acute infections, neutrophils may show vacuolation of the cytoplasm and their granules become coarse and blue-stained. These 'toxic granules' are indicative of severe toxaemia. Heavy granulation is also seen in aplastic anaemias.

Normal Thrombopoiesis

1. Megakaryoblast: Measures 20 to 25 micrones; nucleus single, oval or slightly indented; several nucleoli; cytoplasm scanty, blue and agranular.

Haemocytoblast (primitive multipotential)	Myeloblast (committed)	Promyelocyte	Myelocyte	Metamyelocyte	Polymorph in marrow and blood
% age	< 1	< 5	< 15		
Size (diameter) 15/25 μm	15–18 μm	12–18 μm	12–18 μm	12–15 μm	10–15 μm
Nucleus Spherical; even dispersal of chromatin	Spherical; even dispersal of chromatin	Spherical; chromatin slightly condensed	Ovoid; condensation of chromatin	'Band' of 'stab' shape; chromatin condesed	2–5 lobes; chromatin condensed
Nucleoli Several	2–4	2–4	None	None	None
Cytoplasm Blue (high RNA content)	Blue (high RNA content)	Blue	Less blue	Less blue Glycogen^{++}	Less blue Glycogen^{++}
Granules None	None	Scanty large granules; *myeloper-oxidase* and *hydrolases*	Many small granules; alkaline *phosphatase*, various lytic enzymes	→ → →	→ → →

Fig. 3.11: Stages in the formation of polymorph

2. Promegakaryocyte: Larger than the precursor; nucleus indented with coarser chromatin than that of the precursor; nucleoli present; cytoplasm shows a few purplish red granules at the periphery.
3. Megakarycocyte: Measures 40 to 70 microns; cell border irregular in the form of pseudopods; many nuclei in the form of lobes in a ring; no nucleoli; cytoplasm pale blue and contains purplish-blue granules.
4. Platelets: Non-nucleated round or oval bodies; measure 2 to 3 microns; cytoplasm blue or purple and contains many granules. They are formed by nipping of the pseudopodia of the megakaryocytes.

DISORDER OF PLATELETS

Abnormalities of Platelets (Fig. 3.12)

A significant reduction of platelets (thrombocytopenia) can be judged in the smear. In essential thrombocytopenia, platelets may in addition show morphological abnormalities in the forms, e.g. small size, giant forms or non-granularity of their cytoplasm. Abnormal variation in the size of platelets is a feature of myelosclerosis. Genesis of thrombocytopenia due to different types of platelet disorder is shown in Fig. 3.12.

Idiopathic Thrombocytopenic Purpura (ITP)

Synonyms: Primary or immune thrombocytopenic purpura.

ITP is an autoimmune disorder characterised by thrombocytopenia due to antibody formation.

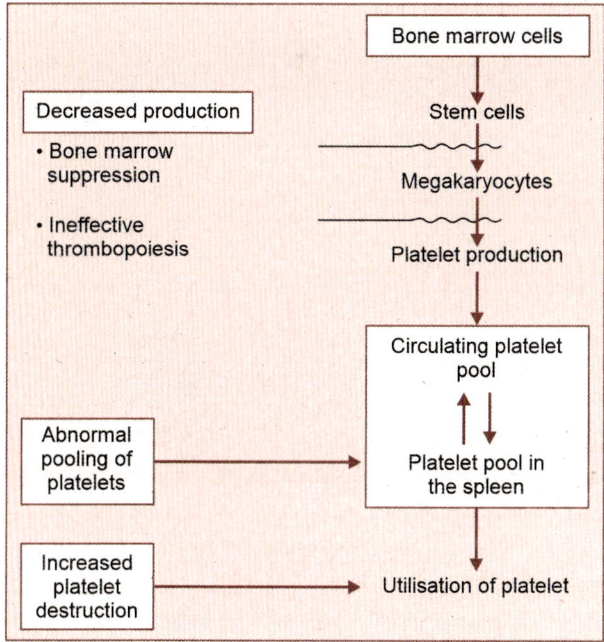

Fig. 3.12: Genesis of thrombocytopenia

Types

- Acute ITP
  - Common in children, rare in adults
  - No sex preponderance
- Chronic ITP
  - Common in adults (20–40 years)
  - No sex preponderance

The difference between acute ITP and chronic ITP is shown in Table 3.1.

Table 3.1: Acute and chronic ITP

	Acute ITP	*Chronic ITP*
Age	Children	Adults (20–40 years)
Duration	<6 months	>6 months
Onset	Sudden appearance of petechial gum bleeding or epistaxis	• No specific signs and symptoms • Petechial gum bleeding, mucosal bleeding or menorrhagia
Platelet count	$<20 \times 10^9$/L	$<1 \times 10^9$/L
Course	Weeks (1–8)	Months/years
M:F ratio	Equal	> in females

Pathogenesis: Patients suffering from ITP develop autoantibody directed against two platelet membrane glycoprotein complex IIb–IIIa and Ib–IX. These antibodies are commonly IgG class but IgM antibodies are also found. These antibodies act in two ways:

- **As opsonins:** The antibodies opsonise the platelets and are then phagocytosed by the phagocytic cells.
- **Impair the platelet function:** Antibodies bind to epitopes on critical region of these glycoproteins and prevent platelet function.

The main site of platelet removal is spleen, which is also the site of autoantibody formation.

Thrombotic Thrombocytopenic Purpora (TTP)

TTP is a syndrome characterised by:

- **Five features:** Thrombocytopenia
  Microangiopathic haemolytic anaemia
  Transient neurological deficit
  Fever
  Renal failure
- **Incidence:** Rare
- **Age:** Adults
- **Sex:** Females

Pathogenesis

The exact initiating cause of TTP is not known. However, immune disorders, infections and chemicals may cause vascular endothelial damage. The damaged endothelium releases unusual large multimers of factor VIII—von Willebrand complex into the circulation. These complexes cause platelet aggregation giving rise to thrombus formation which typically involve terminal arterioles and capillaries. Multiple thrombi consume a large number of platelets causing thrombocytopenia (consumption thrombocytopenia). A large number of RBCs also get involved in the thrombus formation. These RBCs get lysed and cause anaemia (microangiopathic haemolytic anaemia). Thrombus occludes many organs. Occlusion of kidney causes renal failure. The other common organ involved is brain which causes neurological deficit.

Lab Investigations

- **Platelet count:** Typically the count is lowest, in acute ITP (< 20,000/ml) compared to chronic ITP (<1 lakh)
- **Bleeding time:** Pronlonged
- **Platelet autoantibody** is positive (+)
- **Peripheral smear:**
  - Sometimes abnormal platelets can be identified. These are generally large in size
  - Bleeding may lead to anaemia → normocytic normochromic
- **Bone marrow:** Often shows increased number of megakaryocytes some of which appear immature (non-lobulated and single nuclei) with lesser degree of cytoplasmic granularity. All these changes are non-specific and are due to accelerated thrombopoiesis. Bone marrow may also be normal. Marrow examination is essential to rule out aplastic changes causing decrease in platelet count.
- **Splenic changes:**
  - Normal to moderate enlargement of spleen
  - Megakaryocytes may be seen in spleen
  - Congestion of splenic sinusoid.

Anaemias in General and Iron Deficiency Anaemias

Chapter Outline

INTRODUCTION: DEFINITION OF ANAEMIA

Anaemia is a state in which the amount of haemoglobin or the number of red cells in the blood is below the normal limits. The red cell which is the carrier of haemoglobin has a limited life span. To maintain haemoglobin and red cells within the normal limits new fully haemoglobinised red cells must be produced to replace the lost ones. Anaemia will, therefore, necessarily result

1. if the production of red cells is inadequate in quality or quantity,
2. if red cell destruction or blood loss exceeds the production, or
3. if these two factors combine.

Anaemia is thus a symptom or sign of either of the two events mentioned above; it is not a disease. The objective behind investigating a case of anaemia is to unearth the underlying mechanism, to discover the cause of the imbalance between the production and the destruction of the red cell.

Mechanism of Production of Anaemia

The mechanism is threefolds

1. Diminished erythropoiesis (dyshaemopoietic anaemias)
2. Blood loss (haemorrhagic anaemias); and
3. Increased haemolysis (haemolytic anaemias).

Dimished erythropoiesis (dyshaemopoiesis) is either due to nutritional deficiency or due to marrow failure. Nutritional factors essential for erythropoiesis are: Iron, traces of copper, cobalt, vitamin B complex (vitamin B_{12} folic acid, pyridoxine, riboflavin and nicotinic acid), vitamin C, first class proteins, or possibly some internal secretions (thyroid, pituitary, sex hormones) and pigments (bile pigments and chlorophyll). The deficiency of these factors may be dietetic or due to defective absorption, or due to increased demands (pregnancy or period of growth). Dietetic defiency is a common cause of nutritional anaemias in our country. Failure of marrow (resulting in aplastic or hypoplastic anaemias) may be primary (idiopathic) or due to extraneous toxic factors (chemicals, drugs and irradiations). Blood loss may be acute or chronic and brought about by trauma or disease.

Increased haemolysis may be due to hereditary intracorpusular defects (spherocytosis, sickling) reducing the life span of the red cell, or may be acquired and due to the action of haemolytic agents (physical, chemical, bacterial and antibodies).

In the atiological diagnosis of anaemia the following points are important:

- The family history regarding anaemia, jaundice and bleeding in other members of the family;
- The personal history regarding dietary habits, occupation (contact with chemicals), drugs and chronic bleeding from any site;
- The physical examination (to detect lymphadenopathy, hepatosplenomegaly, and evidence of deficiency states);
- Ancillary examinations like roentgenography and laboratory investigations.

Moderate anaemia may not be detectable by the physical examination. Two laboratory screening procedures are available to decide the issue:

1. Estimation of haemoglobin, and
2. Haematocrit determination.

In an adult haemoglobin below 12 gm per 100 ml or PCV below 37 per 100 ml indicates the presence of anaemia. If both haemoglobin estimation and determination of PCV are carried out, they are a check against one another.

The basic study consists of the cytological examination of the blood; this includes the determination of haemoglobin, the enumeration of red cells and leucocytes (with the reticulocyte count and platelet count in special cases), the differential count and the examination of the stained smear. The levels of haemoglobin and red cells will tell about the severity of the anaemic state and the examination of the smear will give information about the size of the red cell, its haemoglobin concentration and the presence of abnormal red cells. To know the morphologic type of anaemia with exactitude the first step is haematocrit determination which gives the corpuscular volume of the packed cell (PCV) per 100 ml of the blood. From PCV, haemoglobin in gram per 100 ml and red cell per cu mm, two values most essential for the morphologic typing of anaemias can be calculated. These are the mean corpuscular volume (MCV) and the mean corpuscular haemoglobin concentration (MCHC).

Anaemias of common morphologic type and their causes are given in Table 4.1.

Classification of anaemias based on pathophysiologic factors is given in Table 4.2.

An approach to case of anaemia is shown in Fig. 4.1.

An approach to a case of neonatal anaemia is shown in Fig. 4.2.

IRON DEFICIENCY ANAEMIA

Iron deficiency anaemia is the most common form of nutritional deficiency in the world. The cause of iron deficiency varies in different sexes, population groups and ages. In India worm infestation is the most common cause of iron deficiency anaemia in children.

Definition of Iron Deficiency Anaemia

The World Health Organization has defined iron deficiency anaemia as haemoglobin less than 14 g/dl for adult men; 12 g/dl for adult non-pregnant women; and 11 g/dl for pregnant women.

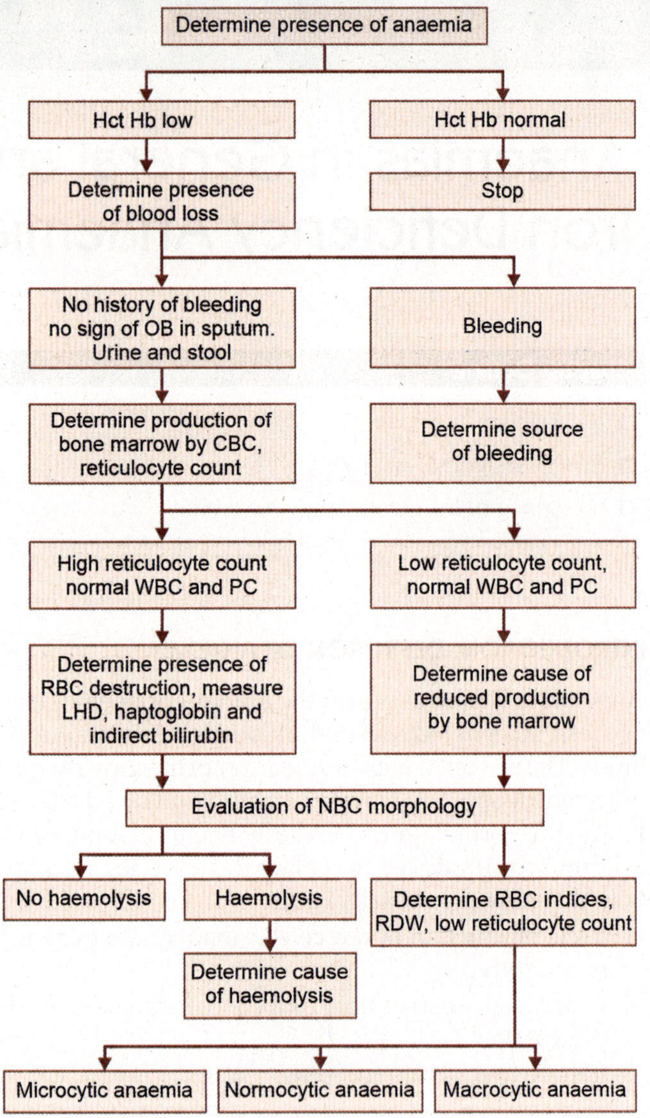

Fig. 4.1: Approach to a case of anaemia

Incidence of Iron Deficiency Anaemia

Incidence of iron deficiency anaemia is high in infants and pregnant women. In India the incidence of iron deficiency anaemia in adult women varies from 35 to 64%; in pregnant women from 56 to 80%; and in adult males 6%.

Table 4.1: Anaemias: Common morphologic types and their causes

Types of anaemia	*MCV (fl) C. microns*	*MCHC percentage*	*Common cause*
1. Macrocytic normochromic	More than 94	More than 30	Deficiency of vitamin B_{12} or of folic acid; some times aplastic and haemolytic anaemia
2. Macrocytic hypochromic	More than 94	Less than 30	Deficiency of vitamin B_{12} or of folic acid plus iron
3. Normocytic normochromic	Between 78 and 94	Between 30 and 33	Haemorrhagic anaemias and haemolytic anaemias; hypolastic and aplastic anaemias
4. Microcytic normochromic	Below 78	Between 30 and 33	Anaemia due to infections
5. Microcytic hypochromic	Below 78	Below 30	Deficiency or lack of iron

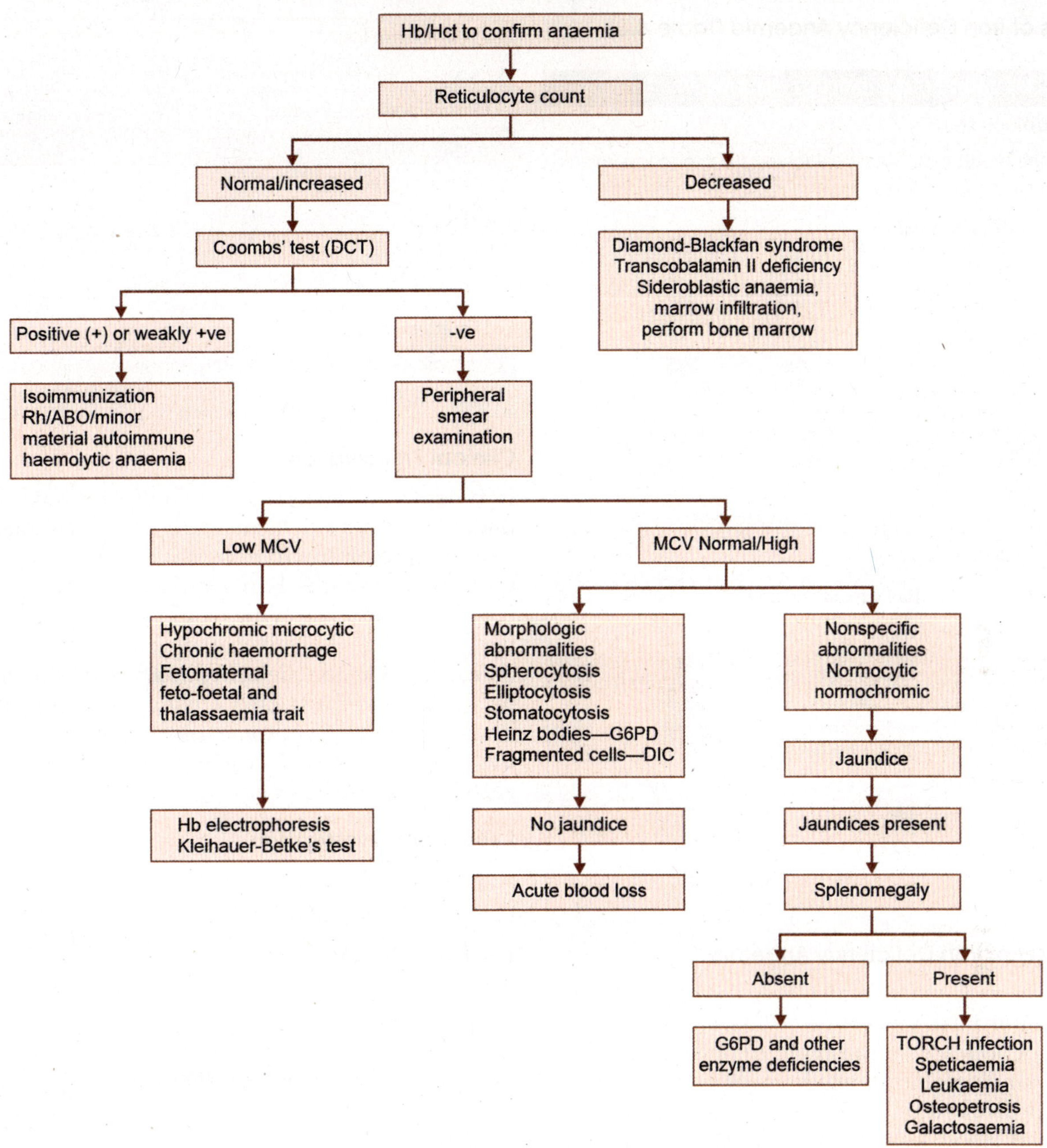

Fig. 4.2: Approach to a case of neonatal anaemia

Table 4.2: Classification of anaemia based on pathophysiologic factors
Anaemia due to blood loss
▪ Acute blood loss (external and internal bleeding)
▪ Chronic blood loss (gastrointestinal, reproductive and urinary tract)
▪ Fetal and perinatal blood loss.
Anaemia due to excessive destruction of red cells
▪ Hereditary (elliptocytosis, spherocytosis, enzyme deficiencies, haemoglobinopathies)
▪ Acquired (isoantibodies, autoantibodies, drug or chemically induced mechanical and traumatic, infection, hypersplenism, poroxysmal nocturnal haemoglobinuria)
Anaemia due to decreased production of red cells
▪ Nutritional deficiencies (inadequate nutritional intake: Fe, vitamin B_{12} folate deficiency; defective absorption)
▪ Bone marrow failure (endocrine, idiopathic, myelophthisic, toxic)

Causes of Iron Deficiency Anaemia (Table 4.3)

Table 4.3: Causes of iron deficiency anaemia
Chronic blood loss
▪ **Ulcerine blood loss:** Menstrual losses and blood loss related to pregnancy and delivery
Gastrointestinal blood loss
Benign conditions
▪ Peptic ulcers (gastric or duodenal)
▪ Esophageal varices
▪ Hiatal hernia
▪ Colonic diverticula or polyps
▪ Hemorrhoids
▪ Chronic aspirin use
▪ Long-distance running that induces mild diffuse
▪ Gastrointestinal bleeding
▪ Hereditary haemorrhagic telangiectasia
▪ Parasites (e.g. hookworm)
Malignancy
▪ Colon and colorectal carcinoma
▪ Gastric carcinoma
▪ Esophageal carcinoma
▪ Gastric carcinoma
▪ Esophageal carcinoma
▪ Small intestinal carcinoma

Aetiology of Iron Deficiency Anaemia

Iron deficiency anaemia results from conditions that decrease iron intake, increase iron loss, increase demand for iron or decrease iron absorption (Table 4.4). In many instances multiple factors may be involved. A marginally adequate dietary iron intake associated with increased menstrual blood loss or a hookworm infection may precipitate anaemia.

Table 4.4 Aetiology of iron deficiency anaemia
Decreased iron intake
▪ Inadequate diet
▪ Impaired absorption
◦ Sprue
◦ Crohn's disease
◦ Post-gastrectomy
◦ Pica
Increased demand for iron
▪ Rapid growth in infancy or adolescence
▪ Pregnancy
▪ Lactation
Increased iron loss
▪ Excessive menstrual flow
▪ Gastrointestinal bleeding
◦ Haemorrhoids
◦ Peptic ulcer
◦ Hookworm
◦ Neoplasms
◦ Ulcerative colitis
▪ Disorders of haemostasis
▪ Chronic renal failure and haemodialysis
▪ Haematuria

Clinical Presentation

Iron deficiency anaemia is not a disease but a sign of underlying disease. Patients manifest with fatigue, pallor and reduced ability to exercise. The patients become symptomatic as the Hb levels goes below 7 gm/dl. Fissures in the angle of the mouth and flattened spoon-like finger nails (koilonychia) develop with severe iron deficiency. Sore tongue with papillary atrophy (tongue becoems smooth) is also a common manifestation. Plummer Vinson syndrome (pharyngeal webs causing dysphagia and iron deficiency anaemia) and atrophic gastritis may also be seen.

Laboratory investigation

Haemoglobin

Low (usually 8 g/dl or lower)

Peripheral Smear (PS)

RBCs are **microcytic hypochromic.** Hypochromia is the presence of > 1/3 pallor. The number of microcytes depends on severity of the anaemia. In very severe case the RBC may appear as rings (Fig. 4.3).

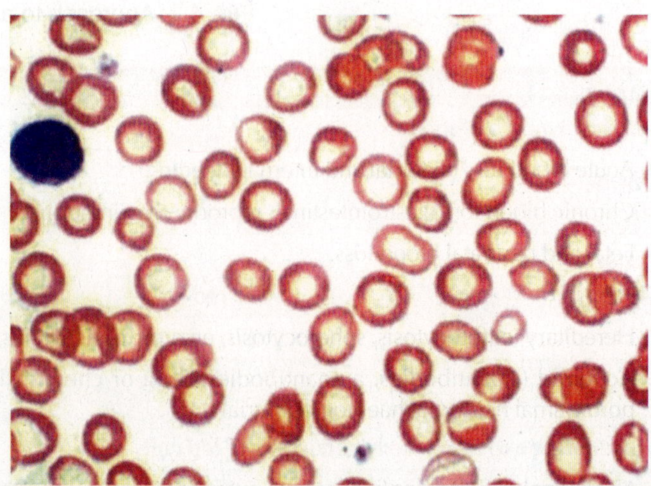

Fig. 4.3: Photomicrograph showing microcytic hypochromic picture (Giemsa × 100).

Poikilocytes: Abnormal shape of RBC may be seen in moderate numbers, such as:

- Elongated (pencil-shaped) and elliptical
- Tailed

WBC: Normal

Platelet: Increased, because of microhaemorrhages

Bone marrow: Erythroid hyperplasia of variable degree (M:E is 2:1 to reversed state of 1:2). A few erythroid cells show karyorrhexis and nuclear budding.

Final diagnosis of *iron deficiency* aneamia is always by laboratory studies described below.

1. **Serum iron:** Serum iron represents the amount of circulating iron bound to transferrin. Serum iron is decreased in iron deficiency anaemia. Normal serum iron value is 50–150 μg/dl.
2. **Total iron-binding capacity (TIBC):** Total iron-binding capacity of transferrin in normal individual is 300–600 μg/dl. In iron deficiency anaemia due to less available iron more transferin is available for binding and thus increase the iron-binding capacity (TIBC). Thus, TIBC is an indirect measure of circulating transferrin.

Transferrin Saturation

In iron deficiency state due to decrease availability of iron the saturation of transferrin (i.e. binding of transferrin with iron) is less, generally below 18%.

Serum Ferritin

Serum ferritin is the best measure of iron store in the body. Serum ferritin estimation is the most useful diagnostic test. However, it lacks sensitivity. The normal value for ferritin varies with age and gender. Normal serum ferritin value varies from 50 to 300 μg/L.

Red Cell Protoporphyrin

Protoporphyrin is an intermediate product in heme synthesis pathway. When iron is deficient heme synthesis is impaired and this intermediate product 'protoporphyrin' accumulates. Thus, in iron deficiency anaemia red blood cell protoporphyrin levels in excess of 100 μg/dl are seen (normal is <30 μg/dl).

Bone Marrow Iron Store

Bodies iron store can be estimated by iron stain of bone marrow RE cells in aspirate or biopsy. Marrow iron stain provides additional information about effective delivery or iron to developing erythroblasts called sideroblasts as they show iron granules. If iron delivery is blocked, the number of sideroblast will be very few (normal value is 40–60% out of total erythroblasts) though iron in RE cells of marrow will be normal.

Red Cell Indices

- MCV (mean corpuscular volume) – ↓(N = 78 – 98 fl)
- MCH (mean corpuscular haemoglobin)– ↓ (N = 26 – 33 pg)
- MCHC (mean corpuscular haemoglobin concentration)– ↓ (N = 30 – 35 g/dl)

The degree of changes in red cells indices depends on duration and severity of anaemia.

Reticulocyte count may be normal of slightly ↑ Platelet count is usually increased.

Differential diagnosis of microcytic hypochromic anaemia

- Sideroblastic anaemia—presence of ring sideroblast
- Thalassaemia—picture of haemolytic anaemia
- Lead poisoning—basophilic stippling
- Anaemia of chronic disorders—iron stores are normal or increased.

Laboratory tests in the differential diagnosis of microcytic hypochromic anaemias are described in Tables 4.5 to 4.7

Table 4.5: Value in iron deficient states

	Normal	*Iron depletion*	*Iron deficiency erythropoiesis*	*Iron deficiency anaemia*
RBC morphology	N	N	N	Microcytic hypochromic
Sideroblasts (%)	40–60	40–60	<10	<10
RBC protoporphyrin (μg/dl RBC)	30	30	100	200
Transferrin saturation (%)	20–50	30	<15	<10
Plasma iron (μg/dl)	65–165	115	<60	<40
Plasma ferritin (μg /dl)	300–360	360	390	410
RE marrow iron	2–3+	0–1+	0	0

Table 4.6: Laboratory tests in different diagnosis of microcytic (MCV <80 fl) and hypochromic (MCHC <30 dl) anaemias

Types of Anaemia	*Serum iron*	*TIBC*	*Transferrin saturation*	*Serum ferritin*	*FEP**	*Marrow haemosiderin*	*Sideroblasts*	*Type of haemoglobin*	*Anaemia*	*RBC count*	*RDW*
Normal values	80–160 μg/dl in men 50–150 μg/dl in women	250–410 μg/dl	20–55%	20–150 μg/dl			30–50%	αα			11.5–14.5
Iron deficiency	D	I	D	D	I	O	D	αα	Hypochromic, normocytic, or microcytic	D	I
Normochromic normocytic, or microcytic of chronic disease	D	D or N	D or N	N or slightly I	I	N or I	D	αα	Normochromic, normocytic, or microcytic	D	N
Thalassaemia Major	I	D	I		N	I	I	20–90% F	Hypochromic Microcytic	I	N
Minor	N or I	N	N or I	I	N	N or I	I	2–8% F, A_2 is I			
Sideroblastic	N or I	D or N	I	I	D	I	I	αα	Hypochromic and/or microcytic with normocytic or macrocytic changes, dimorphic RBC population	D	I

O = absent; D = decreased; I = increased, N = normal.
*FEP = free erythrocyte protoporphyrin is useful to distinguish between iron deficiency and β-thalassaemia
Iron depletion: Early—serum iron is normal; TIBC may be increased. Latter—serum iron decreases; anaemia is often normocytic when mild or of rapid onset; anaemia first becomes microcytic, then hypochromic.
Iron deficiency may occur without anaemia (transferrin saturation < 15% decreased marrow iron and sideroblasts).

Table 4.7: Laboratory features in microcytic and hypochromic anaemias

	Serum iron	*Serum TIBC*	*% Saturation*	*Marrow*		*Serum ferritin*	*FEB*	*HbA₂*	*HbF*
				% Sideroblasts	*Iron stores*				
Iron deficiency	↓	↑	↓	↓	↓	↓	↑	N-↓	N
β-Thalassaemia trait	N(↑)	N	N	N	N–↑	N–↑	N		N–↑
Anaemia of chronic disease	↓	N–↓	↓	↓	N–↑	N–↑	↑	N	N
Sideroblastic anaemia	↑	↓	↑	↑	↑	↑	↑ (↓)	N	N–↑

TIBC = Total iron-binding capacity; FEP = free erythrocyte porphyrins; ↓= decreased; N = normal; ↑= increased

Chapter 5

Megaloblastic Anaemia and Pernicious Anaemia

Chapter Outline

- Megaloblastic Anaemia
- Genesis of Megaloblastic Anaemia
- Types and Features of Megaloblastic Anaemias

Megaloblastic anaemia is a form of anaemia characterized by very large red blood cells and a decrease in the number of those cells. Anaemias are blood disorders that occur when the body has fewer red blood cells than normal. Red blood cells carry oxygen throughout the body using a protein called haemoglobin, if there are not enough of these cells or this protein, anaemia results.

For all types of megaloblastic anaemia, in addition to the red blood cells being large, the inner contents of each cell are not completely developed. This malformation causes the bone marrow to produce fewer cells, and sometimes the red blood cells die earlier than the 120-day life expectancy.

MEGALOBLASTIC ANAEMIA

Genesis of Megaloblastic Anaemia

The main cause of megaloblastic anaemia is impaired DNA synthesis. As a result nuclear development lags behind the cytoplasmic development. Thus, the nucleus is large and immature compared to cytoplasm.

Since DNA synthesis depends on vitamin B_{12} (cyanocobalamin) and folic acid, deficiency of either or both can cause megaloblastic anaemia.

Cobalamin is only present in animal products. During digestion in stomach cobalamin is released from food. It combines with gastric R binder. Gastric R binder is found in gastric secretions. In the duodenum cobalamin R binder is digested releasing cobalamin (Cbl), it then binds to intrinsic factor (IF). The IF is produced by the parietal cells of the stomach. The IF–Cbl complex goes to distal ileum and binds to specific receptor on the epithelial cells of distal ileum. IF acts as carrier for Cbl. IF–Cbl complex is internalised inside the heal epithelial mucosal cells. Inside the epithelium, IF is destroyed and Cbl released. Cbl then combines to transcobalamin (TC) II. Cbl-TC (II) complex is then secreted into circulation. It goes to liver, bone marrow and many other cells where Cbl is picked up. Cbl is stored in liver and other cells.

Megaloblastic anaemia is a type of macrocytic anaemia. An anaemia is a red blood cell defect that can lead to an undersupply of oxygen. Megaloblastic anaemia results from inhibition of DNA synthesis during red blood cell production. When DNA synthesis is impaired, the cell cycle cannot progress from the G2 growth stage to the mitosis (M) stage. This leads to continuing cell growth without division, which presents as macrocytosis. Megaloblastic anaemia has a rather slow onset, especially when compared to that of other anaemias. The defect in red cell DNA synthesis is most often due to hypovitaminosis, specifically vitamin B_{12} deficiency or folate deficiency. Loss of micronutrients may also be a cause.

Figure 5.1 shows genesis of vitamin B_{12} deficiency and IF interactions for development of autoantibodies against IF and parietal cells.

The pathological state of megaloblastosis is characterized by many large immature and dysfunctional red blood cells (megaloblasts) in the bone marrow (Fig. 5.2), and also by hypersegmented neutrophils defined as the presence of neutrophils with six or more lobes or the presence of more than 3% of neutrophils with at least five lobes (Fig. 5.3). These hypersegmented neutrophils can be detected in the peripheral blood (using a diagnostic smear of a blood sample).

Diagrammatic representation of causes of vitamin B_{12} deficiencies is shown in Fig. 5.4.

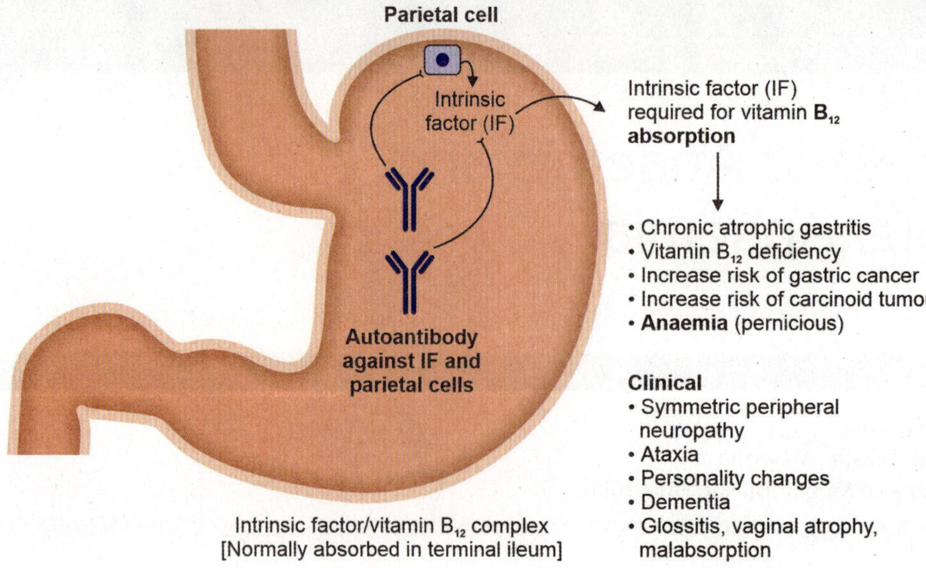

Fig. 5.1: Vitamin B_{12} deficiency genesis and pernicious anaemias

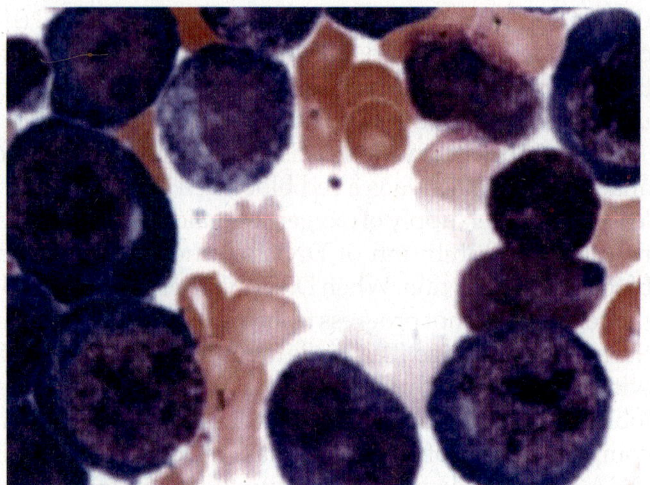

Fig. 5.2: Photomicrograph: Megaloblastic anaemia shows megaloblast bone marrow (Giemsa × 1000)

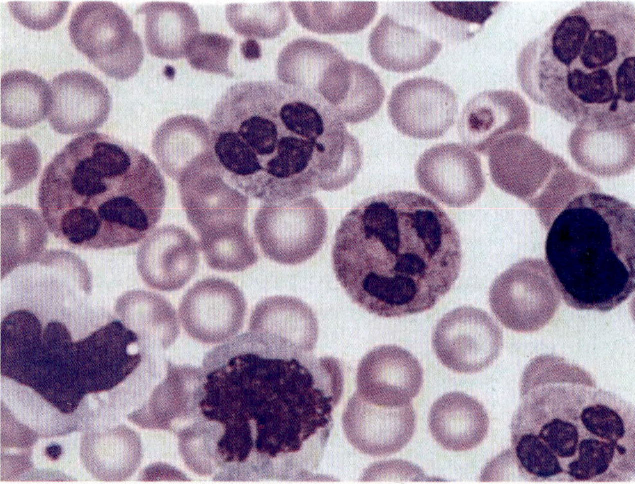

Fig. 5.3: Microphotograph showing hypersegmented polymorph (Giemsa × 1000)

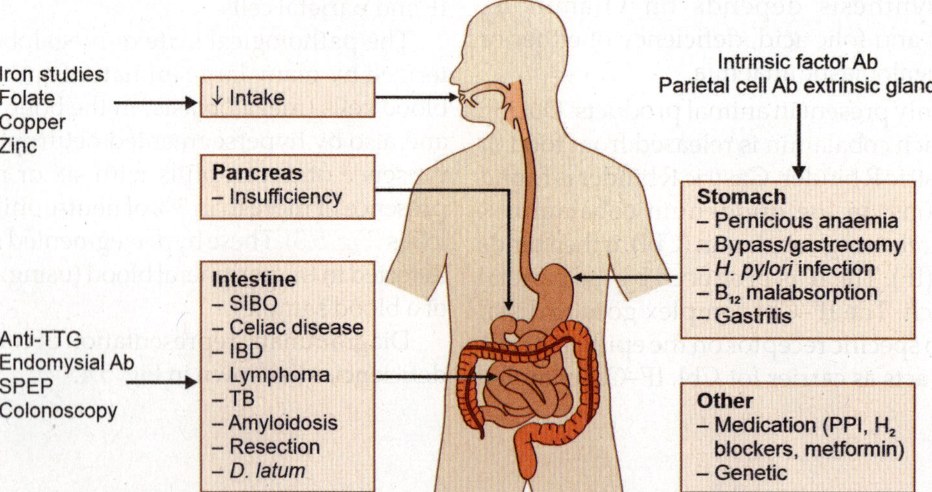

Fig. 5.4: Causes of vitamin B_{12} deficiency diagram representation

Table 5.1 shows known causes of vitamin B_{12} deficiency.

Table 5.1: Known causes of vitamin B_{12} deficiency
Depletion by decreased dietary intake
• Vegans and vegetarians
Poor absorption
Absence of intrinsic factor
• Pernicious anaemia (PA)
• Gastrectomy
• Corrosive chemical damage to stomach epithelium
• Infiltration of the stomach ((by lymphoma or carcinoma)
Increased bacterial utilization of vitamin B_{12} in areas of overgrowth
• Blind-loop syndrome
• Gastrointestinal bypass surgery
• Small bowel (jejunal) diverticula
• Intestinal stasis and obstruction due to strictures
Parasitic infestation
• Fish tapeworm (*Diphyllobothrium latum*)
Pathology in absorption sites
• Tuberculosis of the ileum
• Lymphoma of the small intestines
• Tropical sprue
• Regional enteritis
Others
• Congenital absence of transcobalamin II (TC II) [rare]
• Nitrous oxide abuse (inactivates vitamin B_{12} by oxidation of the cobalt atom)

Types and Features of Megaloblastic Anaemias

Megaloblastic anaemias are of many different kinds, but all of them are ultimately due to deficiency of vitamin B_{12} or folic acid, or of both. The two large groups are:

1. Hereditary constitutional megaloblastic anaemia (Addisonian pernicious anaemia), and
2. A symptomatic megaloblastic anaemia.

The former is due to the absence of the intrinsic factor in the gastric juice a constitutional defect causing defective absorption of vitamin B_{12}. The anaemia is macrocytic (MCV >100) and normochromic (MCHC normal). The leucocytes and platelets are reduced; the nuclei of neutrophils are hypersegmented (6 to 8 lobes). The marrow shows megaloblastic erythropoiesis and giant stab forms juveniles, and promyelocytes. The van den Bergh reaction on the serum is indirectly positive, the serum vitamin B_{12} is reduced below 100 µg/ml and the serum iron is normal. Gastric analysis shows histamine fast achlorhydria. Hereditary constitutional megaloblastic anaemias react to treatment by liver extract, vitamin B_{12} and folic acid. The last drug, however, precipitates the complication of subacute combined degeneration of the cord and is, therefore, not used. The treatment has to be life long, since the defect is constitutional. Among the broad group of symptomatic megaloblastic anaemias the commoner subvarieties are as follows:

a. Nutritional megaloblastic anaemia is due to dietetic deficiency of vitamin B_{12} or folic acid; it may be seen in infants, adult males, non-pregnant females and pregnant females (so called prenicious anaemias of pregnancy)
b. Due to the malabsorption syndrome; in tropical sprue idiopathic steatorrhoea, celiac disease, regional ileitis and patients with gastretomy and with intestinal obstruction.
c. Due to the fish tapeworm *Diphyllobothrium latum* which utilizes vitamin B_{12} in the bowel and deprives the body of the element.
d. Due to anti-convulsant drugs, folic acid anatagonists, and deficiency of ascorbic acid; in these conditions the inadequate utilization of folic acid causes megaloblastic anaemia.

These symptomatic anaemias show the following differences from the herediatary constitutional type. The anaemia may not be macrocytic and it may be hypochromic. In peripheral blood, the presence of hypersegmented neutrophils and megaloblasts are the only diagnostic featuees. The marrow picture is identical. The van den Bergh reaction may be negative. Either vitamin B_{12} or folic acid of the serum, or both may be low; the serum iron may be low. Histamine fast achlorhydria may not be present. Special tests are required to demonstrate specific defects like malasorption, steatorrhoea or the presence of tapeworm. Once the defect is removed the anaemia is cured and life-long maintenance therapy is not required.

Table 5.2 gives causes of folate deficiency.

Table 5.2: Causes of folate deficiency
Reduced intake of folate
Poor nutrition
• Alcoholism
• Anorexia nervosa
• Hyperalimentation
• Poor diet in the elderly
Malabsorption
• Alcoholism
• Loss of normal mucosa
– Celiac and tropical sprue
– Crohn's disease
– Regional ileitis
• Infiltration of submucosa
– Intestinal lymphoma
– Amyloidosis

Contd.

Table 5.2: Causes of folate deficiency (Contd.)
⁎ Loss of absorbing surface through jejunal resection and shunting.
⁎ Anticonvulsant drug therapy
Increased folate requirements
⁎ Pregnancy
⁎ Haemolytic anaemias
⁎ Exfoliative dermatitis and psoriasis
Impaired folate utilization
⁎ Alcoholism
⁎ Administration of folate antagonists trimethoprim and methotrexate.
⁎ Inborn errors of folate metabolism

The aetiology of megaloblasic anaemia is summarised in Table 5.3.

Table 5.3: Aetiology of megaloblastic anaemia	
Deficiency of cobalamin and folic acid	
Inadequate diet	⁎ Phytates in vegetarian diet prevent cobalamin absorption
	⁎ Unbalanced diet in alcoholics and infants
Malabsorption	⁎ Tropical sprue
	⁎ Non-tropical sprue
Increased requirement	⁎ Pregnancy ⁎ Disseminated cancer
Deficiency of cobalamin	
↓ IF production:	⁎ Pernicious anaemia ⁎ Gastrectomy
↓ Absorptive site: Competition for cobalamin:	⁎ Ileal resection ⁎ Bacterial overgrowth in blind loops and diverticula ⁎ Fish tapeworm
↓ Release of cobalamin from food	⁎ Partial gastrectomy ⁎ Achlorhydria ⁎ Drugs that prevent acid secretion
Deficiency of folic acid	
⁎ Increased requirements	⁎ Infancy ⁎ ↑ Haematopoiesis as in haemolytic anaemia ⁎ Haemodialysis
Inhibitors of folic acid metabolism (dihydrofolate reductase)	
	⁎ Methotrexate ⁎ Trimethoprim

Morphology

Peripheral Smear

RBC changes

Anisocytosis: There is a marked variation in the shape and size of the red blood cells. Some RBCs are large (macrocytic) and oval in shape (ovalocytes) filled with haemoglobin and, thus do not have central pallor. These are called macro-ovalocytes (Fig. 5.5).

In severe anaemia occasional megaloblast may be seen in peripheral smear.

Features of dyserythropoiesis:

- Some basophilic stippling
- Cabots ring (pink coloured '8' shaped ring)
- Howell-Jolly bodies: These are nuclear remnants
- Nucleated RBCs

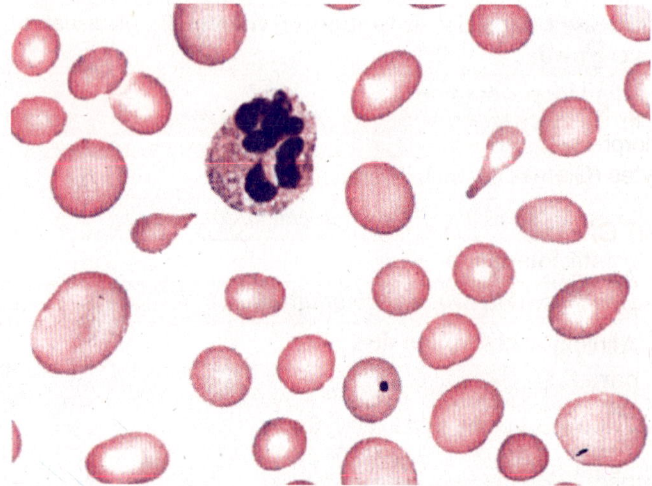

Fig. 5.5: Photomicrograph of peripheral smear showing macrocytes, macro-ovulocytes, poikilocytes and Howell-Jolly bodies

Neutrophillic changes

- Large neutrophils
- Hypersegmented neutrophils with 5 or more than 5 nuclear lobules in at least 3 neutrophils or more than 6 lobes in one neutrophil. It is the first sign of the presence of megaloblastic anaemia (Fig. 5.6).
- Platelet count is diminished

Bone Marrow

Hypercellular marrow (Fig. 5.7)**:** The fat spaces are replaced by erythroid cells. Myeloid: Erythroid ratio becomes 1: 1 (normal is 3:1) with abundant stainable iron.

Genesis of Anaemia

1. Accumulation of a large number of megaloblast with very few mature erythrocyte.
2. Haemolytic destruction: Megaloblasts readily undergo autohaemolysis. They are also phagocytosed by phagocytic cells in the marrow.
3. Ineffective erythropoiesis.

Changes in other Organs

Changes in other organs are generally found in severe megaloblastic anaemia such as pernicious anaemia.

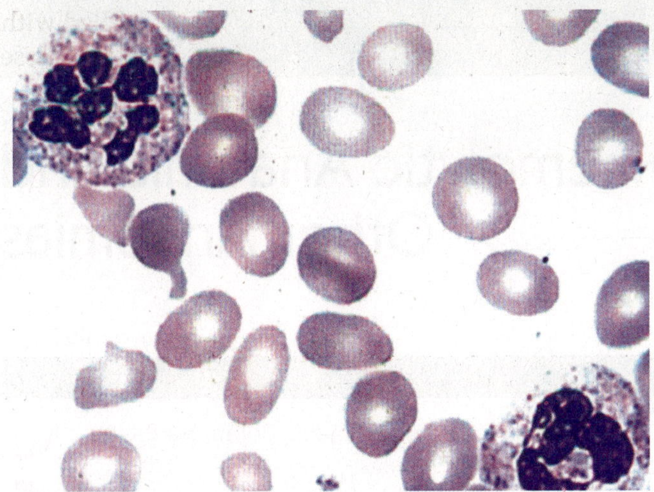

Fig. 5.6: Microphotograph peripheral smear showing polymorphs segmented (neutrophil), macrocytes and macro-ovulocytes (Giemsa × 1000).

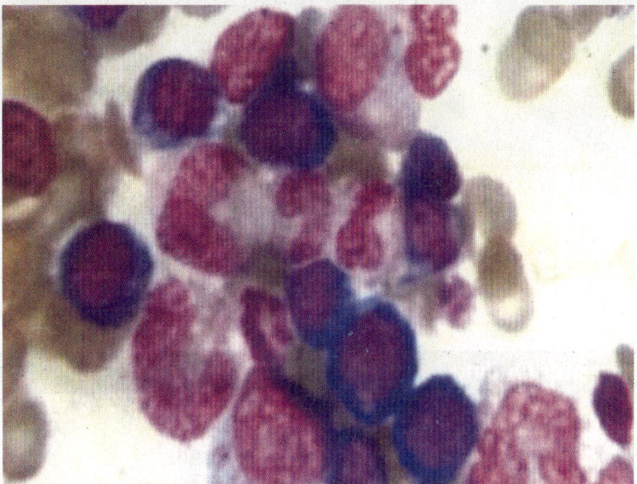

Fig. 5.7: Microphotograph of hypercellular bone marrow showing megaloblasts; blue by cytoplasm (Giemsa × 1000)

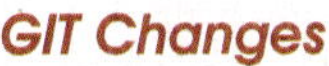

GIT Changes

- Atrophic glossitis. The tongue is shinny, glazed and red.
- Atrophic gastritis. Atrophy of both chief cells and parietal cells with intestinal metaplasia.

CNS Changes

Subacute combined degeneration

- Myelin degeneration of the dorsal and lateral tracts
- Sometimes loss of axons

These changes can involve both the sensory and motor pathways, thus it is called subacute combined degeneration.

Clinical Picture

The patient present with anaemia, atrophic glossitis and in severe cases neurological deficiency attributed to subacute combined degeneration. These are:

- Spastic paraparesis
- Sensory ataxia
- Severe paresthesia

Diagnosis

- Mean corpuscular volume (MCV). Due to macrocytosis the MCV is increased, generally > 100 fl
- Peripheral smear
- Bone marrow changes
- Serum bilirubin increased (as a result of haemolysis)
- Serum cobalamin levels. Value <100 pg/ml indicates megaloblastic anaemia. N is 200–900 pg/ml.

Serum folic acid levels. N is 6–20 ng/ml. A value of ≤4 ng/ml is diagnostic of folate deficiency.

Schilling Test

Schilling test is used to find the cause of cobalamin deficiency. The patient is given radioactive cobalamin orally followed by an intramuscular injection of unlabelled cobalamin. Urinary excretion of the radioactive substance is measured over the next 24 hours and its percentage excretion is calculated. This gives an accurate measurement of cobalamin absorption. If urinary excretion of the radioactive substance is low, then radio labelled cobalamin bound to IF is given orally. If the radioactive substance excretion returns to normal, then there is deficiency of IF.

If the excretion is still not normal, the patient may have diverticula or bacterial infection.

FIGLU Test

Increased excretion in urine occurs in folate deficiency. Serum homocysteine levels are increased.

Haemolytic Anaemia and Other Anaemias

Chapter Outline

- Haemolytic Anaemia
- Haemolytic Anaemia of Cellular Origin
- Glucose-6-Phosphate Dehydrogenase (G6PD) Deficiency
- Paroxysmal Nocturnal Haemoglobinuria (PNH)
- Sideroblastic Anaemias

HAEMOLYTIC ANAEMIA

Introduction

Haemolytic anaemia is a form of anaemia due to haemolysis, the abnormal breakdown of red blood cells (RBCs), either in the blood vessels (intravascular haemolysis) or elsewhere in the human body (extravascular). This most commonly occurs within the spleen but also can occur in the reticuloendothelial system or mechanically prosthetic valve damage.

Haemolytic anaemia accounts for 5% of all existing anaemias. It has numerous possible consequences, ranging from general symptoms to life-threatening systemic effects. The general classification of haemolytic anaemia is either intrinsic or extrinsic. Treatment depends on the type and cause of haemolytic anaemia.

Definition

Haemolytic anaemia is defined by the premature destruction of red blood cells, and can be chronic or life-threatening. It should be part of the differential diagnosis for any normocytic or macrocytic anaemia. Haemolysis may occur intravascularly, extravascularly in the reticuloendothelial system, or both. Mechanisms include poor deformability leading to trapping and phagocytosis, antibody-mediated destruction through phagocytosis or direct complement activation, fragmentation due to microthrombi or direct mechanical trauma, oxidation, or direct cellular destruction. If the rate of erythrocyte destruction is only moderately accelerated, anaemia will not develop because the bone marrow can compensate for the disorder (so called compensated haemolysis). If, however, the destruction takes place at a high rate, anaemia with increased serum bilirubin and serum iron values will develop.

Etiology of Haemolytic Anaemia

There are 2 main types of haemolytic anaemia: Inherited and acquired. Different diseases, conditions, or factors can cause each type.

- Types of Haemolytic anaemia is shown in Fig. 6.1 indicating examples in each of the above 2 types.

Classification

Haemolytic anaemia can be inherited or acquired:

- Inherited haemolytic anaemia happens when parents pass the gene for the condition on to their children.
- Acquired haemolytic anaemia is not something you are born with. You develop the condition later.

Causes

Haemolytic anaemias can be further subdivided into: (i) Intrinsic and (ii) extrinsic causes. According to the means of haemolysis, being either intrinsic in cases where the cause is related to the red blood cell (RBC) itself, or extrinsic in cases where factors external to the RBC dominate. Intrinsic effects may include problems with RBC proteins or oxidative stress handling, whereas external factors include immune attack and microvascular angiopathies (RBCs are mechanically damaged in circulation).

i. Extrinsic Causes

Acquired haemolytic anaemia may be caused by immune-mediated causes, drugs, and other miscellaneous causes.

- Immune-mediated causes could include transient factors as in *Mycoplasma pneumoniae* infection (cold agglutinin disease) or permanent factors as in autoimmune diseases like autoimmune haemolytic anaemia (itself more common in diseases such as systemic lupus erythematosus, rheumatoid arthritis, Hodgkin's lymphoma, and chronic lymphocytic leukaemia).

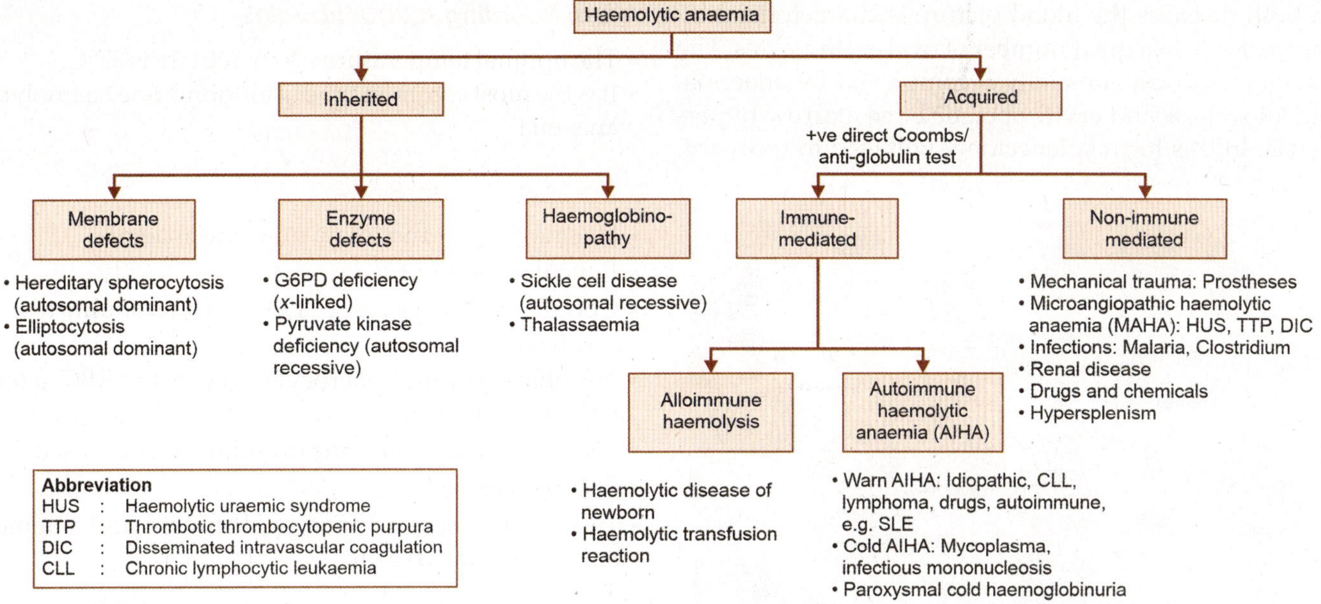

Fig. 6.1: Indicating examples in each of inherited and acquired causes

- Spur cell haemolytic anaemia
- Any of the causes of hypersplenism (increased activity of the spleen), such as portal hypertension.
- Acquired haemolytic anaemia is also encountered in burns and as a result of certain infections (e.g. malaria).
- Paroxysmal nocturnal haemoglobinuria (PNH), sometimes referred to as Marchiafava-Micheli syndrome, is a rare, acquired, potentially life-threatening disease of the blood characterized by complement induced intravascular haemolytic anaemia.
- Lead poisoning resulting from the environment causes non-immune haemolytic anaemia.
- Similarly, poisoning by arsine or stibine also causes haemolytic anaemia.
- Runners can suffer haemolytic anaemia due to 'foot-strike haemolysis', owing to the destruction of red blood cells in feet at foot impact.
- Low-grade haemolytic anaemia occurs in 70% of prosthetic heart valve recipients, and severe haemolytic anaemia occurs in 3%.

ii. Intrinsic Causes

Defects intrinsic to the RBC that can cause haemolysis involve abnormalities of the RBC membrane, cell metabolism, or haemoglobin structure.

Abnormalities include hereditary cell membrane disorders (e.g. hereditary spherocytosis), acquired cell membrane disorders (e.g. paroxysmal nocturnal haemoglobinuria), disorders of RBC metabolism (e.g. glucose-6-phosphate dehydrogenase (G6PD) deficiency), and haemoglobinopathies (e.g. sickle cell disease, thalassaemias). Quantitative and functional abnormalities of certain RBC membrane proteins (alpha- and beta-spectrin, protein 4.1, F-actin, ankyrin) cause haemolytic anaemias.

HAEMOLYTIC ANAEMIA OF CELLULAR ORIGIN

Congenital Spherocytosis

This anaemia, inherited as a dominant autosomal trait, is characterized by small round cells that do not show a central pale area. In the blood smear only a certain number of erythrocytes posses this form. In addition, there is some polychromasia indicating reticulocytosis. The spherocytes are characterized by increased osmotic fragility. They are preferentially destroyed in the spleen, this being the cause of splenomegaly. Splencectomy cures the anaemia: the spherocytes persist and are even more numerous than before, because they no longer undergo an accelerated destruction in the spleen (Fig. 6.2).

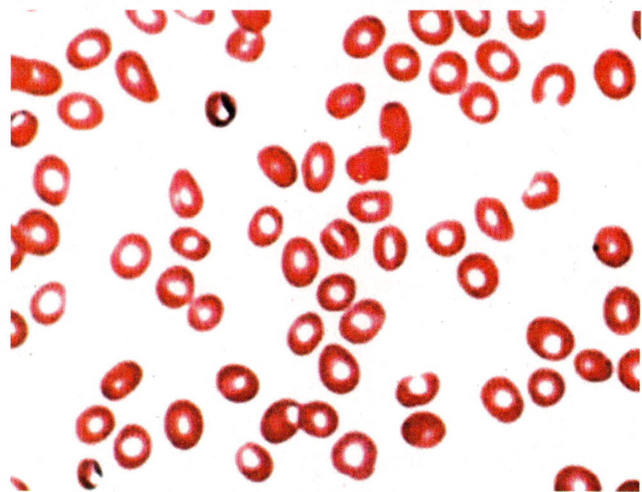

Fig. 6.2: Spherocytes in cases of congenital spherocytosis

Congenital Ovalocytosis (Fig. 6.3)

Congenital ovalocytosis can be present with or without haemolysis. The reason for this difference is not known.

In both diseases the blood picture is characterised by the presence of a great number of oval erythrocytes. The haemolytic form is usually accompanied by anaemia, reticulocylosis and erythropoietic bone marrow hyperplasia. In this form splenectomy will lead to recovery.

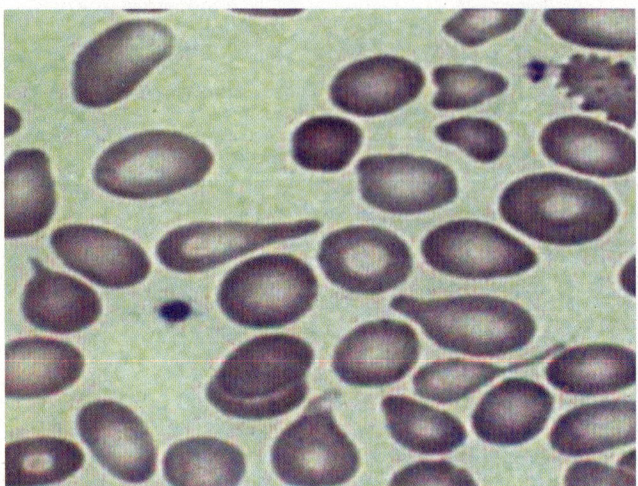

Fig. 6.3: Ovulocytes in blood smear in a case of congenital spherocytosis

Haemolytic Anaemias of Extracellular Origin

Plasmodia directly infest the erythrocytes and lead to their destruction in the reticuloendothelial system.

Industrial poisons and drugs, lead poisoning is characterized by erythrocytes with basophilic stippling. Phenacetin containing drugs, occasionally also sulfonamides, cause an inclusion anaemia if taken in large amounts. The Heinz inclusion bodies consist of denatured methemogiobin and can only be demonstrated as coarse blue dots by means of brilliant cresyl blue supravital staining. The methemoglobin has lost the ability to transport oxygen because the divalent $HbFe^{++}$ has been oxidized to the trivalent Fe^{+++} by the drugs.

Autoimmune Haemolytic Anaemias

On rare occasions the human body forms antibodies against its own erythrocytes. The cells carrying such antibodies can be detected by the direct Coombs' test. They are destroyed at an accelerated rate in the reticuloendothelial system. In the peripheral blood such cells can appear as spherocytes. The number of reticulocytes is always increased. Accordingly one finds an increased number of polychromatic erythrocytes in the peripheral blood. There are two types of autoantibodies.

- Warm reacting autoantibodies
- Cold reacting autoantibodies

Warm Reacting Autoantibodies

- The optimal temperature for its activity is 37°C.
- It is the most common type of autoimmune haemolytic anaemia.

Laboratory Diagnosis

- Haemoglobin—moderate to severe anaemia
- Reticulocyte count ↑
- Coombs test is positive. Direct antiglobulin test is positive.
- Peripheral smear: Spherocytes, nucleated RBC, a few polychromatophils
- Serum bilirubin and urine urobilinogen increased
- SLDH increased
- Haemoglobinemia, haemoglobinuria and haemosiderinuria are present.

Cold-reactive Antibodies

Cold-reactive antibodies are IgM type antibodies and react with red cells at low temperature generally between 0° and 4°C. Rarely the antibody is IgG type, e.g. Donath-Landsteiner antibody of paroxysmal cold haemoglobinuria.

Hereditary haemolytic disorders are given in Table 6.1. Immune haemolytic anaemia and demonstrable autoantibodies, acquired red cells defects are given in Table 6.2 and haemolytic disorders not associated with demonstrable antibodies are summarised in Table 6.3.

Table 6.1: Hereditary haemolytic disorders
Red cell membrane disorders
• Altered phospholipid concentration
• Hereditary elliptocytosis
• Hereditary spherocytosis
• Hereditary stomatocytosis
Enzyme abnormalities
• Defect in Embden-Meyerhof pathway (pyruvate kinase deficiency: Rarely deficiencies of triose isomerase, glucose phosphate isomerase, 2, 3-diphosphoglycerate mutase, glyceraldehyde-3-phosphate dehydrogenase, hexokinase, phosphoglycerate kinase, and phosphofructokinase)
• Defect in pentose phosphate pathway (deficiency of glucose-6-phosphate dehydrogenase, 6-phosphogluconate dehydrogenase)
• Deficiency of glutathione reductase and peroxidase or ATPase
Haemoglobin or haemoglobin synthesis abnormalities
• Erythropoietic porphyria
• Haemoglobinopathies (sickling haemoglobins, haemoglobin C)
• Thalassaemia

Table 6.2: Immune haemolytic anaemia with demonstrable antibodies and acquired red cell defects
Acquired red cell defects
× Paroxysmal nocturnal haemoglobinuria
× Nutritional deficiencies (vitamin B_{12}, folic acid, iron)
Haemolytic disorders and isoantibodies
× Erythroblastosis fetalis (ABO, Rh)
× Most transfusion reactions
Acquired autoimmune haemolytic disease
× Warm-reactive antibodies
× Idiopathic
× Secondary to lymphoma, lupus erythematosus, infectious mononucleosis
× Cold-reactive antibodies
× Cold haemagglutinin disease
× Secondary to pneumonia, lymphoma, infectious mononucleosis
× Paroxysmal cold haemoglobinuria
Drug-dependent antibodies

Table 6.3: Haemolytic disorders not associated with demonstrable antibodies
× Haemolytic disorders not associated with demonstrable antibodies
× Haemolytic disorders caused by chemicals (heavy metals, arsine, naphthalene, phenylhydrazine, oxidant and surface-active compounds, hypotonic solutions)
× Haemolytic disorders caused by infectious agents (bacterial toxins, haemolysins, parasites)
× Haemolytic disorders caused by physical agents (thermal injury, hyperoxemia)
× Haemolytic disorders caused by unknown mechanisms (infections, liver disease, malignancy, renal disease).
× Microangiopathic haemolytic anaemia (associated with cardiac valve prosthesis, carcinomatosis, eclampsia, haemolytic uraemia syndrome, malignant hypertension, thrombotic thrombocytopenic purpura)

Osmotic Fragility Test

Normal red cells, when placed in hypotonic salt solutions, absorb fluid, thus causing the volume to increase and the shape to change from that of biconcave discs to spherical forms. Further expansion of volume leads to cell rupture or haemolysis. Cells which are thicker than normal or spherical cannot expand as much as can normal cells without placing their capsule under tension and, therefore, they haemolyze more readily in low salt concentrations than do normal cells. On the other hand, cells which are thin (leptocytes), sickled cells or cells with surface folds (target cells) are capable of a greater than normal percentile expansion of volume before reaching the spherical shape. These thin cells therefore do not hemolyze in hypotonic salt solutions as readily as do normal cells.

For testing the osmotic fragility of erythrocytes, blood is placed in a series of tubes containing descending concentrations of sodium chloride. The degree of haemolysis or the point of beginning and complete haemolysis is noted. Control tests are always needed for there are many variables such as the criteria used in evaluating haemolysis, the accuracy of measurements of the salt concentrations, the chemical purity of the salt, cleanliness of glassware, the amount of blood in relation to the anticoagulant the final pH, any contamination, and the time elapsed between the drawing of blood and the reading of the rest.

Methods

Qualitative

A stock solution of sodium chloride is prepared by dissolving 1 g of CP sodium chloride, which has been dried in a desiccator, in 100 ml of distilled water. By using varying amounts of this 1% salt solution and making up to 10 ml with distilled water, the desired ranges of salt concentration are prepared. Thus, if a 0.64% solution is desired, 6.4 ml of stock solution are mixed with 3.6 ml of water; for a 0.60% solution, 6.0 ml of stock solution plus 4.0 ml of water, etc.

The usual range is provided by making up a duplicate series of 10 tubes, each set having concentrations 0.64 to 0.28% of intervals of 0.04%. It is important to mix water and saline by inversion of the tube.

After venous blood is collected, 1 drop of blood is added to each tube. If the patient is anaemic, 2 drops are preferred. The blood first may be mixed with EDTA and 0.1 ml or 1 drop from a 1 ml pipette added to each tube. The blood from the control and the patient must be handled in exactly the same way. After thoroughly mixing, the tubes are allowed to stand for several hours, preferably in a refrigerator, until the red cells settle. If more rapid reading is desired, the tubes may be centrifuged.

The point of beginning haemolysis in each series is noted by looking for the tube with the highest concentration in which the pink tinting of the supernatant fluid is detectable. A bright light, a white background, and comparison with other tubes help in determining this end point.

The point of complete haemolysis is indicated by the tube in which there are no red cells left intact. Aids is determining this end point are a slight agitation of the sediment to see if whorls of cells come up from the bottom, or the reading of point through the solutions as a means of detecting turbidity. The solution at the point of complete haemolysis is clear.

Example of report:

	Beginning haemolysis	Complete haemolysis
Patient	0.48% NaCl	0.36% NaCl
Control	0.44% NaCl	0.32% NaCl

A difference of more than one tube is significant.

Quantitative

Principle

Blood in known quantities is added to measure amounts of varying concentrations of sodium chloride buffered to pH 7.4 with sodium phosphates. The degree of haemolysis in each mixture is measured photoelectrically. A stock solution of buffered sodium chloride, which is osmotically equivalent to 10% NaCl, is made by dissolving NaCl 180.0 gm, Na_2HPO_4 27.31 gm and $NaH_2PO_4 . 2H_2O$ 4.86 gm in approximately 1,000 ml of distilled water, after which the solution is made up to a volume of 2,000 ml of distilled water. This stock solution will keep for months if stored in a stoppered bottle. In preparing a series of hypotonic solutions, a working 1% solution is prepared, from a series of final solutions are prepared which are equivalent to 0.85, 0.75, 0.65, 0.60, 0.55, 0.50, 0.45, 0.40, 0.35, 0.30, 0.20, 0.10 and 0.00% NaCl. These final dilute solutions will keep in the refrigerator for several weeks. They should be discarded if they become cloudy owing to growth of molds.

Equipment

1. Test tube rack containing two series of 13 matched colourimeter tubes which are chemically clean and which have been rinsed with distilled water and dried.
2. Calibrated serological pipettes, 10 ml.
3. Sahli pipettes, 20 cu mm.
4. Photoelectric colourimeter, green filter 510 mμ.

Procedure

Five milliliters of buffered salt solution equivalent to 0.85% NaCl are placed in the first test tube of the front row of tubes and a similar amount in the first test tube of the back row. Next 5 ml of the 0.75% solution are placed in the third pair of tubes, and so forth. Distilled water (5 ml) is placed in the last pair of tubes.

The 5 ml blood is collected from the patient and the control at approximately the same period of time. The venous blood may be heparinized or defibrinated. For defibrination place 5 ml blood in a 60 ml Erlenmeyer flask containing one glass bead (size 3 to 1 mm) for each milliliter of blood. The flask should be gently rotated for 5 minutes or until the fibrin collects around the beads.

Using a Sahli pipette, 20 cu mm of blood to be tested are placed in each of the buffered salt solutions in the front series of tubes. After each addition of blood to the respective hypotonic saline solution, the pipette should be rinsed several times and the residual contents blown out forcefully. There is no need of thoroughly drying the pipette each time or using a separate pipette for each specimen. Twenty cubic millimeters of heparinized or defibrinated blood from the normal control patient are now added to each of tile 13 tubes in the back control row of tubes. The blood and saline is mixed and allowed to stand at room temperature for 30 minutes, after which the tubes are centrifuged for 5 minutes at approximately 900 × g. Following this the tubes are in turn placed in a photoelectric colourimeter and the optical density is determined. The supernatant fluid in the 0.85% NaCl tubes serves as a "blank" and the supernatant fluid in the distilled water tube (0.00% NaCl) serves as the tube of reference for complete or 100% haemolysis. The degree of haemolysis as revealed by the scale reading of the dial is noted for each of the tubes. The degree of haemolysis in each tube is expressed in terms of percentage of the scale reading of the completely hemolyzed reference tube. The plotting on graph paper of the per cent of haemolysis of the patient and the control against the varying concentrations of buffered saline is recommended.

The test can be made more sensitive by allowing the blood to remain in contact with the hypotonic salt solutions for 24 hours at 37°C.

Because the quantitative test using multiple tubes is so time consuming, one may perform a screening test by determining the per cent of haemolysis in the 0.50% tube.

Interpretation (Fig. 6.4)

In normal individuals a sigmoid type of curve is obtained in which there is 50% haemolysis in the 0.50 to 0.40% NaCl range.

Clinical Applications

When normal blood is mixed with descending concentrations of hypotonic salt solution, some of the red cells undergo haemolysis within the range of 0.48 to 0.40% NaCl (average 0.44%) and there is complete haemolysis between 0.40 and 0.32% NaCl (average 0.34%).

In hereditary spherocytic anaemia, and in certain patients with acquired haemolytic jaundice, there is partial haemolysis in concentration above the control and often above 0.50% NaCl. In thalassaemia, sicklemia and obstructive (regurgitant) jaundice, haemolysis occurs at levels lower than the control and there is often a greater spread than normal between the tubes in which there is beginning haemolysis and complete haemolysis. In sicklemia and thalassaemia, and perhaps in other conditions, it is thought that the red cells are not only thinner than normal, and, therefore can expand to a greater extent before haemolysis occurs, but that these cells act as poor osmometers and do not imbibe fluids as readily as do nonnal cells.

The fragility test is a fairly time-consuming procedure which is not indicated unless haemolytic jaundice is suspected.

Indications for ordering the test and unexplained jaundice of a haemolytic type, abnormal red cell regeneration and splenomegaly. The test is not needed in the diagnosis of sickle cell anaemia or in obstructive jaundice. In the majority of cases of anaemia in which there is neither evidence of abnormal blood destruction, nor compensatory regenerative signs, the test should not be ordered, for it will be of no value and will add pain, expense and unnecessary labour.

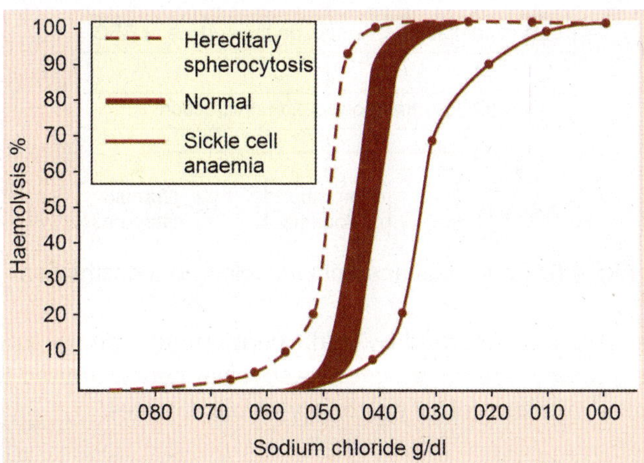

Fig. 6.4: Quantitative osmotic fragility test. Range of normal variation indicated by stippled area

GLUCOSE-6-PHOSPHATE DEHYDROGENASE (G6PD) DEFICIENCY

G6PD deficiency is a defect in the hexose-monophosphate shunt causing failure to protect the red cell membrane from oxidation.

A large number of genetic variants of G6PD deficiency have been described. In most cases the change is a base substitution causing an amino acid replacement. These mutations produce enzymes with different electrophoretic and kinetic characteristics.

Pathogenesis

When normal RBCs are exposed to drugs (Table 6.4) and toxins, which generates oxygen radical, the glucose metabolism via hexose-monophosphate shunt is increased several times. This generates a large amount of reduced glutathione (GSH). The GSH inactivates the oxygen radical produced by the drug or toxin.

Table 6.4: Drugs causing haemolysis in G6PD deficiency
• Antimalarials: Primaquine, quinacrine
• Sulfonamides: Sulfamethoxazole, nitrofurantoin, dapsone, septran
• Analgesics: Acetanilid, acetyl salicylic acid
• Phenacitin
• Nitrofurans: Nalidixic acid, furazolidone

In G6PD deficient state the generation of reduced glutathione (GSH) is impaired (Fig. 6.5). Thus, the oxygen radical accumulates and causes oxidation of the haemoglobin sulfhydryl group of the globin chain. The denatured haemoglobin precipitates within the RBC. This precipitate appears as dark inclusion by crystal violet stain (Heinz body). When these RBCs pass through the spleen, the macrophages remove the Heinz bodies. Removal of the Heinz bodies give rise to red cells that appear to have been bitten of a part. These cells are called bite cells. Multiple bites cause fragment formation (fragmented RBC). The loss of membrane leads to the formation of spherocytes.

G6PD deficiencies generally do not manifest any haemolysis unless exposed to oxidant drugs or toxins.

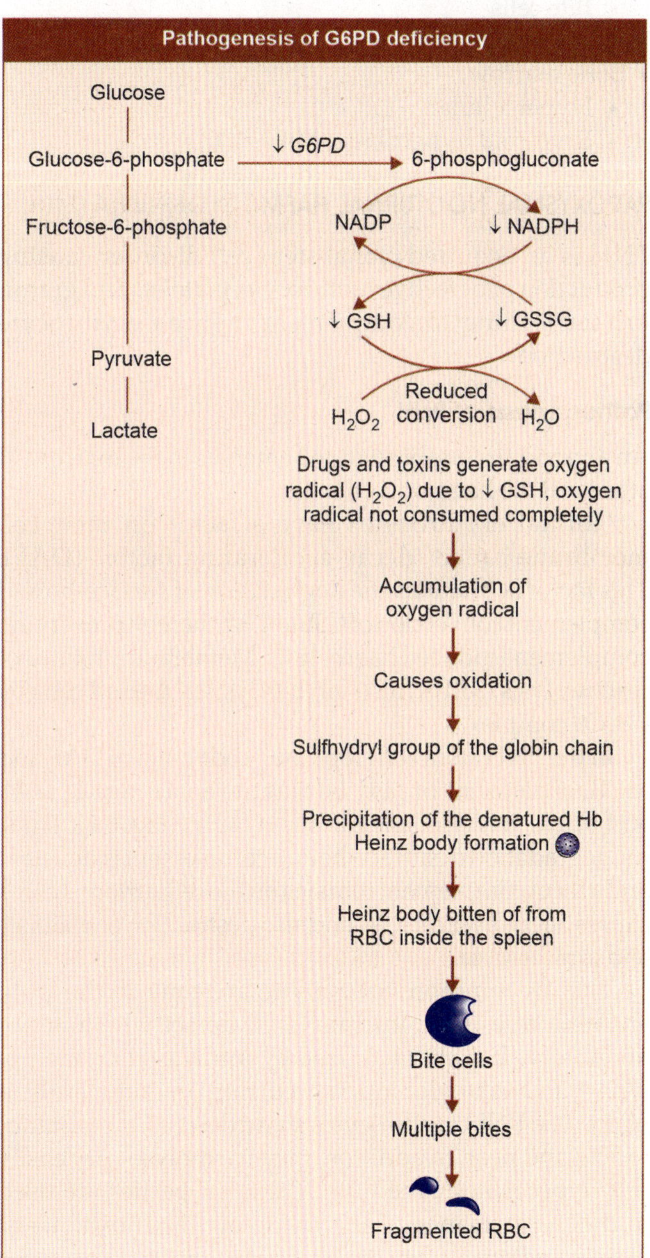

Fig. 6.5: Genesis of G6PD deficiency leading to haemolytic anaemia

However, haemolytic crisis can manifest within hours of drug intake leading to:

- Haemoglobinuria
- Haemoglobinemia
- Peripheral vascular collapse → in severe cases

Diagnosis

Peripheral smear

- Peripheral smear shows:
  - Normocytic normochromic anaemia (Hb↓)
  - Fragmented RBC
  - Nucleated RBC
  - Polychromatophils
- The specific findings are:
  - Heinz body
  - Bite cells
- Spherocytes
- Bone marrow:
  - Hypercellular
  - Erythroid hyperplasia, M:E—1:1

PAROXYSMAL NOCTURNAL HAEMOGLOBINURIA (PNH)

PNH is an acquired clonal stem cell disorder causing production of defective erythrocyte, platelets and granulocytes leading to complement induced erythrocyte destruction.

Pathogenesis of PNH

An abnormal clone of stem cell emerges in the marrow. It affects all the haemopoietic cells.

Normal erythrocytes have a factor on their cell membrane called 'decay-accelerating factor' (DAF). This factor accelerates the degradation of surface-bound complement conversion of C3b to C3d, thereby preventing complement-induced haemolysis. Membrane inhibitor of reactive lysis (MIRL) also inhibits lysis of the red cells by C8–C9 complex.

In the PNH stem cell clone the production of DAF and MIRL is deficient or may be that the anchorage of DAF and MIRL to the cell membrane is faulty (Fig. 6.6). Thus, the degradation of surface-bound complement is deficient and a lot of complement remains on the cell surface, which causes haemolysis of RBC and also destruction of platelets and granulocyte.

This uncommon haemolytic anaemia is the only anaemia due to an intrinisic cell defect which is not hereditary. It is characterized by intravascular haemolysis with haemoglobinuria occurring predominantly at night. The PNH erythrocytes show decreased resistance to acid and heat. In addition, they haemolyse very easily in a hyperosmotic medium. These properties are used in the performance of the following diagnostic tests: Ham's acid serum test, the Maier-Hegglin heat resistance test and the sucrose haemolysis test. The anaemia is

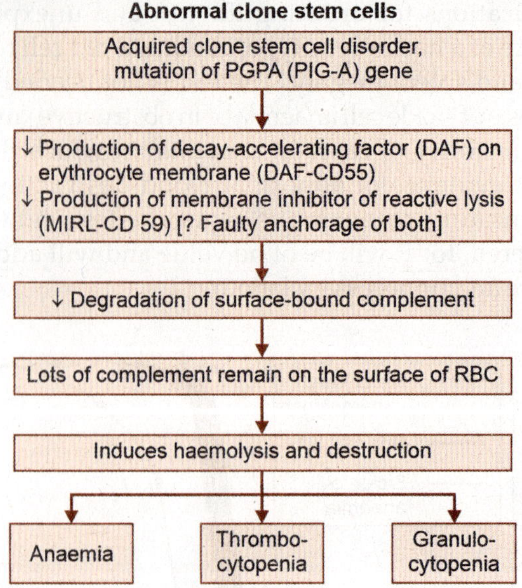

Fig. 6.6: Genesis of anaemia and blood cell destruction

usually accompanied by leukopenia (neutropenia) and thrombocytopenia. In severe cases treatment is limited to the administration of erythrocyte concentrates.

Diagnosis

- ↑Reticulocyte count
- ↓Serum iron
- Thrombocytopenia
- Granulocytopenia
- Peripheral smear: Normocytic normochromic anaemia, a few polychromatophils are seen.
- Bone marrow: Hypercellular, erythroid hyperplasia with normoblastic reaction.
- HAMS test +ve: RBC gets lysed in acidic pH.
- Gel card: CD59 and CD55 are reduced on RBC surface. Can be estimated by Gel cards.
- NAP: ↓ (GPI linked)

Complications

- Thrombosis is a common complication possibly due to complement-mediated activation of platelet, e.g.
  - Abdominal deep vein thrombosis
  - Hepatic venous thrombosis
  - Pancytopenia
  - Myelodysplastic syndrome
  - Acute leukaemia (AML)

SIDEROBLASTIC ANAEMIAS

Miscellaneous group of diseases characterized by increased sideroblasts (erythroblasts containing iron inclusions) in marrow.

Due to drugs (e.g. isoniazid, chloramphenicol, alcohol, lead, cytotoxic drugs such as nitrogen mustard and azathioprine)

Diseases

- Haematologic (e.g. leukaemia, polycythaemia vera, megaloblastic anaemia,. haemolytic anaemia)
- Neoplastic (e.g. lymphoma, carcinoma)
- Inflammatory (e.g. infection, RA, polyarteritis nodosa)
- Miscellaneous (uraemia, myxoedema, thyrotoxicosis, porphyria)
  a. Hereditary
  b. Idiopathic

Hereditary

- Usual onset in young adults but may be in children or infants.
- Anaemia is usually severe, hypochromic, microcytic with anisocytosis, poikilocytosis, target cells, basophilic stippling; dimorphic RBC population.
- WBC and platelets are usually normal.
- Bone marrow shows erythroid hyperplasia with normoblastic maturation; 10–40% of normoblasts are ringed sideroblasts; excessive haemosiderin. Megaloblastic changes indicate complicating folate deficiency.
- Transferrin saturation is increased.
- <50% of patients respond to pyridoxine therapy.

Idiopathic Refractory

- Usual onset in older adults (rarely < 50 years).
- Dimorphic anaemia is usually moderate, normocytic, or macrocytic with a small population of hypochromic RBCs on blood smear, some of which show marked stippling.
- Reticulocytes are usually not increased.
- WBC is variable but usually normal. WBCs may show morphologic changes (hypogranular, Pelger-Huët like neutrophils). Blasts <1%.
- Platelet counts are variable. Abnormal thrombopoiesis with abnormal morphology (e.g. hypogranular, large platelets or fragments, large nuclei).
- Bone marrow shows erythroid hyperplasia. 45–95% of normoblasts are ringed sideroblasts, excessive haemosiderin. Megaloblastic changes due to complicating folate deficiency are found in 20% of patients. Dysgranulopoiesis and dysmegakaryopoiesis may be evident.
- Transferrin saturation is increased (>90% in 33% patients).
- Serum ferritin and iron stores are increased due to ineffective erythropoiesis. Acute leukaemia develops in ~10% of patients.

Secondary: Due to drugs and toxic agents (e.g. chloramphenicol, antituberculosis drugs, lead poisoning, alcoholism) or associated with other diseases such as neoplasms (e.g. lymphomas, myeloma), haematologic diseases (e.g. leukaemia, polycythaemia vera), inflammatory diseases (e.g. SLE, rheumatoid arthritis, polyarteritis nodosa), miscellaneous diseases (e.g. thyroid dysfunction, porphyrias, uraemia).

Pyridoxine-Responsive Anaemia

Severe hypochromic microcytic anaemia is present.

Blood smear shows anisocytosis, poikilocytosis with many bizarre forms, target cells, hypochromia. Polychromatophilia and reticulocytosis are not increased.

Serum iron is increased; TIBC is somewhat decreased; transferrin saturation is markedly increased. Marrow sideroblasts and blood siderocytes are increased.

Marrow and liver biopsy show increased haemosiderin.

Bone marrow usually shows normoblastic hyperplasia, occasionally it is megaloblastic.

Response to pyridoxine is always incomplete. Even when haemoglobin becomes normal, morphologic changes in RBCs persist.

Tryptophan tolerance test demonstrates pyridoxine deficiency. It may be positive in pyridoxine-responsive anaemia, or it may be normal. A positive test produces abnormally large urinary excretion of xanthurenic acid.

Anaemia of Chronic Disorders

The pathogenesis of anaemia appears to be related to the decreased release of iron from macrophages to plasma and so to erythroblasts, reduced red cell life span and an inadequate erythropoietin response to anaemia. The anaemia is corrected by the successful treatment of the underlying disease but does not respond to iron therapy despite the low serum iron. Responses to recombinant erythropoietin therapy may be obtained, e.g. in rheumatiod arthritis or myeloma, but this alone does not correct the anaemia completely. In many conditions this anaemia is complicated by anaemia due to other causes, e.g. iron or folate deficiency, renal failure, bone marrow infiltration, hypersplenism or endocrine abnormality (Table 6.5).

Table 6.5: Causes of anaemia of chronic disorders
Chronic inflammatory diseases
• Infectious, e.g. pulmonary abscess, tuberculosis, osteomyelitis, pneumonia, bacterial endocarditis
• Non-infectious, e.g. rheumatoid arthritis, SLE and other connective tissue diseases, sarcoid, Crohn's disease, cirrhosis
Malignant diseases
• For example, carcinoma, lymphoma, sarcoma, myeloma
• It may be complicated by additional features which may be due to disease affecting particularly one or other system.

The characteristic features are:

1. Normochromic, normocytic or mildly hypochromic indices and red cell morphology.
2. Mild and non-progressive anaemia (haemoglobin rarely less than 9.0 g/dl)—the severity being related to the severity of disease.

3. Both the serum iron and HIBC (total iron-binding capacity) are reduced.
4. The serum ferritin is normal or raised.
5. Bone marrow (reticuloendothelial) storage iron is normal but incorporation of iron into erythroblasts is reduced.

Malignant Diseases (Other than Primary Bone Marrow Diseases)

Anaemia

Contributing factors include anaemia of chronic disorders, blood loss and iron deficiency marrow infiltration often associated with a leucoerythroblastic blood film, folate deficiency, haemolysis and marrow suppression from radiotherapy or chemotherapy.

Microangiopathic haemolytic anaemia occurs with mucin-secreting adenocarcinoma, particularly of the stomach, lung and breast. Less common forms of anaemia with maligant disease include autoimmune haemolytic anaemia with malignant lymphoma and, rarely, with other tumours; primary red cell aplasia with thymoma; and myelodysplastic syndromes secondary to chemotherapy. There is also an association of pernicious anaemia with carcinoma of the stomach.

The anaemia of malignant disease may respond partly to erythropoietin. Folic acid should only be given if there is definite megaloblastic anaemia due to the deficiency; it might 'feed' the tumour.

Anaemia in Pregnancy

Anaemia in pregnancy is widespread throughout the world. However, it is more common and more severe in developing and underdeveloped countries. Most of the time, it is the continuation of anaemia of non-pregnant state. Pregnancy precipitates it prematurely and make the situation bad to worse. It is associated with raised maternal and perinatal mortalily and morbidity rate.

A reduction in haemoglobin and volume of packed red cells occurs during normal pregnancy, this being evident by the 8th week and progressing until the 16th to the 22nd week, when the values become stationary at levels of 11 g haemoglobin and 32 to 34 ml packed red cells per 100 ml blood, or rise somewhat about the 32nd to 34th week. The red cells remain normal in size and haemoglobin content. In the puerperium the blood values return rapidly to normal. The bone marrow gives no evidence of alteration from the normal in the erythroid series; the leukocytic picture suggests hyperplasia. The latter is especially marked in the late months of pregnancy, when megakaryocytic hyperplasia may also be found.

This is not a true anaemia, however, as the total blood volume increases significantly during pregnancy. The total blood volume increases an average of 30%, the plasma volume 40%, the red cell mass 18%. Thus, the 'anaemia' really represents haemodilution. The major change has occurred by the 33rd week of pregnancy, after which the plasma volume remains unchanged but a small increase in red cell mass takes place. Ferrokinetic studies have shown, if anything accelerated erythropoiesis rather than retarded blood formation as once was thought to be the case. The alterations in blood volume during pregnancy provide a protective mechanism which allows large losses of blood during delivery without significant anaemia developing in the puerperium.

In many pregnant women, however, some iron deficiency is present. Measurements of serum iron showed a decrease in the latter part of pregnancy, together with an increase in iron-binding capacity, as occurs in iron deficiency anaemia. It is noteworthy that, in pregnant Bantu women, whose diet is habitually high in iron, no significant change in serum iron was observed and no anaemia developed.

In some pregnant women a clearly defined hypochromic microcytic anaemia, due to iron deficiency, is observed. In this country a reduction in haemoglobin below 10 gm per 100 ml is most often due to this cause. Sometimes other factors, such as infection and anaemia or protein deficiency, play an important part. Macrocytic anaemia of pregnancy is rare except where nutrition deficiency and other factors play a role, as in India.

Chapter 7

Normal and Abnormal Haemoglobin—Haemoglobinopathies

Chapter Outline

- Normal and abnormal haemoglobins
- Haemoglobinopathies
- Estimation of HbA_2
- Estimation of HbF
- Sickle cell disease
- Sickling Phenomenon (Tests for HbS)

NORMAL AND ABNORMAL HAEMOGLOBINS

Normal haemoglobin consists of a haeme component and a globin component which is a glycoprotein. Haemoglobinopathies are disorders of the globin component of haemoglobin. These globin components are coded for by 5 different alleles, namely alpha (α); beta (β); gamma (γ); delta (δ); epsilon (∈).

Each globin component consists of a pair of chains as: αα (α_2): ββ (β_2); γγ (γ_2); δδ (δ_2); ∈∈ ($\in_2$).

Normal Haemoglobin

Structure

The structure of haemoglobin is shown in Fig. 7.1. The molecule has two components:

1. Heme moiety, which contains one ferrous iron atom (Fe^{2+}) carried in a porphyrin ring (the structure and synthesis of porphyrin are described).
2. Globin tetramer, which is bound to the heme moiety and is composed of two alpha- (α-) globin chains and two non-α globin chains (the structure and synthesis of the globin chains are described).

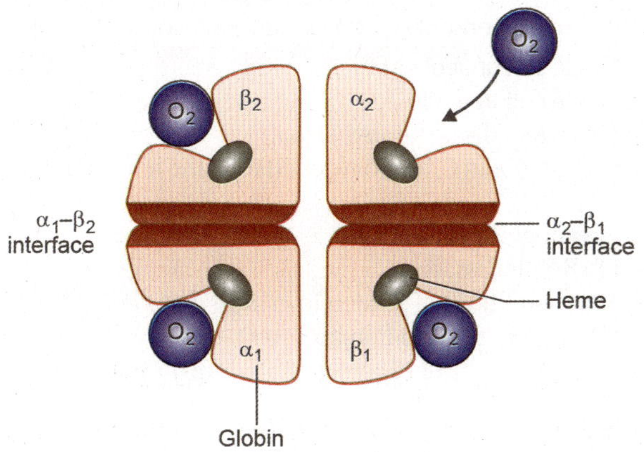

Fig. 7.1: Structure of HBA

Differentiation

The type of haemoglobin is determined by the globin chains that comprise it. The types of globin chains available for haemoglobin synthesis depend on the developmental stage of the individual:

1. **Embryonic haemoglobin:** Red cell synthesis begins in the yolk sac of 19-day-old embryos, continues in the liver by 6 weeks, and begins in the bone marrow by 4–5 months gestation. The main embryonic haemoglobins present in the first 3–6 months in utero are:
   a. *Gower I* ($\zeta_2\varepsilon_2$), which is composed of two-like globin chains called zeta (ζ) chains and two epsilon (ε) chains, a type of globin closely related to the prominent non-α-globin in adults called the beta (β) globin.
   b. *Gower II* ($\alpha_2\varepsilon_2$), which is composed of two α-globin chains and two ε-globin chains.
   c. *Portland* ($\zeta_2\gamma_2$), which is composed of two ζ-globin chains and two chains of gamma (γ) globin, another β-like globin that is a successor to the ε-globin.
2. **Fetal haemoglobin ($\alpha_2\gamma_2$):** Fetal haemoglobin (*HbF*) is composed of two α-globin chains and two γ-globin chains and represents 90–95% of the *in utero* haemoglobin from 8–35 weeks gestation until the switch from fetal to adult haemoglobin occurs.
3. **Adult haemoglobin ($\alpha_2\beta_2$)** is composed of two α- and two β-globin chains, is designated HbA, and accounts for 96–98% of all adult haemoglobin. Adult haemoglobin ($\alpha_2\delta_2$) composed of two α-globin chains and two chains of delta (δ) globin, another, β-like globin, is *designated* HbA_2 and represents 1.5–3% of all adult haemoglobin. Small amounts of *HbF* (0.5–1%) also remain in the adult (Fig. 7.1).

Normal and abnormal haemoglobins are given in Table 7.1.

Table 7.1: Normal and abnormal haemoglobins
Various normal haemoglobins include:
1. Normal adult haemoglobin (HBA)$\alpha_2\beta_2$—95–98% of adult haemoglobin.
2. Fetal haemoglobin (HbF) $\alpha_2\,\gamma_2$ — 70–90% of fetal haemoglobin at birth.
3. HB A-2 — $\alpha_2\delta_2$ —2–3% of normal adult haemoglobin.
4. $\alpha_2\ \in_2$—Gower II (present at 6–8 wk of IU life)
5. $Z_2\varepsilon_2$ Embryonic Hb—Gower I.
Abnormal haemoglobins may be due to
1. Qualitative defects: Result in Hb C, D, E, H, S, e.g. sickle cell anaemia (structural).
2. Quantitative defects result in normally increased or decreased production of globin chains, e.g. thalassaemias.
3. Mixed defects. Sickle thalassaemias.

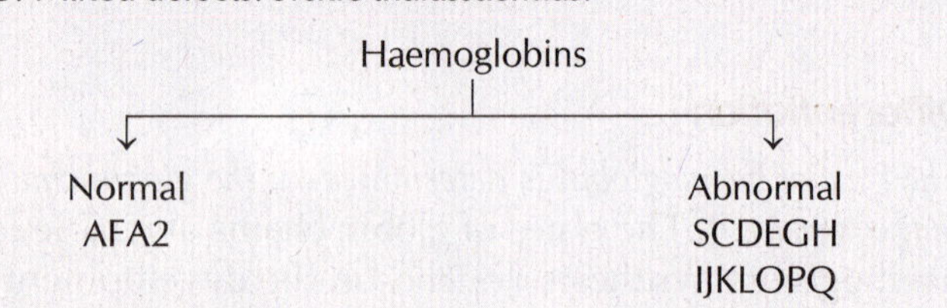

HAEMOGLOBINOPATHIES

Introduction

Definition: Haemoglobinopathies are inherited disorders in which *mutations* in or near the globin genes alter the structure (amino acid sequence) or the rate of synthesis of a particular globin chain. Most pathologic genetic variants result from a single amino acid substitution in one of the normal globin chains.

Nomenclature: The haemoglobin tetramers formed by the variant globin plus the normal globin are designated or named by a letter or after the city in which the discovery was first made; a more informative system is to name them according to the actual amino acid substitution.

Classification: The haemoglobinopathies can be classified according to the effects of the genetic mutations

a. Solubility abnormalities
b. Oxygen transport malfunction
c. Oxidation—reduction abnormalities
d. Abnormal monomeric states.

Classification of haemoglobinopathies is given in Table 7.2.

Table 7.2: Classification of haemoglobinopathies	
Classification: The haemoglobinopathies can be classified according to the effects of the genetic mutations	
a. Solubility abnormalities:	
1. Globin chain synthesis: α-Thalassaemia	Thalassaemias: • Hydrops fetalis • Hb H disease • α-Thalassaemia trait • α-Thalassaemia carrier
β-Thalassaemias:	• β-Thalassaemia major (β°β°) • β-Thalassaemia intermedia (β°β° or $\beta^+\beta^+$) • Hb lepore disease • β-Thalassaemia trait (ββ° or $\beta^+\beta^+$) • β-Thalassaemia minor (β-thalassaemia) • Hereditary persistence of fetal haemoglobin
2. Formation of precipitates or intracellular inclusion bodies: • Hb-Geneva • Hb-Gun Hill • Hb-Seattle • Rb-Tacoma • Hb-Torino • Hb-Zurich	
b. Oxygen transport malfunction:	
• Hb-Chesapeake • Hb-Hiroshima • Hb-Gun Hill • Hb-Rainer • Hb-Tacoma • Hb-Zurich	
c. Oxydation–reduction abnormalities:	
1. Congenital methemoglobinemia	
Hb-M	
Methemoglobin reductase deficiency (NADH-cytochrome (b) 5 reductase deficiency)	
2. Acquired methemoglobinemia	
• Well water contaminated with nitrates and inorganic nitrites. • Drugs—acetanilide, phenacetin, acetaminophen, nitroprusside, sulphonamides. • Local Anesthetics—lidocaine, benzocaine.	
d. Abnormal monomeric states: Common conditions include:	
• Sickle cell anaemia (Hb-SS) • Sickle cell trait (Hb-AS) • Sickle that disease (Hb-S-D thal) • Haemoglobin C, homozygous (HbC) and heterozygous (Hb AC) • Haemoglobin SC disease • Hb-S-K-thalassaemia • Rare conditions of academic interest include: • Hb-SD, Hb-SO, Hb-Punjab, Hb-D, Hb-O, Hb-Arab (B121glu-gln) (B-121glu-lys)	

Thalassaemia (Mediterranean Anaemia)

The anaemia, which frequently affects inhabitants of Mediterranean countries, is being increasingly encounter in Northern Europe with the influx of labour from Southern countries. The homozygous form is designated as thalassaemia major and the heterozous is thalassaemia minor.

Thalassaemia occurs in the Mediterranean countries and extends through Middle East, Pakistan, India to South-East Asia. It probably spreads to India during the Western invasion.

There are two types of thalassaemia:

1. **β-Thalassaemia:** There is deficient synthesis of β chain of haemoglobin.
2. **α-Thalassaemia:** This is characterised by deficient synthesis of the α chain of haemoglobin.

Classification of β-thalassaemia

β-Thalassaemia is classified according to the severity of anaemia and the genetic defect (Table 7.3) into:

1. Thalassaemia major
2. Thalassaemia intermedia
3. Thalassaemia minor or thalassaemia trait

Table 7.3: Classification of β-thalassaemia

1. Thalassaemia major	β°β° (homozygous) $\beta^+\beta^+$ (homozygous) $\beta°\beta^+$ (double heterozygous)
2. Thalassaemia intermedia	β°β° (heterozygous with a normal gene) $\beta^+\beta^+$ (homozygous)
3. Thalassaemia minor or thalassaemia trait	β°β $\beta^+\beta$

β° = no β globin synthesis, β^+ = variable β globin synthesis, β = normal globin synthesis

Thalassaemia major is a severe anaemia with considerable enlargement of liver and spleen, already manifesting itself in early childhood. The peripheral blood shows pronounced anisocytosis with hypochromic erythrocytes and a clear tendency to microcytosis. Apart from microcytes one encounters poikilocytes. Target cells and erythrocytes with basophilic stippling. The appearance of erythroblasts in the peripheral blood is a characteristic finding. In most cases treatment is limited to blood transfusions. Despite this, life expectancy does not extend beyond childhood or adolescence.

Thalassaemia minor usually follows an asymptomatic course. In most cases diagnosis is made accidentally or on checking family members of known thalassaemia cases. In the blood smears one finds purely erythrocytic changes which are less marked than in thalassaemia major (hypochromasia, microcytes, target cells and basophilic stippling) (Table 7.4); there are no erythroblasts in the peripheral blood. Characteristic is at first glance, the paradoxical discrepancy of hypochromic blood picture with increased serum iron. This finding can be explained by a defect in haemoglobin synthesis (hypochromic erythrocytes) and by an increased rate of erythrocyte destruction (increased serum iron). Thalassaemia minor requires no treatment.

To diagnose thalassaemia the abnormal proportion of the three physiological haemoglobins is used (normal values in the adult: $HbA_0 \geq 96\%$ $HbA_2 < 3\%$. HbF Fetal Hb ≤0.75%). In thalassaemia major HbA_2 and HbF are increased and in thalassaemia minor only HbA_2.

Table 7.4: Blood cells in thalassaemia major, thalassaemia minor, and iron deficiency anaemia

	Thalassemia major	*Thalassemia minor*	*Iron deficiency anaemia*
Peripheral blood			
Anisocytosis	2–4+	1–2+	1–2+
Hypochromic Microcytosis	2–4+	1–3+	2–4+
Poikilocytosis	2–4+	1–2+	0–1+
Polychromasia/ basophilic stippling	2–3+	1–2+	No
Target cells	3–4+	2–3+	0–1+
Howell-Jolly bodies	Occasional	No	No
Normoblasts	Occasional	Seldom	Seldom
Reticulocytes	Significantly increased	Moderately increased	Decreased
Platelets	Normal to increased	Normal	Normal to increased or decreased
White blood cells	Normal to increased	Normal	Normal to decreased
Bone marrow			
Erythroid hyperplasia	3–4+	Normal to 2+	1–4+
Haemosiderin	3–4+	Normal to 2+	Absent

Investigation of the Haemoglobinopathies

Collection of Blood and Preparation of Haemolysates

Blood can be collected into any anticoagulant, but if the samples have to be transported, ACD is the most suitable.

For routine analysis wash the red cells three times in 9.0 g/L NaCl (saline) and then lyse them by adding to the packed cells 2 volumes of water and 1 volume of toluene or carbon tetrachloride (CCl_4). Both of these solutions are toxic and should be used with care. Mouth pipetting must be avoided. After shaking in a mechanical agitator, centrifuge the mixture at 3000 rpm (1200 g) for 30 min and pipette off the clear Hb solution. Preferably, however since organic solvents precipitate unstable Hbs and free globin chains, better results are obtained by lysing the cells in 2 volumes of water (without toluene) and centrifuging at 20,000 rpm (18000 g) at 4°C for 20 min.

In a routine laboratory, if many samples are to be analysed, a practical rapid alternative is to lyse the once washed packed cells with a few drops of a solution containing 20 g/L saponin plus 10 g/L KCN. However, this type of haemolysate does not keep for more than 1–2 days at 4°C at room temperature, as it tends to gel.

Storing specimens prepared by either procedure at –20°C is satisfactory only a few weeks, but lysates can be stored indefinitely in liquid nitrogen.

When it is suspected that a patient is suffering from a haemoglobinopathy, the clinical history and ethnic group, family history, the physical findings and the blood picture provide important information. However, for a definitive diagnosis, an abnormal Hb and/or the laboratory features of thalassaemia have to be demonstrated.

The International Committee for Standardization in Haematology (ICSH) Export Panel on Abnormal Haemoglobins and Thalassaemia have proposed a recommended procedure for the identification of haemoglobinopathies. The proposals have been incorporated in the recommendations in this chapter.

The laboratory investigations should be carried out in several stages (Table 6.3):

1. **Preliminary tests**
   a. Blood count and film.
   b. Zone electrophoresis of Hb at an alkaline pH on cellulose acetate.
   c. Tests for sickling and/or solubility.
   d. Quantitation of HbA_2.
   e. Quantitaive and qualitative distribution of HbF.
2. **Identification of abnormal haemoglobins:** If indicated, further electrophoresis techniques to identify abnormal Hbs.

Blood Count and Film

A full blood count, including red-cell count, haemoglobin level, mean cell volume and mean cell haemoglobin, provide valuable information in the diagnosis of both α and β thalassaemias, whilst examination of blood films may show characteristic red cell changes, e.g. target cells and HbC and sickle cells with HbS.

Cellulose Acetate Electrophoresis at Alkaline pH

For routine work, the best method for separating abnormal Hbs is by electrophoresis on cellulose acetate membrane. This method is simple and generally satisfactory for distinguishing the common types of Hb. Various buffers can be used for Hb electrophoresis at an alkaline pH, with a continuous or discontinuous system.

Continuous buffer system

Tris-EDTA-borate, pH 8.9. Tris-(hydroxymethyl)-aminomethane 14.4 g; EDTA (disodium salt) 1.5 g; boric acid 0.9 g; water to 1 litre.

Discontinuous buffer system

Tris-EDTA-borate, pH 9.1 (anode chamber). Tris-(hydroxymethyl)-aminomethane 25.1 g; EDTA (disodium salt) 2.5 g; boric acid 1.9 g; water to 1 litre.

Barbitone, pH 8.6 (cathode chamber). Sodium diethylbarbiturate 25.75 g; barbitone (diethyl barbituric acid) 4.6 g; thiomersal (preservative) 0.25 g; water to 5 litre.

Method

Soak cellulose acetate membrane strips in the buffer used (a mixture of equal volumes of the two buffers in the discontinous system) and, after blotting, place them across the bridges of the electrophoresis tank. Secure the strips using wicks of Whatmar No. 1 filter paper, soaked in buffer.

Apply the haemolysate near to the cathode bridge. A variety of applicators are available commercially, or a fine pen or fine capillary tube may be used.

Then carry out electrophoresis at 200–300 V (approximately 1 mA/cm width of strip). Separation should be complete within 30 min. Then stain the strips for C_2 min in 0.2% ponceau S in 3% trichloracetic acid. Remove excess stain with 7% acetic acid, made up in tap water.

The relative electrophoretic mobility of some Hbs at pH 8.9 is shown in **Fig. 7.2**.

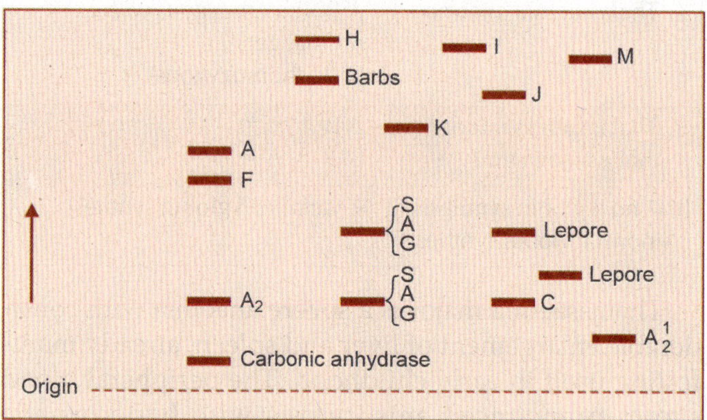

Fig. 7.2: Relative electrophoretic mobility

Control Preparation

It is advisable to electrophorese a known control sample with each electrophoresis.

The following method is recommended for preparing a control haemolysate containing Hbs A, F, S and C:

1. Obtain the following fresh blood samples (in any anticoagulant): AC: SS: F (cord blood).
2. Wash the cells three times with saline. Lyse the cells with a half volume of water and add 1 volume of CCl_4. Mix vigorously and then centrifuge for 10 min at 3000 rpm (1200 g).
3. Add a few drops of 0.3 mol/L KCN (2 g/dl) to the haemolysate to stabilise the Hb as cyanmethaemoglobin (HiCN).
4. Adjust the Hb concentrations of the haemolysates with water to within 20 g/L.
5. Mix equal volumes of the three haemolysates.
6. Check the mixture by electrophoresis.
7. Dispense in 0.5 ml volumes. If stored at 4°C, they should be stable for several weeks; however, if stored in liquid nitrogen, they should be stable for several months.

ESTIMATION OF HbA_2

The International Committee for Standardization in Haematology has made recommendations for two methods suitable for HbA_2 estimation. The first uses separation of HbA_2 by electrophoresis on cellulose acetate membrane, based on the method of Marengo-Rowe. The second method is the microcolumn technique of Efremov, et al. The microcolumn method is simpler and more precise, but the electrophoretic method provides a useful screen for the presence of some abnormal Hbs; it is more suitable for the laboratory performing tests only intermittently.

Electrophoresis

Reagent

Buffer, 0.13 mol/L tris-EDTA-borate, pH 9.1. Trishydroxy-methyl)-aminomethane 82.5 g; EDTA (disodium salt) 7.8 g; boric acid 4.6 g; water to 5 litre.

Method

Soak two cellulose acetate strips per sample in buffer and blot. Place the strips across the bridges of the tank. Secure with buffer-soaked filter paper wicks.

Apply approximately 10 µl of a haemolysate (approximately 10 g/dl) between the cathode bridge and mid-point of the strip, leaving not less than a 0.5 cm gap at each side of the strip. A glass capillary tube is a suitable applicator. Apply 200 V until there is a clear separation, which normally takes place within 60–100 min. Then cut-out the HbA and HbA_2 zones and elute them in 20 ml and 4 ml, respectively, of buffer, for a minimum of 30 min. Set up a normal control with each batch of samples.

Read the absorbance (A) at 413 nm and determine the percentage of HbA_2 by the equation below. Treat a Hb-free piece of cellulose acetate similarly, and use as a blank.

Calculation

$$\%\ HbA_2 = \frac{A^{413}HbA_2}{\left(A^{413}HbA \times 5\right) + A^{413}HbA_2} \times 100$$

Normal range 1.8–3.5%.

ESTIMATION OF HbF

HbF may be estimated by several methods, all of which are based on its resistance to denaturation at alkaline pH.

For small amount of HbF the method of Betke et al is most reliable, whilst for levels of over 50%, and in cord blood, the method of Jonxis and Visser is preferable.

Method of Jonxis and Visser

Add 0.1 ml of blood or haemolysate (approximately 100 g/L) to 10 ml of water, then add 2 drops of 10% NH_4OH solution. Measure the absorbance at 576 nm (A_B), then add 0.1 ml of the same blood or lysate to 10 ml of 0.06 mol/L NaOH; add 2 drops of 10% NA_4OH solution at room temperature. Mix thoroughly and measure the absorbance every min for 15 min at 37°C for 15 min, cool to room temperature and measure the absorbance (A_E). The ratio A_8:A_E should be constant.

Calculate the percentage of undentured Hb at each minute:

$$\frac{A_T^{576} - A_E^{576}}{A_B^{576} - A_E^{576}} \times 100$$

Then plot the percentage on the logarithmic scale of semilogarithmic paper, against time. This should produce a straight line from which the original amount of HbF, i.e. that at zero time, can be found by extrapolation.

Quantitative alkali denaturation method for estimation of fetal haemoglobin

1. Take 9.5 ml of Drabkin's solution in a test tube, add 0.5 ml of haemolysate. Cyanmethaemoglobin (HiCN) is formed. Mix well.
2. Transfer 2.8 ml of HiCN solution in a tube and keep at 20°C. To this add 0.2 ml of 1.2 N NaOH solution. Mix rapidly, incubate for 2 minutes at 20°C. Mix again and let stand for 5–10 minutes. Filter through Whatman filter paper mumber 3.
3. Prepare the total haemoglobin by adding 0.4 ml of the original HiCN solution to 6.5 ml of distilled water.
4. Using Drabkin's solution as blank at 540 nm, read the total haemoglobin and filtrate.
5. The optical density should fall between 0.05 and 0.5. If it is beyond 0.5, dilute the haemolysate with distilled water and repeat the said procedure.
6. Calculate as:

   Haemoglobin F percentage or HbF

$$= \frac{\text{OD of filtrate}}{\text{OD of total haemoglobin}} \times \frac{100}{10}$$

Significance

In infants aged 1 year the level of HbF should not be more that 1%. The normal range for adults is 0.5–0.8%.

Increased levels are found in many disorders, notably in β-thalassaemia trait and sickle cell disease. But any haematological condition, congenital or acquired, may be associated with a slight increase.

HbF and HbS concentration of various haemoglobinopathies are summarised in Table 7.5.

Table 7.5: HbF and HbS concentration as percentage of total Hb concentration in various disorders

Disorder	*HbF%*	*HbS%*
Normal	<1% (in adults)	Not present
Sickle cell trait (AS)	Normal	30–40%
Sickle cell anaemia (SS)	1–20%	75–95%
HbS β-thalassaemia [Sβ⁺ (some β chains present)] [Sβ° (no β chains present)]	 2–10% 5–30%	 60–85% 76–90%
HbS-C (SC)	1–5%	50–55%
HbS-D (SD)	1–5%	95% (S + D)
β-Thalassaemia major	10–98%	—
α-Thalassaemia	Reduced	—

SICKLE CELL DISEASE

Sickle cell disease is a type of hereditary haemoglobinopathy caused by a mutation in the β-globin gene forming a characteristic sickle-shaped RBC. The mutant (3-globin gene) forms haemoglobin 'S' (Hb-S) leading to sickling of the red cell.

Epidemiology

Sickle cell anaemia is common among the Blacks. This is also found in parts of the Mediterranean basin, the Middle East and India.

Pathogenesis

Sickle cell anaemia is caused by a mutation in the β-globin gene which substitutes valine for glutamic acid at the sixth position of the β-globin chain

The haemoglobin produced by this mutant gene is HbS. When HbS is deoxygenated it undergoes polymerisation and aggregation. This is a reversible change and on oxygenation it reverses to depolymerised state.

The polymerisation and aggregation forms a gelatinous network of fibrous polymers. This makes the red cell membrane stiff. It changes the free flowing liquid haemoglobin to a viscous gel. Red cell loses potassium and water, and calcium influxes. This causes dehydration of the red cell. These changes produce sickle shape. The extent of sickling change will depend on the concentration of HbS and its interaction with other haemoglobins. In heterozygous state (HbSA) there is larger amount of adult haemoglobin (HBA ~60%) compared to HbS. Thus, during deoxygenation and gelatinisation of HbS, HBA takes a weak part. So there is very little tendency to sickle.

This is called sickle cell trait. However, in homozygous state (HbSS) the haemoglobin is almost totally of HbS type. Thus, this shows a full-blown picture of sickle cell anaemia (sickle cell disease).

Double heterozygotes: One gene is HbS and the other gene may be either HbD or HbE or HbC or α-thalassaemia gene or β-thalassaemia gene.

Morphology

- Hb↓
- Peripheral smear shows normocytic normochromic to microcytic hypochromic cells with sickled red cells. (Figs 7.3 and 7.4)

There may be a few fragmented red cells, target cells and ovalocytes.

- Howell-Jolly bodies
- Reticulocyte count— increased (5 to 20%)
- ESR—decreased (due to decreased rouleaux formation)

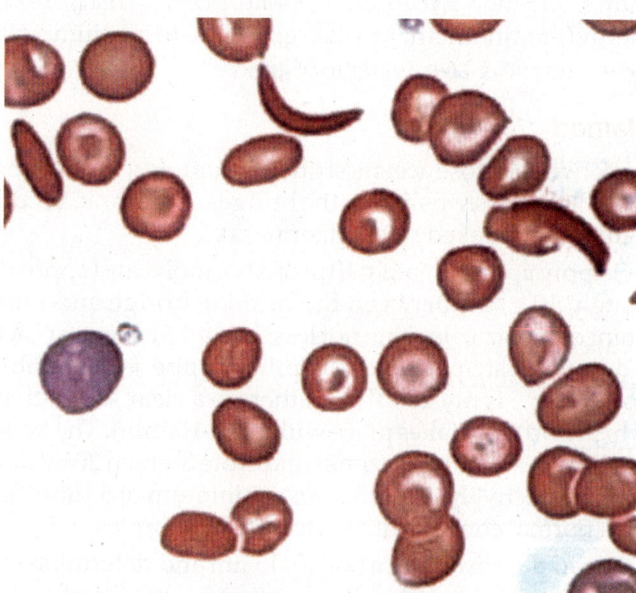

Fig. 7.3: Sickle cells *in vivo* peripheral blood sugar

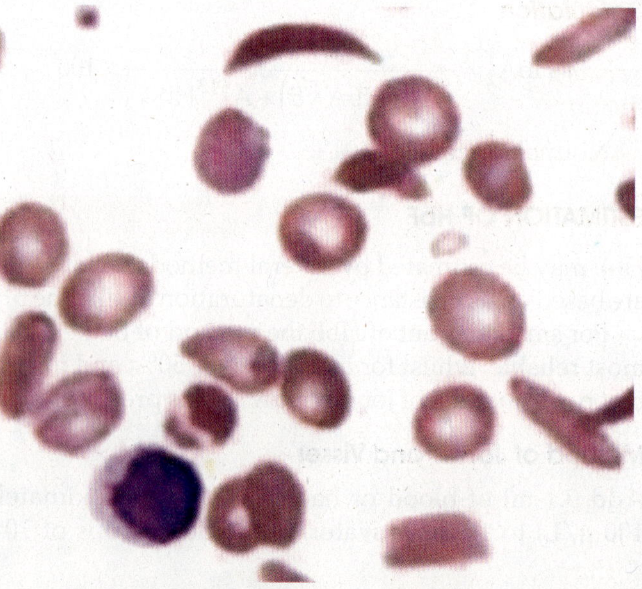

Fig. 7.4: Sickle cells in PS

- Bone marrow is hyperplastic. There is increase in normoblasts. There is secondary new bone formation.
- Extramedullary haematopoiesis may appear in spleen and liver.

Iron status: ↑ iron deposition in different organs.

Complications

Most of the complication arises because of blockage of blood vessels by sickled RBCs causing ischaemia.

- Growth retardation
- **Thrombosis or infarction of spleen:** Spleen suffers from marked hypoxia and scarring. This makes the person susceptible to infection. Progressive scarring will cause shrinkage of spleen.
- **Occlusion of retinal vessels:** This can cause retinal haemorrhage and ultimately retinal detachment.
- **Kidney:** In kidney vascular occlusion can produce renal papillary necrosis and renal failure.
- **Bones and joints:** Ischaemia of bones and joints particularly femoral or humeral heads.
- **Hepatomegaly:** Sinusoids gets distended by sickle cells causing enlargement of liver.
- **Infection:** Prone to infections
- **Osteomyelitis** due to salmonella infection.
- **Ulcer lower leg:** Ulcer in lower leg arises due to vascular occlusion leading to ischaemia and super added infection.
- **Occlusion of pulmonary vessels:** This may lead to cor pulmonale.
- **Gallstone formation:** Haemolysis leads to hyperbilirubinemia and bile stone formation.
- **Priapism:** Accumulation of blood in corpora cavernosa.

SICKLING PHENOMENON (TESTS FOR HbS)

Tests for HbS

Tests to detect the presence of HbS depend on the decreased solubility of the abnormal Hb at low oxygen tensions.

Sickling in Whole Blood (Figs 7.5 and 7.6)

The sickling phenomenon may be simply demonstrated in a thin wet film of blood sealed between slide and coverglass by means of a petroleum jelly-paraffin wax mixture. Sickling develops in the various types of sickle-cell disease and also in HbS trait. In homozygous HbS disease (or HbS C disease or Hb S/β-thalassaemia) marked sickling is usually visible after incubation for 1 hour or less at 37°C and filamentous forms are conspicuous. In HbS trait the process is slower and the changes are less severe and incubation for as long as 12 hours may be necessary for the changes to develop.

They can, however, be hastened by the addition of reducing agents to the blood, e.g. sodium dithionite.

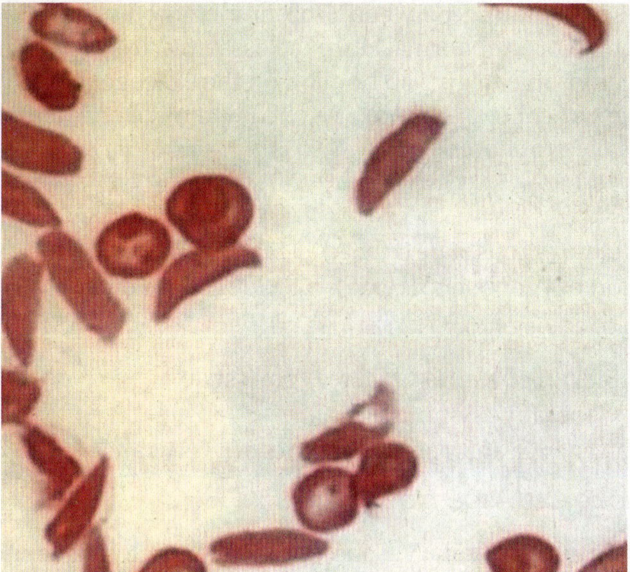

Fig. 7.5: *In vitro* demonstration sickle cells

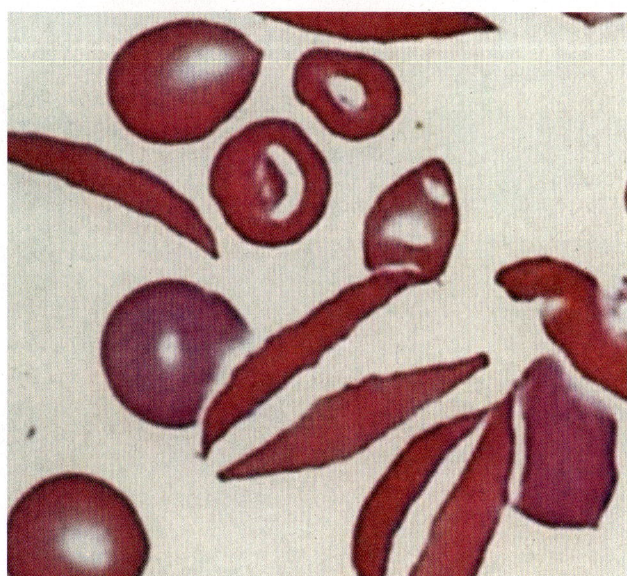

Fig. 7.6: Sickling phenomenon

Method using Reducing Agent

Reagents

A. Sodium dithionite (Na_2Sp_4), 0.114 mol/L; 19.85 g/L. Prepare freshly just before use.
B. Disodium hydrogen phosphate (Na_2HPO_4), 0.114 mol/L 16.2 g/L. For use, mix 2 volumes of A with 3 volumes of B to obtain a final pH of 6.8.

Add 5 drops of the freshly prepared reagent to 1 drop of anti-coagulated blood on a slide. Cover immediately with a cover-glass and seal with petroleum jelly–paraffin wax mixture. Sickling takes place almost immediately in HbS disease and should be obvious in HbS trait within 1 hour.

Qualitative Solubility Test

Hb solubility tests provide rapid method for the detection of HbS. They are particularly useful for tentatively discriminating between HbS homozygotes and HbS with A or an abnormal Hb or thalassaemia. It is, however, inadvisable to give an opinion on the exact genotype of the patient (e.g. Hb AS, SS or SC) without confirmation by electrophoresis.

Clinical Picture

Heterozygous state (HbSA) → Sickle cell trait
Homozygous state (HbSS) → Sickle cell anaemia

Sickle Cell Trait

- Sickle cell trait is a heterozygous state
- Generally asymptomatic
- Anaemia and painful episodes are very rare

Sickle Cell Anaemia

Painful ischaemia: Vasoocclusion in connective tisue and musculoskeletal structures produce ischaemia causing acute pain, tenderness, fever and tachycardia. These painful crises are the most common manifestation. The frequency and seventy of these crises varies. These crises can be precipitated by infection, fever, exercise, anxiety and sudden change in temperature.

Diagnosis

- **Clinical picture:** Intermittent episodes of ischaemic pain
- **Peripheral blood picture** with sickled red blood cells.
- **Haemoglobin electrophoresis:** Haemoglobin S can be detected by its specific band formation. (HbS is a slow moving band.)
- **HbSS:** HbS : 70–90%
  HbF : 10–30%
  HBA : absent
- **HbSA:** HbS : 25–40%
  HBA : 60–75%
- **Sickling test**
- **Genetic analysis:** To find out the type of globin chain.

Chapter 8

Aplastic Anaemia

Chapter Outline

INTRODUCTION

Aplastic anaemia (AA) is a rare life-threatening disorder which is characterized by bi- or tricytopenia and hypoplastic or aplastic bone marrow. AA can present as an acquired or congenital disorder. In recent years it was noted that a subgroup of patients with seemingly acquired AA with onset in adulthood carry mutations which cause or at least predispose to bone marrow failure, e.g. mutations in the genes of the telomerase complex. Options for the first-line treatment are allogeneic stem cell transplantation or immunosuppression.

Bone marrow does not create enough blood cells. People with aplastic anaemia may experience fatigue, bruising or shortness of breath. For many people, medications effectively treat these symptoms.

A rare and serious condition, aplastic anaemia can develop at any age. It can occur suddenly, or it can come on slowly and worsen over time. It can be mild or severe.

Definition

- Pancytopenia with hypocellularity (aplasia) of bone marrow
- Aplastic anaemia is a severe, life-threatening syndrome in which production of erythrocytes, WBCs, and platelets has failed.

Causes of Aplastic Anaemia

1. Congenital or inherited causes of aplastic anaemia (20%)
   - Patients usually have dysmorphic features or physical stigmata. On occasion, marrow failure may be the initial presenting feature.
   - Fanconi anaemia
   - Dyskeratosis congenita
   - Cartilage-hair hypoplasia
   - Pearson syndrome
   - Amegakaryocytic thrombocytopenia (thrombocytopenia-absent radius [TAR] syndrome)
2. Acquired causes of aplastic anaemia (80%)
   - Idiopathic factors
   - Infectious causes: Hepatitis virus, EBV, HIV, parvovirus, and Mycobacteria
   - Toxic chemical: Benzene, lindane, glue vapers, and radiation.
   - Idiosyncratic drug reactions: Chloramphenicol, gold, NSAID (phenylbutazone, indomethacin), sulfonamides, AEDs (felbamate), arsenicals.
3. I. Primary (idiopathic) 70–80%: Immune-mediated disease.

   II. Secondary drugs
   1. Unpredictable (idiosyncratic reaction)
      - Antiepileptic drugs (hydantoins)
      - Oral antidiabetic agents (tolbutamide, chlorpropamide)
      - Tranquillizers (chlorpromazine, chlordiazepoxide)
      - Antirheumatic drugs (gold, indomethacin, phenylbutazone)
      - Antibacterial agents (sulfonamides, isoniazid, steptomycin, tetracyclines, chloramphenicol)
   2. Unpredictable hypersensitivity (immune reaction)
      - Many drugs

AETIOLOGY OF APLASTIC ANAEMIA

It is summarised in Table 8.1

Stem cells in the bone marrow produce blood cells—red cells, white cells and platelets. In aplastic anaemia, stem cells are damaged. As a result, the bone marrow is either empty (aplastic) or contains a few blood cells (hypoplastic).

Table 8.1: Aetiology of aplastic anaemia	
Category	*Specific agents (examples, not all-inclusive)*
Autoimmune	Antibody-induced, eosinophilic fasciitis, GVHD, SLE
Chemicals	Benzene (organic solvent), lindane (insecticide), inorganic arsenicals, pentachlorophenol (wood preservative), toluene (glue)
Drugs (dose-dependent)	Alkylating agents (carboplatin) antibiotics (chloramphenicol, sulfonamides), anti-metabolites (methotrexate), ticlopidine
Drugs (idiosyncratic)	Antiepileptics (carbamazepine, hydantoins), anti-thyroid (methimazole, propylthiouracil), chloramphenicol, gold salts, NSAIDs (indomethacin, phenylbutazone), organic arsenicals (arsenic trioxide), penicillamine
Hereditary	Amegakaryocytic thrombocytopenia, dyskeratosis congenita, Fanconi anaemia, Shwachman-Diamond-Oski syndrome, telomerase defects
Idiopathic	Acquired stem cell defects
Infections	Sepsis, viral (CMV, EBV, seronegative hepatitis, HHV-6, HIV, VZV)
Miscellaneous	Anorexia nervosa/starvation, hypopituitarism, PNH, pregnancy, thymoma
Radiation	Accident (Chermobyl, 5-Mile Island), therapy (whole body irradiation)
CMV: Cytomegalovirus; EBV: Epstein-Barr virus; GVHD: Graft-versus-host disease; HHV-6: Human herpesvirus 6; HIV: Human immunodeficiency virus; NSAIDs: Non-steroidal anti-inflammatory drugs, PNH: Paroxysmal nocturnal hemoglobinuria; SLE: Systemic lupus erythematosus; VZV: Varicella-zoster virus	

RISK FACTORS

Aplastic anaemia is rare. Factors that can increase risk include:

- Treatment with high-dose radiation or chemotherapy for cancer
- Exposure to toxic chemicals
- The use of some prescription drugs such as chloramphenicol, which is used to treat bacterial infections, and gold compounds used to treat rheumatoid arthritis
- Certain blood diseases, autoimmune disorders and serious infections.
- **A viral infection:** Viral infections that affect bone marrow can play a role in the development of aplastic anaemia. Viruses that have been linked to aplastic anaemia include hepatitis, Epstein-Barr, cytomegalovirus, parvovirus B19 and HIV.
- **Autoimmune disorders:** An autoimmune disorder, in which your immune system attacks healthy cells, might involve stem cells in your bone marrow.
- **Pregnancy:** Your immune system might attack your bone marrow during pregnancy.

The most common cause of aplastic anaemia is from your immune system attacking the stem cells in your bone marrow. Other factors that can injure bone marrow and affect blood cell production include:

- **Radiation and chemotherapy treatments:** While these cancer-fighting therapies kill cancer cells, they can also damage healthy cells, including stem cells in bone marrow.
- **Unknown factors:** In many cases, doctors are not able to identify the cause of aplastic anaemia (idiopathic aplastic anaemia).

Substances associated with aplastic anaemia is given in Table 8.2.

Table 8.2: Substances associated with aplastic anaemia
Analgesics
Antiseizure agents (mephenytoin, trimethadione*)
Antihistamines
Antimicrobials*
Antineoplastic agents (alkylating agents, antitumor antibiotics, antimetabolites)
Antithyroid medications
Benzene*
Chloramphenicol*
Gold compounds*
Heavy metals
Hypoglycemic agents
Insecticides
Organic arsenicals*
Phenylbutazone*
Phenothiazines
Sulfonamides*
Sedatives

*Most common

Why does aplastic anaemia develop?

It is summarised in Table 8.3.

Table 8.3: Causes and risk factors of aplastic anaemia
Exposure to radiation (e.g. atomic bomb victims)
Structural chromosomal abnormalities
Exposure to carcinogens or chemicals
Viral infections
Previous chemotherapy or radiation therapy
Long-term exposure to toxic chemicals such as benzene
Other drugs including antibiotics. Anti-epileptic drugs herbal medications.
Folk remedies without known ingredients
Autoimmune disease
Paroxysmal nocturnal hemoglobinuria

Two types of aplastic anaemia

- Inherited aplastic anaemia occurs because of a random gene mutation. It is most common in children and younger adults.

- Acquired aplastic anaemia occurs because of an immune system problem. It is most common in older adults, but can occur in younger adults.

Aplastic Anaemia—Forms of Disease

- **Inevitable:** Dose related, e.g. cytotoxic drugs, ionizing radiation. The timing, duration of aplasia and recovery depend on the dose. Recovery is usual except with whole body irradiation.
- **Idiosyncratic:** Unpredictable to drugs, e.g. anti-inflammatory antibiotics anti-epileptic, these agents usually do not produce marrow failure in the majority of persons exposed to these agents.

Aplastic anaemia is classified as severe according to blood counts. Most of the discussion that follows relates to severe aplastic anaemia. There are two types of aplastic anaemia.

Signs and Symptoms

Symptoms vary from person to person, depending on which type of blood cells are most affected and the cause of the disorder.

- Fatigue
- Shortness of breath
- Rapid or irregular heart rate
- Pale skin
- Frequent or prolonged infections
- Unexplained or easy bruising
- Nosebleeds and bleeding gums
- Prolonged bleeding from cuts
- Skin rash
- Dizziness
- Headache
- Fever
- Red or purple spots on the skin caused by bleeding under the skin.

Incidence of Aplastic Anaemia

Overall incidence of 2.35 (95% CI: 2.06–2.64) cases per million inhabitants per year. Median age was 60 years (range: 2–92), and median follow-up was 76 (0–193) months. Primary treatments included immunosuppressive therapy (63%), allogenic stem cell transplantation (10%), or single-agent cyclosporine/no specific therapy (27%). The 5-year survival was 90. 7% in patients aged 0–18 years, 90.5% in patients aged 19–39 years, 70. 7% in patients aged 40–59 years, and 38.1% in patients aged ≥60 years.

Myelodysplastic Syndrome (MDS) and Aplastic Anaemia

MDS: Most cases of MDS are linked to changes to the DNA in stem cells in the bone marrow, but the exact cause is usually not known. Aging may play a role, because as your age increases, your stem cells get older and are more likely to develop abnormalities that can lead to MDS. Certain environmental or health conditions, such as radiation and chemotherapy treatment, exposure to certain chemicals, and smoking are also associated with MDS.

Acquired Aplastic Anaemia

Acquired aplastic anaemia is usually considered an autoimmune disease. Normally, your immune system attacks only foreign substances. When your immune system attacks your own body, you are said to have an autoimmune disease. Other autoimmune diseases include rheumatoid arthritis and lupus.

Acquired aplastic anaemia can begin at any time in life.

Aplastic anaemia can be acquired, meaning it develops after birth, or it can be inherited, meaning it is passed down in genes from your parents. Acquired aplastic anaemia is more common than the inherited disorder. With inherited aplastic anaemia, it is important that siblings also be tested for the disease so that it can be treated as early as possible.

Acquired aplastic anaemia is a rare, serious blood disorder, which leads to failure to produce blood cells due to failure of the bone marrow.

When your immune system attacks your own body, you are said to have an autoimmune disease. Other autoimmune diseases include rheumatoid arthritis and lupus. Acquired aplastic anaemia can begin at any time in life. About 75 out of 100 cases of acquired aplastic anaemia are idiopathic.

PNH arises in the setting of autoimmune acquired aplastic anaemia and bone marrow failure. Individuals affected with acquired aplastic anaemia are also at risk that it will evolve into another similar disorder known as myelodysplasia. In a minority of cases, acquired aplastic anaemia may eventually develop leukaemia.

Diagnosis and Investigations

Blood tests: Normally, red blood cell, white blood cell and platelet levels stay within certain ranges. In aplastic anaemia all three of these blood cell levels are low (Fig. 8.1).

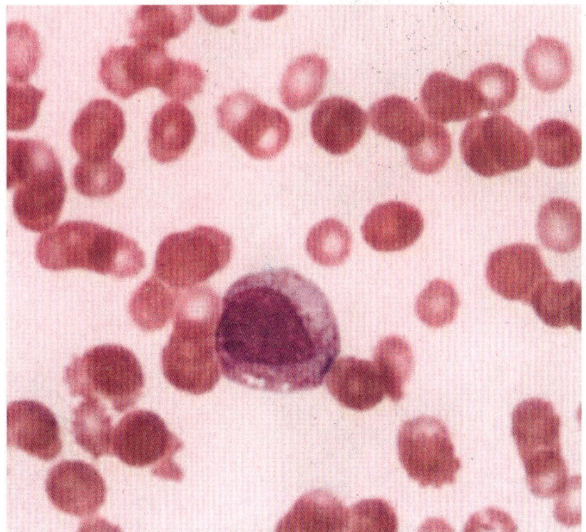

Fig. 8.1: Peripheral blood showing normocytic RBCs, pancytopenia, no abnormal cells and no platelets

Lab Diagnosis of Aplastic Anaemia

The sample is examined under a microscope to rule out other blood-related diseases. In aplastic anaemia, bone marrow contains fewer blood cells than normal. Confirming a diagnosis of aplastic anaemia requires a bone marrow biopsy.

Peripheral Blood

- Normochromic: Normocytic RBCs (normal MCV and MCH)
- Pancytopenia
- No abnormal cells

Plus at least two of the following peripheral blood findings:

- Neutrophils less than 0.5 × 10.
- Platelets less than 20×10^9 /L
- Reticulocytes less than 20×10^9/L

Bone Marrow Biopsy (Figs 8.2 and 8.3)

Bone marrow contains fewer blood cells than normal. Marrow cellularity < 25% (or 25–50% with <30% residual hematopoietic cells).

Hypocellular bone marrow with increased:

- Fat spaces
- Lymph cells
- Plasma cells
- Macrophages
- Mast cells

Recent Advances and Management of Treatment

Treatment plan depends on several factors, such as your age, overall health and symptoms. Aplastic anaemia treatment may include:

- **Immunosuppressants:** These medicines suppress your immune system. Aplastic anaemia symptoms improve in about 2 out of 3 people who take immunosuppressive medications.
- **Bone marrow stimulants:** Certain types of drugs can stimulate your bone marrow to produce more blood cells. You may take sargramostim (Leukine®), filgrastim (Neupogen®) or epoetin alfa (Epogen®).
- **Blood transfusion:** Transfusions replace red blood cells and platelets. Transfusions are not a cure for aplastic anaemia, but they can treat symptoms like fatigue or bruising easily.
- **Supportive antibiotics:** Depending on the severity.

Recent advances in the treatment of aplastic anaemia (AA) made most of patients to expect to achieve a long-term survival. Allogeneic stem cell transplantation (SCT) from HLA-matched sibling donor (MSD-SCT) is a preferred first-line treatment option for younger patients with severe or very severe AA, whereas immuno-suppressive treatment (IST) is an alternative option for others. Horse anti-thymocyte globulin (ATG) with cyclosporin A (CsA) had been a standard IST regimen with acceptable response rate.

Recently, horse ATG had been not available and replaced with rabbit ATG in most countries.

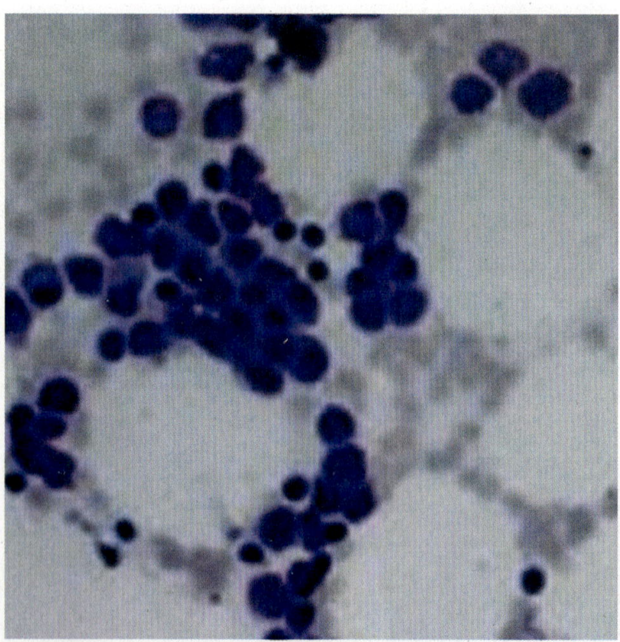

Fig. 8.2: Bone marrow showing decrease precursor cells, hypocellular bone marrow with increase lymph and plasma cell, macrophages

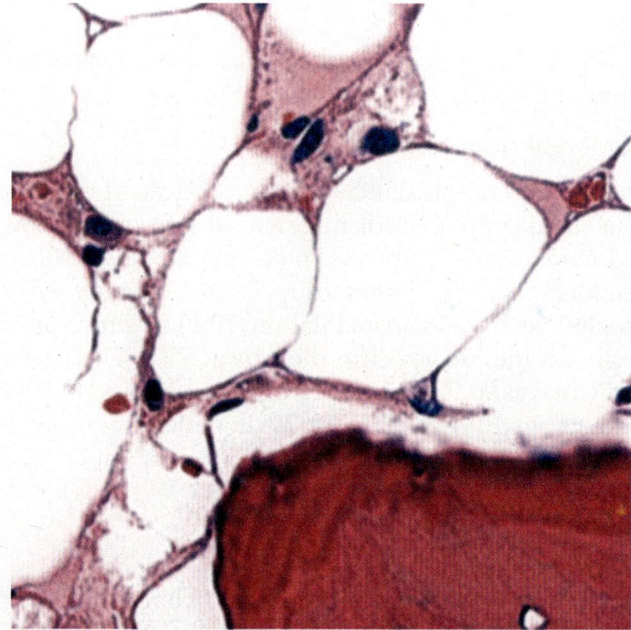

Fig. 8.3: Bone marrow biopsy showing increase fat cells

Subsequently, recent comparative studies showed that the outcomes of patients who received rabbit ATG/CsA were similar or inferior compared to those who received horse ATG/CsA. Therefore, further studies to improve the outcomes of IST, including additional eltrombopag, are necessary. On the other hand, the upper age limit of patients who are able to receive MSD-SCT as first-line treatment is a current issue because of favourable outcomes of MSD-SCT of older patients using fludarabine-based conditioning.

In addition, further studies to improve the outcomes of patients who receive allogeneic SCT from alternative donors are needed. However, decision depends on severity of the disease, age and comorbidity of the patient and availability of a matched stem cell donor. Probability of survival after HLA-identical sibling transplantation exceeds 90% in young patients with bone marrow as the stem cell source and conditioning with an ATG-containing regimen. Results of matched unrelated donor transplantation have improved substantially over the last 10 years.

Since the introduction of immunosuppressive therapy and allogeneic stem cell transplantation, the outcome has improved considerably, and the 5-year survival is reported to be 70–80% in selected patient cohorts.

Chapter 9

Bone Marrow Examination (BME) and Diagnostic Significance of Peripheral Blood Examination

Chapter Outline

INTRODUCTION

Bone marrow is the sponge-like tissue in the interior of bones which produces red blood cells, white blood cells, and platelets. In adults, few bones still contain this important tissue: hip bones, shoulder bones, ribs, breastbone, vertebrae, and the skull. In infants, all bones contain active bone marrow.

Bone marrow is a soft, spongy tissue found in the center of most bones. Bone marrow makes different types of blood cells, including:

- Red blood cells (also called erythrocytes), which carry oxygen from your lungs to every cell in your body.
- White blood cells (also called leukocytes), which help you fight infections.
- Platelets, which help with blood clotting.

There are two types of procedures used to collect bone marrow samples for testing:

- **Bone marrow aspiration** removes a small amount of bone marrow fluid and cells.
- **Bone marrow biopsy** removes a small piece of bone and bone marrow.

One or both of these procedures may be performed. Bone marrow aspirate is usually done first, and is performed by inserting a special needle into the bone, typically the hip bone in adults, and removing a small sample of liquid marrow. A bone marrow biopsy is performed in a similar manner. A small cylindrical sample of solid bone marrow, known as a core biopsy, is removed. The samples are then sent to the laboratory for examination.

A bone marrow examination provides more detailed information about the structure, production, and maturity of blood cells. Bone marrow examination is helpful in the diagnosis of many conditions including leukaemia, lymphoma, myeloma, myelodysplastic syndromes, and myeloproliferative disorders. Bone marrow examination may also be used to determine the stage of a disease or to monitor treatment.

Bone marrow contains immature cells, called stem cells. Many people with blood cancers, such as leukaemia and lymphoma, sickle cell anaemia, and other life-threatening diseases, rely on bone marrow or cord blood to survive.

Healthy bone marrow and blood cells are needed in order to live. When the disease affects bone marrow so that it can no longer function effectively, a marrow or cord blood transplant could be the best treatment option; for some patients, it is the only potential cure.

Bone marrow examination is used in the diagnosis of a number of conditions, including leukaemia, multiple myeloma, lymphoma, anaemia, and pancytopenia. The bone marrow produces the cellular elements of the blood, including platelets, red blood cells, and white blood cells.

While much information can be obtained by testing the blood itself (drawn from a vein by phlebotomy), it is sometimes necessary to examine the source of the blood cells in the bone marrow to obtain more information on hematopoiesis; this is the role of bone marrow aspiration and biopsy.

Frequently, a trephine biopsy is also obtained, which yields a narrow, cylindrically shaped solid piece of bone marrow, 2 mm wide and 2 cm long (80 μL), which is examined microscopically (sometimes with the aid of immunohistochemistry) for cellularity and infiltrative processes. An aspiration, using a 20 mL syringe, yields approximately 300 μL of bone marrow. A volume greater than 300 μL is not recommended, since it may dilute the sample with peripheral blood.

Bone marrow aspiration and bone marrow biopsy procedures are usually done at the same time. A health care provider will collect the marrow samples for testing. Usually, the samples can be collected in about ten minutes (Fig. 9.1).

BONE MARROW EXAMINATION

Bone marrow examination is an important and widely used investigation in the diagnosis of haematologic disease. Normal marrow is soft and semifluid during life and can be aspirated easily using a sternal puncture needle with adjustable guard.

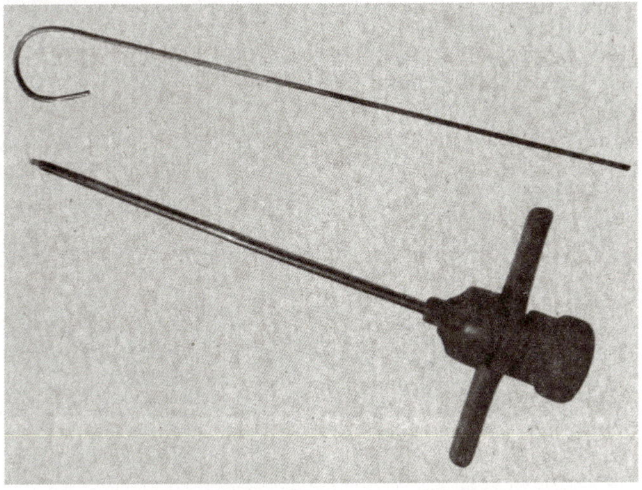

Fig. 9.1: Bone marrow aspiration needle

BONE MARROW SMEARS

Significance of Bone Marrow Smears and Indications (Fig. 9.2)

The red cells, white cells, and platelets are manufactured in the bone marrow. If the manufacturing process is abnormal, it may indicate disease. The manufacturing process may be studied by obtaining a smear of the bone marrow and evaluating the cells.

The normal values for bone marrow smears are given in Table 9.1.

What is the M:E ratio? The M:E stands for myeloid–erythroid. Thus, the M:E ratio is the myeloid–erythroid ratio. It is the ratio of white cells to nucleated red cells.

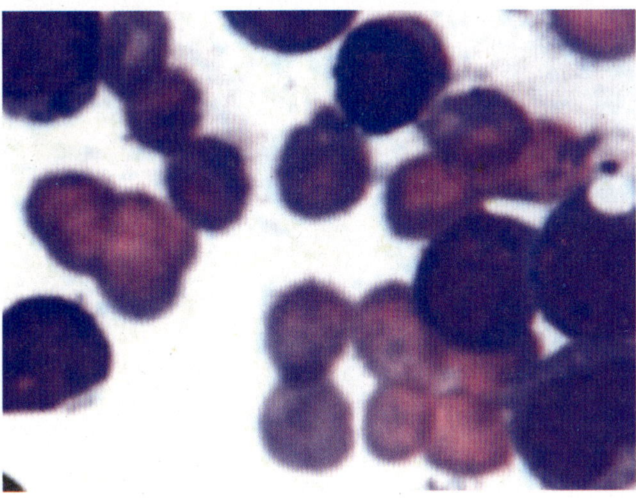

Fig. 9.2: Bone marrow smear

For example, if a bone marrow smear shows 80% white cells and 20% nucleated red cells, the M:E ratio is 4: 1.

The M:E ratio is often referred to as the WBC: Nucleated RBC ratio.

The average M:E ratio is 4:1, with a normal range of 6:1 to 2:1.

An increased M:E ratio (7:1 or more) may be found in infections, granulocytic leukaemia, leukemoid reactions, and a decrease in the number of nucleated red cells.

A decreased M:E ratio (I: 1 or less) may be encountered in either a decrease in the production of white cells or an increase in the production of red cells.

Bone marrow smears are of particular interest to the physician in the following diseases: Aplastic anaemia; pernicious anaemia, leukaemia, purpura haemorrhagica, agranulocytosis, and multiple myeloma (Table 9.2).

INDICATIONS FOR BONE MARROW

- **Absolute indications**
  - Megaloblastic macrocytic anaemia.
  - Aleukaemic or subleukaemic leukaemia.
- **Diagnostic importance**
  - Multiple myeloma
  - Aplastic anaemia
  - Gaucher's disease
- **Confirmatory importance**
  - Leukaemias of all types
  - Haemolytic anaemia
  - Idiopathic thrombocytopenic purpura
  - Idiopathic granulocytopenia
  - Leishmaniasis
  - Disseminated lupus erythematosus
  - Metastatic diseases
  - Myeloproliferative disorders
  - Lipid storage
  - Sideroblastic anaemia
  - Iron deficiency anaemia
  - Lymphoma (staging).

Preparation and Staining of Bone Marrow Smears

1. Place a small amount of bone marrow a glass slide.
2. Make a bone marrow smear in the same manner that you would make a blood smear.
3. Make about 5 more bone marrow ·smears.
4. Make a finger puncture on the patient.
5. Make two blood smears for a differential white cell count.
6. Write the patient's name and date on both the bone marrow smears and blood smears.
7. Allow the bone marrow smears and the blood smears to dry. (It takes about 20 minutes for bone marrow smears to dry.)

Table 9.1: Cell distribution in bone marrow and peripheral blood

	Marrow%		*Peripheral blood%*	
Types of cells	***Average***	***Range***	***Average***	***Range***
Myeloblasts	2.5	0.5–5 0	0	
Promyelocytes	6	1–8	0	
Myelocytes	15	8–20	0	
× Neutrophilic	12	5–19	0	
× Eosinophilic	1.5	0.5–3.0	0	
× Basophilic	0.3	0.0–0.3	0	
Metamyelocytes	29	14–36	0	
× Neutrophilic	26.4	13–32	0	
× Eosinophilic	2.0	0.5–3.0	0	
× Basophilic	0.3	0.0–0.3	0	
Segmented granulocytes	32	17–43		
× Neutrophils	27	15–35	60	50–70
× Eosinophils	4	1–7	2	1–4
× Basophils	1	0.5–1.5	0	0–1
Monocytes	2	0.4–4.0	5	2–10
Lymphocytes	13	5–20	30	20–40
Pronormoblasts	0.6	0.2–4	0	
Early normoblast	2.4	1.5–5.8	0	
Intermediate normoblast	10.6	5.0–20.0	0	
Late normoblast	6.6	3.0–20.0	0	
Megaloblasts	0.2	0–0.5	0	
Megakaryocytes	0.4	0.04–2.0	0	
Reticulum cells	1.0	0.2–3.0	0	
Plasma cells	0.6	0–2.0	0	
M:E ratio	3–4 : 1			

Table 9.2: The more significant bone marrow abnormalities in various diseases

Disease	***Abnormality***	***Normal values***
Aplastic anaemia	Hypoplastic (defective and incomplete development of cells)	Normoplastic
Iron deficiency anaemia	Hyperplastic (overactive): Increase in nucleated red cells (30–60%)	Normoplastic
Pernicious anaemia	Increase in nucleated red cells (30–50%): Presence of "pernicious anaemia type" nucleated red cells	8–30%
Hereditary spherocytic anaemia	Increase in nucleated red cells (30–60%)	8–30%
Sickle cell anaemia	Increase in nucleated red cells (40–70%)	8–30%
Thalassaemia major	Increase in nucleated red cells (30–60%)	8–30%
Acute granulocytic leukaemia	Increase in myeloblasts (15–50%)	0–5%
Chronic granulocytic leukaemia	Increase in myeloblasts (5–15%); increase in myelocytes and metamyelocytes	0–5%
Acute lymphocytic leukaemia	Increase in lymphoblasts (15–75%)	0%

Contd.

Table 9.2: The more significant bone marrow abnormalities in various diseases (Contd.)

Disease	*Abnormality*	*Normal values*
Chronic lymphocytic leukaemia	Increase in lymphocytes (30–90%)	5–15%
Monocytic leukaemia	Increase in monocytes (20–60%)	0–5%
Plasmacytic leukaemia	Increase in plasmacytes (15–75%)	0–1%
Purpura haemorrhagica (idiopathic thrombocytopenic purpura)	Number of megakaryocytes is normal or increased; platelet formation is decreased	0–3%
Polycythaemia vera	Hyperplastic; percentage of white cells, red cells, and platelets is normal	Normoplastic
Agranulocytosis	Granulocytes are decreased during height of disease but increased during recovery: percentage of nucleated red cells is normal: percentage of megakaryocytes is normal	8–30% 0–3%
Infectious mononucleosis	Increase in lymphocytes (15–35%)	5–15%
Multiple myeloma	10–90%	0%
Hodgkin's disease	Presence of Reed-Sternberg cells	0%
Gaucher's disease	Presence of Gaucher' s cells	0%

8. Then stain both the marrow smears and blood smears with Giemsa stain and buffer solution.
9. After staining the bone marrow smears and blood smears, allow them to dry. (It requires about 10 min.)
10. Make the study of bone marrow cells which is given below.

The procedure given below is recommended for studying the marrow films:

1. Naked eye inspection of the slides to select the smear-containing particles.
2. With 10X objective survey the particles whether they are normoplastic, hypoplastic or hyperplastic.
3. Select a cellular area (usually in the tail portion of the film around particles). Study the cytologic details by high power 40X and oil immersion 100X objectives.

Note the under-mentioned points

Cellularity: Normo-hypo-hyperplastic marrow particles. Cellularity is better defined by studying histologic sections of aspirated particles, though crude estimates can be given on films. The normal cellularity of the marrow varies with age being more in infants and least in elderly individuals.

Next look for *reaction of erythropoiesis*, whether it is normoblastic, megaloblastic or micro-normoblastic. Look for maturity of leukopoietic cells. The M:E ratio is based on a count of 500–1000 marrow cells. In the normal adult, the reaction is normoblastic, leukopoietic maturity is normal and **M:E ratio** is about 3 or 4:1. The M:E ratio at birth is 1.85:1, during the first two weeks it reaches its peak of 11:1. It then gradually drops to the (years 1 to 20) average of 3:1 (Table 9.3).

LASTLY, TO ANSWER THE QUESTIONS

Q. Why is a bone marrow examination performed and what are they used for?

Ans. In brief:

- A bone marrow examination provides more detailed information about the structure, production, and maturity of blood cells. Bone marrow examination is helpful in the diagnosis of many conditions including leukaemia, lymphoma, myeloma, myelodysplastic syndromes, and myeloproliferative disorders. Bone marrow examination may also be used to determine the stage of a disease or to monitor treatment.
- Bone marrow tests are used to:
  - Find out the cause of problems with red blood cells, white blood cells, or platelets
  - Diagnose and monitor blood disorders, such as:
    - Anaemia (when the cause is unknown)
    - Polycythaemia vera
    - Thrombocytopenia
  - Diagnose bone marrow disorders
  - Diagnose and monitor treatment for certain types of cancers, including leukaemia, multiple myeloma, and lymphoma
  - Diagnose the cause of an unexplained fever, which could be from an infection in the bone marrow.

DIAGNOSTIC SIGNIFICANCE OF PERIPHERAL BLOOD SMEARS

Apart from the search for blood parasites, examination of the stained smear is screening of formed elements of the blood. Valuable information can be collected in cases of anaemias and definite diagnosis can be established of

Table 9.3: Conditions in which various types of reaction may be observed, as demonstrated by bone marrow aspiration

1. **M:E ratio increased** Myeloid forms of leukaemia The majority of infections Leukemoid reaction Decrease in nucleated red cells	
2. **M:E ratio normal** Normal marrow Myelosclerosis Multiple myeloma, etc. Aplastic anaemia	
3. **M:E ratio decreased** Decrease in myeloid cells (agranulocytosis) Increase in erythroid cells due to either	
Normoblastic hyperplasia	***or Megaloblastic hyperplasia***
- Haemorrhagic anaemias	- Pernicious anaemia
- Iron deficiency anaemia	- Sprue, idiopathic
- Haemolytic anaemias	- Steatorrhea, resection of small intestine (certain cases)
- Thalassaemia	- Tropical macrocytic anaemia
- Cirrhosis of the liver	- Non-tropical nutritional macrocytic anaemia
- Polycythaemia vera	- Macrocytic anaemia with *Diphyllobothrium* infestation
- Plumbism	- Megaloblastic anaemia of infancy
- Anaemia of chronic renal disease	- Megaloblastic anaemia of pregnancy
	- "Refractory megaloblastic" anaemia
	- "Achrestic" anaemia
4. **Non-myeloid cells increased** - Other forms of leukaemia - Multiple myeloma - Metastases from carcinoma, etc. - Gaucher's disease, Niemann-Pick disease - Aplastic anaemia (usually relative increase only) - Infectious mononucleosis	

the nature of some of them, like megaloblastic anaemia and sickle cell anaemia. Infectious mononucleosis and frank leukaemias can also be easily spotted out. Lastly examination of the smear, used as a baseline study, can prompt one about further examinations to be undertaken for the diagnosis.

In patient care, diagnostic formulations rest on a tripod consisting of clinical history, physical examination and laboratory investigations. The literature reveals that as much as 70% of clinical decisions and diagnoses are supported by laboratory medicine.

Peripheral blood film (PBF) is a basic and a highly informative haematological tool at the clinician's disposal in screening, diagnosis and monitoring of disease progression.

Despite advances in haematology automation and application of molecular techniques, the PBF has remained a very important diagnostic test to the haematologist. A good quality smear, thorough examination and proper interpretation in line with patient's clinical state should be ensured by the haematopathologist. Clinicians should be abreast with its clinical utility and proper application of the reports in the management of patients.

Examination of the peripheral blood smear should be considered, along with review of the results of peripheral blood counts and red blood cell indices, an essential component of the initial evaluation of all patients with hematologic disorders. The examination of blood films stained with Wright's stain frequently provides important clues in the diagnosis of anaemias and various disorders of leukocytes and platelets.

The diagnostic relevance of a PBF is enormous. The PBF exposes the morphology of peripheral blood cells, which ensures its place in the morphologic diagnosis of various primary and secondary blood and blood related diseases. It is diagnostic relevance has not been lessened by advances in haematology automation and molecular techniques.

Morphology of the blood cells on a PBF smear is best discussed in line with each haemopoietic cell lineage. The distribution, size, shape, colour, cellular inclusions of the red blood cell (RBC) and morphology of the other major cell lines should be carefully assessed. However, some abnormalities such as broken cells (smear or smudge cells) may be artefacts and should be taken into consideration when reporting.

For estimating total leucocyte count, the smear cells seen must be included in the counts to avoid spurious results. Blood film should be interpreted alongside patient's clinical details (history and physical examination). Results of other routine laboratory work-ups including full blood count, erythrocyte sedimentation rate, red cell indices should be part of the interpreting framework for reporting a PBF.

A manual review of automated counts with peripheral blood film should be performed when flagging occurs due to excess counts. Falsely elevated leucocyte count may be generated by the automated or manual counts due to circulating nucleated red cells. A PBF examination can be used to correct the error.

Indications for a Peripheral Blood Film (PBF)

Initiation of a PBF is often a clinical request by the attending clinician on account of a clinical suspicion or less frequently initiated by the laboratory. The laboratory may initiate peripheral blood film based on abnormal findings from an automated count or patients clinical information whose diagnosis may be supported by a peripheral blood film. The latter is guided by individual laboratory policies or local regulating guidelines.

Common clinical indications for peripheral blood film analysis inlude unexplained cytopenia: anaemia, leucopenia or thrombocytopenia; unexplained leukocytosis, lymphocytosis or monocytosis; unexplained jaundice or haemolysis; features of congenital haemolytic anaemias such as splenomegaly, jaundice or bone pains; suspected chronic or acute myeloproliferative disease, e.g. chronic myeloid leukaemia; suspected organ failure such as renal disease, liver failure; features of hyperviscosity syndrome.

A blood smear can be used to help diagnose or check on many conditions, such as:

- Anaemia
- Jaundice
- Sickle cell disease
- Thrombocytopenia
- Malaria
- Sudden kidney failure
- G6PD deficiency
- Certain cancers, etc.

Abnormalities of Erythrocytes

Size: With some experience it is possible to say if the red cells are of normal size (normocytosis), diminished in size (microcytosis) or increased in size (macrocytosis). One judges the size by the diameter (normal average: 7.2 microns). In severe anaemia there is variation in the size of cells; this is anisocytosis. Megalocytes are large oval cells found in megaloblastic anaemias.

Shape: Red cells with an irregular shape are called poikilocytes. The commonest irregularity is a pear-shaped cell. Poikilocytosis, like anisocytosis, is non-specific phenomenon found in all severe anaemias. In haemolytic anaemias the red cells are abnormally thick; they look like densely stained microcytes; the abnormality is known as microspherocytosis. Target cells are thin red cells with a relatively large diameter and resemble the concentric circles of a rifle target; they are seen in various anaemias, in obstructive jaundice and after splenectomy. Sickle cells may be seen in stained smears; their presence, diagnostic of sickle cells disease due to the abnormal haemoglobin S, is best demonstrated by a special *in vitro* technique. Burr cells are red cells with a spiny periphery; they are seen in large numbers in uraemia. Schistocytes are red cell fragments found in many blood diseases with increased haemolysis.

Spherocytes are round, densely staining red cells that lack central pallor and have a smaller than normal diameter. In *stomatocytes*, the area of central pallor is elliptical rather than round, giving the cell the appearance of the opening of a mouth (stoma).

Echinocytes are also cells with cytoplasmic projections, but in contrast to acanthocytes, the projections are typically evenly spaced on the cell surface, more numerous (often 10 to 15), and frequently have sharper points.

Schizocytes (schistocytes) are fragmented erythrocytes appearing in a variety of morphologic forms such as small triangular erythrocytes, helmet cells, and normal size erythrocytes with 2–3 pointed surface projections (keratocytes, or "horn cells").

Furthermore, the arrangement of the cell may generate some clinical suspicion. Rouleaux formation (stacking of the red cells like coins) in the presence of a bluish background suggests paraproteinaemia/plasma cell dyscrasia. Rouleaux are also seen in macroglobulinaemias. Agglutination of the red cells may be seen in cold haemagglutinin disease (CHAD) and Waldenström's macroglobulinaemia while erythrophagocytosis is seen in paroxysmal cold haemoglobinuria.

Erythrocyte shape abnormalities and the conditions where they are observed are shown in Table 9.4.

Table 9.4: Red cell shape abnormalities and their differentials

Red cell shapes	*Differential diagnosis*
Irreversibly sickled red cells (drepanocytes)	Sickle cell syndromes (SS, SC, S β-thalassaemia)
Target cells (codocytes, Mexican hat cells)	Sickle cell disease, haemoglobin C trait, haemoglobin CC disease, the liver disease (cholestasis), asplenia
Fragmented red cells (schistocytes, helmet cells, keratocytes)	Thrombotic micro-angiopathic haemolytic anaemias such as disseminated intrevascular coagulation (DIC), thrombotic thrombocytopenic purpura, haemolytic anaemia
Burr cells (echinocytes crenated red cells)	*In vitro* artifact following prolonged storage or slow drying of the smear due to uraemia malnutrition
Spur cells (acanthocytes)	Liver disease, renal failure, abetalipoproteinaemia, spur cell anaemia

Colour: The intensity of the red colour of the erythrocyte in a stained smear is a rough indication of corpuscular haemoglobin concentration. In a hypochromic red cell the normal central pallor is increased. Hypochromasia indicates iron deficiency.

Significant differences among erythrocytes in the amount of central pallor is referred to as *anisochromia*. *Polychromatophilia* means the erythrocytes have a blue-gray hue to the colour of their cytoplasm.

Immature Red Cells

Immature red cells in the peripheral blood can only come from the marrow. The correct significance of immature red cells in the peripheral blood can be best realised by studying their source—erythropoiesis in the marrow by means of marrow biopsy. Normal erythropoiesis is described as "normoblastic". Abnormal erythropoiesis is called "megaloblastic" and is due to the deficiency of vitamin B_{12} or folic acid, or both.

Only common findings are referred to in what follows. Polychromasia (polychromatophilia) is diffuse bluish-grey staining of the red cell. Basophil stippling is the presence of multiple coarse granules in the red cell. Cells which show polychromatophilia and basophil stippling are reticulocytes and their presence is indicative of active erythropoiesis, as in haemolytic anaemias. Pappenheimer bodies are small scanty basophilic granules in the red cell: Unlike the granules of basophilic stippling, these bodies give a positive Prussian blue reaction; they are siderophilic granules. Pappenheimer bodies are characteristically present after splenectomy. Cells with Pappenheimer bodies or siderophil granules are known as siderocytes. Cabbot's rings are reddish purple rings or like the figure of eight. Howell-Jolly bodies are reddish blue nucleated fragments. Cabbot's rings and Howell-Jolly bodies are seen in severe anaemias and after splenectomy. They have no specific significance.

The nucleated red cell commonly encountered in the peripheral blood is the normoblast. An occasional normoblast is a normal finding in the newborn. A few normoblasts—2 to 5 per 100 leucocytes—may be present in any severe anaemia. If present in large numbers, a haemolytic anaemia with an actively regenerating marrow is suspected. The presence of a megaloblast in the peripheral blood means that erythropoiesis must be megaloblastic and that the patient must be suffering from a megaloblastic anaemia. The common red cell abnormalities are summarised in Table 9.5.

Neutrophilia is commonly a response to bacterial infections especially pyogenic infections. Other associations of neutrophilia include any form of acute inflammation (such as myocardial infarction), burns, corticosteroid use (inhibits neutrophil margination), malignancy, chronic myelogenous leukaemia.

These mainly consist of the presence of immature leucocytes and granulocytes with toxic granulations. Normally an occasional metamyelocyte or juvenile (about 1%) are present. In pyogenic infections (with leucocytosis) their count goes up. A few myelocytes are common in the blood of infants and children. In adults a few myelocytes and an occasional myeloblast (without leucocytosis) may be found in severe anaemias and when the marrow is the seat of metastatic deposits of a carcinoma.

However, in chronic myeloid leukaemia, the blood shows a large number of myelocytes (10–50%) and fewer myeloblasts (2–5%). In acute myeloid leukaemia the myeloblast is the predominant cell in the blood (up to 90%).

Neoplastic lymphoid blasts when seen on blood film are also large with a size comparable to activated lymphocytes but have a high N:C ratio. Lymphoma cells are seen in leukaemic phase of non-Hodgkin's lymphomas and usually show varying sizes and various nuclear morphologies. Some have single deep nuclear cleavage (follicular cells), some have multiple indentations and clefts (mantle cells).

Causes of absolute lymphocytosis include reactive conditions like infectious mononucleosis, hepatitis, cytomegalovirus infections, pertussis, chronic intracellular bacterial infections (such as tuberculosis or brucellosis), chronic lymphocytic leukaemia, acute lymphoblastic leukaemia and leukaemic spills of lymphomas.

Eosinophils are slightly larger than polymorphs and the nucleus is usually bilobed. Their defining characteristic is the presence of orange-red granules. Lymphoplasmacytoid lymphocytes have eccentric nucleus, blue cytoplasm and some perinuclear halo.

In chronic lymphatic leukaemia the predominant cell in the blood is the small lymphocyte, forming 85–99% of leucocytes; lymphoblasts are rare. In acute lymphatic leukaemia the lymphoblast is the predominant cell. In monocytic leukaemia 50–90% of leucocytes are monocytes and their precursors (monoblasts); a few myelocytes and myeloblasts are also encountered. In infectious mononucleosis (grandular fever) 40–80% of leucocytes are ordinary lymphocytes, ordinary "abnormal cells". The last is primitive monocytes.

Morphologically, infectious mononucleosis can be confused with monocytic leukaemia; in the former the patient's serum contains agglutinins for sheep's red cells (Paul-Bunnel's test).

In severe acute infections neutrophils may show vacuolation of the cytoplasm and their granules become coarse the blue-stained. These, "toxic granules" are indicative of severe toxaemia. Heavy granulation is also seen in aplastic anaemias.

Significant eosinophilia may be seen in allergies and parasites infections. However, marked eosinophilia (>1500/ml) suggest hypereosinophilic syndrome (especially with associated tissue damage) or a neoplastic entity especially when there is an associated cellular dysplasia as in chronic eosinophilic leukaemia.

ABNORMALITIES OF PLATELETS

A significant reduction of platelets (thromobocytopenia) can be judged in the smear. In essential thrombocytopenia platelets may in addition show morphological abnormalities in the forms of small size, giant forms or non-granularity of their cytoplasm. Abnormal variation in the size of platelets is a feature of myelosclerosis.

Platelet Size

- **Increased in**
  - Bernard-Soulier syndrome
  - Grey platelet syndrome (X-storage pool deficiency)
- **Decreased in**
  - Essential thrombocytopenia
  - Wiscott-Aldrich syndrome
  - Isolated storage pool deficiency

Table 9.5: Peripheral blood smear in differential diagnosis of anaemias and other conditions	
The smear may also confirm the RBC indices or indicate leukaemia or other conditions	
I. RBC inclusions	
Basophilic or polychromatophilic macrocytes	⁎ Increased erythropoiesis in haemorrhage, or haemolysis
Microcytes with stippling	⁎ Thalassaemia, lead or heavy metal poisoning
Cabbot's ring	⁎ Occasionally in severe haemolytic anaemias and pernicious anaemia
Howell-Jolly bodies (dark purple spherical bodies)	⁎ Occasionally in severe haemolytic anaemias and pernicious anaemia ⁎ Occasionally in leukaemia, thalassaemia, postsplenectomy state
Pappenheimer bodies (siderotic granules) (purple coccoid granules at periphery)	⁎ Anaemias with defect of incorporating iron into haemoglobin (e.g. sideroblastic anaemia, thalassaemia, lead poisoning, pyridoxine—unresponsive and responsive anaemias)
Heinz-Ehrlich bodies	⁎ Congenital G6PD deficiency ⁎ Other drug-induced haemolytic anaemias ⁎ Unstable haemoglobin disorders after splenectomy
Plasmodium trophozoites	⁎ Malaria
II. Abnormally shaped RBCs	
Round	
⁎ Macrocytes	⁎ Increased erythropoiesis ⁎ Oval in megaloblastic anaemia ⁎ Round in liver disease
⁎ Microcytes, spherocytes	⁎ Hereditary spherocytosis ⁎ Immunohaemolytic anaemia
⁎ Stomatocytes	⁎ Acute alcoholism (transient) ⁎ Certain drugs (e.g. phenothiazines) ⁎ Neoplastic, cardiovascular, hepatobiliary diseases ⁎ Congenital stomatocytosis ⁎ Artifactual
⁎ Target cells	⁎ Haemoglobin C disease or trait ⁎ Thalassaemia minor ⁎ Iron deficiency anaemia ⁎ Liver disease ⁎ Postsplenectomy state ⁎ Artifactual
Elongated	
⁎ Ovalocytes (elliptocytes)	⁎ Hereditary (>25% in smear) ⁎ Microcytic anaemia (<25% in smear) ⁎ Megaloblastic anaemia
⁎ Teardrop (dacrocyte)	⁎ Spent polycythaemia ⁎ Myelofibrosis ⁎ Thalassaemia (especially homozygous beta)
⁎ Sickle cells	⁎ Sickle cell disorders (not in S trait)
⁎ Haemoglobin C crystalloids	⁎ Haemoglobin C trait or disease
Speculated	
⁎ Acanthocytes	⁎ Abetalipoproteinemia (many are present) ⁎ Postsplenectomy state (a few are present) ⁎ Fulminating liver disease (variable number)
⁎ Burr cells (echinocyte; crenated RBC)	⁎ Usually artifactual ⁎ Uremia, GI bleeding, stomach carcinoma

Contd.

Table 9.5: Peripheral blood smear in differential diagnosis of anaemias and other conditions (Contd.)	
• Schistocytes (helmet, triangle)	• Microangiopathic haemolytic anaemia (e.g. disseminated intravascular coagulation [DIC), thrombotic thrombocytopenic purpura [TTP])
• "Bite" cells	• Prosthetic heart valves or severe valvular heart disease • Severe burns • Snakebite • Haemolysis due to certain drugs with or without G6PD, deficiency
RBC fragmentation (seen on peripheral blood smear [>10/1000 RBCs] and on histogram of RBC size with automated cell counters)	• Cytotoxic chemotherapy for neoplasia • Autoimmune haemolytic anaemia • Severe iron deficiency • Megaloblastic anaemia • Acute leukaemia • Myelodysplasia • Inherited structural abnormality of RBC membrane protein spectrin

Parasites in Blood

The malarial parasite and microfilariae are the commonest in our country. The former is seen in the red cell and takes various forms, depending upon the species and the stage of development. The latter is found free in the blood and a special technique has to be followed for its demonstration. The other blood parasites are the Leishman-Donovan bodies (in kala-azar), trypanosomes (in sleeping sickness of Africa) and spirochaetes (in relapsing fever). You will be learning about these parasites in detail in parasitology chapter.

Chapter 10

Leukaemias, Myelodysplastic Syndromes, and Myeloproliferative Disorders

Chapter Outline

LEUKAEMIAS

Leukaemoid reaction is a morbid condition characterised by widespread hyperplasia of leucopoietic tissue, either myeloid or lymphatic, which is usually associated with qualitative and quantitative changes in the white cells of the circulating blood.

Leukaemias are classified as (Fig. 10.1):

1. Myeloid leukaemia (acute and chronic)
2. Lymphatic leukaemia (acute and chronic)

Acute Leukaemias

Two main forms of acute leukaemias are recognised: Myeloid (AML), more frequent in adults (more than 20 years), and lymphoblastic (ALL), predominantly in children (<15 years).

A typical laeukemias:

a. Aleukaemic leukaemia
b. Chloroma
c. Plasma cells leukaemia
d. Eosinophilic, basophilic, mast cell leukaemias
e. Megakaryocytic leukaemia, etc.

Acute Myeloid Leukaemia

Acute myeloid leukaemias are heterogeneous group of neoplastic disorders of haemopoietic stem cells. Since these stem cells can give rise to granulocytes, monocytes, erythrocytes and megakaryocytes, any of these lineage of cells may be affected.

Incidence: 20% of all the leukaemias are AML.

- **Age:** Mainly in adults between 15 and 39 years. It is 85% of all leukaemias in adults.
- **Children:** 20% of all childhood leukaemias
- **Sex:** Higher in males compared to females

Aetiology

- **Genetic disorders:** Certain genetic disorders are associated with an increased incidence of AML, such as:
  1. Chromosomal aneuploidy (total number of chromosomes not exact multiple of haploid).
     - Down syndrome (trisomy 21)
     - Klinefelter's syndrome (XXY)
     - Patau syndrome (trisomy 13)
  2. Increased chromosomal fragility
     - Fanconi anaemia
     - Ataxia telangiectasia
     - Bloom syndrome

Radiation: There was increased incidence of AML in survivors of atomic bomb explosion in Japan. In fact, when radiation exposure exceeds 100 rad, a linear relationship between ionising radiation dose and the development of AML can be seen.

Myelotoxic chemicals: Numerous chemicals are associated with an increased incidence of AML. These are:

1. Benzene: Used as solvent in plastic, rubber and pharmaceutical industries
2. Smoking
3. Exposure to petroleum products
4. Paint
5. Ethylene oxide
6. Herbicides
7. Pesticides

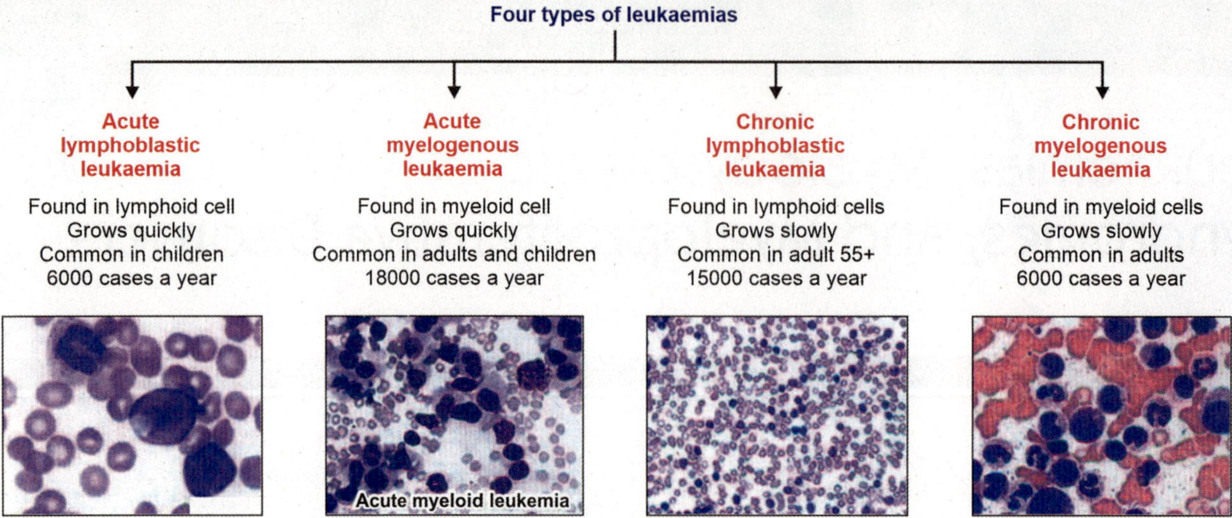

Fig. 10.1: Four types of leukaemias

Drugs: Antineoplastic drugs like alkylating agents used for the treatment of different malignancy can cause secondary cancer 4–6 years after the drug therapy.

Some drugs cause bone marrow failure which evolve into AML. Some of these important drugs are:
- Chloramphenicol
- Phenylbutazone
- Chloroquine

Chronic clonal haematological diseases: Many chronic clonal haematological diseases have an increased risk of AML, such as:
- Aplastic anaemia
- Myeloproliferative disorders
- Myelodysplastic syndromes
- Paroxysmal-nocturnal haemoglobinuria

Classification: AML has been classified according to the criteria proposed by the French, American and British (FAB) groups. Thus, it is known as FAB classification (Fig. 10.2).

A blood film of acute leukaemia (AML) is given in Fig. 10.3.

Recently, the World Health Organization has proposed a classification which takes into account molecular, cytogenetic, morphologic and clinical features (Table 10.1). This classification has given a lot of importance to cytogenetic and molecular features as these are becoming an important guidelines to choose therapeutic modalities. It subclassifies AML based on recurrent chromosomal rearrangements, therapy-related changes or changes due to myelodysplastic syndrome.

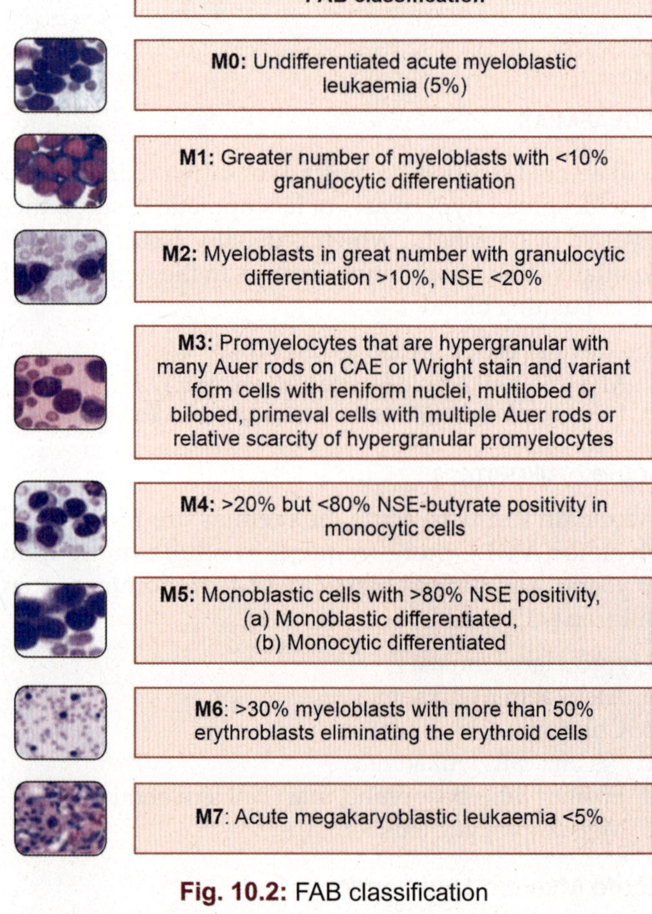

Fig. 10.2: FAB classification

Molecular Changes in AML

Most of the molecular changes are linked to cytogenetic abnormalities. These molecular changes involve numerous chromosomes. Thus, WHO proposed a new classification of AML where they have taken into consideration the molecular and cytogenetic changes. Chromosome 17 has retinoic acid receptor-α (RARA) gene which gets translocated near the promyelocytic leukaemia (PML) gene in chromosome 15. This leads to the formation of various fusion proteins. The PML-RARA fusion protein tends to suppress gene transcription and blocks differentiation of the myeloid cells.

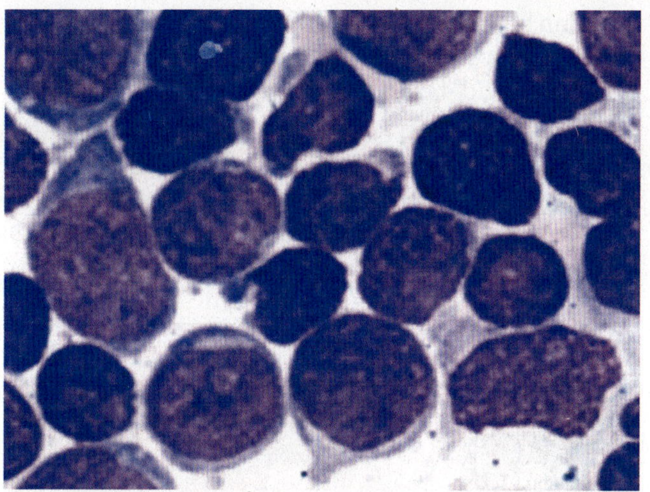

Fig. 10.3: Microphotograph: Blood film of acute myeloid leukaemia (AML)

Complex core-binding factor (CBF) is a transcription factor complex. It is involved in the expression of a number of genes in myeloid cells, which are myeloid cell differentiation dependent. The complex core-binding factor has two subunits, a core-binding factor α (CBFA) and a core-binding factor β (CBFB). The inv(16) in acute myelomonocytic leukaemia (M4EO) causes fusion of CBFB gene with myosin heavy chain gene. This results in blockage of its transcription action. Similarly, in t(8;21) in AML with maturation (M_2) the CBFA gene on chromosome 21 fuses with the ETO gene, which gets translocated from chromosome 8.

The CBFA/ETO protein blocks transcription of the genes which are controlled by CBFA–CBFB genes.

Monocytic leukaemias often show 11q23 rearrangement. This region has myeloid-lymphoid or mixed-lineage leukaemia gene (MLL gene).

Table 10.1: World Health Organization classification

I. AML with recurrent cytogenetic translocations	
* AML with t(8; 21) (q22; q22); AML 1 (CBFA)/ETO 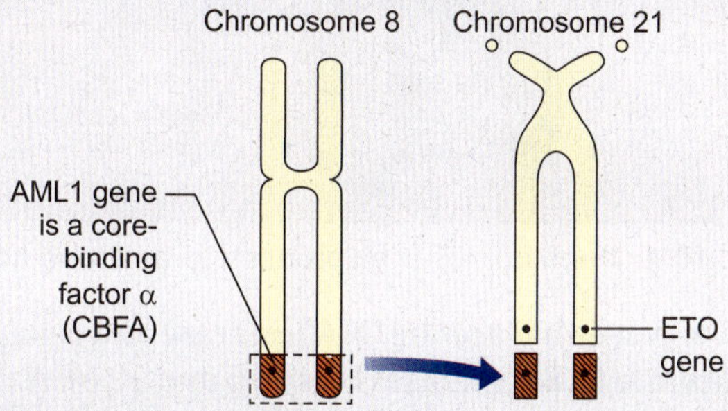 Chromosome 8 · Chromosome 21 AML1 gene is a core-binding factor α (CBFA) ETO gene	II. AML with multilineage dysplasia * With prior myelodysplastic syndrome * Without prior myelodysplastic syndrome III. AML and myelodysplastic syndrome, therapy related * Alkylating agent-related * Epipodophyllotoxin-related * Others
* Acute promyelocytic leukaemia—AML with t(15;17) (q22; q12) and variants; PML/RARA 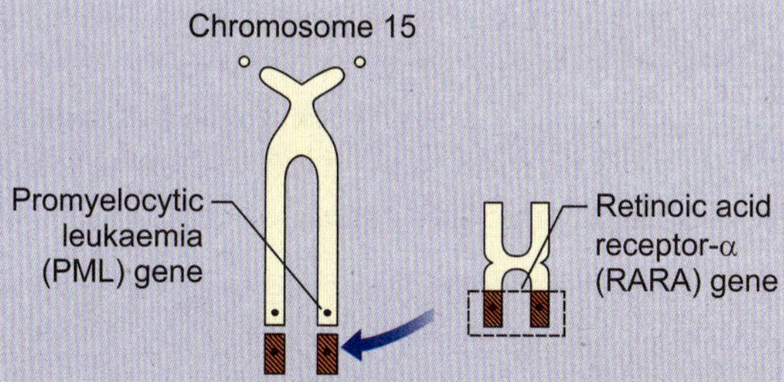 Chromosome 15 Promyelocytic leukaemia (PML) gene Retinoic acid receptor-α (RARA) gene	IV. AML not otherwise categorised * AML minimally differentiated * AML without maturation * AML with maturation * Acute myelomonocytic leukaemia * Acute monocytic leukaemia * Acute erythroid leukaemia * Acute megakaryocytic leukaemia * Acute basophilic leukaemia * Acute panmyelosis with myelofibrosis
* AML with abnormal bone marrow eosinophils → inv(16) (p1.3q22) or t(16;16) (p13;q22) CBFB/MYH1 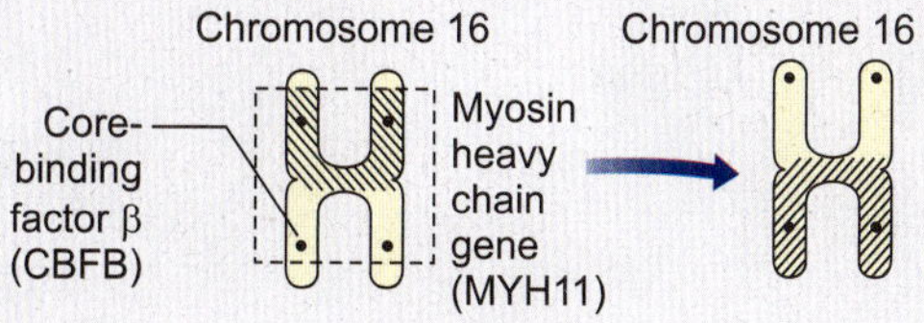 Chromosome 16 · Chromosome 16 Core-binding factor β (CBFB) Myosin heavy chain gene (MYH11)	
* AML with 11q23 (myeloid-lymphoid or mixed-lineage leukaemia gene) abnormalities	

Chromosomal Changes in AML

AML shows numerous chromosomal changes. They provide important prognostic indicators (Table 10.2).

Table 10.2: Chromosomal changes and prognosis

Cytogenetic change	*FAB class*	*Prognosis*	
t(q;22) (q34;q11) is Ph chromosome	M_1	Poor	
t(8;21) (q22;q22) t(15;17) (q22;q21)	M_2 M_3	Favourable Intermediate DIC	Young age
Inversion (16)(P13;q22) del(16) (q22)	$M_4 E_0$	Favourable	
t(9;11) (p22;q23) 11q-	M_5	Poor	
del(5q) del(7q)	Varies	Poor Commonly seen in secondary leukaemia	Older age

CYTOCHEMISTRY OF AML

Certain cytochemical reactions are essential in distinguishing AML from undifferentiated forms of ALL (e.g. L_2). This is particularly so in cases where the cells are immature, e.g. in M_1 (myeloblastic leukaemia poorly differentiated). The peroxidase, Sudan black B and chloroacetate esterase reactions reveal granulocytic differentiation in M_1, M_2, M_3 and M_4 types of AML. Whilst the nonspecific esterases nephthol acetate (NASDA) and alphanephthol acetate esterase (ANAE) ± sodium fluoride (NaF) and the acid phosphatase and lysozyme reactions, demonstrate monocytic differentiation. Nonspecific esterase reactions are usually weak or negative in M_3. In erythroleukaemia (M_6) the PAS (periodic acid–Schiff) reaction may be strongly positive.

Cytochemical reactions are usually done to detect the deficiency of enzyme contents of mature neutrophils in AML, particularly in M_2 and M_6. The NAP scores are usually normal and high in ALL and M_5.

In acute megakaryoblastic leukaemia, the blast cells appear undifferentiated, and may resemble lymphoblasts. The cytochemical profile of these cells is similar to that of megakaryocytes, i.e. positive reactions with PAS, acid phosphatase and ANAE (NaF-sensitive as in monocyte). The cytochemical classification of some leukaemias is possible by use of 7 different tests.

1. Naphthol AS-D chloroacetate (NASDCA) esterase activity.
2. Alpha-naphthyl acetate (NA) esterase.
3. Alpha-naphthyl butyrate (NB) esterase activity.
4. Myeloperoxidase (MP) activity.
5. Sudan black B (SBB) reaction.
6. Acid phosphatase (AP) activity.
7. Periodic acid–Schiff (PAS) stain.

The cytochemical classification of some leukaemias is possible by use of 7 different tests (Figs 10.4 to 10.10).

A. **Naphthol AS-D chloroacetate** (NASDCA) **esterase** (Fig. 10.4) activity is exhibited by cells of granulocytic lineage. NASDCA activity appears at differentiated myeloblast/progranulocytic stage of cellular development.

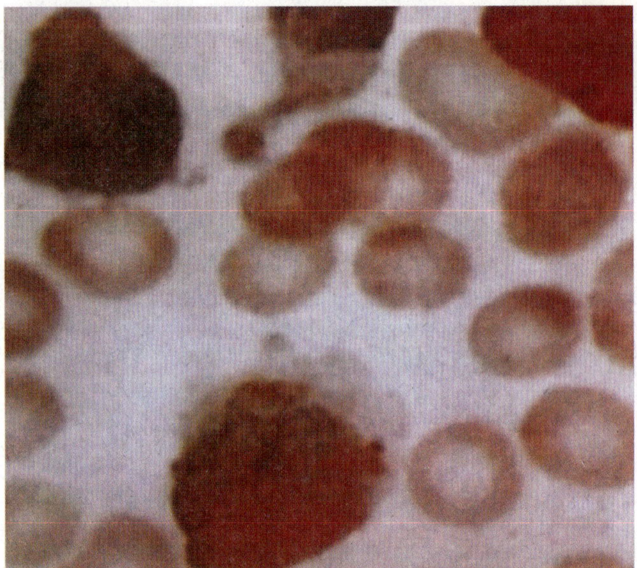

Fig. 10.4: Naphthol AS-D chloroacetate-esterase activity

B & C. **α-Naphthyl acetate (NA) esterase and α-naphthyl butyrate (NB) esterase** (Figs 10.5 and 10.6). Activities are used to recognize cells of monocytic origin. At pH 7.6 NA is seen almost exclusively in monocytes and histiocytes, with occasional granules in polymorphonuclear leukocytes and lymphocytes. At this pH, megakaryocytes and erythroblasts exhibit intense NA activity. Sodium fluoride inhibits monocytes enzymes and is used to distinguish monocyte activity from other esterase activity.

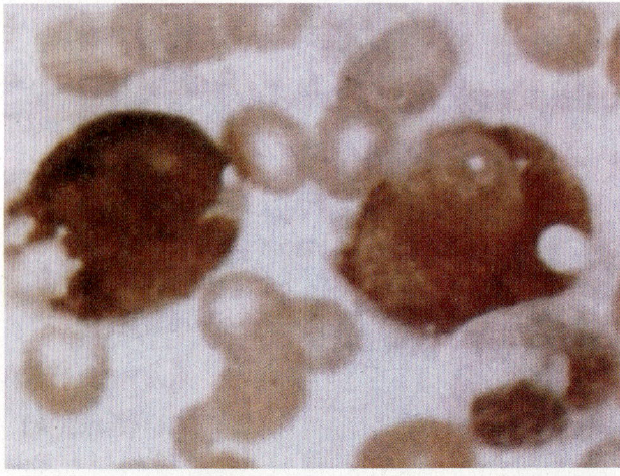

Fig. 10.5: α-Naphthyl acetate (NA) esterase activity

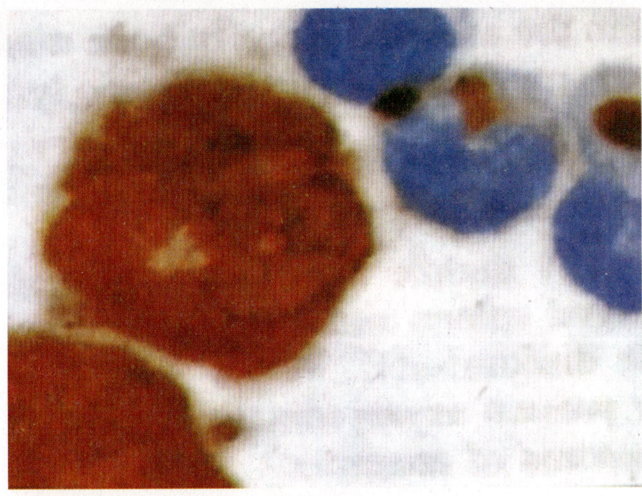

Fig. 10.6: α-Nephthyl butyrate (NB) esterase activity

D. **Myeloperoxidase** (MP) (Fig. 10.7) is normally confined to primary granules of myeloid and monocytoid cells.

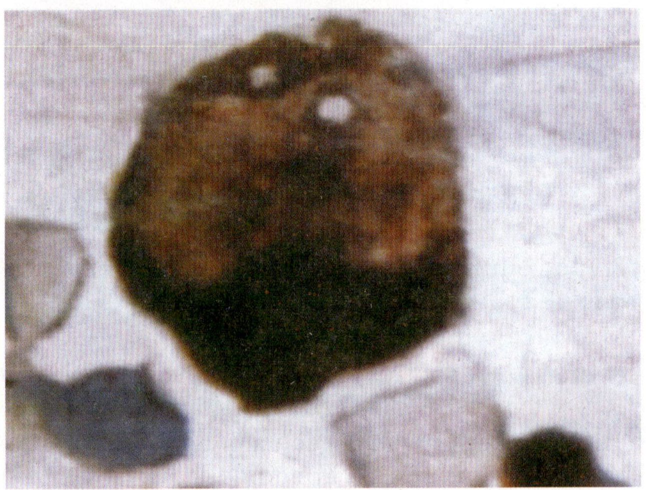

Fig. 10.7: Myeloperoxidase (MP) activity

However, primitive blasts committed to myeloid path exhibit MP activity in the endoplasmic reticulum, paranuclear area and Golgi apparatus.

E. **Sudan black B** (SBB) (Fig. 10.8) reacts with lipid deposits in cells, paralleling the MP pattern of cellular distribution. The parallelism is not invariant since SB-positive blasts sometimes exceed those exhibiting MP. SBB-positive and MP-negative blasts have been reported.

F. **Acid phosphatase** (AP) (Fig. 10.9) is useful for differentiating sub-groups of acute lymphoblastic leukaemia and delineating hairy cell leukaemia from other chronic lymphoid neoplasias.

G. **Periodic acid–Schiff (PAS)** (Fig. 10.10) stains glycogen and other 1,2-glycol-containing carbohydrates. The earliest myeloid precursors are not PAS reactive, but staining increases with maturation along myeloid pathways. Normal erythroid precursors are negative while megakaryoblasts, megakaryocytes and platelets

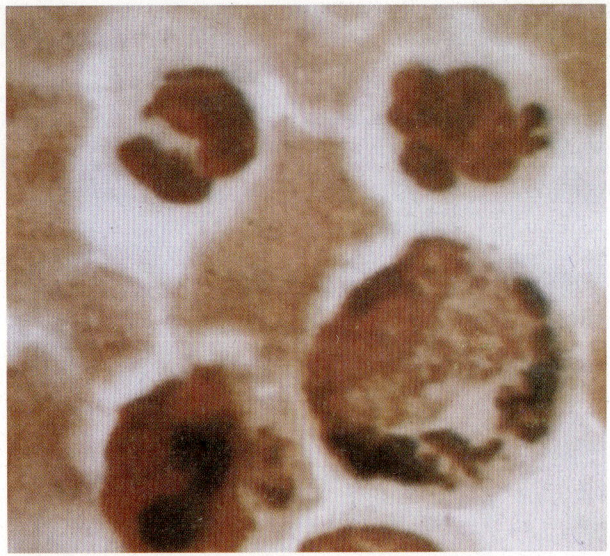

Fig. 10.8: Sudan black (B) reacts with lipid deposits

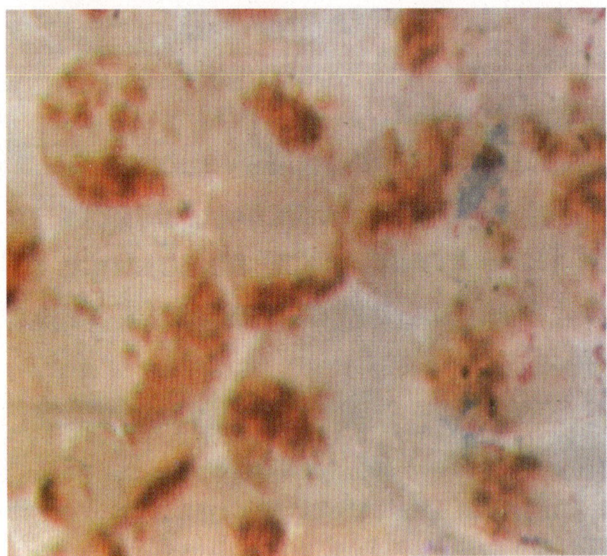

Fig. 10.9: Acid phosphatase (AP) reaction

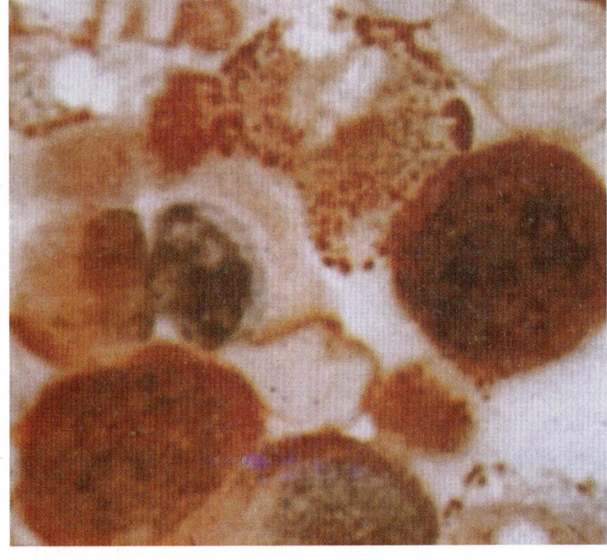

Fig. 10.10: Periodic acid-Schiff (PAS) stain: Positive

Table 10.3: Cytochemical reactions in normal blood cells and blast cells of acute leukaemia

	Peroxidase Sudan black B	*α-Naphthyl acetate*	*α-Naphthyl butyrate*	*Naphthol ASD chloroacetate*	*PAS*	*Acid phosphatase*
Promyelocyte	+/+ +	–/±	–	+/+ +	±/+	+/+ +
Neutrophil	+ +	–/±	–	+/+ +	+ + +	+
Monocyte	–/±	+ + +	+ +/+ + +	–/±	±	+ +
Lymphocyte	–/±	–/±	–/±	–	–/±	–/+ +
Erythroblast	–	–±	–	–	–	±/–
Megakaryocyte	–	+ + +	±	–	+ +	+ +
ALL	–	–/+	–	–	+/+ +	–/+
AML (M_1)	+	–	–	+	+	–
AML (M_2)	+ +	–/±	–/±	+ +	+	+
APL (M_3)	+ + +	–/± +	–	+ + +	±/+ +	+ +
AMML (M_4)	+ +	+ +/+ + +	+	+ +	–/+ +	+ +
AMoL (M_5)	–/±	+ + +	+ + +	–/±	+ +	–
EL (M_6)	–	+ +	+	–	+ +	–
MegL (M_7)	–	+	–/±	–	+ +	+
AUL	–	–	–	–	–	–

– = negative; ± = weak or a few positive cells; + = moderate; ++ = moderately strong; +++ strongly positive (most cells)

stain intensely. Diffuse or granular PAS patterns are exhibited by monocytes.

The characteristics and interpretations are shown in Table 10.3.

Changes in other organs (AML)

- Spleen shows prominent myeloid metaplasia
- Liver shows foci of myeloid metaplasia in the sinusoids.
- Lymph node: Myeloid metaplasia may initially involve the sinuses and the paracortex but later obliterates the nodal architecture.
- Bone:
  - Expansion of medullary space
  - Infiltration of periosteum
- Joint: Infiltration of synovium
- Orbit: In rare situation leukemic cells can form discrete tumour masses in soft tissue adjacent to the orbit. This can infiltrate the orbit and cause proptosis. These tumour masses are called chloroma (meaning green colour which is due to myeloperoxidase).

Clinical presentation

- Fatigue
- Malaise
- Bleeding (because of thrombocytopenia)
- DIC (AML M_3 because of release of procoagulant factor)
- Gum hypertrophy (leukaemia infiltration → M_4, M_5)
- Bone pain
- Hepatosplenomegaly

Bone Marrow (AML) (Table 10.4)

- Hypercellular: Marked increase in myeloid cell (Fig. 10.11)
- Myeloid: Erythroid ratio 10 : 1 to 50 : 1
- Myeloblasts and promyelocytes together form less than 10% of the total nucleated cell population.
- The blast percentage is generally normal or slightly raised but less than 10% in chronic phase.
- Basophilia +
- Eosinophilia +
- Monocytosis +
- Megakaryocytes are numerous with features of dysmegakaryopoiesis. Marrow fibrosis may be present.

Table 10.4: Normal adult and AML bone marrow

Normal adult bone marrow	*AML bone marrow*
Fat : cell = 1: 1	Fat spaces markedly ↓ and replace by cells, mainly blasts
Myeloid : erythroid = 2–7 : 1	Myeloid : erythroid ratio is severely altered due to proliferation of myeloid cell
Granulocytic series 40–60% of surface area	Normal granulocytic precursors markedly ↓
Lymphocytes <20%	Lymphocyte N/↓
Fibrosis — nil	Myelofibrosis may be present
Megakaryocyte 2–5/high power	Megakaryocyte ↓
Erythroid cells 10–20% of surface area	Erythroid cells ↓

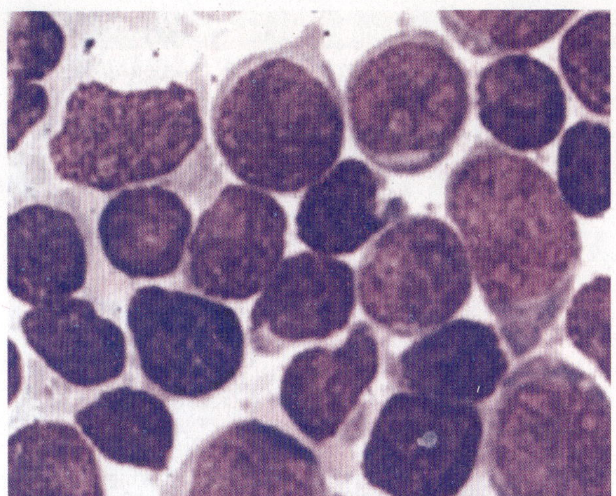

Fig. 10.11: Bone marrow micrograph (AML)

ACUTE LYMPHOCYTIC LEUKAEMIA (ALL)

Three morphological types have been described by the FAB group: L_1, L_2 and L_3. The differences in age incidence (L_1 is more common in children and L_2 is more frequent in adults), the strong correlation of L_3 with B-ALL (with monoclonal membrane immunoglobulins) and the difference in prognosis between L_1 and L_2 (worse in L_2) within similar age groups together suggest that the three morphological types may reflect true biological differences. L_1 lymphoblasts tend to be small and have scanty cytoplasm; the nucleo-cytoplasmic (N:C) ratio is high in the majority and they have a small and not easily visible nucleolus; the nuclear membrane is often regular. L_2 lymphoblasts, in contrast to L_1 are larger, have more abundant cytoplasm (low N:C ratio) and have one or more prominent nucleoli; the nuclear outline is irregular in over 25% of cells. The differences between L_1 and L_2 can be more easliy resolved in borderline cases by the simple scoring system proposed by the FAB group. L_3 (or Burkitt type) cells, because of their resemblance to cells of the endemic African lymphoma, are uniformly large, have finely stippled nuclear chromatin and, characteristically, a deep basophilic cytoplasm often associated with prominent vacuolation.

Three cytochemical tests are useful in the study of ALL; the PAS, acid phosphatase and ANAE reactions. They do not correlate with the L_1, L_2 or L_3 morphological types but they do show a relationship to the imunological subtypes of ALL (Table 10.5).

In cases in which the cells are undifferentiated (usually L_2 blast cells in adult patients), it is important to exclude AML (usually M_1 and M_{5a}). For this, the peroxidase, Sudan black B and NASDA reactions should be shown to be negative. ANAE can show in ALL a granular reaction, but this is not the strong diffuse pattern (NaF-sensitive) seen in M_5. The PAS reaction is often positive in ALL—at least, in a proportion of blasts, as shown by coarse granules or blocks of positively-reacting material (usually glycogen).

Table 10.5: Cytochemistry and the immunological classification of ALL

Method	*Common ALL*	*Null ALL*	*T-ALL*	*B-ALL*
Morphology	L_1–L_2	L_1–L_2	L_1–L_2	L_3
PAS	+ or + + coarse granules	– or + +	– or +	–
Acid phosphate	– or +	– or + +	+ + or + + +	–
ANAE	–	– or +	+ or + +	–
Peroxidase Sudan black B Lysozyme }	–	–	–	–

This pattern of reaction, particularly with a negative background, is rarely seen in AML; it is more typical of the common form of childhood ALL which can be defined by immunological tests for the ALL antigen described as non-B, non-T ALL (negative B and T markers) or common ALL.

In T-ALL (positive T cell markers), the PAS reaction is negative in two-thirds of cases; in B-ALL it is negative in the majority. The differences shown by the PAS reaction probably reflect the different proliferation kinetics of the immunologically-defined subtypes of ALL. For example, in B-ALL (PAS-negative) a greater number of cells are in cycle; this is also reflected in the numerous mitotic figures seen in bone marrow with L_3 morphology. The acid phosphatase test gives a consistently localized positive reaction in T-ALL and pre-T-ALL blast cells.

Immunophenotypic markers are useful for diagnosis and classification. However, there are morphological features which can to some extent distinguish myeloblast from lymphoblast (Tables 10.6 and 10.7).

Table 10.6: Immunologic subtyping of ALL

Subtype	*Frequency of cases*	*FAB classification*	*Cytogenetic changes*	*Prognosis*
Early pre-B	60%	L1 and L2	–	Very good
Pre-B	20%	L1 and L2	t(9;22), t(4;11), t(1;19)	Intermediate
B cell	5%	L3	t(8;14), t(8:22), t(2; 8)	Poor
T cell	15%	L1 and L2	14q11 or 7q34	Intermediate

Table 10.7: Differences between ALL and AML

Morphology	ALL	AML
Folded nucleus		+
Clefted nucleus	+	
Nucleoli	1 (except L2 and L3)	2–5
Auer rods	–	+
Cytochemistry		
Myeloperoxidase	–	+
Sudan black B	–	+
Periodic acid–Schiff (PAS)	+ (block positivity)	–
Nonspecific esterases	–	+ (M_4 and M_5)
Immunologic markers		
Common ALL antigen	+	–
Terminal deoxynucleotidyl transferase (TdT)	+	–

Table 10.8: Prognostic indicators of ALL

Prognostic indicators	*Favourable prognosis*	*Unfavourable prognosis*
FAB classification	L1	L2 and L3
Immunological type	Pre-B type	B cell and T cell types
t(4:11)	–	+
t(9;22)	–	+
Hyperdiploidy	+	–
Pseudoploidy	–	+
Age	2–10 years	<1 year and >10 years
TLC	<10,000/µl	<50,000/µl
CNS	–	Involved +
Lymphadenopathy	–	+
Mediastinal mass	–	+

Differences between ALL and AML are shown in Table 10.7 and Fig. 10.12A and B and prognostic indicators of ALL in Table 10.8.

The prognostic indicators of ALL are shown in Table 10.8.

CHRONIC LEUKAEMIAS

Definition: Primary malignancies of haemopoietic cells in which the clinical course is measured in months and years in contrast to the acute leukaemias.

Many of the malignant cells are differentiated and these relatively mature cells appear in large numbers in the peripheral blood, giving rise to leucocytosis which may be very marked.

Classification

I. **Myeloid origin**
  1. Chronic granulocytic (synonymous myeloid)—CGL or CML.
  2. Chronic myelomonocytic (CMML).
  3. Chronic erythroleukaemia (Di Guglielmo syndrome).

II. **Lymphoid origin**
  1. Chronic lymphocytic (B cell or T cell).
  2. Prolymphocytic (B cell or T cell).
  3. Hairy cell (leukaemic reticuloendotheliosis).

Chronic Myeloid Leukaemia (CML)

Chronic myeloid leukaemia is a neoplastic disorder of haematopoietic stem cell possessing a reciprocal translocation between chromosomes 9 and 22 → Philadelphia chromosome (Ph) (Fig. 10.13).

- **Incidence:** CML constitutes 20% of all leukaemias
- **Age:** Incidence of CML rises slowly with age. It becomes common in middle and elderly age group. However, the most common age group is 40–50 years.
- **Sex:** Higher in men than in women.

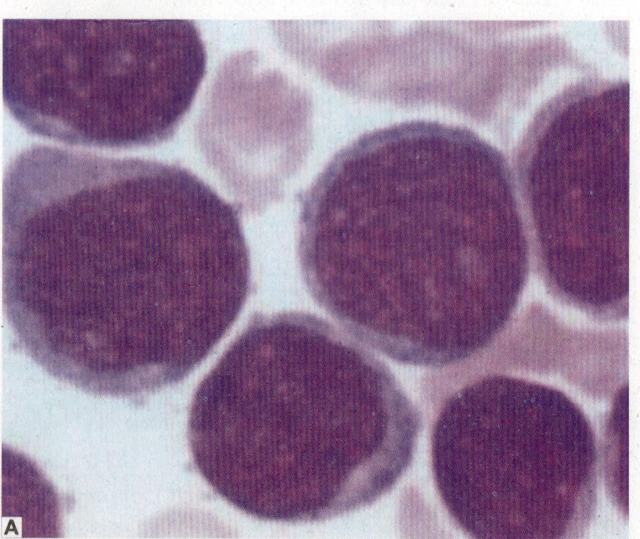

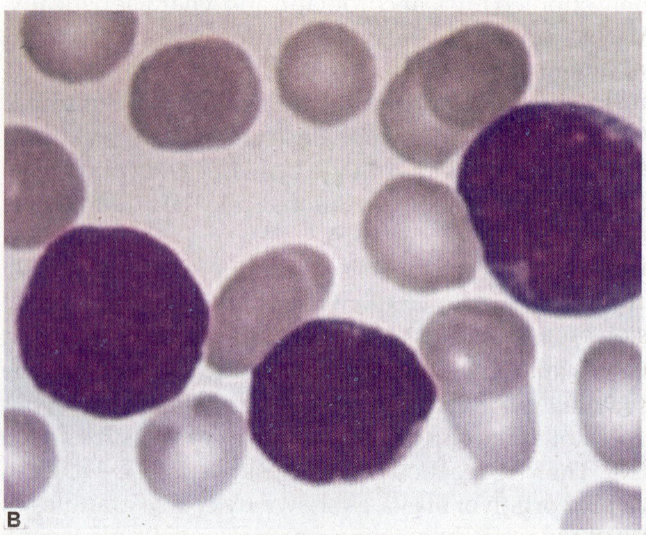

Fig. 10.12A and B: Microphotograph: (A) ALL and (B) AML

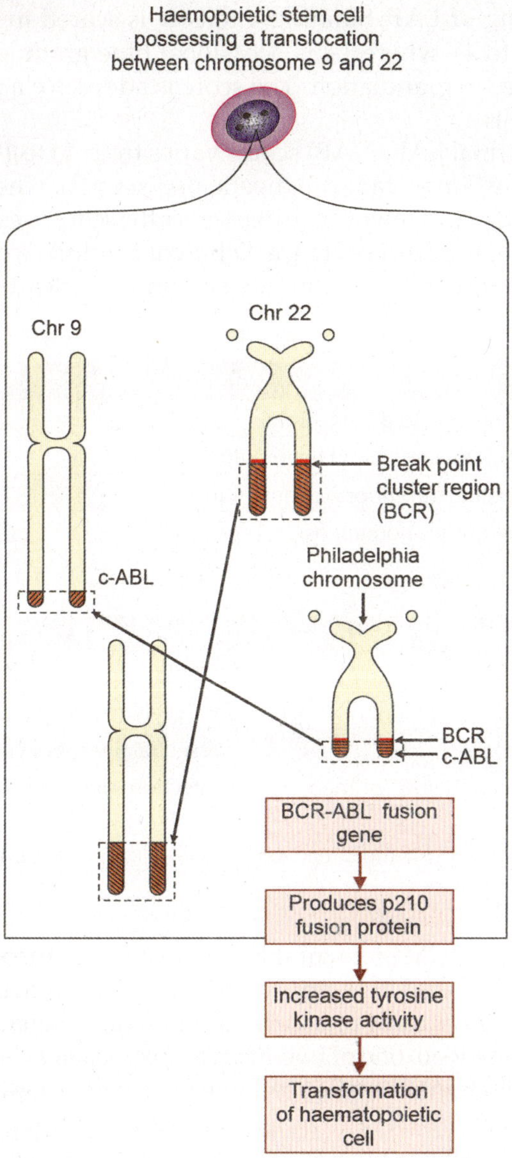

Haemopoietic stem cell possessing a translocation between chromosome 9 and 22

Chr 9

Chr 22

Break point cluster region (BCR)

c-ABL

Philadelphia chromosome

BCR

c-ABL

BCR-ABL fusion gene

Produces p210 fusion protein

Increased tyrosine kinase activity

Transformation of haematopoietic cell

Fig. 10.13: Philadelphia chromosome. Role of t(9; 22) in the genesis of CML

CML is thought to arise from malignant transformation of a haematopoietic stem cell which has chromosome 9;22 translocation. This plays a central role in the development of CML. As a result of this translocation, the protooncogene c-ABL (named after the Abelson murine leukaemia virus) located on chromosome 9 is translocated adjacent to break point cluster region (BCR) gene on chromosome 22. The translocated chromosome 22 is called Philadelphia (Ph) chromosome. The fusion of these two genes produces a fusion protein known as p210. This has enhanced tyrosine kinase activity. This can transform haematopoietic progenitor cells to leukaemic cells.

Aetiopathogenesis

Exact aetiology of CML is not known. However, large dose of radiation can cause CML. Such increase in CML incidence was found in survivors of atomic bomb in Japan and also in patients who were treated with spinal irradiation for ankylosing spondylitis.

Benzene is also known to cause CML.

Clinical presentation

1. Typically middle age, but seen in all age groups.
2. Enlarged spleen and liver (splenomegaly may be massive and cause discomfort).
3. May present asymptomatically on routine blood count.
4. Symptoms of anaemia.
5. Abnormal bleeding.
6. Weight loss, anorexia, sweats, fever, 2° amenorrhoea.
7. Hyperviscosity syndrome from leucostasis.
8. Gout.
9. *De novo* 'blast transformation' clinically indistinguishable from acute leukaemia.

Severe infection is rare in untreated CGL (unlike all other types of leukaemia) as the relatively mature myeloid cells seen in the blood have some bacteriocidal capabilities.

Clinical signs

1. Splenomegaly; may vary from just palpable to masive and may have audible rub or bruit.
2. Hepatomegaly.
3. Pallor, emaciation (if advanced).
4. Bruising (seldom petechial, except in blast transformation).
5. Fever (low grade, even in absence of infection).
6. Fundal haemorrhages, tortuous veins, papilloedema (leucostasis).
7. Bone tenderness, especially sternum.
8. Lymphadenopathy (rare).
9. Skin infiltration (uncommon).

Investigations

Blood count

1. Leucocytosis may be very marked, often well over 100 $\times 10^9$/L. Degree of leucocytosis tends to correlate with size of spleen and degree of anaemia.
2. Differential leucocyte count; whole spectrum from neutrophils (around 50%) to blast (usually >5%). Myelocytes common. Eosinophils and basophils increased.

   Nucleated RBCs often seen.
3. Anaemia: Normochromic, normocytic, may be mild or severe.
4. Thrombocytosis sometimes $>1000 \times 10^9$/L. Platelets occasionally low—may herald blast transformation.

The diagnosis is often obvious from the clinical signs and the blood count alone, in classical CGL.

Bone marrow

1. Grossly hypercellular (Fig. 10.14).
2. May be difficult to aspirate.
3. Gross granulocytic hyperplasia with all degrees of differentiation seen, and increased megakaryocytes.

4. Examination for Ph[1] and other chromosome anomalies.
5. Marrow trephine to assess fibrosis, may also show pockets of blasts not detected on aspirate, in early transformation.

☞ **Note:** If Ph[1] chromosome detected in peripheral blood cells, it may not always be necessary to perform a bone marrow.

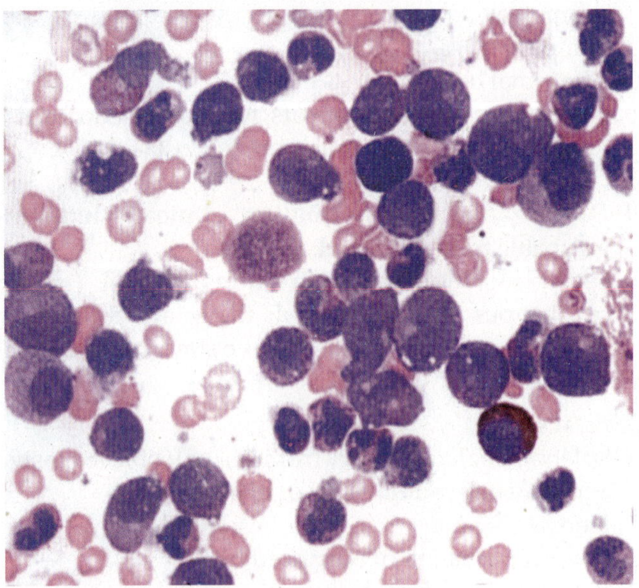

Fig. 10.14: Chronic myeloid leukaemia (CML)

Additional investigations (once diagnosis made or suspected):

1. Urate—often very high.
2. NAP score—neutrophil alkaline phosphatase zero or very low in untreated CML, in contrast to other causes of leucocytosis. Tends to rise after control of WBC, or before blast transformation.
3. Liver function—deranged enzymes and mildly raised bilirubin common.
4. Renal function—as baseline.
5. Serum vitamin B_{12} level and binding proteins if available. (Transcobalamin secreted by leucocytes is raised in CML and other myeloproliferative diseases, giving rise to high serum vitamin B_{12} level.)

LAP (NAP) SCORE

Leucocyte alkaline phosphatase (LAP) or neutrophil alkaline phosphatase (NAP) enzyme is present in the cytoplasm of mature neutrophils and also to some level in metamyelocytes. LAP activity first appears in myelocytes and then rapidly increases with the maturation of the cell to the neutrophil.

Method: Naphthol AS phosphate is used as substrate for the leucocyte alkaline phosphatase enzyme. The enzyme liberates naphthol. Naphthol combines with the azo-dye (fast blue BB) to give blue colour, which appears in the cytoplasm as granules.

Scoring of LAP: Staining intensity is scored in a scale of 1+ to 4+ where 1+ is occasional blue granule and 4 + is heavy granulation. The score is added for a total of 100 cells.

Normal LAP (NAP) scores varies from 40 to 100. It is the most important diagnostic use in CML, where it is around zero. However, in blast crisis the score rises giving it a prognostic importance. Different conditions causing low and high LAP score are shown in Tables 10.9 and 10.10.

Table 10.9: Causes of low LAP (NAP) score
Chronic myeloid leukaemia
Paroxysmal nocturnal haemoglobinuria
Idiopathic thrombocytopenic purpura
Infectious mononucleosis
Sarcoidosis

Table 10.10: Causes of high LAP (NAP) score	
Newborn	Myelofibrosis
Children	Polycythaemia vera
Pregnancy	Essential thrombocythaemia
Premenopausal women	Infection—leukaemoid reaction
Infection leukaemoid reaction	

Disease Progression

At present, CML is incurable by conventional techniques. Median survival is approximately three years. After the initial chronic phase disease in which the patient is clinically well, one of two main terminal states develop:

1. **Blast transformation:** A more malignant clone appears which gives rise to progeny which are primitive blast cells. The result is a slow or abrupt transformation to an acute leukaemia of particularly resistant type, with appearance of increased number of blasts in marrow and peripheral blood.

   Blasts often have additional chromosome anomalies as well as Ph[1]. May be of any phenotype, i.e. AML, ALL, undifferentiated or megakaryoblastic. Some CML patients present for first time in this phase.

   Treatment is that of acute leukaemia. Remission rates and duration less than straightforward. ALL and patients who respond revert back to chronic phase disease. Grafting with autologous buffy coat cells (obtained at diagnosis by leucapheresis and cryopreserved), after intensive chemotherapy or radiotherapy, has been used, but long-term results poor.
2. **Bone marrow failure:** Some patients do not enter a discernible blast crisis but develop insidious marrow failure with progressive anaemia, thrombocytopenia and splenomegaly. Marrow often very fibrotic. May be natural disease process or related to chemotherapy, particularly busulphan. Patients often emaciated and hypercatabolic. Treatment is supportive only.

Juvenile Chronic Myeloid Leukaemia

Adult-type CGL does occur occasionally in childhood, usually in older age group. Juvenile chronic myeloid leukaemia is a distinct rare disease.

Clinical features

1. Age <2 years.
2. Mild splenomegaly.
3. Lymphadenopathy.
4. Facial rash.

Laboratory features

1. Thrombocytopenia.
2. Increased monocytes and blasts in blood and marrow.
3. Many nucleated RBC.
4. High HbF level.
5. Absence of Ph^1 chromosome.

Chronic Myelomonocytic Leukaemia

It may be classified either as a type of myelogenous leukaemia or as a myelodysplastic syndrome.

Clinical and laboratory features

1. Elderly patient.
2. Chronic course often over several years.
3. Leucocytosis with absolute increase in monocytes and some abnormal forms in blood and bone marrow.
4. Splenomegaly.
5. Anaemia and thrombocytopenia.

FAB: Classification of CML is shown in Table 10.11.

Treatment

1. Treatment is generally supportive, and many patients do relatively well.
2. Gentle chemotherapy, e.g. 6-mercaptopurine or hydroxyurea may be useful in controlling very high WBC count and splenomegaly, and may improve anaemia and thrombocytopenia.

Chronic Erythroleukaemia

(Synonyms of Di Guglielmo's syndrome is chronic erythraemic myelosis)

A chronic variation of which the acute counterpart is M6-AML.

Clinical features: Chronic form usually presents with anaemia and runs a course over months and years. Splenomegaly may be present.

Laboratory features

1. Anaemia.
2. Increased reticulocytes.
3. Numerous nucleated RBC in blood.
4. Gross erythroid hyperplasia in marrow.
5. PAS + ve erythroblasts in marrow.
6. Variable dysmyelopoiesis.
7. May terminate as AML.

CHRONIC LYMPHOID LEUKAEMIAS

These can be classified:

1. Clinically.
2. Morphologically.
3. Immunologically.

Generally the malignant clone has a normal counterpart in lymphocyte development, but the cells have aberrant features and are functionally defective.

B Cell Chronic Lymphocytic Leukaemia (B-CLL)

Commonest form of leukaemia in United Kingdom. Affects mainly elderly—very rare below thirty. Often detected on routine blood count as an absolute lymphocytosis. CLL is the most common cause of persistent lymphocytosis in a middle-aged or elderly patient.

Clinical features (B-CLL)

1. Often asymptomatic with no abnormal physical signs.
2. Lymphadenopathy—all areas, soft, may be very extensive.
3. Hepatosplenomegaly.
4. Weight loss, night sweats, fatigue, recurrent infections.

Laboratory features

1. Absolute lymphocytosis $>15 \times 10^9$/L. WBC may be very high $500–600 \times 10^9$/L.
2. 'Smudge' cells or smear cells (lymphocytes ruptured on spreading film) characteristic.
3. Anaemia, neutropenia and thrombocytopenia develop as the disease progresses.

Staging: Three main staging systems based on clinical and haematological parameters. All assume diagnosis based on minimum criteria of:

1. Peripheral blood lymphocytosis $>15 \times 10^9$/L.
2. Bone marrow lymphocytosis >40%.

Table 10.11: FAB classification of CML

	Basophils	*Blasts*	*Monocytes*	*Dysplasia*	*Immature granulocytes*
Classical chronic granulocytic leukaemia	≥2%	<2%	<3%	–	>20%
Atypical CML	<2%	>2%	3–10%	+ +	10–20%
Chronic myelomonocytic leukaemia (CMML)	<2%	<2%	>3–10%	+	<10%

The simplest classification is as follows:

- Stage A: Hb >10 g/dl. Platelets >100 × 10^9/L
  < 3 lymphoid areas involved.
- Stage B: Hb >10 g/dl. Platelets >100 × 10^9/L
  3 or more lymphoid areas involved.
- Stage C: Hb <10 g/dl, or platelets
  <100 × 10^9/L. Regardless of lymphoid areas involved.

☞ NB:

1. A lymphoid area includes liver, or spleen or a single group of nodes, e.g. neck, axillae, groins.
2. Level of lymphocyte count not considered prognostically important although counts tend to rise as disease progresses.
3. Anaemia and thrombocytopenia excludes that caused by a definite autoimmune process.

Investigations

1. Full blood count and reticulocytes, film, direct antiglobulin test.
2. Peripheral blood for lymphocyte markers, 'mouse rosettes' and 'sIg' (surface immunoglobulin), if available.
3. Bone marrow aspirate and trephine. A 'nodular' pattern of lymphocyte infiltration on trephine may suggest better prognosis than diffuse infiltrate.
4. Renal and liver function.
5. Uric acid.
6. Protein electrophoresis and immunoglobulin levels.
7. Chest X-ray

Prognosis

1. Related to stage of disease.
2. Overall median survival six years.
3. Death usually associated with bone marrow failure or infection.
4. Acute transformation analogous to CGL is very rare.

T-Cell Chronic Lymphocytic Leukaemia (T-CLL)

Much less common than B-CLL in United Kingdom. Generally, greater splenomegaly for the same stage of disease. May occur in younger age group.

Prolymphocytic Leukaemia

- Less common than CLL.
- May have B or T cell characteristics.
- Diagnosis based on peripheral blood appearances and immunology.

Clinical and laboratory features

1. Splenomegaly prominent.
2. Lymphadenopathy slight or absent.
3. Elderly males predominate.
4. Often very high WBC.

Prognosis: Much worse than CLL.

Hairy Cell Leukaemia (Leukaemic Reticuloendotheliosis)

Typically 'hairy cells' are found in peripheral blood, but may not always be apparent on light microscopy.

Clinical features

1. Usually elderly—male > female.
2. Pancytopenia.
3. Splenomegaly prominent.
4. Recurrent infections common.

Hairy Cell Leukaemia (Fig. 10.15)

Hairy cell leukaemia is a rare form of B cell leukaemia showing characteristic cells having fine hair-like projections in peripheral blood.

- Age: Elderly people
- Sex: Male preponderance

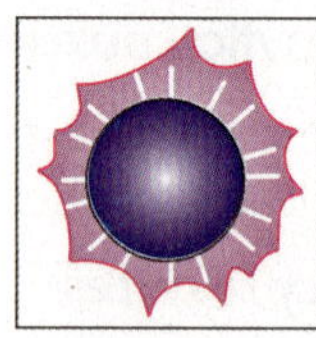

Fig. 10.15: Hairy cell leukaemia fine hair like projection B-cells

Blood Smears

- Pancytopenia
- TLC—leucopenia
- Hb decreased
- Neutrophils <5 × 10^9/µl
- Platelet count <50,000/µl
- Presence of characteristic hairy cells. These are 10–20 nm in diameter. Characteristically they have fine, irregular cytoplasmic projections.

Laboratory features

1. 'Hairy cells'—lymphocytes with spiky projections from cytoplasm.
2. Pancytopenia and especially monocytopenia.
3. Bone marrow aspiration often difficult. Usually hypocellular with lymphoid cells showing staining with tartrate resistant acid phosphatase.
4. Trephine biopsy often needed for diagnosis and shows excess fibrosis.

ALEUKAEMIC LEUKAEMIA AND LEUKAEMOID REACTIONS

Aleukaemic Leukaemia

Aleukaemic leukaemia is also referred to as aleukaemic lymphadenosis and aleukaemic myelosis.

Aleukaemic leukaemia means white blood without white blood. It is a phase of leukaemia in which the white cell count is normal or below normal and the differential white cell count may show only a few immature white cells.

Aleukaemic leukaemia occurs in 10–20% of all cases of leukaemia. Its significance lies in the fact that, during this phase, the disease may easily be confused with other diseases such as aplastic anaemia or agranulocytosis.

With the exception of the white cells, the laboratory findings and clinical picture are the same as those which have just been described for the various leukaemias.

Because the white cell count is normal or below normal, the white cells in the differential white cell count are relatively few. These white cells may be concentrated, however, and the differential white cell count run on the concentrated specimen. The concentrated specimen of white cells is called buffy coat preparation.

As previously stated, in aleukaemic leukaemia, the differential white cell count may not show many immature white cells. A bone marrow examination then becomes the more significant laboratory examination. This examination usually reveals large numbers immature white cells.

Leukaemoid Reactions

Leukaemoid reactions are reactions which resemble leukaemia. Thus, the white cell count is high and the differential white cell count shows immature white cells. But the patient does not have leukaemia.

The distinction between a leukaemoid reaction and true leukaemia is usually made by (1) careful clinical observation of the patient, (2) a continual check for changes in laboratory examinations, and (3) a bone marrow examination.

The more commonly encountered leukaemoid reactions are neutrophilic leukaemoid reactions and lymphocytic leukaemoid reactions. These reactions are briefly discussed below.

Neutrophilic leukaemoid reactions

A neutrophilic leukaemoid reaction is accompanied by a white cell count of 20,000 to 100,000 per cubic millimetre and a differential white cell count showing immature neutrophils such as neutrophilic metamyelocytes and neutrophilic myelocytes.

Thus, from a laboratory viewpoint, a neutrophilic leukaemoid reaction may resemble granulocytic leukaemia.

A neutrophilic leukaemoid reaction may be found in the following conditions: Tuberculosis, meningitis, diphtheria, lobar pneumonia, malaria, syphilis, haemorrhage, haemolytic anaemia, severe burns, tumours, Hodgkin's disease, myeloid metaplasia, mercury poisoning, and eclampsia.

If it is difficult to distinguish between a neutrophilic leukaemoid reaction and granulocytic leukaemia, the alkaline phosphatase stain may be used.

The alkaline phosphatase stain reveals values above normal in a neutrophilic leukaemoid reaction and values below normal in granulocytic leukaemia.

Lymphocytic leukaemoid reactions

A lymphocytic leukaemoid reaction is accompanied by a white cell count of 20,000 to 150,000/cu mm and a differential white cell count showing 35–95% lymphocytes.

Thus, from a laboratory viewpoint, a lymphocytic leukaemoid reaction may resemble lymphocytic leukaemia.

A lymphocytic leukaemoid reaction may be found in the following conditions: Mumps, measles, chickenpox, whooping cough, infectious lymphocytosis, and infectious mononucleosis.

Of the above conditions, infectious mononucleosis probably gives the most trouble, for it is often difficult to differentiate between infectious mononucleosis and lymphocytic leukaemia.

Causes of leukemoid reactions are shown in Table 10.12.

Table 10.12: Causes of leukaemoid reactions
• Bacterial infections
• Infectious mononucleosis
• Cytomegalovirus
• Pertusis
• Tuberculosis
• Acute haemolytic anaemia
• Malignancy

Differences between leukaemoid reaction and leukaemia are given in Table 10.13.

MYELODYSPLASTIC SYNDROMES

Myelodysplastic syndromes are heterogeneous group of haematologic disorders characterised by hypercellular bone marrow with peripheral blood showing pancytopenia of varying severity.

The term myelodysplastic syndromes was suggested. This term encompasses a variety of other syndromes, such as smoldering leukaemia, subacute myeloid leukaemia, Di Guglielmo's syndrome and hypocellular leukaemia.

Definition: Myelodysplastic syndromes are a group of clonal haemopoietic disorders characterized by abnormalities of stem cell and progenitor cell, abnormal bone marrow and peripheral blood morphology, various and frequently progressive cytopenias and a propensity in some cases for transformation to acute myelogenous leukaemia.

Classification: French-American-British (FAB) classification divides myelodysplastic syndromes into five subtypes (Table 10.14).

Table 10.13: Differences between leukaemoid reaction and leukaemia

	Leukaemoid reaction	*Leukaemia*
Clinical picture	Presents with infection. The exact picture depends on the causative aetiology	Commonly present with splenomegaly, lymphadenopathy and haemorrhage
TLC	Generally up to 100,000/μL	May be > 100,000/μl
Immature cells	Blast ≤5% in peripheral blood	Blast count is usually high
Toxic granules	Usually seen	Generally not seen
Anaemia	Slight or absent	Generally present and progressive
Nucleated RBC	Often	Infrequent
Neutrophil alkaline phosphatase	N/↑	↓
Platelet	N/↑	↓
Bone marrow	Hyperplasia is less severe	• Severe hyperplasia
	• Blast count low	• Blast count >30%

Table 10.14: FAB classification of myelodysplastic syndromes

1.	Refractory anaemia (RA)	<5%	<1%		
2.	Acquired idiopathic sideroblastic anaemia (AISA)	<5%	<1%		+
3.	RA with excess blasts (RAEB)	5–20%	<5%	–/+	–/+
4.	Chronic myelo-monocytic leukaemia (CMML)	<20%	<5%	+	–/+
5.	RAEB in transfor-mation (RAEBT)	>20–30%	≥5%	–/+	–/+

1. Refractory anaemia (RA), with erythroid hyperplasia and/or dyserythropoiesis.
2. RA with ring sideroblasts, also designated as acquired idiopathic sideroblastic anaemia (AISA), the main feature being the presence of ring sideroblasts in at least 15% of erythroblasts.
3. RA with excess blasts (RAEB) which shows dyspoiesis in the three bone marrrow cell lineages, dysgranulopoiesis being always conspicuous. The percentage of bone marrow blasts is between 5% and 20%; these cells may have a few or no azurophil granules.
4. Chronic myelomonocytic leukaemia (CMML), with many features of RAEB plus a significant peripheral blood monocytosis (usually over 1×10^9/L).
5. RAEB in transformation, a group close to AML, and defined by the presence of blasts in the peripheral blood (over 5%) and between 20% and 30% in the bone marrow.

In addition to staining for iron, the other cytochemical methods used in AML may be useful for the study of the MDS. They may help to define the monocytic component in CMML or the type of blasts in RAEB and they are particularly useful in demonstrating dysgranulopoiesis,, e.g. by the presence of neutrophils negative for peroxidase and/or Sudan black B reactions or giving extremely low NAP scores.

WHO classification of MDS is given in Table 10.15.

Table 10.15: WHO classification of MDS (myelodysplastic syndrome)

Refractory anaemia	Anaemia	• Dysplasia in erythroid cells • <5% Blasts
Refractory anaemia with ringed sideroblasts	Anaemia	• >15% Ringed sideroblasts
Refractory cytopenia with multi-lineage dysplasia	Bicytopenia/pancytopenia No blasts	• Dysplasia >10% of the cells of 2 or more myeloid series • <5% Blasts • <15% Ringed sideroblasts
Refractory cytopenia with multi-lineage dysplasia and ringed sideroblasts	• Bicytopenia/pancytopenia • No/rare blasts	• >15% Ringed sideroblasts • <5% Blasts • Dysplasia >10% of cells in 2 or more myeloid series

Contd.

Table 10.15: WHO classification of MDS (myelodysplastic syndrome) (Contd.)

Refractory anaemia with excess blasts 1	• <5% Blasts bicytopenia/pancytopenia	• 5–9% Blasts show unilineage/multilineage dysplasia
Refractory anaemia with excess blasts 2	• Cytopenia • 5–19% Blasts; Auer rods +ve	• Unilineage/multilineage blasts • 10–19% Blasts; Auer rods +ve
$5q^-$ syndrome	• Anaemia • <5% Blasts • Normal/increased platelet count	• <5% Blasts • Megakaryocytes normal or increased with hypolobated forms

AETIOPATHOGENESIS

Different aetiological factors are tabulated in Table 10.16. However, myelodysplastic syndrome is a clonal proliferation of abnormal stem cells. Thus, there is increased haematopoiesis in the marrow however, the haematopoiesis is ineffective and disorderly causing pancytopenia. The abnormal stem cell clone in the bone marrow is genetically unstable and frequently undergoes transformation to acute myeloid leukaemia.

Table 10.16: Aetiology of myelodysplastic syndrome
1. Environmental exposure of
• Benzene
• Radiation
2. Radiation therapy
3. Chemotherapy
• Busulfan
• Nitrosourea
4. Immunosuppressive treatment
5. Fanconi's anaemia
6. Paroxysmal nocturnal haemoglobinuria
7. Aplastic anaemia
8. Mutation of N-ras, p53 and Bcl-2

Clinical findings: MDS is a disease found principally in the higher age group. The average age is 65 years and male sex is predominant. About 10–15% patients are below the age of 50 years and MDS patients are diagnosed even in children. Anaemia is the change most frequently found at diagnosis (Table 10.17).

Table 10.17: Important clinical findings in patients with MDS (Pooled Data)

Age (years)	65 (16–92)
Sex (M : F)	1.6:1
Anaemia	83%
Thrombocytopenia	54%
Leukopenia	48%
Leukocytosis	15%
Splenomegaly	15%

Laboratory diagnosis (Table 10.18)

Peripheral blood smears show the following abnormalities:

a. Anaemia, macrocytosis, tear drop formations and moderate poikilocytosis. Reticulocyte count is low. 'Megaloblastoid' nucleated red cells are frequently detected. MCV normal or slightly increased. Basophilic stippling, polychromatophils and Howell-

Table 10.18: Peripheral blood and bone marrow findings in the myelodysplastic syndromes

	RA	*RARS*	*RAEB*	*RAEBIT*	*CMML*
Anaemia	+	+	+	+	+/–
Granulocytopenia	+/–	+/–	Usually +	Usually +	+/–
Thrombocytopenia	+/–	+/–	Usually +	Usually +	+/–
Marrow dysplasia:					
• erythroid	+	+	Usually +	Usually +	+/–
• myeloid	+/–	+/–	Usually +	Usually +	+/–
• megakaryocytic	+/–	+/–	Usually +	Usually +	+/–
• Auer rods	–	–	–	+/–	–
Ringed sideroblasts >15%	–	+	+/–	+/–	+/–
Peripheral blood blasts	≤1%	≤1%	<5%	Maybe >5	<5%
Abnormal marrow blasts	<5%	5%	5–20%	20–30%	≤5
Peripheral blood monocytosis (>.1 × 10^9/L)	–	–	–	–	+

Jolly body may be seen. A characteristic finding is dimorphic picture, with a combination of normocytic and macrocytic or erythrocyte and macrocyte.

b. Neutrophils may display decreased lobulation (the Pelger-Hüet anomaly) and the neutrophil granules are frequently absent or very large. Grossly hypersegmented or polyploid neutrophils may be seen.
c. 'Giant' platelets may be seen. Circulating megakaryocyte fragments or micromegakaryocytes may also be seen.
d. Nuclei may be sausage-shaped or trilobed in monocytes; promonocytes (fine azurophilic granulation) may be seen.
e. Blasts of either type I or type II.

Bone Marrow Findings

1. Bone marrow cellularity is usually normal to increased.
2. Excessive reticulin is found in most of the cases.
3. Dysmorphology may be present in one, two or (most frequently) all three cell lines.

MYELOPROLIFERATIVE DISORDERS

Myeloproliferative disorders have been defined as a group of interrelated neoplastic diseases having similar pathophysiology. They all arise due to clonal expansion of multipotent haematopoietic progenitor cell giving rise to overproduction of one or more lineage of mature cells, that is, erythroid, granulocytic, monocytic and megakaryocytic cells (Table 10.19). There is uncontrolled proliferation of these cells allowing their accumulation. Depending on the type of cell involved, four subtypes are recognised:

1. Idiopathic thrombocythemia
2. Polycythaemia vera
3. Myelofibrosis
4. Chronic myeloid leukaemia

Evolution of Myeloproliferative Diseases

Origin and progression of myeloproliferative diseases are given in Fig. 10.16.

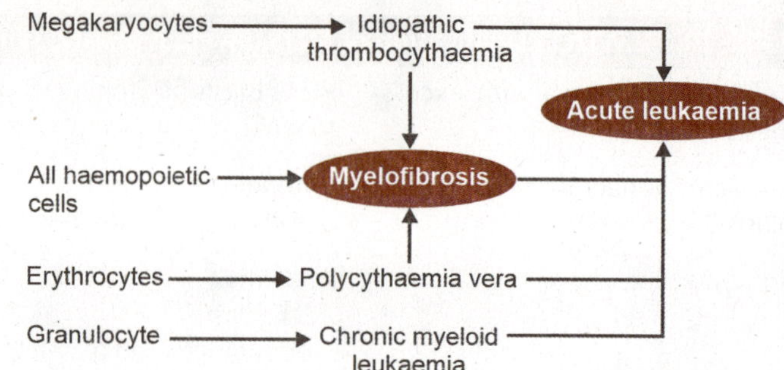

Fig. 10.16: Origin and progression of myeloproliferative disease

Cell origin and cell types of myeloproliferative disorders are given in Table 10.19.

POLYCYTHAEMIA

Polycythaemia is defined as increased concentration of circulating red cells above normal limits. The term polycythaemia is often used interchangeable with erythrocytosis. However, the term polycythaemia is specifically used when two or more types of haematopoietic cells are increased. Polycythaemia is classified as **relative** or **absolute**. In relative polycythaemia the total red cell mass is normal but due to decreased plasma volume the cell count is high (haemoconcentration). In absolute polycythaemia there is an increase in total red cell mass.

Relative Polycythaemia

In relative polycythaemia the increase in red cell mass is only relative due to decrease in plasma volume (dehydration). This may be seen in middle-aged, overweight males who are heavy smokers (Table 10.20).

Absolute Polycythaemia

Absolute polycythaemia is subdivided into primary and secondary. In primary polycythaemia a clone of cell continuously proliferate in the absence of growth stimulating factors. Thus, this is a clonal stem cell disorder and is called polycythaemia vera (Table 10.20).

Main cause of secondary polycythaemia is hypoxia. Hypoxia causes stimulation of erythropoietin produc-

Table 10.19: Cell-cell Origin and types of myeloproliferative disorders

Cell	Disorder
1. Megakaryocytes	Idiopathic thrombocythemia
2. Erythrocytes	Polycythaemia vera
3. All haemopoietic cells	Myelofibrosis. The platelets produce platelet-derived growth factor, which causes deposition of reticulin and fibrous tissue in myelofibrosis
4. Granulocytes	Chronic myeloid leukaemia (CML): Though CML share similar phenotypic characteristics but genetically it is distinctly different from other types of leukaemias. It is a type of leukaemia showing chromosomes 9 and 22 translocation with differentiation into a large number of mature forms, which is different than acute myeloid leukaemia where there are a large number of immature blast. However, all the subtypes of myeloproliferative disorders can progress to acute leukaemia.

Table 10.20: Classification of polycythaemia

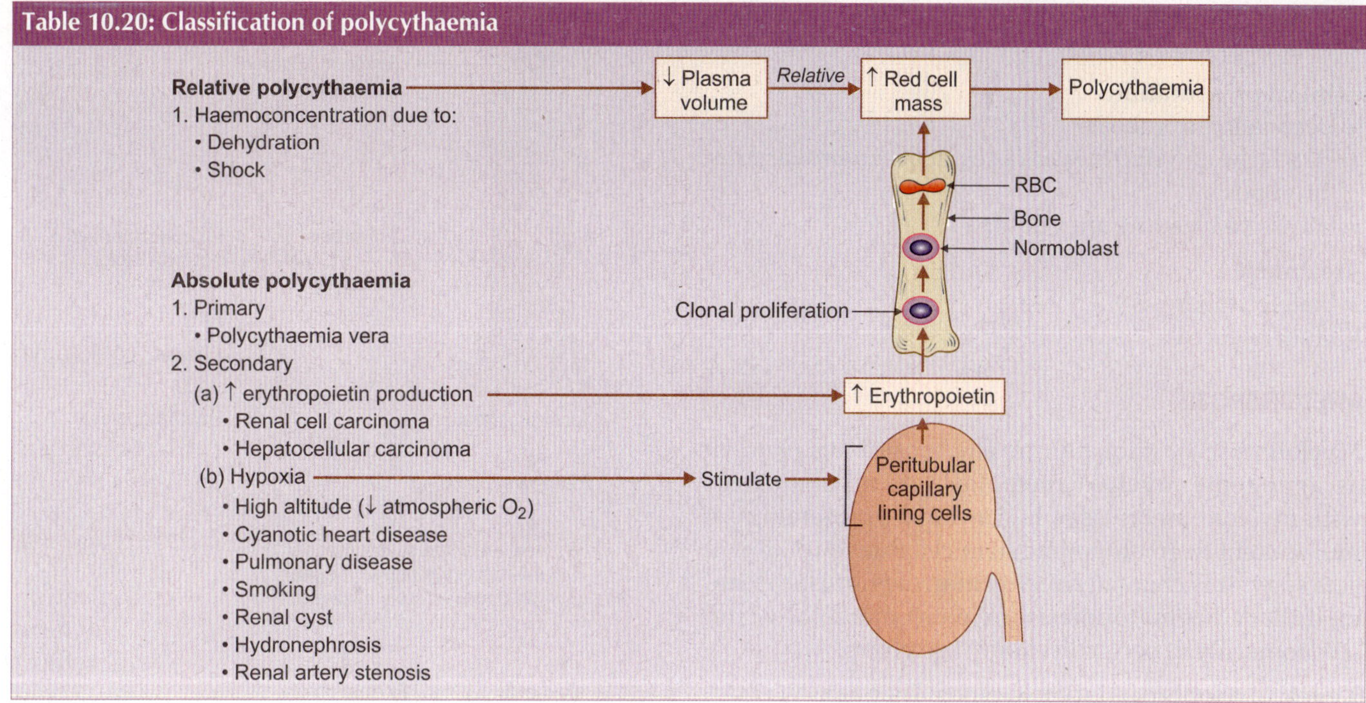

tion. Erythropoietin stimulates red cell production and secondary polycythaemia. The various causes are listed in Table 10.20. However, secondary polycythaemia can occur in the absence of hypoxia. Renal lesions such as hydronephrosis or cyst may produce compression effect on kidney causing localised hypoxia. This may result in production of erythropoietin by kidney. Some of the tumours can also produce erythropoietin and stimulate RBC production.

Laboratory investigation

- Haemoglobin—raised, often above 20 g/dl.
- RBC count—raised > 6 million/cu mm
- TLC—raised
- Haematocrit—raised >55% in males and >48% in females
- Arterial O_2 saturation > 92% in polycythaemia vera and < 92% in secondary polycythaemia
- Neutrophil count—raised
- NAP score raised in polycythaemia vera but is normal in secondary polycythaemia
- Platelet count—raised (400–700 × 10^9/µl)
- Bone marrow:
  - Hypercellular
  - Erythroid hyperplasia
  - Myeloid hyperplasia
  - Megakaryocyte hyperplasia
  - Marrow reticulin normal in initial stages and later fibrosis occurs.
- Biochemical
  - S. uric acid
  - S. LDH

  These are increased in polycythaemia vera but is normal in secondary polycythaemia

Clinical features

Skin is dusky red in colour with cyanosis.

- The patient suffers from headache, lethargy, dizziness and vertigo due to hyperviscosity of blood.
- Conjunctiva is congested with dimness of vision.
- Large mass of cells produce high uric acid level on destruction. This produces acute gout.
- On examination, spleen may be palpable due to congestion and extramedullary haematopoiesis.
- There is pruritus which gets aggravated by bathing in hot water.

Treatment: Repeated venesection for removal of blood or use of cytotoxic drug or radiophosphorus has been used for treatment.

Prognosis: Polycythaemia may progress to myelofibrosis or acute myeloid leukaemia.

ESSENTIAL THROMBOCYTHAEMIA

- Essential thrombocythaemia is a chronic myeloproliferative disorder.
- Age group 49–70 years
- Hb—normal
- TLC—increased
- Platelet count—increased (>600 × 10^9/µl)
- Peripheral smear shows normocytic normochromic picture with large aggregates of platelets. Some of which are large and hypogranular.
- NAP score—increased
- Bone marrow:
  - Hypercellular
  - Megakaryocytic hyperplasia with a few giant megakaryocytes. Some show features of dysmega-

karyopoiesis. Myeloid and erythroid series are normal.

Clinical presentation

- Deep vein thrombosis
- Headache and dizziness as a result of cerebrovascular thrombosis.
- Excessive bleeding after trauma

Treatment

- Platelet apheresis
- Hydroxyurea

MYELOFIBROSIS

Myelofibrosis or idiopathic myelofibrosis is also known as agnogenic myeloid metaplasia or myelofibrosis with myeloid metaplasia. It is a clonal proliferation of multipotent haematopoietic stem cell due to unknown aetiology. It is characterised by marrow fibrosis, extramedullary haematopoiesis, myeloid metaplasia and splenomegaly. It occurs in elderly age group.

Types: Myelofibrosis is of two types. They are:

- Idiopathic myelofibrosis:
  - Cause is unknown
  - Chronic myeloproliferative disorder
- Secondary myelofibrosis:
  - Hodgkin's lymphoma involving bone marrow
  - CML
  - Hairy cell leukaemia
  - Metastatic carcinoma

Pathogenesis: The aetiology of idiopathic myelofibrosis is unknown. It arises from malignant transformation of a single multipotent haematopoietic stem cells that has not committed to any particular cell type. Thus, idiopathic myelofibrosis is a clonal proliferation (Fig. 10.17).

The proliferation occurs in the bone marrow, from here it goes to other organs such as spleen and liver. Thus, spleen and liver become the sites of myeloid cell proliferation (myeloid metaplasia) with extramedullary haematopoiesis. The megakaryocytes or platelets secrete growth factors—platelets derived growth factor (PDGF) and transforming growth factor β (TGF-β). These growth factors cause fibrosis of the marrow.

Laboratory findings

Peripheral blood picture

- **RBC changes**
  - Tear drop-shaped red cell
  - Nucleated red cell
  - Poikilocytes (variation in shape)
- **WBC changes**
  - Myelocytes
  - Promyelocytes
  - Myeloblast

These changes suggest extramedullary haematopoiesis.

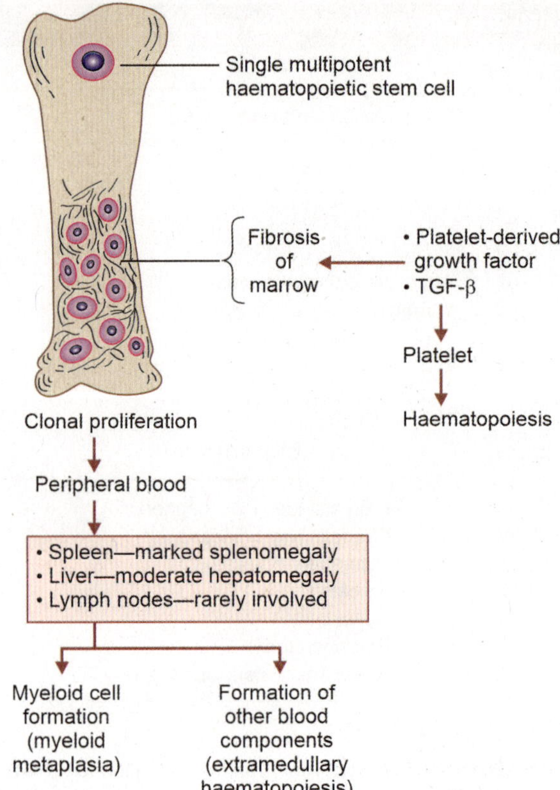

Fig. 10.17: Pathogenesis of idiopathic myelofibrosis

- **Platelet changes**
  - ↑ platelets (thrombocytosis)
  - Large size and bizarre looking platelets

This type of blood picture is called leukoerythroblastic and this is typical of myelofibrosis.

- NAP score—raised

Bone marrow changes: Due to fibrosis of marrow, bone marrow aspiration often fails. Bone marrow biopsy (trephine biopsy) shows:

- Hypercellular marrow
- All the three types of cell lineages that are erythroid, myeloid and megakaryocytes show hyperplasia (trilineage hyperplasia in early phase).
- Megakaryocytes are large, dysplastic and are present in small groups.
- ↑ reticulin fibres (fibrosis). With progressive fibrosis marrow becomes hypocellular.

Clinical presentation

- Massive splenomegaly
- Malaise and lethargy due to anaemia
- Mild hepatomegaly
- Bleeding
- Idiopathic myelofibrosis generally presents with progressive anaemia or with a dragging sensation in the left upper quadrant due to severe splenomegaly.
- Expanded mass of myeloid cells causes increased metabolism with symptoms of fatigue, night sweats and weight loss.

Progression of the disease

- Idiopathic myelofibrosis progresses to marrow failure with transfusion-dependent anaemia and increasing organomegaly.
- Like CML, idiopathic myelofibrosis can also progress from a chronic phase to an accelerated phase with constitutional symptoms and a progressive marrow failure.

PLASMA CELL NEOPLASIA

Synonym: Monoclonal gammopathies, paraproteinemias, plasma cell dyscrasias and dysproteinemias

This is a group of monoclonal neoplasms arising from common progenitors in the B lymphocytic series. The diseases belonging to this group are:

- Multiple myeloma
- Waldenström's macroglobulinaemia
- Primary amyloidosis
- Heavy chain disease

Multiple Myeloma

Multiple myeloma is malignant proliferation of a single clone of plasma cell.

- Age incidence
  - Peak age between 50 and 60 years
  - Rarely under 40 years
- Sex incidence: No sex preponderances

Aetiopathogenesis

- **Ionising radiation:** Long-term survivors of nuclear bomb in Japan suffered a five times increased incidence of multiple myeloma.
- **Oncogenes:** Overexpression of myc or ras oncogene has been found in multiple myeloma.
- **Mutation of suppressor oncogenes:** Mutation of p53 and Rb-1 (retinoblastoma 1) suppressor oncogene has been noted in multiple myeloma.
- **Occupational hazard:** Increased incidence of multiple myeloma has been seen in:
  - Woodworkers
  - Leather workers
  - Workers exposed to petroleum products
- **Chromosomal changes:** A large number of chromosomal changes have been found in multiple myeloma. The most common is t(11 ; 14) (q13; q32).
- **IL-6:** IL-6 acts on plasma cell causing its proliferation. It then replaces the normal haematopoietic elements of the bone marrow. The plasma cells cause the stromal cells to secrete IL-1β which act on osteoclasts leading to osteolytic lesions in bone. Further plasma cell secrete immunoglobulin causing M band on electrophoresis.

Whatever may be the aetiologic factor they cause transformation of a pluripotent stem cell (clonal transformation) which differentiates predominantly along the B cell–plasma cell pathway. Interleukin-6 (IL-6) may cause proliferation of neoplastic myeloma cells. The proliferation of myeloma cells occurs in multiple bones:

- Vertebral bones—most common
- Ribs
- Skull
- Pelvis
- Femur
- Clavicle
- Scapula

The proliferating myeloma cells erode and destroy the cortical bone causing pathological fractures.

Morphology

- Anaemia—Rb is decreased
- Peripheral smear shows rouleaux formation due to high concentration of immunoglobulin. Occasionally, an abnormal plasma cell is seen. RBCs are normocytic normochromic.
- ESR—increased due to rouleaux formation.
- Bleeding time—increased (platelet aggregation is impaired as they get coated by M component)
- Bone marrow (Fig. 10.18)
  - Hypercellular
  - Marrow elements are replaced by diffuse sheets or nodular aggregates of plasma cells. Plasma cell constitutes almost 30–90% of all cells. Neoplastic plasma cells may appear normal or may show morphological features of undifferentiated blast with pleomorphism and nucleoli. The cells are large with eccentric nucleus and blue cytoplasm. Some of them can show multiple nucleoli.
  - Russell bodies are immunoglobulin inclusion in the cytoplasm of the plasma cells.
  - Flame cells—the periphery of the cytoplasm of these plasma cells shows a pink-coloured flare.
  - Erythroid
  - Myeloid
  - Megakaryocytes

  } ↓ leading to anaemia and thrombocytopenia

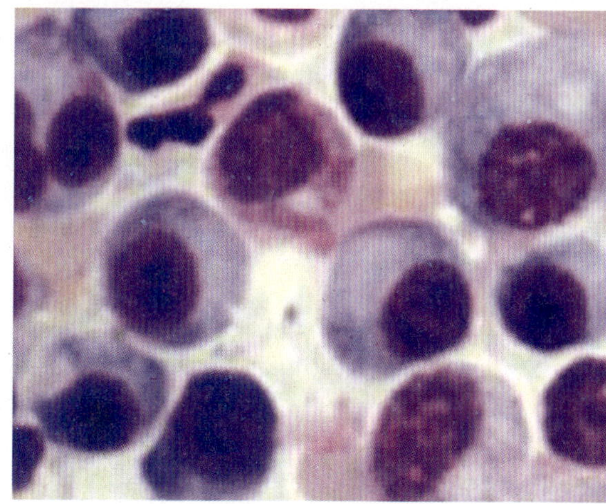

Fig. 10.18: Microphotograph of multiple myeloma. Aggregates of plasma cells

Laboratory Diagnosis

M Spike

Multiple myeloma produces increasing amount of immunoglobulin. Multiple myeloma being a monoclonal disorder produces a single type of immunoglobulin, a sharp spike in the immunoglobulin region at electrophoresis. This sharp spike is called M spike (M stands for monoclonal) or M component (Fig. 10.19).

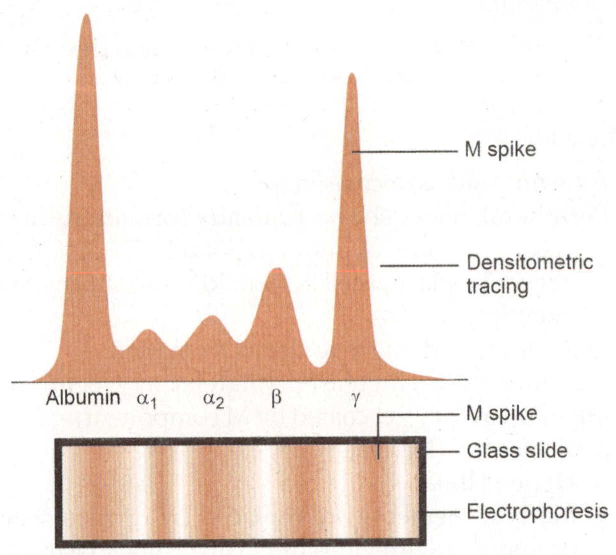

Fig. 10.19: Serum electrophoresis showing high level monoclonal antibody also called M spike

Bence-Jones Proteins

Bence-Jones proteins are globulin of either the κ (kappa) or λ (lambda) immunoglobulin light chain. Characteristically, this protein precipitates at 60°C and remains till 80°C and beyond 80°C it again disappears. Conditions producing Bence-Jones protein are:

- Multiple myeloma
- Macroglobulinemia

X-ray

Numerous osteolytic lesions in skull, ribs, pelvis and vertebrae.

Biochemical

- Serum calcium increases (because of extensive osteolytic lesions)
- Serum β_2-microglobulin increases (high level indicates poor prognosis)
- Serum creatinine increases } Because of impairment of kidney functions
- Serum uric acid increases } Because of impairment of kidney functions
- Urea increases

PLASMA CELL LEUKAEMIA

- Plasma cells in the peripheral blood are >20% of the differential count.
- Present with hepatosplenomegaly and hypercalcema
- Prognosis is poor

Monoclonal Gammopathy of Undetermined Significance (MGUS)

- Age group—elderly
- Bone marrow plasma cells <10%
- M spike IgG <3 g/dl
- Light chain in urine <1 g/24 hours
- No lytic lesions
- No treatment is required
- May progress to multiple myeloma in some patients.

Waldenström's Macroglobulinaemia

- Age group >60 years
- B cell neoplasm with IgM type M spike
- Morphology:
  - Anaemia
  - M spike—IgM type (10–30 g/L)
  - Peripheral smear shows rouleaux formation and lymphocytosis, some of which are a typical plasma cytoid type.
  - Bone marrow: Replacement of marrow by atypical plasmacytoid lympocytes. These cells are large with eccentric nucleus and light blue cytoplasm. These are PAS positive cells. In later stage erythroid, myeloid and megakaryocytes are suppressed.

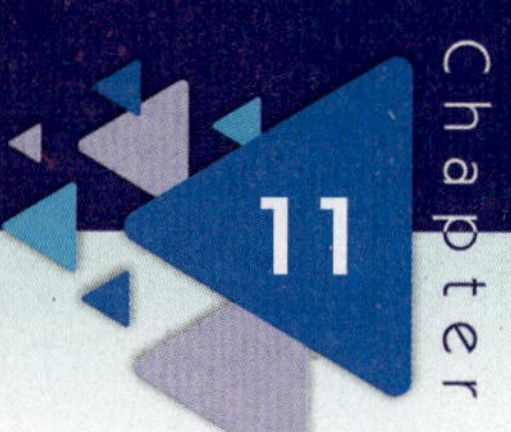

Normal Haemostasis and Haemostatic Disorders

Chapter Outline

- Introduction: Haemostasis
- Process of Haemostasis
- Haemophilia B
- von Willebrand Disease
- Acquired Coagulation Disorders
- Disseminated Intravascular Coagulation
- Liver Disease
- Vitamin K Deficiency

INTRODUCTION: HAEMOSTASIS

Haemostasis is the process by which bleeding at any site is arrested by formation of a haemostatic plug. This is followed by removal of the plug so that normal flow of blood through vessels is maintained.

Spontaneous arrest of bleeding is a complicated process. The first event after injury to a vessel is bleeding for sometime. This is followed by prompt retraction and reflex vasoconstriction of damaged vessels lasting for a few minutes; simultaneously the normal tissue tone and the increased pressure on the vessel wall from without by the extravasated blood tend to halt the further escape of blood. The third event is the settling of platelets on damaged sites in the vessel wall and their agglutination. Agglutinated platelets release serotonin which causes a prolonged vasoconstriction of both damaged and surrounding vessels. Meanwhile a firm fibrin clot has formed in the wound and seals the vessel so that even with dilatation of the vessel, there is no further bleeding.

Haemorrhagic disorders are characterised by bleeding into tissues, either spontaneous or after slight injury. They are due to failure of the normal haemostatic mechanism.

Components of Haemostasis

There are 5 components of haemostasis:

1. Blood vessels
2. Platelets
3. Coagulation
4. Fibrinolytic system and
5. Inhibitors of coagulation.

1. Blood Vessels

Blood vessels are lined by endothelial cells which rest on subendothelial connective tissue.

A. Endothelium

Endothelial cells play an important role in haemostasis (Fig. 11.1) by forming a continuous monolayer which is non-thrombogenic.

Thus, endothelial cells are capable of activating coagulation systems, fibrinolytic system, protein C system and release von Willebrand's factor (vWF).

B. Subendothelial collagen

Subendothelial collagen is exposed when endothelial damage occurs (Fig. 11.2).

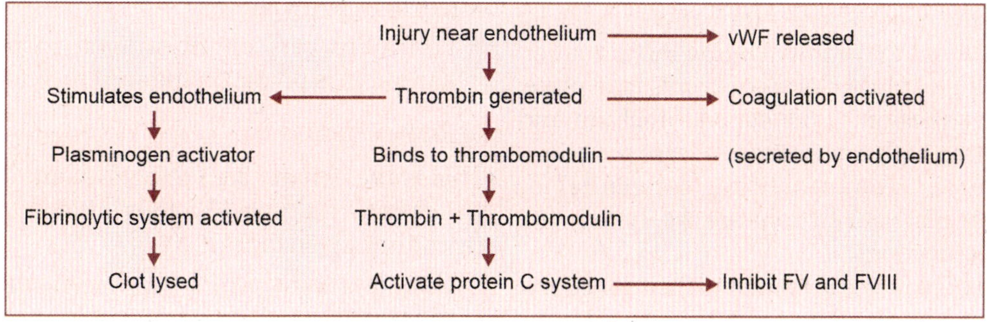

Fig. 11.1: Role of endothelial cells in haemostasis

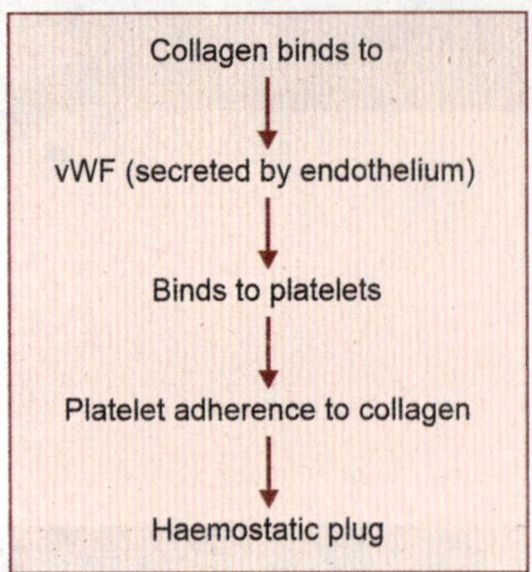

Fig. 11.2: Platelets adhere to collagen by binding first to vWF which attaches itself to subendothelial collagen

C. Vasoconstriction

Vessels, after injury, contract, arresting blood loss.

2. Platelets

The process of haemostasis (following injury) begins by adherence of platelets to subendothelial collagen. Adhered platelets undergo release reaction resulting in aggregation (Fig. 11.3).

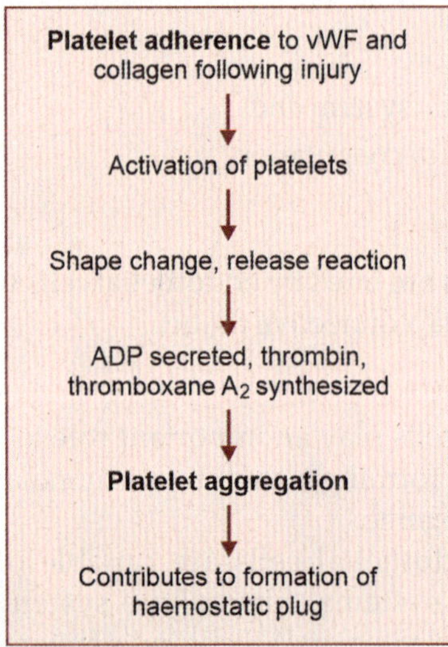

Fig. 11.3: Haemostatic plug platelet adherence is followed by activation of platelets, secretion of ADP and platelet aggregation

Role of platelets in haemostasis

An adequate number of normally functioning platelets is necessary for normal haemostasis. Platelets play two distinct roles in the haemostasis—formation of platelet plug and contribution to clotting. During the formation of hemostatic platelet plug a series of events take place, namely platelet adhesion to the subendothelium and platelet aggregation with concomitant release of various platelet substances. Abnormalities (congenital or acquired) of these platelet reactions are associated with impaired platelet functions.

The structure of platelets is related to their functions. Morphologically the platelets have peripheral zone (cell membrane), sol-gel zone and organelle zone. The peripheral zone is primarily involved for adhesion and the sol-gel zone which contains microtubules and microfilaments and is responsible for contraction. The organelle zone which consists of granules dense bodies and mitochondria and is involved with secretion. The storage granules are a source of ADP and 5-HT. Stimulation of platelets with ADP, collagen, thrombin, aggregated immunoglobulins, etc. is associated with platelet shape change from disc to sphere and formation of surface projections which finally results in release of various substances from the storage granules.

Prostaglandins play an important role in the platelet function. With the stimulation of platelet there is formation of various prostaglandin derivatives which stimulate (e.g. prostaglandin endoperoxides and thromboxanes) or inhibit the platelet aggregation (e.g. PGE_2 and prostacyclin). *In vivo,* there appears to be a balance between these two systems and normal haemostasis is maintained.

3. Coagulation

Nomenclature for blood coagulation factors

Factor	*Synonym*
I	Fibrinogen
II	Prothrombin
III	Thromboplastin (tissue)
IV	Calcium
V	Proaccelerin, labile factor Entity not defined
VII	Proconvertin
VIII	Antihaemophilic factor (AHF)
IX	Christmas factor, plasma thromboplastic component (PTC)
X	Stuart-Prower factor
XI	Plasma thromboplastin antecedent (PTA)
XII	Hageman factor
XIII	Fibrin stabilising factor, Laki-Lorand factor Prekallikrein High molecular weight Kininogen

The main event of coagulation is production of thrombin by:

- Intrinsic pathway and
- Extrinsic pathway.
- Thrombin acts on fibrinogen to produce fibrin. Thrombin is pivotal in the amplification process.

A. Intrinsic pathway

This is the contact activation system initiated by FXII which in turn acts on FXI, thus initiating the coagulation cascade as given in Fig. 11.4.

The mechanism of coagulation, the intrinsic and extrinsic pathway and inhibitors are shown in Fig. 11.5 and fibrinolytic system in Fig. 11.6.

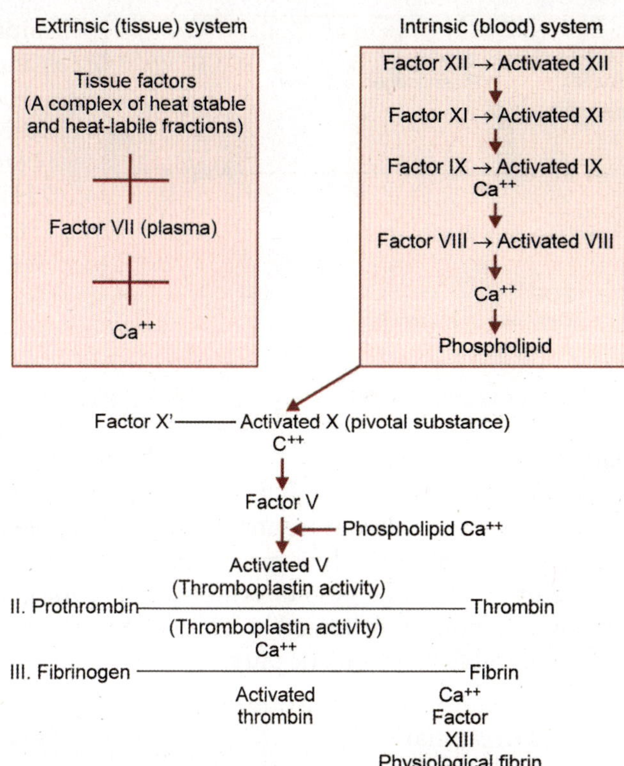

Fig. 11.4: The development of thromboplastic activity: Coagulation cascade

B. Extrinsic pathway

Tissue factor is released following tissue injury and is the co-factor for the extrinsic pathway and initiator of coagulation.

4. Fibrinolytic System

Removal of fibrin from a clot is controlled by fibrinolytic system. Fibrinogen and fibrin are acted upon by plasmin, thus cleaving them and forming fibrin degradation products (FDPs), so that the minor clots which are formed in vessels are cleared and blood flow is restored. Physiologic control of the fibrinolysis is such that plasmin action is limited to the site of injury and formation of clot/thrombus and systemic action of plasmin does not occur (Fig. 11.6).

5. Inhibitors of Coagulation

A number of mechanisms are responsible for limitation of the clotting process at the site of injury so that it does not become generalized. Some of the important mechanisms are:

a. **Antithrombin III:** It binds to thrombin forming inactive thrombin–antithrombin complex. It is also anti-Xa.

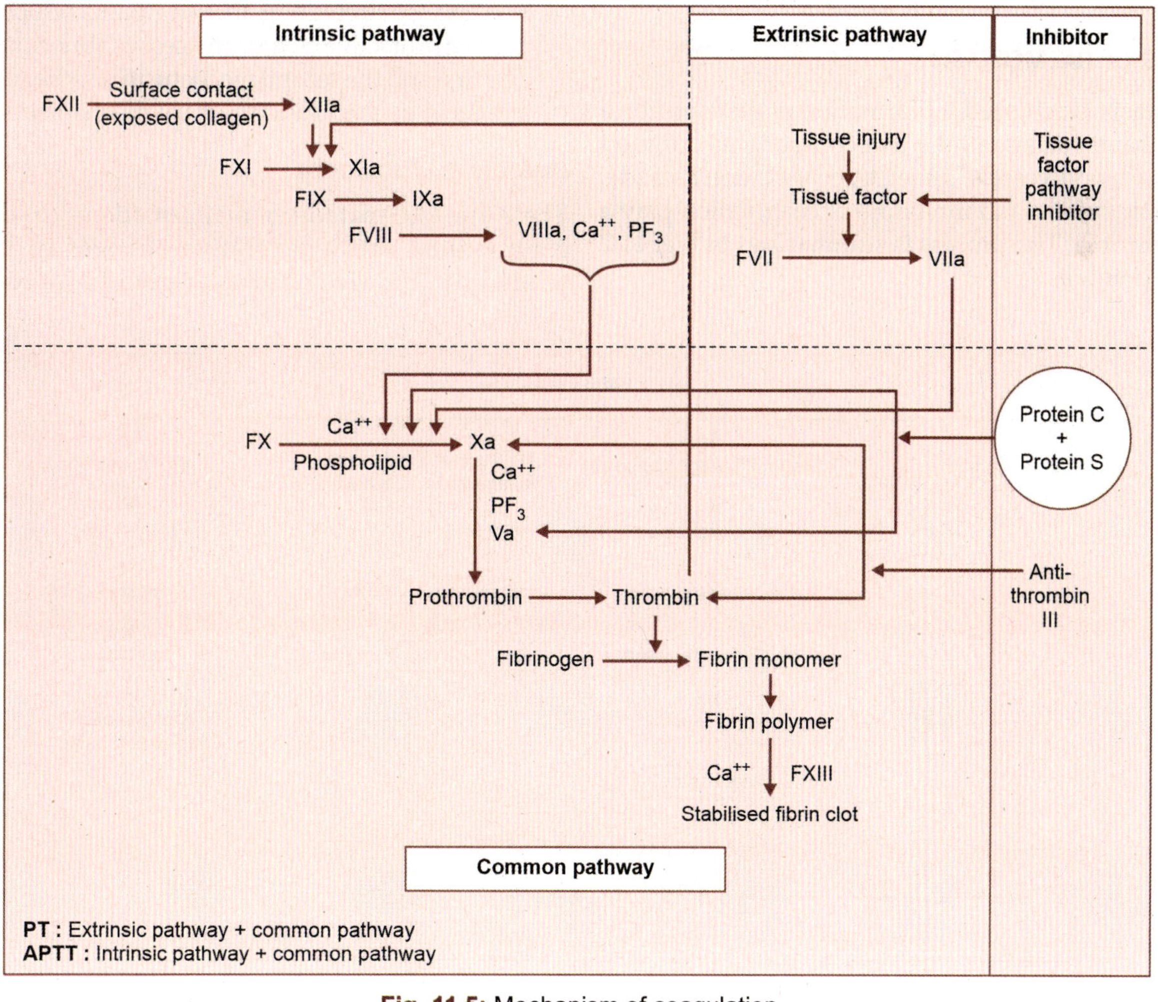

Intrinsic pathway | Extrinsic pathway | Inhibitor

FXII —Surface contact (exposed collagen)→ XIIa
FXI → XIa
FIX → IXa
FVIII → VIIIa, Ca^{++}, PF_3

Tissue injury
Tissue factor ← Tissue factor pathway inhibitor
FVII → VIIa

FX —Ca^{++}, Phospholipid→ Xa
Ca^{++}
PF_3
Va
Protein C + Protein S
Prothrombin → Thrombin ← Anti-thrombin III
Fibrinogen → Fibrin monomer
Fibrin polymer
Ca^{++} FXIII
Stabilised fibrin clot

Common pathway

PT : Extrinsic pathway + common pathway
APTT : Intrinsic pathway + common pathway

Fig. 11.5: Mechanism of coagulation

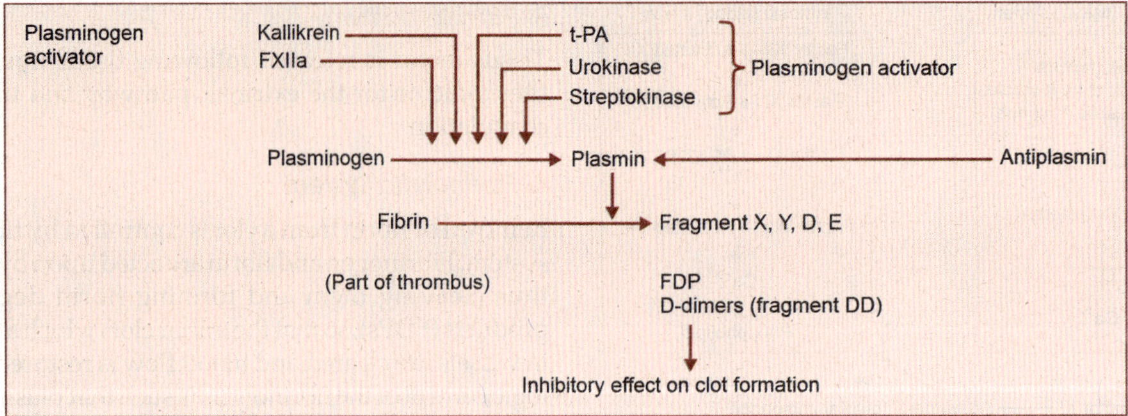

Fig. 11.6: Fibrinolytic system

b. Protein C inactivates FVa and FVIIIa. Protein C requires protein S as a co-factor for its action.

c. **Fibrinolytic mechanism** acts as a further check on uncontrolled clot formation.

Almost all of the coagulation factors and inhibitors are synthesized in liver and therefore, liver disease is an important cause of abnormal bleeding. Factors II, VII, IX and X require vitamin K for synthesis in their completed form. Vitamin K inhibitors coumarins (warfarin) are important anticoagulant drugs in use.

PROCESS OF HAEMOSTASIS

Haemostasis is achieved by formation of platelet-fibrin plug. In haemostasis, all the five components outlined above, i.e. blood vessels, platelets, coagulation cascade, fibrinolytic system and inhibitors of coagulation play a significant role. The process is summarised in Fig. 11.7 and two points as:

1. Inhibitors of coagulation are antithrombin III, protein C, protein S and fibrinolytic mechanism.
2. Platelet adherence to subendothelial collagen following injury is followed by platelet aggregation and eventually haemostatic plug.

Defective haemostasis may be due to:

1. Defects in capillaries
2. Defects in platelets
3. Defects in plasma factors responsible for the clotting of blood
4. Presence of circulating anticoagulants which may be normal protective factors in excess or abnormal factors.

The first and the second mechanism may be combined, as also, the second and the third mechanism.

Defects in Capillaries

These are: (a) Anatomical malformations, (b) defective contractility, (c) degenerative changes in the wall produced by old age, and (d) damage to the wall caused by

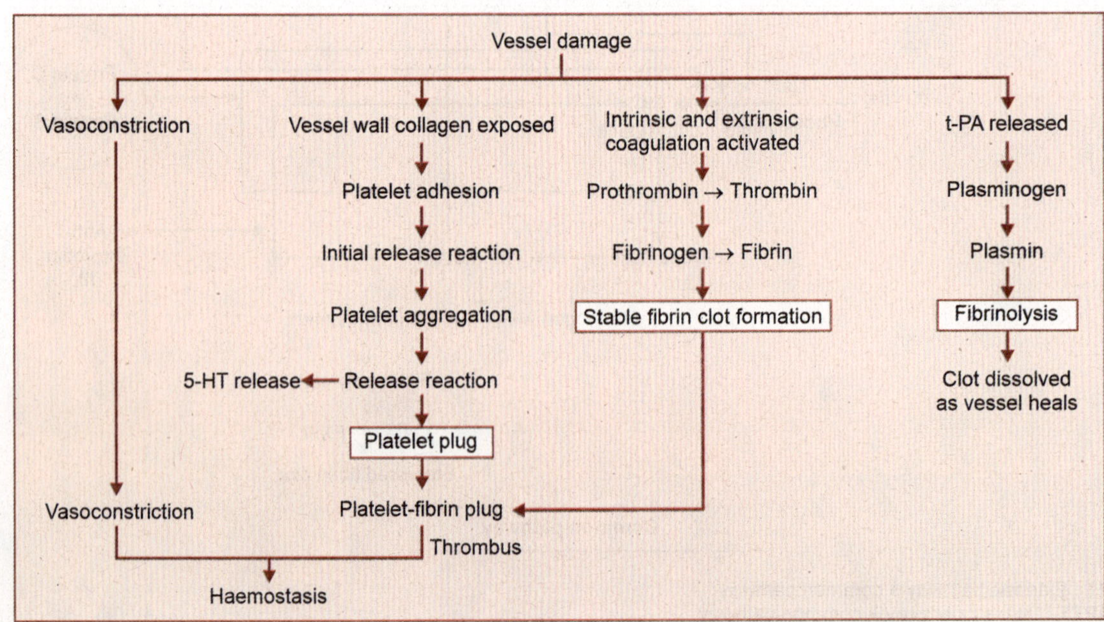

Fig. 11.7: Formation of a platelet-fibrin plug in normal haemostasis

deficiency of vitamins C and P, bacterial toxins, chemicals, drugs and products generated during hyper-sensitivity reactions. The manifestations of capillary damage may be purpura (spontaneous pin-point haemorrhages in the skin and mucous membranes), ecchymosis (large purple areas of haemorrhage, which later become bluish, in the skin) and haemorrhages into tissues of internal organs. Hess' capillary resistance test (described below) is used to demonstrate capillary defects.

Defects in Platelets

Normally the number of platelets is 250,000 to 500,000/cu mm. The lifespan of the platelet is 3 to 4 days. The spleen is their main graveyard but some destruction also occurs all over the reticuloendothelial system. Possibly they have many functions, the chief one being haemostasis. They mechanically seal off defects in vascular endothelium. On coming into contact with a water-wettable surface larger than themselves, they adhere to it and disintegrate (only in the presence of Ca ions) liberating thromboplastin (ethanolamine-phosphatid) which converts prothrombin into thrombin. A small number of platelets suffices for this reaction. However, plentiful platelets must be present to cause retraction of the fibrin clot. Platelets also contain serotonin (5-hydroxytryptamine) and epinephrine and norepinephrine which can cause vasoconstriction of small vessels. A heparin-neutralising factor has also been demonstrated in them.

Defects in platelets may be quantitative or qualitative (Table 11.1). Reduction in platelets (thrombocytopenia) below 40,000 is usually associated with purpura; there is also an increase in the bleeding time and the capillary resistance test is positive, but the coagulation time is not altered unless the reduction is extreme. The clot, however, will not retract well. The decrease in the number may be due to insufficient production in the marrow (hypoplasia or ·aplasia of the marrow) or due to splenic action (hypersplenism) restricting their release into circulation, or due to consumption of a large number in closing-gaps in bleeding blood vessels, or due to an antiplatelet antibody (produced as an immunologic response) destroying platelets rapidly. The qualitative defect consists of an undue stability (thrombasthenia) which will lengthen the coagulation time, or of reduction in their adhesive property (possibly due to the splenic influence).

Table 11.1: Qualitative and quantitative platelet disorders

Platelet Disorders
I. Quantitative Platelet Disorders
A. Thrombocytopenia
1. Congenital
i. Deficient/ineffective thrombopoiesis Fanconi syndrome. Congenital hereditary thrombocytopenias, neonatal infections, maternal ingestion of drugs like thiazides
ii. Accelerated platelet destruction or utilisation Neonatal idiopathic thrombocytopenic purpura. Isoimmune neonatal thrombocytopenia due to platelet group incompatibility, drug sensitivity, giant haemangiomas
2. Acquired
i. Deficient/ineffective thrombopoiesis Aplastic anaemia, marrow infiltration, ionising radiation, myelosuppressive drugs, deficiency of vit B_{12} and folic acid. Viral infections (measles, dengue), paroxysmal nocturnal haemoglobinuria.
ii. Accelerated platelet destruction or utilisation Idiopathic thrombocytopenic purpura, drug-induced thrombocytopenia, SLE, disseminated intravascular coagulation, thrombotic thrombocytopenic purpura, haemolytic uraemic syndrome
iii. Thrombocytopenia due to platelet sequestration, hypersplenism, hypothermia
B. Thrombocytosis
a. Primary (essential) thrombocythemia, and other myeloproliferative disorders
b. Secondary (reactive): Chronic and acute inflammatory disorders. Acute haemorrhage, iron deficiency, postsplenectomy.
II. Qualitative Platelet Disorders
1. Congenital i. Defects of adhesion: Bernard-Soulier syndrome, von Willebrand syndrome ii. Defects of ADP aggregation: Thrombasthenia (Glanzmann's), afibrinogenemia iii. Defective release reaction: Storage poor disease, cyclo-oxygenase deficiency
2. Acquired: Drug-induced (aspirin, nonsteroidal anti-inflammatory agents), uraemia, liver diseases, myeloproliferative disorders, dysproteinemias

Disorders of Coagulation: Inherited and Acquired

The three common inherited disorders of deficiency of coagulation factors are: haemophilia A, haemophilia B and von Willebrand disease. Majority of patients of coagulation disorders bleed into muscles, joints and bony cavities. Acquired coagulation disorders are DIC, vitamin K deficiency and liver disease.

Haemophilia A: Factor VIII Deficiency

Factor VIII is a glycoprotein and a critical component of clotting cascade. It is deficient in haemophilia A. It has 2 components

- VIIIc—the smaller, procoagulant fraction is synthesized in liver.
- vWF—the larger fraction: von Willebrand factor is a carrier for F VIIIc and is reduced in von Willebrand disease (Table 11.2).

- vWF is synthesized by endothelial cells and megakaryocytes.

Table 11.2: Factor VIII and its subunits vWF and VIIIc		
FVIII =	*vWF+*	*VIIIc*
	Synthesized by - Endothelial cells - Megakaryocytes	Synthesized in liver
	Under control of gene on chromosome 12 ↓	Under control of X-linked gene ↓
	Responsible for platelet adhesion (and aggregation to ristocetin *in vitro*) ↓ Essential for formation of haemostatic plug	Responsible for intrinsic pathway ↓ Deficient in haemophilia A

Pathogenesis: It is due to deficiency of FVIIIc—the procoagulant fraction of FVIII.

Severity of disease is based on the amount of FVIII activity (Table 11.3).

Inheritance

- X-linked recessive disease and the gene is present on X chromosome.
- As males have only one X chromosome and the X^h gene is defective, therefore, synthesis of FVIII is reduced.
- Males are the sufferers and females are the carriers, rare female homozygous cases are encountered (Fig. 11.8).

Laboratory investigations

- Bleeding time—normal
- Clotting time—prolonged (not a sensitive test)
- Platelet count—normal
- Prothrombin time—normal
- Activated partial thromboplastin time (APTT)
  - Increased (normal 30–35 seconds).
  - Prolongation of APTT is dependent upon the severity of deficiency of FVIIIc.
  - APTT gets corrected on addition of normal plasma.
- Fibrinogen assay—normal
- FDP—negative
- Factor VIII assay—to assess the FVIII levels and severity of disease.

The difference between haemophilia A vs von Willebrand disease is shown in Table 11.4.

Table 11.3: Classification of severity of haemophilia A

Severity	*FVIII activity of normal*	*Incidence*	*Age of presentation*	*Clinical features*	*Joint bleeds*
Mild	5–25%	70%	Adolescence and young	Post-traumatic or surgery bleeding (severe injury)	Rare
Moderate	1–5%	15%	Children 1–5 years	Bleeding episodes + on slight injury	Some
Severe	<1%	15%	At birth	Spontaneous frequent bleeding episodes	Frequent

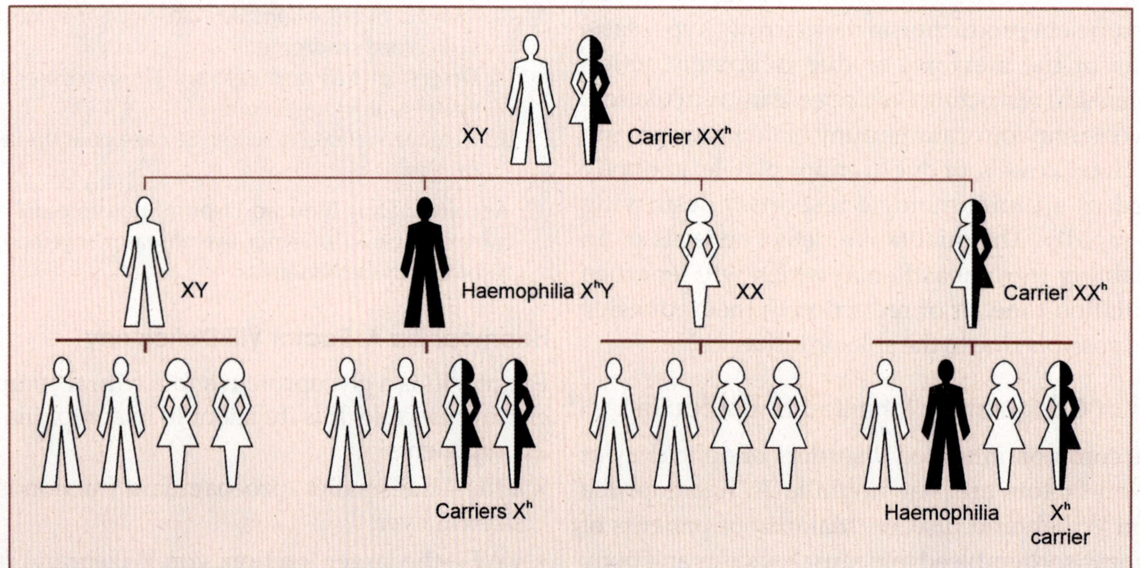

Fig. 11.8: Family tree in a case where mother is carrier for haemophilia (XX^h) and father (XY) is normal. Male child X^hY is the sufferer

Table 11.4: Haemophilia A vs von Willebrand disease

Test	*Haemophilia A*	*von Willebrand disease*
Skin, mucosa! bleeding	–	+
Haemarthrosis	++	+
Bleeding time	Normal	↑
Hess test	–	+
Clotting time	↑	↑
Prothrombin time	Normal	Normal
APTT	↑	↑
FVIII assay	↓	Normal or reduced
vWF: Ristocetin co-factor assay	N	↓

Complications of Haemophilia

1. **Hepatitis:** Patients who have received multiple transfusions of FFP or cryoprecipitate are likely to get viral hapatitis B, C, D or G and especially those who received these blood products in eighties when screening for hapatitis B, C and G was not mandatory.
2. **AIDS:** Patients who have received FFP or cryoprecipitate in eighties may get AIDS since screening for HIV was not available then.
3. **Contractures:** Contractures in muscles develop due to organisation and fibrosis of intramuscular haematomas.

HAEMOPHILIA B

Haemophilia B is due to deficiency of FIX. Haemophilia B has a prevalence of 1 in 40,000 males. It is an X-linked recessive disease.

Clinical features: Clinical features are usually milder than those of haemophilia A. In both the diseases, haemarthrosis in the age group of 5–15 years is the common presentation.

Laboratory diagnosis: Similar as for haemophilia A

- PT—normal.
- APTT—↑ (normal 30–35 seconds)
- FIX—reduced.

VON WILLEBRAND DISEASE

von Willebrand disease is the most common bleeding disorder characterised by:

1. A platelet function defect
2. A coagulation defect affecting nearly 1% of the population. It is a group of multiple disorders with variable clinical picture and modes of inheritance.

Inheritance: Inherited as autosomal codominant condition, one variant is autosomal recessive, and the other is sex-linked.

Pathogenesis: Factor VIII is made up of 2 units—the larger one is vWF and the smaller one is VIIIc.

A. Defective haemostasis

- There is deficiency of von Willebrand factor (vWF).
- Platelet adhesion: vWF mediates platelet adhesion via glycoprotein Ib (GPIb) adhesion receptor. vWF acts as a bridge between platelets and subendothelial collagen.
- Since vWF is deficient, there is defect in the adhesion of platelets to collagen affecting the formation of haemostatic plug (Fig. 11.9).

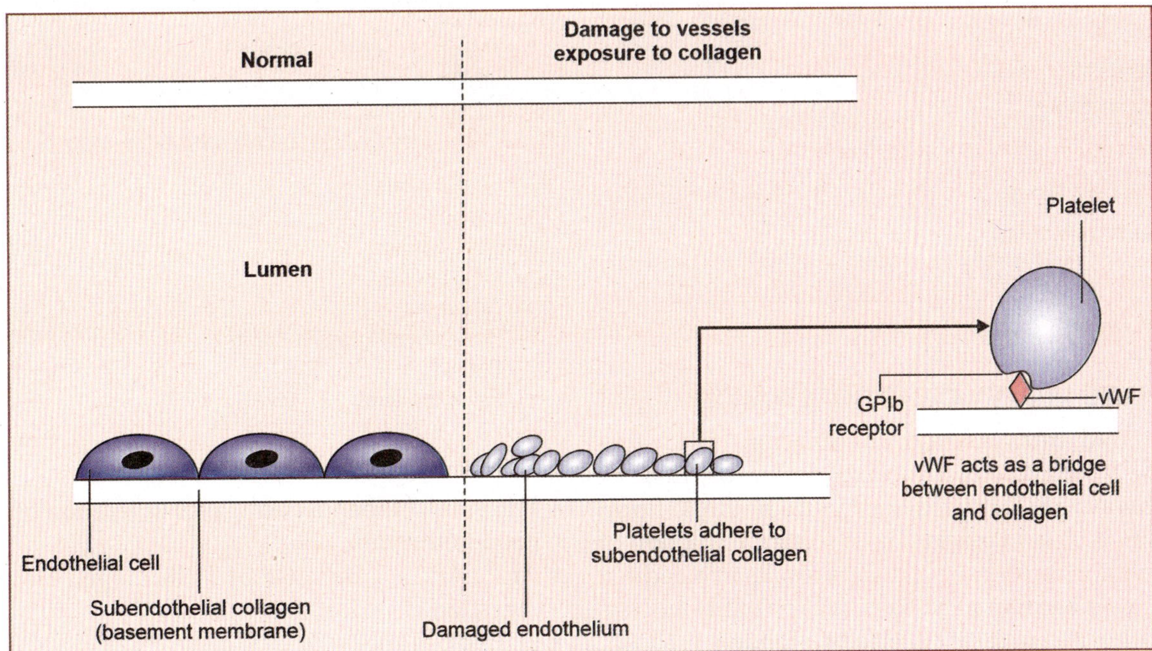

Fig. 11.9: von Willebrand factor. vWF acts as a bridge between the platelet and subendothelial collagen and is essential for platelet adherence

B. Coagulation defect

- vWF is a *carrier of VIIIc in plasma*. VIIIc is synthesized normally but has a short half-life because of reduced vWF (carrier) levels. Therefore, VIIIc deficiency in plasma results accounting for the coagulation defect.

Laboratory findings

- Tourniquet test (Hess test) is positive because of defective platelet adhesion.
- Bleeding time—prolonged because of platelet function defect.
- APTT—slightly prolonged because of secondarily reduced VIIIc activity.
- vWF assay—↓ levels
- Platelet function tests—ristocetin-induced aggregation is defective and is diagnostic of vWD.
- Platelet count—normal.

ACQUIRED COAGULATION DISORDERS

Vitamin K is required by liver to synthesize FII, VII, FIX, FX, protein C and protein S. Deficiency of Vitamin K or chronic liver disease affects the synthesis of coagulation factors. In certain diseases like DIC, widespread coagulation results in severe deficiency of coagulation factors leading to bleeding. Acquired coagulation disorders are classified in Table 11.5.

Table 11.5: Acquired coagulation disorders
1. Deficiency of Vit. K dependent factors
• Haemorrhagic disease of the newborn
• Malabsorption of vitamin K
• Biliary obstruction
• Anticoagulant therapy
+ Coumarins
+ Indanediones
2. Disseminated intravascular coagulation
3. Miscellaneous group
• Multiple myeloma
• Massive transfusion
• Liver disease

DISSEMINATED INTRAVASCULAR COAGULATION

Disseminated intravascular coagulation (DIC) is a syndrome in which either the extrinsic or intrinsic or both pathways are activated to produce multiple fibrin clots in small blood vessels. The resultant reduction of the coagulation factors and platelets results in bleeding. This process is accompanied by activation of fibrinolysis which further accentuates the bleeding tendency. Most of the DIC syndromes are acute and generalised. It is a complex systemic thrombohaemorrhagic disorder involving the generation of intravascular fibrin and the consumption of procoagulants and platelets.

Mechanism of DIC

The various aetiological factors activate:

- Extrinsic and intrinsic pathways of coagulation which result in widespread clotting in small blood vessels.
- As the fibrin monomers polymerise in the microvascular system, there is platelet entrapment in the thrombus resulting in thrombocytopenia in addition to marked reduction of clotting factors (*consumption coagulopathy*).
- Fibrinolytic system is activated simultaneously, resulting in lysis of fibrin, forming split products—fibrin degradation products (FDP) which further inhibit clot formation (Fig. 11.10) resulting in widespread bleeding.

Etiology

The various causes of acute DIC are given in Table 11.6.

Acute DIC: DIC develops acutely when sudden exposure of blood procoagulants occurs. Compensatory haemostatic mechanisms are quickly overwhelmed (Table 11.6).

Table 11.6: Causes of acute DIC
1. Obstetric complications • Amniotic fluid embolism • Eclampsia • Premature separation of placenta • Retained dead fetus/placenta
2. Malignancies • AML-M_3 (acute promyelocytic leukaemia) • Metastatic mucus secreting adenocarcinoma
3. Infections • Meningococcal septicemia • Septic abortion • *Clostridium welchii* septicemia • Gram –ve sepsis (*E. coli* and Pseudomonas)
4. Miscellaneous • Snake bite • Severe burns • Heat stroke • Anaphylaxis • Post-surgery/massive trauma • PNH • Fat embolism

Lab findings in DIC

- Thrombocytopenia because of utilization of platelets in microthrombi.
- PT ↑, APTT ↑ because of ↓ fibrinogen and plasmic digestion of various factors.
- FDP +, D-dimer +
- Thrombin time (TT) ↑ because of ↓ fibrinogen
- Presence of fragmented RBCs in the peripheral smear.

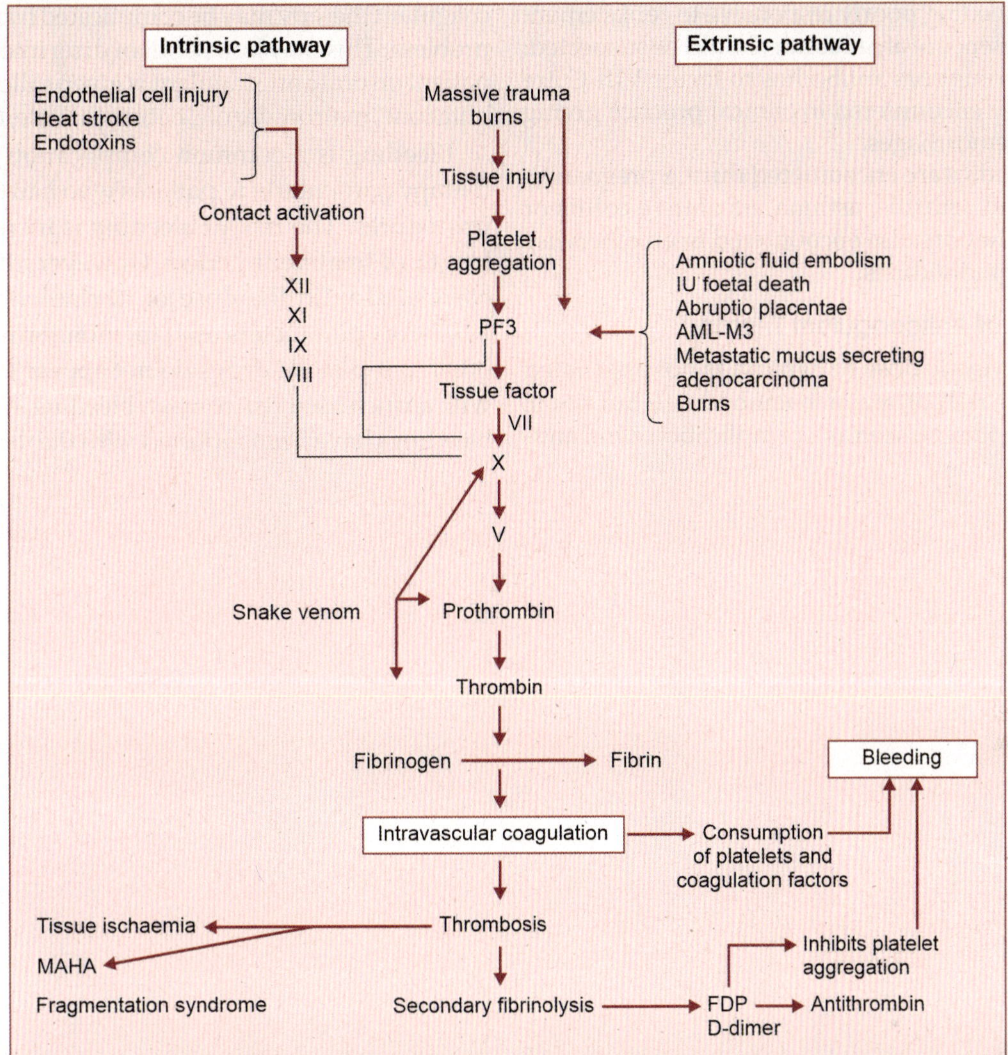

Fig. 11.10: Mechanism of DIC. Various etiological factors activate intrinsic and extrinsic coagulation cascades leading to widespread coagulation in small blood vessels resulting in consumption of coagulation factors and thrombocytopenia which promote bleeding. Bleeding is further accentuated by FDPs which inhibit platelet aggregation. (MAHA: Microangiopathic haemolytic anaemia)

LIVER DISEASE

Hepatic disease results in deficiency of factors synthesized in liver like II, VII, IX and X. Severe liver disease leads to low levels of FV and fibrinogen also. These factors are required for both extrinsic and intrinsic pathways and therefore

- PT—prolonged
- APTT—prolonged

VITAMIN K DEFICIENCY

One of the important causes of neonatal hemorrhagic disease is severe deficiency of one or more of the four vitamin K dependent coagulation factors II, VII, IX, X in the newborn the plasma level of these factors are normally lower than in adults, perhaps because vitamin K is in short supply due to lack of intestinal flora. This deficiency is augmented in some neonates, due to poor content of vitamin K in the mother's breat milk. Immaturity of the liver may also play some role. This defect is largely but not wholly, corrected by the administration of vitamin K.

In adults, it is a rare disorder and may occur due to long-term therapy with broad spectrum antibiotics which kill intestinal flora or due to long-term treatment with parenteral ailmentation without addition of vitamin K. Sometimes vitamin K deficiency may be seen in obstructive jaundice and fat malabsorption.

The bleeding seen in this group of patients varies in severity with the degree of the deficiency state and consists mainly of large cutaneous ecchymosis, petechial haemorrhages, gastrointestinal bleeding or bleeding from the nose, gums and hematuria.

Bleeding due to Presence of Inhibitors

Antibodies interfering with the haemostatic mechanism occur under a wide variety of conditions in all cases of unexplained bleeding poorly responsive to replacement therapy the presence of an inhibitor should be suspected. Among these inhibitors antibodies to factor VIII C are most frequently encountered in clinical practice giving rise to severe hemorrhages.

These antibodies are encountered during pregnancy. SLE rheumatoid arthritis, asthma, ulcerative colitis or drug allergy. They are also encountered in an otherwise healthy elderly individuals.

Complication of Anticoagulant Therapy

Usually prophylactic dose of heparin is not associated with increased risk of major haemorrhage but some minor bleeding may be seen as a complication. Oral anticoagulant therapy may be complicated by major bleeding problem. This may be a result of drug interaction when a patient on oral anticoagulant is given salicylates, phenylbutazone, metronidazole, cotrimoxazole, cimetidine, etc.

Bleeding is a common complication of fibrinolytic therapy particularly in patients who had recent invasive procedures. The risk of bleeding is increased with the length of treatment period. However, the risk is never correlated with the dose of fibrinolytic drugs or the laboratory parameters used for monitoring. Daxtran and other anti-platelet drugs do not appear to be associated with an increased risk of major bleeding. However, minor bleedings have been reported with the use of dextran.

Chapter 12

LE Cell Phenomenon and Systemic Lupus Erythematosus

Chapter Outline

INTRODUCTION

The LE cell was discovered in bone marrow in 1948 by Malcolm McCallum Hargraves (1903–1982), a physician and practising histologist at the Mayo Clinic. Hargraves may have gained priority by suppressing a publication draft of John R Haserick, who credits Dr Dorothy Sundberg, chief haematologist at the University of Minnesota Hospitals, with first identifying LE cells.

LE CELL PHENOMENON

Systemic lupus erythematosus affects women most commonly and is characterized by a skin rash, arthralgia; fever, renal, cardiac, and vascular lesions, anaemia, leukopenia, and often thrombocytopenia. There is a factor in the serum that has the ability to cause depolymerization of the nuclear chromatin of polymorphonuclear leucocytes and this depolymerized material is subsequently phagocytosed by an intact polymorph, giving rise to the "LE cell". This antinuclear material may be found in other collagen disorders, in some cases of rheumatoid arthritis, and in some cases of chronic discoid lupus erythematosus, which is a relatively benign form of the disease limited to the skin. The serum factor is an immunoglobulin and may be of the IgG, IgM, or IgA class, or combinations of them. IgG is most commonly present. There does not appear to be any relationship between the immunoglobulin class and the clinical status.

Demonstration of LE cells: A variety of methods exist, all of which can be used. The rotary technique is considered the most sensitive cellular technique. In practice, most laboratories perform a latex test and anti-DNA antibody test. If these are both negative, the LE cell preparation is not performed (vide infra).

Clotted blood: This is the simplest method and gives good results. 10 ml of clotted blood is placed in the water bath at 32°C for 1 to 2 hours. After incubation the supernatant and loose cells are withdrawn (the clot may first have to be 'ringed', or separated) and buffy coat smears made.

Alternatively, the whole clotted specimen after incubation may be mashed through a fine, wire sieve and buffy coat smears made from the resultant cell suspension.

Defibrinated blood: Defibrinated blood gives good preparations. The blood is defibrinated immediately after withdrawal and the blood incubated for 2 hours at 37°C. Smears are made as with clotted blood.

Citrated or heparinized blood: Citrated or heparinized blood may be used and incubated, as for clotted and defibrinated blood. The preparations obtained in this manner are satisfactory, but inferior to those from clotted or defibrinated blood. Also, heparin tends to produce bluish staining.

Incubated serum: The patient's serum may be incubated with washed normal leucocytes, even after storage of the serum at 20°C for months.

Rotary method: Five glass beads 3 mm in diameter are added to a heparinized sample of blood. The tube is then rotated at 50 rpm for 30 minutes at 37°C. Buffy coat smears are subsequently prepared.

THE LE CELL

A lupus erythematosus (LE) cell, also known as Hargraves cell, is a neutrophil or macrophage that has phagocytized (engulfed) the denatured material is an absorbed haematoxylin body (also called an LE body).

This is usually a neutrophil polymorph (occasionally a monocyte or eosinophil) that has ingested the altered nucleus of another polymorph. The bulk of the cell is occupied by a spherical, homogeneous mass that stains purplish-brown. The lobes of the polymorph are usually seen at the periphery of the mass. The smears (LE cells are most numerous at the edges and end of the smear), are searched and a minimum of 500 polymorphs are counted before a negative result is given. Frequently, dead nuclei will be seen lying free; if numerous, these may heighten suspicion, but they are never diagnostic. Occasionally, a group of polymorphs will collect around altered nuclear material and will form a 'Rosette'.

With the rotary technique, free extracellular altered nucleoprotein may be seen and this again will increase the suspicion of LE cells being present. LE cells must be differentiated from 'tart' cells which are usually monocytes that have phagocytosed another whole cell or nucleus (often alymphocyte). The ingested nuclear material is well preserved in contrast to the LE cell inclusion body, and may be found in normal people. Its significance, if any, is unknown.

The LE cell are a characteristic of lupus erythematosus, but also found in similar connective tissue disorders or some autoimmune diseases like in severe rheumatoid arthritis. LE cells can be observed in drug-induced lupus, e.g. following treatment with methyldopa.

Classically, the LE cell is analyzed microscopically and to differentiate from Tart cells (Figs 12.1 and 12.2), LE cells are shown in Figs 12.3 and 12.4.

LE cells should not be confused with tart cells which have engulfed nuclear material, but with a visible chromatin rather than homogeneous appearance.

Sensitivity and specificity of LE tests: The simplest test to perform is the latex nucleoprotein test. This test is specific when positive, but will detect only 45–50% of possible positives. The LE cell test is moderately sensitive and specific but both false positive and false negative results occur. Attention to technique is important and serial examinations should be performed before a patient can be considered as negative for LE. The fluorescent technique for antinuclear antibody (ANA) is a highly suitable screening procedure because of its sensitivity. It

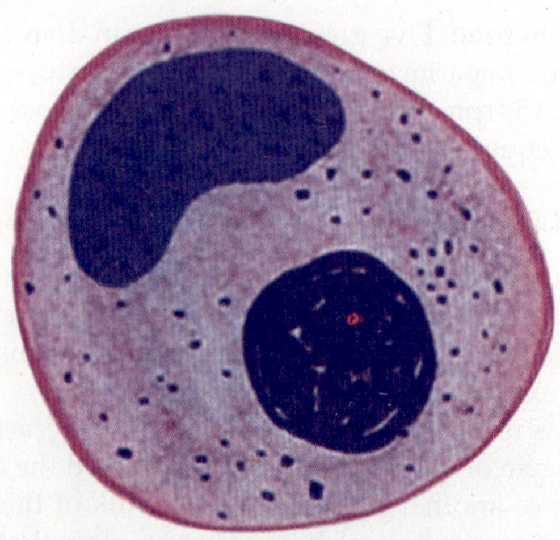

Fig. 12.1: Tart cell

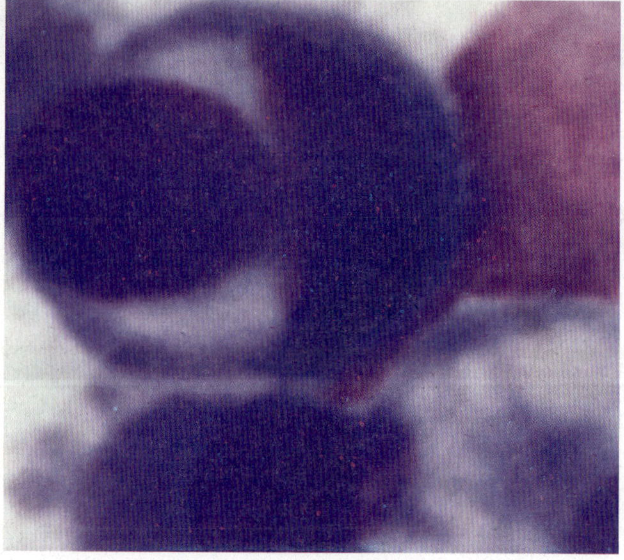

Fig. 12.2: Tart cell

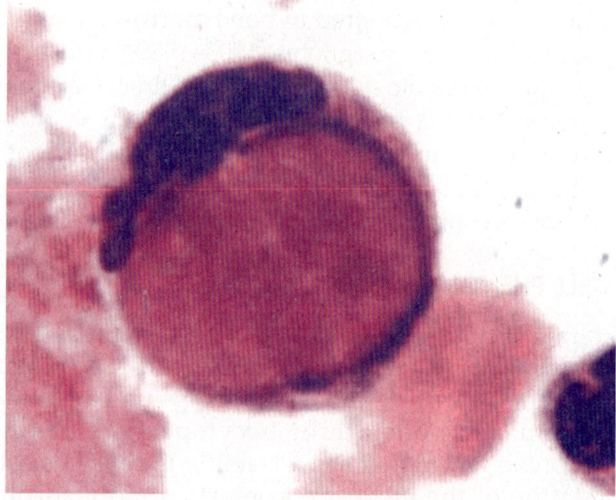

Fig. 12.3: LE cell

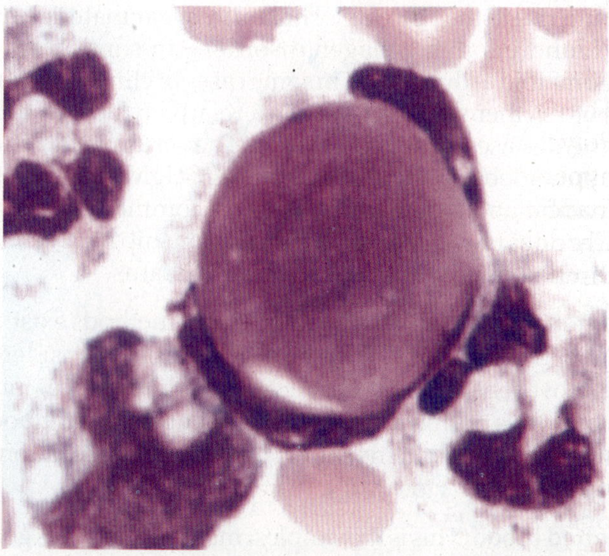

Fig. 12.4: LE cell

does, however, lack specificity and positive results can be obtained in other autoimmune and collagen diseases. A negative ANA virtually eliminates a diagnosis of LE.

SYSTEMIC LUPUS ERYTHEMATOSUS (SLE)

Definition

- Lupus erythematosus (LS) is an autoimmune disease of unknown cause involving the skin and/or other organs.
- LE is the designation of a spectrum of diseases that are linked by distinct clinical findings and distinct pattern of polyclonal B cell immunity.
- It ranges from life-threatening manifestations of systemic LE (SLE) to the limited and exclusive skin involvement in chronic cutaneous LE (CCLE).
- Lupus erythematosus is a complex and highly variable disease in which a combination of genetic, immunologic and environmental factors acts in concert with the production of the disorder.
- Systemic lupus erythematosus (SLE) is a systemic autoimmune disease with multisystem involvement and is associated with significant morbidity and mortality. Genetic, immunological, endocrine, and environmental factors influence the loss of immunological tolerance against self-antigens leading to the formation of pathogenic autoantibodies that cause tissue damage through multiple mechanisms.

PATHOGENESIS AND AETIOLOGY

Systemic lupus erythematosus (SLE) is a systemic autoimmune disease with multisystemic involvement. The condition has several phenotypes, with varying clinical presentations from mild mucocutaneous manifestations to multiorgan and severe central nervous system involvement. Several immunopathogenic pathways play a role in the development of SLE. Hargraves described the lupus erythematosus (LE cell) in 1948. Several pathogenic autoantibodies have since been identified.

- SLE results from tissue damage caused by pathogenic subsets of autoantibodies and immune complexes.
- The abnormal immune responses.
- Polyclonal and antigen-specific T and B lymphocyte hyperactivity.
- Inadequate regulation of that hyperactivity.
- Chronic multisystem inflammatory autoimmune disease.
- Associated with abnormalities of immune system.
- Results from interactions among genetic, hormonal, environmental, and immunologic factors.

Etiology: SLE is a multisystemic disease with an unknown aetiology. However, several genetic, immunological, endocrine, and environmental factors play a role in the etiopathogenesis of SLE.

Familial segregation and high concordance rates in identical twins suggest a strong genetic contribution in SLE, although there is no obvious inheritance pattern. Concordant rates for identical twins have been reported as high as 50%. Over 100 gene loci with polymorphisms (or rarely, copy numbers or mutations) have been identified to be associated with polygenic SLE (majority of cases), and more than 30 genes causing monogenic forms of SLE or SLE-like phenotype have been identified. These genes are associated with activation of the immune system in response to foreign antigens, self-antigen generation, and activation of innate and adaptive immune systems. Some gene mutations that are rare but are considered very high risk for the development of SLE include deficiencies of early complement components C1q, C1r, C1s (>90% risk), C4 (50%), C2 (20%), and TREX1.

Pathophysiology: The pathogenesis of SLE is complex, and the understanding of SLE pathogenesis is constantly evolving. A break in the tolerance in genetically susceptible individuals on exposure to environmental factors leads to the activation of autoimmunity. Cell damage caused by infectious and other environmental factors exposes the immune system to self-antigens leading to activation of T and B cells, which become self-sustained by a chronic self-aimed immune response (Fig. 12.5).

Cytokine release, complement activation, and autoantibody production lead to organ damage.

Both innate and adaptive immune systems play a role in the pathogenesis of SLE. The innate immune system activation is either toll-like receptor (TLR) dependent or independent. The cell membrane-bound TLRs (TLRs 2, 4, 6) are activated on exposure to the extracellular DNA and RNA from dying cells, which leads to downstream activation of the interferon regulatory family identified. Despite recent advances in technology and understanding of the pathological basis and risk factors for SLE, the exact pathogenesis is still not well known. Diagnosis of SLE can be challenging, and while several classification criteria have been posed, their utility in the clinical setting is still a matter of debate. Management of SLE is dictated by organ system involvement.

Despite several agents shown to be efficacious in treating SLE, the disease still poses significant morbidity and mortality risk in patients.

T-lymphocytes and B-lymphocytes play a significant role in the pathogenesis of SLE. Apoptotic and damaged cell-derived antigens are presented to T cells by antigen-presenting cells. T cells in SLE display a distorted gene expression leading to the production of several cytokines. These T cells produce less IL-2, which leads to altered regulatory T cell production. Increased IL-6, IL-10, IL-12, and IL-23 increase mononuclear cell production, while increased IL-17 and IL-21 lead to increased T cell production.

Further, the sautoreactive B cells in SLE, stimulated by self-antigens, are not readily eliminated due to a deficiency of the process involved in the functional neutralization of autoreactive B cells. The B cells can also

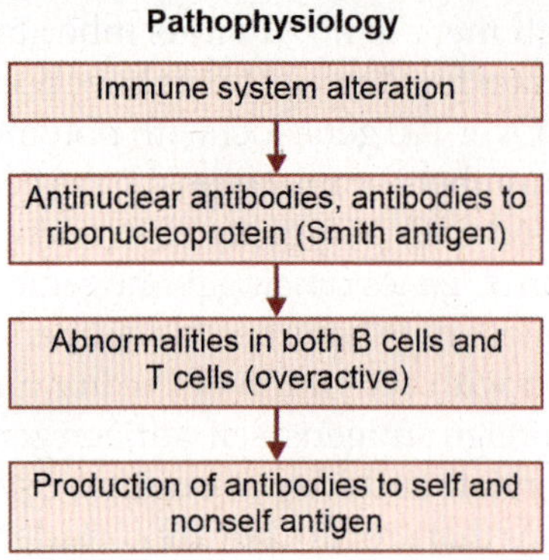

Pathophysiology

Immune system alteration
↓
Antinuclear antibodies, antibodies to ribonucleoprotein (Smith antigen)
↓
Abnormalities in both B cells and T cells (overactive)
↓
Production of antibodies to self and nonself antigen

Fig. 12.5: Pathophysiology—production of Ab to self and nonself antigen

serve as antigen-presenting cells and activate T cells by presenting internalized soluble antigens to T cells. This creates a loop where both B and T cells activate each other, leading to more autoimmunity.

Clinical features

- A chronic autoimmune disease with variable tissue, injury in multiple organs, including kidney, brain, skin, joints, heart, lungs, muscles and blood.
- Strong genetic predisposition MHC and non-MHC immune response genes, females >> males (>10/1).
- The onset may be insidious or fulminant, typically appearing in a previously healthy person in adolescence or young adulthood.
- The course is characterized by multiple flares and remissions.
- Therapy involves intensive use of high dose corticosteroids and alkylating agents or other non-specific immunosuppressive drugs.

DIAGNOSTIC TOOLS FOR SLE

Laboratory Tests

- Tests for autoantibodies:
  - Antinuclear antibody test (ANA)—major serological feature of lupus.
  - Other autoantibody test (anti-dsDNA, anti-Sm, anti-RNP, anti-Ro[SSA], anti-La[SSB])
  - Anticardiolipin antibody
- Tests for disease activity
  - Complement levels (C3, C4), anti-dsDNA
- Routine labs to monitor 'silent involvement':
  - Complete blood count
  - Erythrocyte sedimentation rate (ESR)
  - Urinalysis
  - Blood chemistries
- Kidney biopsy
- Skin biopsy

Diagnosis

- No single test establishes the diagnosis of systemic lupus.
- It is based on clinical and laboratory criteria.
- The most useful lab test is the antinuclear antibody (ANA).
- The American College of Rheumatology (ACR) recommends ANA testing in patients who have two or more unexplained signs or symptoms listed in the earlier slide.

Section 2

Body Fluids Examination

13. Urine Analysis
14. Stool Examination
15. Gastric Analysis
16. Cerebrospinal Fluid (CSF) Examination
17. Semen Analysis (Seminal Fluid Examination)
18. Examination of Sputum
19. Synovial Fluid (SF) Analysis—Synovia
20. Pericardial Fluid Analysis
21. Pleural Fluid Examination
22. Peritoneal Fluid Examination
23. Amniotic Fluid Examination

Chapter 13

Urine Analysis

Chapter Outline

- Indication for Examination of Urine
- Composition of Urine
- Qualitative Tests for Proteins in Urine
- Quantitative Tests for Albumin
- Evaluation of Renal Function Tests

INTRODUCTION

Indication for Examination of Urine

Examination of the urine is an invaluable procedure in the detection of anatomical and functional abnormalities of the kidney and the 'urinary tract'. It is one of the most important screening procedures in clinical medicine because it can give diagnostically important information about the presence of diseased states even outside the urinary tract. For example, the presence of diabetes mellitus, acidosis or jaundice can be so easily detected. Urinalysis becomes a basic investigation in conditions characterised by derangements of metabolism. Cultural examination of the urine is done for the diagnosis of enteric fevers, as also, for the detection of urinary carriers of these infections. So widespread is the utility that basic examination of the urine may be considered as part of the physical examination of a patient.

Composition of Urine

Although about 98 to 99% of the water in the glomerular filtrate is reabsorbed in the tubules, it still constitutes about 95% of the urine. The other 5% (Table 13.1) is 2% urea, and the remaining 3% is divided into small amounts between a number of inorganic and organic substances—principally sodium chloride, potassium, calcium, magnesium, ammonia, uric acid, phosphates, sulphates and creatinine. Variations in diet, work and exercise influence the relative amounts of these various constituents to a considerable degree. The blood serum level of many of these materials is preferred clinically. Therefore, the chemical determination of only those materials that are clinically significant will be considered in the examination of urine. Also, as previously indicated, the chemical composition of an individual's urine varies during different parts of the day, in relation to meals, work and sleep. Normally the total solids excreted in the urine vary from 60 to 75 g with no sugar and no protein.

A rough but valuable estimation of the total solids can be made by the following techniques:

1. The last two figures of the 24 hours specimen specific gravity × 2.33.
2. This figure × the number of ml in the 24-hour specimen.
3. This figure divided by 1000 = total solids in gm.

Table 13.1: Average normal composition of urine

Constituents	*Grams/Liter*
Inorganic	
Chloride (as NaCl)	9.0
Phosphorus (as P_2O_5)	2.0
Total sulphur (as SO_3)	1.5
Sodium (as Na_2O)	4.0
Potassium (as K_2O)	2.0
Calcium (as CaO)	0.2
Magnesium (as MgO)	0.2
Iron	0.003
Organic	
Urea	25.0
Uric acid	0.6
Creatinine	1.5
Ammonia	0.6
Undetermined N	0.6
Sugar (insufficient for positive Benedict's test)	Trace
Ketone bodies	Trace
Carbonates, bicarbonates, and free carbonic acid	Trace
Pigments	
Mucin and mucin-like substances	
Diastase	

Collection of Urine

The sample should be fresh and should be examined immediately. This is because, on keeping at room temperature, the reaction might change (from acidic to alkaline), casts might disintegrate, crystalline precipitate—not originally present—may appear and bacterial growth may make the specimen turbid. General preservation of the specimen, is done by addition of chemicals (boric acid 0.5 g per 60 ml; formaldehyde, 2 to 4 drops per 30 ml; thymol, 0.1 g per 100 ml; and toluol, enough to cover the surface on which it floats) or by keeping the specimen in a refrigerator. Special preservatives are to be used for special tests; for example, concentrated hydrochloric acid in estimations of calcium and nitrogen. Obviously, no preservatives can be added if a bacteriological (culture or animal inoculation) examination is to be done. Specimen meant for examinations, other than bacteriological, can be collected in a bottle of suitable size, cleaned with soap and water. The specimen must be properly labelled.

1. For routine examination the usual practice is to collect the early morning sample, the quantity required being about 100 ml. This sample, being the night's collection, is the most concentrated and will show casts best. On the other hand, if the objective is to determine the presence of albumin or sugar, a specimen collected 2–3 hours after a meal is preferable.
2. For any quantitative test a specimen obtained from a mixed 24 hours collection is absolutely necessary; a quantitative estimation on a random sample has no meaning.

The patient empties the bladder (say at 8 am) and this sample is discarded. Thereafter, he preserves all the urine he voids till 8 am the next day; he must empty the bladder at this time (8 am) and this sample must be added to the total collection. The collection is done in a large bottle of suitable size; a preservative may be added. The whole quantity is thoroughly mixed, its volume measured and about 150 to 200 ml submitted for examination.

Preservation of Specimen

Urinary decomposition occurs quickly in warm temperatures. Hence, fresh specimens should be examined, if not, then it should be refrigerated. As far as possible, the need for preservation should not arise. However, the following preservatives can be used:

1. **Tolunol:** Best for preservation of chemical constituents. Add 2 ml toluol/100 ml urine.
2. **Thymol:** A small floating lump of thymol can preserve the urine for several days in a bottle. Thymol may, however, cause a false positive reaction for protein.
3. **Formalin:** 1 drop/30 ml urine is good for preserving formed elements. It can precipitate proteins and can reduce Benedict's solution.
4. **Boric acid:** 0.3 g/120 ml of urine. However, yeasts can still grow and urine acid crystals get precipitated.

Routine Examination of Urine

Physical Examination

1. Total volume

The quantity of the urine passed in 24 hours varies inversely with the amount of fluid eliminated by the lungs, the skin and the bowels, and is influenced by physiological factors like fluid intake; diet (a high protein diet having a diuretic effect), exercise, environmental temperature and humidity, body-weight and age. Infants and children excrete for their weight, 3–4 times more urine than adults.

Polyuria increases in the output of urine and is seen in diabetes mellitus, diabetes insipidus, early stage of chronic nephritis and during recovery from oedema. In renal insufficiency the night urine may exceed the day urine (nocturia). *Oliguria* is diminution in the urinary output; this is seen in acute and chronic glomerulonephiritis, congestive cardiac failure, shock fevers and dehydration from any cause. *Anuria* is suppression of urine formation, the output falling to less than 100 ml. It is seen commonly in acute glomerulonephiritis, in chronic renal disease (terminally), crushed injury and after a mismatched blood transfusion.

Serial measurement of the total urinary excretion is an important procedure in gauging the efficacy of the treatment of oedema.

2. Specific gravity

A twenty-four hours sample is to be preferred. The urine should be taken in a cylindrical or conical urine-glass and the urinometer floated in it freely. Urinometers are usually calibrated for 20°C. So the observed figure has to be corrected for the difference between this temperature and the room temperature in the proportion of 0.001 to every 3°C.

In health the specific gravity of urine is directly proportional to the concentration of dissolved solids and inversely to the volume. This relationship between the volume and the specific gravity is lost in disease; in diabetes mellitus the volume is increased as also the specific gravity over (1040) due to presence of sugar), while in the late stage of chronic glomerulornephritis the urine passed is of low specific gravity (below 1010) despite the low total volume. Proteinuria (albuminuria) raises the specific gravity (as in the nephrotic syndrome). The fixity of the specific gravity round about 1010—inability of the kidney to lower the specific gravity (or raise the volume) on a high fluid intake, or raise the specific gravity (or lower the volume) on a restricted fluid intake—is an indication of renal insufficiency or defective resorptive power of the renal tubule. The dilution and concentration tests for renal efficiency are based on this principle.

3. Colour

Under normal conditions the colour of the urine varies directly with the concentration because *urochrome*, the chief normal pigment, is a product of endogenous metabolism and excreted in constant quantities independent of the diet. Another yellow pigment normally present in the urine, *urobilin*, is derived from the urobilinogen formed in the intestinal tract and absorbed into the blood stream. With increased blood destruction, as in pernicious anaemia or haemolytic icterus, increased quantities of urobilin are formed, resorbed, escape from the liver into the general circulation and are excreted in the urine. In liver damage increased amounts of urobilin likewise may appear in the urine. A positive test for urobilin, therefore, indicates increased blood destruction or pathologic changes in the liver.

Other pigments (Table 13.2) that may colour the urine include bilirubin or its oxidation product *biliverdin*. Bile pigments are present in the urine only when some obstruction within the duct system or hepatocellular damage prevents their normal excretion by the liver.

Table 13.2: Abnormal colour of urine

Substance	*Colour*	*Pathological states occurring in*
Bilirubin	Yellowish foam	Obstructive lesion of bile duct system or severe hepatocellular damage
Biliverdin	Greenish foam	Oxidation product from bilirubin
Increased urobilin	Yellow to amber	Increased blood destruction or pathological changes in liver
Porphyrins	Reddish	Congenital porphyria, lead and barbital poisoning, pernicious anaemia, and haemolytic jaundice
Haemo-globin	Clear red to reddish brown	Paroxysmal haemoglobinuria, malaria, transfusion reaction, arsenic poisoning
Blood	Smoky red to brown	Acute nephritis, intaremcts in kidneys, bleeding lesions in urogenital tract
Melanin	Brown to black	Malignant melanoma, leukaemia, ochronosis, and carcinoma of liver
Homo-gentisic acid	Black	A congenital anomaly, alkapto-nuria
Methylene blue	Blue	Administered for renal function test
Pyridium	Orange to red	Administreed as urinary analgesic
Acriflavine	Greenish fluorescence	Administered as urinary anti-septic
Phenol	Dark, smoky	Poisoning
Phenolsul-fonphthalein	Red in alka-line urine	Administration as laxative or for renal function test
Bromsul-phalein	Red in alka-line urine	Administration as liver function test

4. Turbidity

Freshly voided acid urine is clear. However, when alkaline it may be cloudy due to the presence of phosphates. Pus and blood also may cause turbidity, the former being white, whereas the latter produces a red smoky appearance. Upon standing urine may show clouding to the point of sediment formation from bacterial decomposition or precipitation of alkaline salts, mostly amorphous phosphates, or a white to pinkish sediment of amorphous urates in acid urine. A faint cloud of mucus, leukocytes and epithelial cells may become visible. All these must be differentiated by microscopic examination.

5. Odour

The normal odour is due to volatile aromatic acids and urinoid. An ammoniacal odour, in a freshly passed sample, is due to decomposition from stasis in the bladder, and is present in cystitis. Fruity odour is present when the urine contains acetone bodies.

Chemical Examination

Reaction: This is tested by means of red and blue litmus papers. It is recorded as acidic, alkaline or amphoteric. The reaction has diagnostic significance. The pH of the urine in health varies between 5 and 7.5. This can also be tested by pH-papers.

QUALITATIVE TESTS FOR PROTEINS IN URINE

Heat and Acetic Acid Test

Procedure: In a 6 × 5/8 inch test tube place about 10 ml of urine; make acidic with a few drops of 30% v/v acetic acid. Heat the top inch of the urine in a small Bunsen flame. If a cloudy precipitate appears in the heated portion of the urine, add a few more drops of 30% v/v acetic acid and reheat. If the precipitate persists, proteins are present.

Methods for recording reactions: A wide diversity of methods for reporting qualitative tests is in use which accounts, in large part, for discrepancies in reports from different laboratories. A uniform method and terminology are urgently needed. The following are recommended:

− = negative

± = *very slight trace*. Cloudiness or ring can just be seen against a black background (0.01% or less).

+ (1) = *slight trace*. Cloud is distinct but not granular; no definite flocculation, or the ring is sufficiently definite to be seen without a black background (0.01 to 0.05%).

+ + (2) = *moderate trace*. Cloud is distinct and granular without definite flocculation, or the ring is dense but not wholly opaque when viewed from above (0.05 to 0.2%).

+ + + (3) = *heavy cloud*. Cloud is dense with marked flocculation or the ring is heavy, wholly opaque and sometimes curdy (0.2 to 0.5%).

+ + + + (4) = *very heavy cloud*. Heavy precipitate to boiling solid; or very dense ring. Represents 0.5 or higher per cent of albumin: 3% albumin boils solid.

Sulphosalicylic Acid Test

Procedure: Layer onto about 3 ml of urine in a test tube an equal quantity of 10% w/v sulphosalicylic acid in 50% methanol. If proteins are present, a cloudy precipitate will appear at the junction of the two fluids.

Heller's Ring Test

Reagent: Nitric acid, concentrated, or 1 part of concentrated nitric acid + 5 parts of a saturated aqueous solution of magnesium sulphate (Robert's reagent).

Take 2 to 3 ml of the reagent in a test tube, and allow filtered urine to run slowly down the inside of the tube from a pipette so as to form a layer on top of the acid. Note whether a ring appears or not.

When the test is positive, a sharply defined white ring of varying density appears where the two fluids come into contact. If only trace of albumin is present, the ring appears after a few minutes.

Uric acid, urea, thymol, and resinous drugs, when present in urine in high concentrations, may give a white crystalline precipitate which however disappears on dilution, and when due to resinous drugs, dissolves in alcohol.

Robert's Test

Reagent: To 5 parts of a saturated solution of magnesium sulphate add one part of pure nitric acid.

Place a few ml of the reagent in a test tube and gently layer the urine on the reagent. Albumin gives a white ring which varies in density with the amount of albumin present. When only traces of albumin are present, the white ring may not appear 2–3 minutes.

QUANTITATIVE TESTS FOR ALBUMIN

Esbach's Test

Prepare the reagent by dissolving 5 g of picric acid and 10 g of citric acid in 500 ml of water. Or, the reagent may be prepared by diluting 100 ml of trichloracetic acid with 900 ml of water.

Fill an Esbach's albuminometer with urine to the mark "U". Add reagent to the mark "R". Close with a rubber stopper, invert several times and set aside in a cool place for 18 to 24 hours. Read off the results according to the markings on the tube which show albumin in grams per litre; to express the per cent, divide by 10.

Bence Jones Protein Test

Bence Jones protein is particularly pathognomic of multiple myeloma. Proteins with somewhat similar characteristics have been observed in leukaemia, osteomalacia and in young persons with high blood pressure. The protein is characterized by the formation of a precipitate when urine is heated at 50° to 60°C. It disappears wholly or partially as the temperature approaches the boiling point and reappears upon cooling. It is markedly influenced by the acidity and salt-concentration.

Technique: It is advisable to put up three tubes of different acidity . Filter the urine if it is not clear, and adjust to a pH just faintly acid to litmus. Put a few ml of this urine into each of three tubes. To the second and third add respectively 1 and 2 drops of 33% acetic acid. Place the tubes in a water bath with a thermometer and heat very slowly and gently. Turbidity will begin to appear at about 40°C and precipitates will be visible at 60°C. Now raise the temperature to 100°C. The precipitate now partly or totally disappears. Allow to cool, and the precipitate will reappear.

Urine containing albumin should be filtered at or near the boiling point and the filtrate is tested for Bence Jones protein.

When only small amount of Bence Jones protein is present, electrophoresis is particularly useful.

Toluenesulfonic acid test: Add 1 ml of TSA reagent to 2 ml of urine, let the reagent flow slowly by the side of the test tube. Mix. A precipitate appearing within 5 minutes, indicates presence of Bence Jones protein. A negative test excludes.

Bence Jones proteins are microglobulins and like haemoglobin are synthesised by plasma cells, both normal and neoplastic (myeloma cells). Bence Jones proteinuria is seen most commonly in multiple myelomatosis (in 50% of cases); uncommonly, it is also seen in leukaemias and other malignant lymphomas, metastatic carcinoma of bone, senile osteomalacia and primary amyloidosis. In multiple myelomatosis combined serum and urine electrophoresis for Bence Jones protein is the procedure of choice.

Test for Mucin

Principle: The exact chemical nature of mucin has not been determined but it appears to be a glycoprotein. Traces may be present in normal urine. It is frequently increased in irritations and inflammations of the mucous membrane of the urinary tract or vagina. Upon boiling with an acid or alkali, as in Fehling test, it may yield a carbohydrate which reduces copper. Mucin must be differentiated from the Bence Jones protein.

Procedure

1. Dilute the urine with about 3 volumes of water and make strongly acid with glacial acetic acid. Do not heat.
2. The presence of turbidity indicates a positive reaction. Albumin is not precipitated by this concentration of acetic acid.

Reducing Substances in Urine

Normally, detectable amounts of reducing substances are not found in urine, except in renal glycosuria. The reducing substance most commonly found in urine is glucose, and its presence there indicates either renal glycosuria, diabetes mellitus, miscellaneous endocrine disorders, intravenous infusion of glucose, or increased intracranial pressure. Other sugars sometimes appears in the urine, e.g. lactose, fructose, pentose, and galactose.

In pregnancy lactosuria occurs at some time in about one-half, glycosuria in about one-fifth, and both sugars together in about one-sixth of the patients, on the average.

Other Reducing Substances

A number of reducing substances other than sugars may be present in urine. Dextrins from ingested pastry, homogentisic acid, and glucuronates reduce Benedict's reagent, although the reduction by homogentisic acid is atypical, ultimately forming a black colour. Preservatives, such as chloroform and formaldehyde, indican, santonin, rhubarb, ascorbic acid, creatinine, and protein may react with Benedict's reagent producing a false positive reaction.

Tests for Reducing Substances in Urine

Benedict's Qualitative Test (Table 13.3)

This test is not specific for sugars and is affected by most reducing substances if they occur in large quantities.

Procedure: In a Pyrex test tube place 0.5 ml (10 drops) of urine and 5.0 ml of Benedict's qualitative reagent. Mix and place in a boiling water bath for five minutes. Allow to cool to room temperature and read as follows:

Table 13.3: Benedict's qualitative tests

Colour	*Observation*	*Result*
Blue	–	Negative
Greenish blue	Tr.	Trace
Green	+	Approximately 0.5% reducing substance
Greenish brown	+ +	Approximately 1.0% reducing substance
Yellow	+ + +	Approximately 1.5% reducing substance
Brick red	+ + + +	Approximately 2.0% reducing substance

Benedict's Quantitative Method

Reagents:

Copper sulphate (pure crystallized)	18 g
Sodium carbonate (crystallized)	200 g
Sodium or potassium citrate	200 g
Potassium ferrocyanide solution (5%)	5 ml
Potassium sulfocyanate	125 g
Distilled water to make	1000 ml

With the aid of heat dissolve the carbonate, citrate, and sulphocyanate in about 700 ml of water and filter. Dissolve the copper sulphate in 100 ml of water stirring constantly. Add the ferrocyanide solution, cool and dilute to 1 litre. The solution now is of such strength that the copper sulphate in 25 ml is reduce by 0.05 g of dextrose.

Technique: Take 25 ml of the reagent in a small flask, add 10 to 20 g of sodium carbonate crystals, and a small quantity of powdered pumice stone. Boil and add the urine a little at a time, but rapidly, from a burette until a chalk-white precipitate forms and the blue colour of the reagent begins to fade. At this point, add urine in drops, until the last trace of blue just disappears. During the period of titration, the mixture must be kept boiling vigorously. Loss of evaporation must be made good by adding sufficient water. Note the quantity of urine required to discharge the blue colour; this amount of urine contains exactly 0.05 g of dextrose.

Thus if 'x' ml of urine is required to reduce 25 ml of Benedict's solution, 0.05 g of dextrose is then present in 'x' ml of urine. Or 100 ml of urine contains $(0.05/x) \times 100$ g of dextrose, i.e. $(5/x)$ g.

If the sugar is shown to be mainly lactose, the following figure may be used in the calculations:

25 ml of reagent = 67 mg of lactose.

Acetone Bodies (Ketone Bodies)

The acetone bodies are acetoacetic acid (diacetic acid) acetone and β-hydroxybutyric acid. A state in which these substances are present in increased amounts in the blood and urine is called *ketosis* and is one type of acidosis. Ketonuria indicates abnormal fat metabolism. Acetoaceric acid and β-hydroxybutyric acid, from which acetone is derived, are normal intermediate products of fat metabolism. When greater amounts of fatty acids are utilized with the production of more acetoacetic acid and β-hydroxybutyric acid than can be oxidized by the tissues, these materials accumulate in the blood and are excreted in the urine. Thus ketosis develops in any of the clinical states of deficient carbohydrate metabolism. The most important of these is diabetes mellitus. A ketosis develops with starvation as the carbohydrate stores are depleted and metabolism of fat predominates. A special type of starvation ketos develops with prolonged vomiting or diarrhea. An interesting but rare condition described by van Creveld associated with a ketos is von Gierke's diseases, in which carbohydrate is stored to an excessive degree in the liver and other organs, but the mobilization is poor. The level of blood sugar is subnormal.

Tests for Acetone Bodies in Urine

Rothera's Test for Acetone and Acetoacetic (Diacetic) Acid

Principle: Both acetone and diacetic acid give a purple colour with alkaline sodium nitroprusside. The test will detect acetone in a dilution of 1 in 10, 000 and diacetic acid in a dilution of 1 in 125, 000.

Procedure: In a test tube place a small crystal of sodium nitroprusside; add about 2 g of ammonium sulphate and about 10 ml of the urine under examination. After shaking well, add about 2 ml of concentrated ammonium hydroxide solution (sp gr 0.88). A deep purple colour indicates the presence of excessive amounts of acetone or diacetic acid or both. A pale purple colour or no colour at all is a negative reaction.

Gerhardt's Test for Acetoacetic (Diacetic) Acid

Principle: Diacetic acid gives a Bordeaux red colour with ferric chloride solution. Many other substances give coloured products with this reagent and it is important to determine whether the colour obtained with a particular urine is the result of the presence of diacetic acid or of some other substance. The excreted derivatives of aspirin are the most common substances that interfere with this test.

Procedure: Place about 5 ml of urine in a test tube and to it add drop by drop, 10% w/v ferric chloride solution until no more precipitate forms; then add two more drops. In the presence of excessive quantities of diacetic acid a Bordeaux red colour will develop. Aspirin gives a purple colour with this reagent, but it may be confused with the diacetic acid reaction. Therefore, the presence of diacetic acid must be confirmed as follows: Place about 5 ml of urine in a Pyrex test tube and boil it over a Bunsen flame for 3 minutes, or place it in a boiling water bath for 15 minutes. This will convert all the diacetic acid to acetone which will then be volatilized. After it cools, the urine is treated as before with ferric chloride solution. If diacetic acid was present, the test will now be negative. If aspirin or other similar drugs are present, the test will still be positive.

Causes of Ketonuria

1. **Diabetic:** Ketonuria indicates ketoacidosis and if unchecked may go on to coma. Juvenile diabetics are more susceptible to develop this. Whenever glycosuria is more than 2 +, always test for ketone bodies also.
2. **Non-diabetic:** In infants and children in
   - Acute febrile states.
   - Toxic states with vomiting, diarrhoea, etc.
   - Hyperemesis gravidarum.
   - Cachexia with vomiting.
   - Post-anaesthesia vomiting.
   - Conditions where there is limited availability of glucose, e.g. glycogen storage disease.
   - Sometimes following exposure to cold or severe exercise.

Urobilin and Urobilinogen

Urobilinogen, urobilin, stercobilinogen, and stercobilin are decomposition products of bilirubin, normally present in the faeces. In conditions in which there is increased excretion of bile by the liver, e.g. haemolytic jaundice, increased amounts of these substances are absorbed from the intestine and are excreted in the urine. Although it is customary to refer to the substances in the urine as urobilinogen and urobilin, stercobilinogen and stercobilin are usually present in higher concentrations than the former.

Schlesinger's Test for Total Urobilinogen and Urobilin

Principle: Urobilinogen is oxidized with iodine to urobilin. The urobilin is then reacted with an alcoholic solution of zinc acetate and a green fluorescent complex is formed.

Procedure: If bilirubin is present, it is removed by adding a few ml of 10% w/v barium chloride solution to about 20 ml of urine and filtering. Place about 10 ml of urine or bilirubin-free filtrate of urine in a test tube and add two or three drops of Lugol's iodine solution. In another test tube place about 1 g of solid zinc acetate and add about 10 ml of ethyl alcohol; mix by shaking. Pour the urine into the zinc acetate solution and shake thoroughly. Filter through a Whatman No. 1 filter paper into a clean dry test tube. Examine the filtrate for green fluorescence, using either daylight or an ultraviolet lamp. Normal urine shows a faint green fluorescence. A definite green fluorescence indicates an increased output of urobilin (ogen).

Ehrlich's test: Nitrites and bilirubin interfere with this test. Sulfonamide and procaine cause yellowish colour reactions. Pyridium, indole, porphobilinogen and PAS yield pink-red colour not different from that produced by urobilinogen.

To 10 ml of fresh sample at room temperature add 1 ml of Ehrlich's reagent, invert several times and let stand for 5 minutes. A pink colour is normal; cherry or darker red colour indicates abnormal amount of urobilinogen. Dilutions may be used. Colour reactions are normal in dilutions up to 1:20 (sensitivity ≥1.3 mgm%).

Bile

The constituents or derivatives of bile that may appear in the urine are the bile pigments bilirubin and biliverdin; bile acids, chiefly glycocholic acid; urobilin and urobilinogen. The presence of bile pigments and acids together is associated with obstruction to the outflow of bile from the liver. This may be either intra- or extrahepatic. Urinary excretion of bilirubin alone is seen in conditions of excessive haemolysis. Increased amounts of urobilin point to functional incapacity of the liver. Urobilinogen normally is present in the urine in amounts sufficient to give a positive test in dilutions of 1:10 to 1:20. Its absence indicates complete biliary obstruction while increased amounts are associated with excessive blood destruction.

Detection of Bile Pigment (Bilirubin and Biliverdin)

Foam test: A yellow or brownish colour of the foam produced by vigorous shaking of a sample of urine is suggestive evidence of the presence of bilirubin and usually bile acids in the urine.

Gmelin's test: To a few ml of urine in a test tube add a small amount of concentrated nitric acid in such a manner that two layers are formed. The formation of a rainbow band of colours at the junction of the layers shows the presence of bilirubin. The colours result from the oxidation of bilirubin.

Iodine ring test: A sensitive cum reliable test. Layer a solution 10%, alcoholic iodine on urine in a test tube. A green ring indicates presence of bile.

Fouchet's Test

Principle: Barium chloride solution is added to the urine. A precipitate of barium sulphate is produced onto which the bilirubin is adsorbed. The barium sulphate adsorbed bilirubin is filtered off and a drop of Fouchet's ferric chloride solution added to the precipitate. The ferric chloride oxidizes the bilirubin to biliverdin, producing a greenish blue spot.

Procedure: Take 10 ml of the urine in a test tube and add 5 ml of barium chloride solution (10% aqueous) to precipitate bilirubin. Mix and filter through Whatman No. 2 filter paper, unfold the paper and invert it on another paper to gently transfer the precipitate. To the second paper now add 1–2 drops of Fouchet's reagent (25 g of trichloroacetic acid. 100 ml of water and 10 ml of 10% ferric chloride solution). Fouchet's reagent oxidises bilirubin to produce a green or blue colour.

Test for Bile Salts (Hay's Sulphur Test)

Take 5 ml of the urine in a test tube and sprinkle on the surface flowers of sulphur. If bile salts are present, sulphur particles sink to the bottom of the tube because bile salts have lowered the surface tension. The urine sample must be fresh and a control with the normal urine should also be done.

In hepatocellular jaundice (infectious hepatitis) there are bile pigments in urine even before jaundice becomes clinically detectable choluria is also present in obstructive jaundice. In haemolytic jaundice there is acholuria, though the urinary urobilinogen is raised.

Blood

Blood present in the urine may be in the form of either intact cells, haematuria, or haemoglobin, haemoglobinuria. Haematuria may be detected by microscopic examination and haemoglobinuria by chemical test.

Haemoglobin, unaccompanied by red cells, appears in the urine with excessive haemolysis in a number of toxic states; notably, in mushroom poisoning, in poisoning by beans of the species *Vicia fava* (favism), following severe burns, in the black-water fever of falciparum malaria, and following reaction from mismatched transfusion. Poisoning by certain chemicals, notably arsine potassium chlorate and pyrogallic acid produce haemolysis with presence of haemoglobin in the urine. *Paroxysmal* haemoglobinuria may occur with exposure to cold and is associated usually with syphilis and the development of specific haemolysins as shown by the Donath-Landsteiner test. In a second type (nocturnal paroxysmal haemoglobinuria) the attacks are not associated with chilling and usually come on at night. In the march variety, haemoglobinuria appears with severe muscular exertion.

Detection of Blood

Benzidine test: Dissolve a small amount (knife-point full) of benzidine base in 2 ml of glacial acetic acid and add an equal volume of 3% hydrogen peroxide. Add 2 ml of urine and mix. The appearance of blue colour indicates the presence of haemoglobin. Inferior grades of benzidine may require the addition of larger amounts to obtain a positive reaction.

Guaiac test: Acidify a portion of urine with glacial acetic acid. Add a fresh alcoholic solution of gum guaiac, drop by drop, until there is a slight turbidity. Add a few ml of 3% hydrogen peroxide solution. Development of a blue colour indicates the presence of haemoglobin.

Pus will produce the blue colour but not if the urine is previously boiled.

A thin film of copper left in the tube after testing for sugar will give a positive reaction as will bromides and iodides.

If minute amounts of blood cells are present, the tests are best performed on the sediment from a centrifuged specimen.

Test for Homogentisic Acid

Alcaptonuria is an inborn error of metabolism characterised by a failure to oxidise completely tyrosine and phenylalanine and the resulting excretion in the urine of homogentisic acid.

Technique

1. **Alkali test:** Addition of 10%. NaOH solution to alcaptonuric urine produces a brown colour in 1 to 2 minutes.

2. **Ferric chloride test:** Upon the addition of dilute ferric chloride solution to the sample of urine, a deep blue colour appears for a moment until oxidation is complete.

Phenylketonuria

Phenylketonuria is a hereditary metabolic defect due to the lack of the enzyme phenylalanine hydroxylase. This results in blocking the conversion of phenylalanine, an essential amino acid, into tyrosine. The accumulation of phenylalanine and/or some of its abnormal metabolites early, perhaps by age 4 to 6 months, results in brain damage and mental retardation. The disease phenylpyruvic oligophrenia develops characterized by severe mental deficiency with elevated serum phenylalanine and a large amount of phenylpyruvic being excreted in the urine. Early detection and proper dietary regime can prevent the development of this disease.

Detection of Phenylpyruvic Acid

Ferric chloride diaper test: A drop of 5 or 10% ferric chloride is placed on the diaper which is wet with urine. A gray green or blue-green spot indicates phenylketonuria.

Ferric chloride tube test: Five drops of 5% ferric chloride are added to acid urine or to urine which has been acidified with dilute sulfuric acid. A dark green colour indicates phenylpyruvic acid.

Test for 5-Hydroxyindoloacetic Acid (HIAA)

In the malignant carcinoid syndrome excessive amounts 5 of HIAA are excreted in the urine . This can be detected as follows:

Technique: 0.2 ml of urine, 0.8 ml of distilled water, and 0.5 ml of 1-nitroso-2-naphthol solution are mixed in a test tube. Add 0.5 ml of freshly prepared nitrous acid solution and let stand for 1 minute. Add 5 ml of ethylene dichloride and shake.

Reagents

1. 1 g of 1-nitroso-naphthol in 100 ml of 95% ethyl alcohol.
2. Nitrous acid (0.2 ml of 2.5% sodium nitrite added to 5.0 ml of 2 N H_2SO_4).

A normal urine should be tested as a control. A purple colour of the top layer indicates increased 5-HIAA excretion.

Calcium

Before the estimation of urinary calcium the patient should be on low calcium diet for 3 days. An aliquot of a 24-hour urine collection is utilized.

Sulkowitch Test

Reagent

Oxalic acid	2.5 g
Ammonium oxalate	2.5 g
Glacial acetic acid	5.0 ml
Distilled water q.s	150 ml

Procedure: To 3 ml of clear urine are added 3 ml of Sulkowitch reagent and they are mixed. After 2 minutes the degree of turbidity is estimated by a scale of 0 (no precipitate) to 4 + (a flocculent precipitate).

Interpretation: A zero test indicates hypocalcemia with a serum level below 7.5 mg per 100 ml, the renal threshold. With a normal serum calcium of 9.5 to 11.5 mg per 100 ml there is a moderate amount of turbidity. A 3 or 4 + test indicates hypercalcuria and suggests hypercalcemia, such as in hyperparathyroidism.

Cystine

To 5 ml of urine add 2 ml of 5% sodium cyanide solution and let them react for 10 minutes. Add 5 drops of 5% sodium nitroprusside solution and mix thoroughly. Cystine produces a magenta colour. If no cystine is present, a pale brown or pale pink colour results. All solutions should be freshly prepared. Also examine the urinary sediment for cystine crystals. Urinary cystine is raised in cystinurias.

Fat in urine

Take equal parts of urine and ether; cloudiness due to fat disappears, decant ether onto a watch glass, evaporate; fat leaves a greasy deposit. Fat may be seen microscopically.

Porphyrins

The porphyrin nucleus is a structural component of haemoglobin, myoglobin, cytochromes, catalases, oxidases and peroxidases. Characteristic magenta fluorescence is seen when acidic solutions of porphyrins are irradiated with ultraviolet light.

In *porphyria* increased amounts of uroporphyrin or protoporphyrin are present in urine. Coproporphyrins also may be present. All are derived from prophobilinogen. The porphyrias are of two types, *porphyria erythropoietica* and *porphyria hepatica,* depending upon the pathway of synthesis. Porphyria erythropoietica has its onset in infancy or childhood. Bullous skin lesions appear on exposure to light. The urine is a burgundy-red colour which darkens with standing. Laboratory identification of uroporphyrins but no porphobilinogen confirms the diagnosis. Porphyria hepatica may be of the intermittent acute type, a chronic disease of adults in which gastrointestinal and neurological symptoms predominate; the cutanea tarda type, in which photosensitivity becomes manifest in adult life, and the mixed type in which symptoms of both are combined. Porphobilinogen is characteristic of the disease but its identification in the urine is difficult. Porphobilinogen in urine exposed to air will be converted into the dark red coloured porphobilin.

In *porphyrinuria* coproporphyrins predominate in the urine. Coproporphyrinuria III may occur after exposure to metals (lead poisoning is a prominent example), sedatives, sulfonamides, alcohol and various organic substances in hypermetabolic states with hepatic disease in various haematological conditions and in pellagra and riboflavin deficiency. In lead poisoning the amount of coproporphyrin III excreted in the urine is markedly increased. Small or moderate increases are to be interpreted with caution.

Methods for identification and quantitative estimation of porphyrins are based upon solubility differences in organic solvents and chromatographic or spectrophotometric analysis. Qualitative testing of urine for porphobilinogen is simple procedure.

Watson-Schwartz Porphobilinogen Test

Ehrlich's reagent

Para-dimethylaminobenzaldehyde	0.7 g
Concentrated hydrochloric acid	150 ml
Distilled water	100 ml

Procedure: Add 3 ml of Ehrlich's reagent to 3 ml of urine and mix. Add 6 ml of saturated solution of sodium acetate. If a reddish colour develops, add 3 ml of chloroform. Shake for 2 minutes, then let stand. Persistence of the reddish colour in the aqueous supernatant indicates porphobilinogen. However, many substances can cause a false positive reaction. Notable are the anticonvulsant drugs, pyridium, urorosein or indoxyl.

Tests for Porphyrins

Principle: Porphyrins are substituted tetrapyril methenes. Small amounts may be found in normal urine. Urine containing large amounts (porphyrinuria) may be dark red or a "port wine" colour. Darkening of a light coloured urine upon standing hours or longer is suggestive of porphyrinuria.

Procedure

1. To 25 ml of urine in a separatory funnel, add 10 ml of glacial acetic acid. Extract this mixture twice with 50 ml portions of ether and combine the extracts. Wash the combined extracts with 10 ml of 5% hydrochloric acid.
2. Examine the washings under ultraviolet light. If there is a strong red fluorescence, a large amount of coproporphyrin is present, suggestive of porphyria. Examine the urine residue after ether extraction under ultraviolet light. A discernible red fluorescence is indicative of the presence of uroporphyrin. These tests should be confirmed spectroscopically as follows:
   i. To 100 ml of urine add 20 ml of a 10% solution of sodium hydroxide.
   ii. Filter or centrifugalize off the precipitate.
   iii. Wash the precipitate with water and with alcohol.
   iv. Add 5 ml of alcohol and 5 to 10 drops of concentrated hydrochloric acid.
   v. Dissolve, filter until absolutely clear, and examine spectroscopically for the adsorption bands of acid haematoporphyrin (Fig. 13.1).

An acetic acid test, which is much less reliable, consists in adding 5 ml of glacial acetic acid to 100 ml of urine and allowing the mixture to stand 48 hours. The pigment exists in the form of a precipitate.

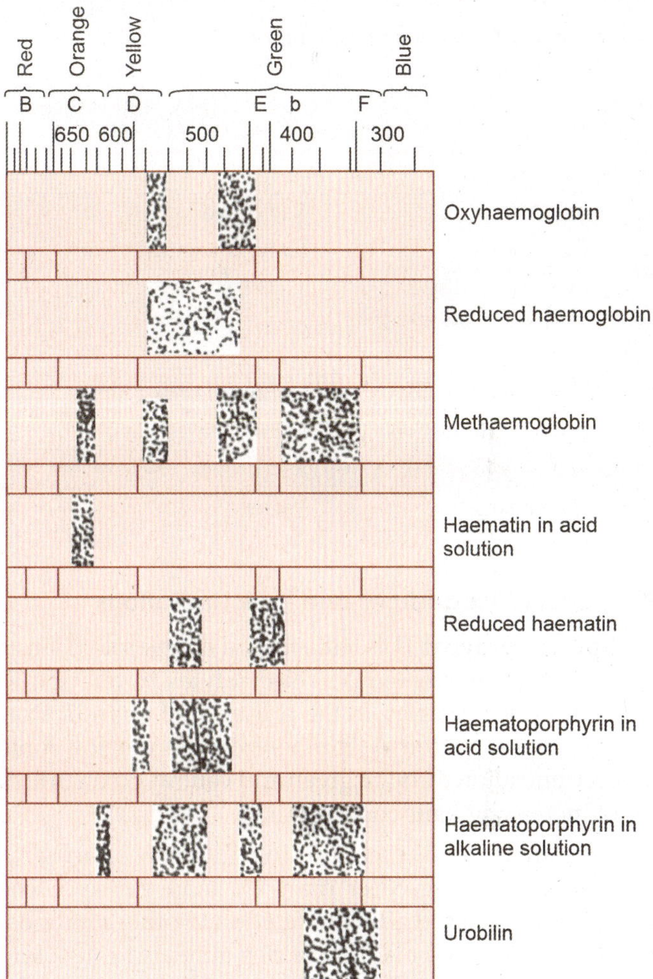

Fig. 13.1: Absorption spectra

Ferric Chloride Testing (Table 13.4)

Many amino acids react with ferric chloride to give distinctive colours. Ferric chloride testing is screening test not only for aminoacidurias but also for many abnormal metabolities and drug excretion products. Definitive diagnosis requires specific identification and measurement of the relevant materials in blood or urine.

Strip Technology

Nowadays strips are available commercially which can be used for the following tests—specific gravity, pH, protein, glucose, ketone (aceto-acetic acid), bilirubin, blood and urobilnogen in urine. The strips are firm plastic strips to which are affixed various separate reagent areas.

Table 13.4: Ferric chloride testing results

Substance	*Colour alteration*
Amino acids	
α-Ketobutyric acid	Purple, fading to red brown
Homogentisic acid (alkaptonuria)	Rapidly fading blue or green
p-Hydroxyphenylpyruvic acid (tyrosinosis)	Rapidly fading green
Valine, leucine, and isoleucine (maple syrup disease)	Blue
Phenyl pyruvic acid (phenylketonuria)	Stable green or blue green
Other metabolites	
Acetoacetic acid	Red or red-brown
Melanin	Gray, changing to black
Indican (Hartnup disease, intestinal stasis, malabsorption)	Violet or blue
Drugs	
Aspirin, salicylates	Stable red-wine colour
Phenothiazine derivatives	Immediate purple-pink
p-Aminosalicylic acid (PAS)	Red-brown
Phenol derivatives	Violet

Principles of Procedures and their Limitations

1. **Specific gravity:** This test is based on the pKa change of certain pretreated polyelectrolytes in relation to ionic concentration. In the presence of an indicator, colours, range from deep blue-green urine of low ionic concentration through green and yellow-green urines of increasing ionic concentration.

   Limitations: Urine containing glucose or urea at concentration greater than 1% may cause a low specific gravity reading in relation to other methods. Highly buffered alkaline urines may also cause low readings. Elevated specific gravity reading may be obtained in the presence of moderate (100–750 mgm/dl) quantities of protein.
2. **pH:** This is based on double indicator principle which gives a broad range of colours covering the entire urinary pH range. Colours range from orange through yellow and green to blue.
3. **Protein:** At a constant buffered pH, the development of any green colour is due to the presence of protein. Colours range from yellow for negative through yellow-green and green to green-blue for positive reactions.

   Limitations: False positive results may be obtained with highly buffered, alkaline urine. Contaminating ammonium compounds may also cause false positive results.
4. **Glucose:** Glucose oxidase enzyme catalyzes the formation of gluconic acid and hydrogen peroxide from oxidation of glucose. Second enzyme peroxidase, catalyzes the reaction of hydrogen peroxide, with a potassium iodide chromogen to oxidize the chromogen to colours ranging from green to brown.

   Limitations: Ascorbic acid concentration of 75 mgm/dl or greater may cause false negative results for specimen containing small amounts of glucose (100 mgm/dl).
5. **Ketone:** It is based on the development of colours ranging from buff-pink, for a negative reaching, to maroon when acetoacetic acid reacts with nitroprusside.

   Limitations: False positive result may occur with highly pigmented urine.
6. **Bilirubin:** This is based on the coupling of bilirubin with diazotized dichloroaniline in a strongly acidic medium. The colour ranges through various shades of tan.

   Limitations: Metabolites of drugs which give a colour at low pH may cause false positive results. Ascorbic acid may cause false negative results.
7. **Blood:** This is based on the peroxidase like activity of haemoglobin.

   Limitations: Elevated specific gravity or proteins may reduce the activity of the test.
8. **Urobilinogen:** This is based on Ehrlich reaction in which paradimethylaminobenzaldehyde reacts with urobilinogen in a strongly acidic medium to produce a brown orange colour.

Procedure

1. Collect fresh urine in a clean, dry container.
2. Remove strip from bottle and replace cap. Completely immerse reagent areas of the strip in fresh urine and remove immediately.
3. Remove excess of urine and hold the strip in horizontal position.
4. Compare test areas to corresponding colour charts on the bottle label at the specific time, match carefully.

Microscopic Examination of Urine

If possible, urine deposits should be examined within 8 hours of collection, preferably within 1 to 2 hours.

Procedure

1. Mix the urine thoroughly and place about 12 ml in a conical centrifuge tube. Centrifuge for 5 minutes at 1500 to 2500 rpm; pour off the supernatant fluid; resuspend the deposit in the few drops of urine that remain by flicking the end of the tube with the finger; then place a drop on a microscope slide; cover with a cover glass.
2. Examine with the low power objective to obtain an overall picture of the deposit. Use the higher power objectives to examine objects more closely. In order

not to miss casts cut the light to a minimum by means of the rheostat, or by lowering the condenser, or by closing the iris diaphragm.

Substances appearing in the urine deposits are of three main types: Cells, casts and crystals (including amorphous chemical deposits).

Cells (Microsediments Urine)

Epithelial Cells

Squamous epithelial cells: These large cells with small round or oval nuclei are derived from the ureters, bladder and urethra. In urine from female patients not obtained by catherization, vagina epithelial cells may also be present. This is normal and of no significance.

Polyhedral epithelial cells: Small round cells slightly larger than leukocytes, and caudate epithelial cells, which are smaller than the squamous cells and have a tail-like process, may also be present. These are derived mainly from the upper tract.

Red cells: In hypertonic urine the red cells may be crenated and smaller than normal. In hypotonic urine they are swollen and larger than usual, losing their typical "double ring" appearance. The presence of red cells in the urine indicates bleeding in some part of the urinary tract. It is important that contamination from menstrual flow be avoided when urine from females is to be examined.

Leukocytes: The normal excretion rate for leukocytes in the urine is up to 3 per µl, i.e. 3000 per ml or up to about 200, 000 per hour.

Microscopy of uncentrifuged urine is better, but the only accurate method is to make quantitative WBC counts on a timed (2–4 hours) specimen of urine, using a Fuchs-Rosenthal or equivalent, hemocytometer, and taking the average of four to six counts on the mixed, fresh specimen.

Spermatozoa: Spermatozoa may be present in the urine of a male after ejaculation or in female urine as a vaginal contaminant after coitus. They are easily recognized.

Bacteria: Bacteria are not normally present in urine. Contamination can easily occur if the urine is not collected by catheterization, however, and if the urine is allowed to stand at room temperature for any length of time, it may be swarming with bacteria. They are of no significance unless the urine has been collected by an aseptic technique and placed in a sterile container.

Casts (Fig. 13.2)

Casts are of many types: They are formed by the solidification of protein in the nephron tubule, often with trapped cells, granular debris, and so forth.

- **Hyaline casts:** Hyaline casts are cylindrical, transparent bodies that are difficult to see unless the illumination is cut a minimum.

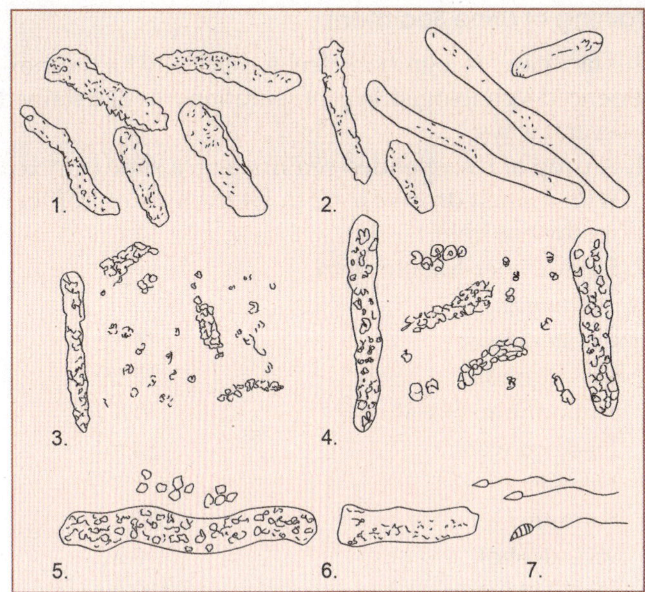

Fig. 13.2: Labelled 1–7: 1. Fine and coarse granular casts; 2. Hyaline casts; 3. Leucocyte casts; 4. Epithelial casts; 5. Blood casts; 6. Waxy casts; 7. Spermatozoa

- **Finely granular casts:** These casts are similar to hyaline casts but contain fine granules.
- **Coarsely granular casts:** These have larger granules than the finely granular casts but are similar in appearance.
- **Leukocyte casts:** Leukocyte casts are composed mainly of leukocytes.
- **Blood casts:** These are easily recognized because they are almost entirely composed of red cells and often have a bright orange colour.
- **Fatty casts:** These casts are any casts that contain fat droplets. Examination by polarized light may show anisotropic lipids, especially in lipid nephrosis.
- **Waxy casts:** Waxy casts are similar to hyaline casts but are more opaque and often have a curled end or 'tail'.
- **Renal failure casts:** In the late stages of many renal diseases residual nephrons often become dilated. Casts developing in these nephrons tend to have large diameters. If they are numerous, they indicate a grave outlook or "end-state" kidney.

Cylindroids: Cylindroids are long ribbon-like formations that resemble hyaline casts but are much longer and are often tapered.

Mucus threads: Mucus threads may be mistaken for hyaline casts, but they are usually much longer, less regular, and wavy, and they have tapered ends. Amorphous urates or phosphates may form aggregates on mucus threads which resemble casts but they seldom have the parallel sides and smooth ends of true casts.

The presence of casts in urine, especially if albumin is also present, usually indicates kidney disease.

Staining of Urine Sediment

This facilitates recognition of cells, especially for the inexperienced technologist. Wet preparations may be stained in several ways:

1. A drop of resuspended sediment on a slide is mixed with a small drop of a 1:2 to 1:4 dilution of Löffler's methylene blue.
2. Sternheimer-Malbin stain

   Solution A:

Crystal violet	3.0 g
95% alcohol	20 ml
Ammonium oxalate	0.8 g
Distilled water	80 ml

   Solution B:

Safranin O	0.25 g
95% alcohol	10 ml
Distilled water	100 ml

   - *Working stain:* Mix 3 volume of solution A with 97 volume of solution B and filter. This will last up to three months.
   - *Procedure:* To the resuspended sediment in a centrifuge tube add 1 drop of the working stain and let stand 3 minutes after mixing. Then place a drop on a microscope slide, cover and examine.
   - *Results:* Normal polymorphonuclear nuclei take up both dyes and stain orange-purple. Glitter cells tend to take only the crystal violet and appear pale blue or colourless. Hyaline casts are stained pink to purple; RBCs, lavender; cellular casts, dark purple; and *Trichomonas* and nuclei of bladder and vaginal epithelia, light blue, blue and purple, in that order.
3. **Oil Red O:** If a drop of sediment is mixed with a drop of saturated solution of oil red O in isopropanol, fatty casts and fat droplets will be stained, but most of the latter, if present, will be found floating on the surface of the urine.

Ova and Parasites in Urine

Trichomonas is occasionally seen, especially in fresh specimens. Ova in urine are usually derived from fecal contamination except in cases of *Schistosoma haematobium infestation*.

Crystals

Crystals are not normally present in freshly passed urine and are precipitated from solution as the urine cools. Generally speaking, crystals in the urine are of no significance, except crystals of sulfonamides, cystine, oxalate in persons with a history of ureteral colic or stone formation, and, possibly, urates in those with gout.

Crystals Appearing in Acid Urine (Fig. 13.3) *and Alkaline Urine* (Fig. 13.4)

- **Calcium oxalate:** These are colourless, octahedral crystals and, appear as small square crossed by two diagonal lines. In another form calcium oxalate crystals are dumbbell-shaped. They vary greatly in size.
- **Uric acid:** Uric acid crystallizes in many forms (e.g. plates, prisms, sheaves, and hexagons). The crystals are usually coloured and are easily dissolved by heating. They are soluble in sodium hydroxide but insoluble in hydrochloric acid.
- **Urates:** Urates often appear as an amorphous sediment which dissolves when heated. Sodium urate crystals are often in the form of thorn apples.
- **Cystine:** These crystals are highly refractile hexagonal plates, similar to the plate form of uric acid crystals; however, they may be differentiated from uric acid crystals by their solubility in hydrochloric acid. They are rarely found, but when present are diagnostic of a rare inborn error of metabolism termed cystinuria, in which the patient excretes excessive amounts of the amino acid in the urine. Cystine crystals are soluble in alkali and are not found in alkaline urine.
- **Tyrosine:** Tyrosine is usually in the shape of fine needles or sheaves. It is seldom found except in acute liver failure.
- **Leucine:** The occurrence of leucine crystals in urine is open to question.

Crystals Appearing in Alkaline Urine (Fig. 13.4)

- **Phosphates:** Phosphates often appear as an amorphous sediment which is soluble in acetic acid.

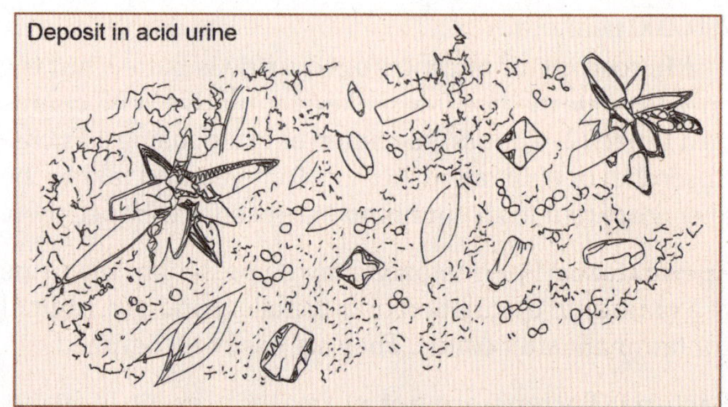

Fig. 13.3: Crystals in acidic urine

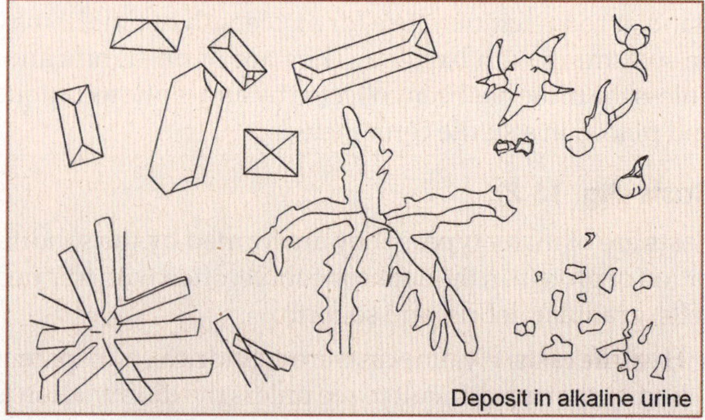

Fig. 13.4: Crystals in alkaline urine

- **Triple phosphates:** The usual forms of these crystals are 'prisms' and 'coffin lids'. They are soluble in acetic acid.
- **Calcium carbonate:** These crystals can appear as dumbbells, spheres, or amorphous granules. They are soluble in acetic acid.
- **Ammonium urate:** These crystals can appear in round, oval or thorn-apple form. They are soluble in acids (Fig. 13.4).

Other Crystals

- **Sulfonamide:** Crystals of the sulfonamides often appear in the urine after administration of these drugs. They are of many forms and may be confused with some of the naturally occurring crystals. If there is any doubt as to the identity of crystals, and if the patient is being treated with sulfonamides, the following test may be applied:
  - Test for sulfonamides: Deposit the crystals by centrifuging the urine in a Pyrex centrifuge tube. Decant the supernatant urine and add to the deposit 0.5 ml of 50% v/v hydrochloric acid. Mix and place the tube in a boiling water bath for about 30 minutes. Cool the solution and then dilute to 10 ml with distilled water.

The presence in the urine of excreted radiographic contrast media, e.g. iodopyracet (Diodrast), occasionally will produce masses of needle-like crystals accompanied by a very high specific gravity.

Various types of epithelial cells and crystals are given in Fig. 13.5 (A–F).

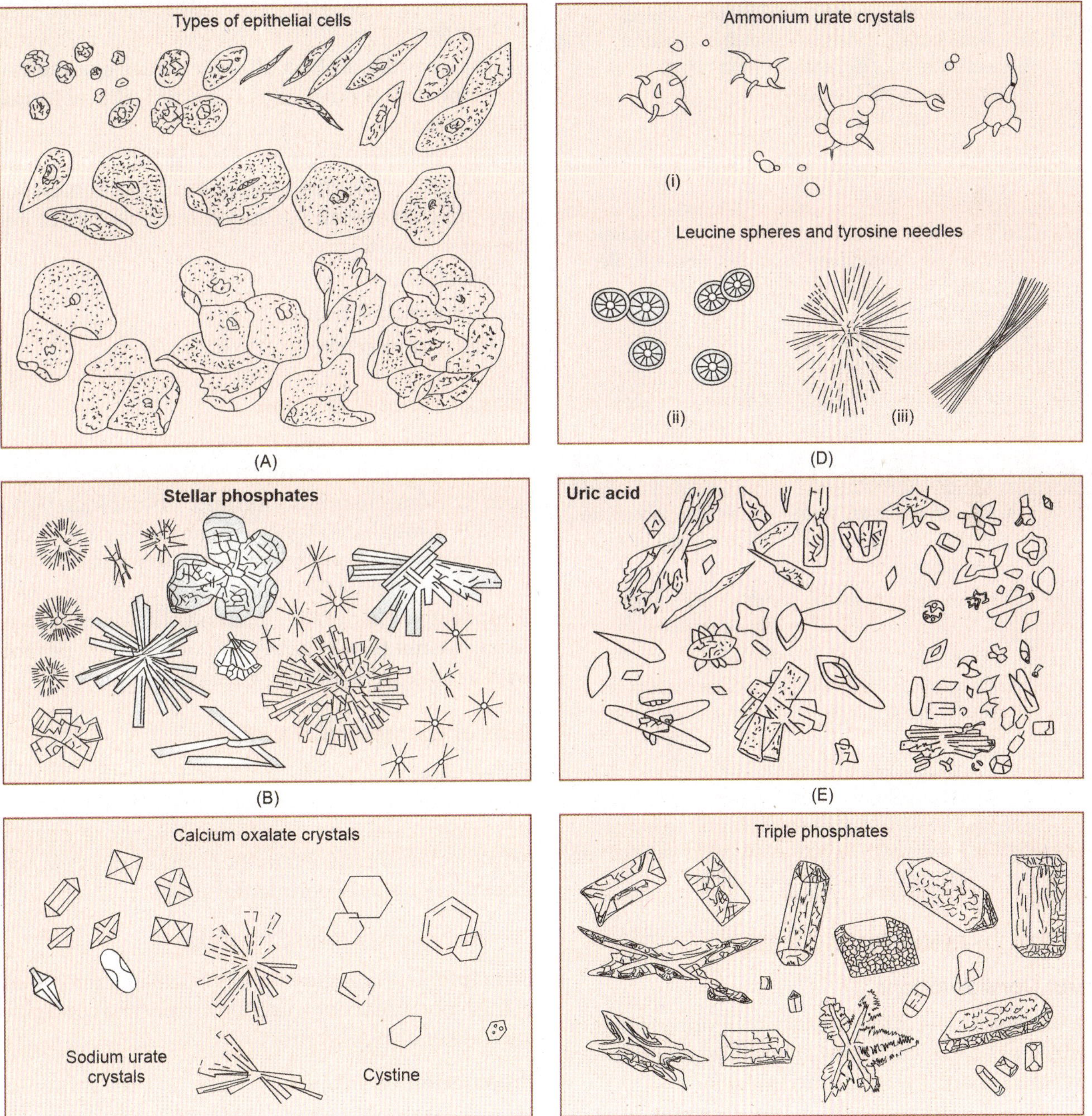

Fig. 13.5 (A–F): (A) Types of epithelial cells; (B) Stellar phosphates crystals; (C) Calcium oxalate crystals; (D) (i) Ammonium urate crystals, (ii) Leucine spheres, (iii) Tyrosine needles, (E) Various shapes of uric acid crystals; (F) Types of triple phosphates

In acidic and alkaline urine various types of chemical sediments are given in Table 13.5 along with chemical composition of sediments.

Table 13.5: Chemical sediments in urine

Reaction of urine	*Character of sediment*	*Chemical composition of sediment*
Acid	i. Yellow or reddish-brown crystals, variable size and shape; most characteristic forms are rosette-like clusters of 'whetstones' or prisms; often rhombic (paler colour).	Uric acid; soluble in sodium hydroxide solution
	ii. Colourless, glistening, octahedral crystals, so-called envelope crystals. Variable size. Unusual forms are: Colourless dumb-bells, sphere. (May be encountered in alkaline urine.)	Calcium oxalate; soluble in hydrochloric acid.
	iii. Fine, yellowish granules, sometime colourless; rarely, slender prisms arranged in fanlike or sheaf-like structure.	Sodium and potassium urates; heat-soluble.
Alkaline	i. Colourless crystals, "coffin-lid" like; sometimes feathery, star-like or leaf-like.	Ammonio-magnesium phosphate; soluble in acetic acid.
	ii. Colourless prisms, arranged in stars or rosettes (stellar phosphate).	Dicalcium phosphate; soluble in acetic aicd.
	iii. Colourless granules.	Amorphous phosphates; soluble in acetic acid.
	iv. Colourless granules; rarely, spheres or dumb-bells.	Calcium carbonate; soluble in acetic acid with liberation of gas.
	v. Opaque yellow crystals, usually spheres with fine or coarse spicules.	Ammonium biurate: Soluble in acetic acid; (rhombic plates of uric acid appear on acidification)

EVALUATION OF RENAL FUNCTION TESTS

General Considerations

A clear understanding of the mechanism of kidney function is essential for a complete appreciation of the significance of urinary findings and the renal function tests.

The kidneys, fortunately, have, like the liver, a tremendous reserve functional capacity. Normal life activities easily can be sustained by only one kidney and while many lesions, infections, tumors, or traumatic injuries may be unilateral, kidney disease, such as glomerulonephritis or nephrosclerosis, is bilaterial. The functions of the kidneys are:

1. To rid the body of waste products of metabolism
2. To rid the body of foreign and nonendogenous substances
3. To maintain salt and water balance
4. To maintain the acid–base equilibrium of the body.

The formation of urine involves three separate activities of the nephron:

1. An adequate flow of blood to the nephron
2. Filtration of the plasma of this blood by the glomerulus
3. Reabsorption and secretion of substances by the renal tubules.

The quantity of fluid ultimately reaching the bladder under normal conditions is 1, 200 to 1, 500 ml during the 24-hour period.

All three primary functions of the nephron can be measured by various tests, and in fact renal function tests are conveniently grouped into these three general classes—those testing:

1. Renal blood flow,
2. Glomerular filtration, and
3. Renal tubular activity.

Tests of Renal Blood Flow

Renal blood or plasma flow is measured by means of substances which are completely cleared from the plasma, both by glomerular filtration and tubular secretion, in its passage through the kidney. Phenolsulfonphthalein lends itself to a simple, convenient, rapid, semiquantitative test. *p*-Aminohippurate (PAII) is utilized in an accurate, more complicated quantitative method. The normal value for renal plasma flow is approximately 650 ml per minute with a range from 500 to 800 ml per minute.

Tests of Glomerular Filtration

Three clearance tests—urea, inulin, and creatinine—often are used to examine for impairment of glomerular filtration. Urea and creatinine are more commonly employed in clinical evaluation and inulin clearance for more meticulous experimental studies.

Determination of Urea Clearance

Principle: The urea clearance is calculated upon the basis of the blood urea concentration, urine urea concentration and rate of urine excretion.

Preparation of subject: No special preparation of the subject is necessary other than giving two glasses of water one-half hour before beginning of the test and one at the end of the first hour to promote free flow of urine.

Procedure

1. Have the patient empty his bladder completely. This specimen is discarded. Accurately record the time of completion of urination.
2. At the end of approximately 1 hour, have the patient void completely and again note accurately the time of voiding. Save this specimen.
3. Have the patient drink a glass of water. Collect a blood specimen for urea determination.
4. At approximately the end of the second hour, have patient void completely and accurately record the time of voiding. Save this specimen.
5. Measure accurately (within 1%) the volume of urine in each specimen by using the smallest graduate cylinder that will completely contain the specimen. Calculate the per minute excretion of urine for each specimen by dividing the total number of milliliters by the number of minutes lapsed between voidings.
6. Determine the blood urea concentration and the urine urea concentration for each separate urine specimen.

Calculation: If the per minute excretion of urine is 2 ml or more, use the formula:

$$\frac{U}{B} \times V = C_m \text{ (maximum clearance)}$$

If the per minute excretion of urine is under 2 ml, use the formula:

$$\frac{U}{B} \times \sqrt{V} = C_s \text{ (standard clearance)}$$

U = Urine urea mg per cent
B = Blood urea mg per cent
V = Volume of urine excreted as ml per minute

$$\frac{C_m}{75} \times 100 \text{ or } \frac{C_s}{54} \times 100 = \text{per cent of normal clearance}$$

Creatinine Clearance

Creatinine is also useful for measuring the glomerular filtration rate and, as little is transferred across tubular cells, its clearance rate is much higher than that of urea and approaches that of inulin. Measurement of the 24-hour excretion of endogenous creatinine is convenient. This longer collection period minimizes timing errors.

Procedure

1. An accurate 24-hour urine specimen is collected ending at 7.00 am and its total volume is measured.
2. Collect a blood sample for serum creatinine determination.
3. Determine serum and urine creatinine concentrations.

Calculation

$C_{creatinine} = (U/P) \times V$

U = Urine creatinine concentration in gm per liter
P = Serum creatinine concentration in mg per cent ÷ 100
V = 24-hour urine volume in ml ÷ 1, 000

The average normal 24-hour endogenous creatinine clearance is 170 litres.

Interpretation: Normal values for men and women corrected to 1.73 sqm body surface area range from 140–180 litres/24 hours (100–150 ml/minute). To correct clearance to standard 1.73 sqm body surface area.

$$\text{Clearance observed} \times \frac{1.73 \text{ sqm}}{\text{Estimated surface area}} = \text{Corrected clearance}$$

(This test is superior to urea clearance).

Creatinine clearance test

Normal range: 110–150 ml/min (males)
105–132 ml/min (females)

Effect of age on normal function: Ages 50–75, subtract 5 ml for each 5-year interval. Age 75 and above, subtract 8 ml for each 5-year interval.

Artifacts that lower calculated figure

- Incomplete urine collection.
- Bacterial multiplication in collecting vessel.
- Ketones, barbiturates, PSP in urine at higher levels than is plasma.

Causes for reduced creatinine clearance

- **Acute:** Shock, hypovolemia, nephrotoxic chemicals, acute glomerulonephritis, malignant hypertension, eclampsia.
- **Chronic:** Glomerulonephritis, pyelonephritis, hypertensive nephrosclerosis, polycystic kidneys.

Since shock, severe dehydration, circulatory failure, and obstruction in the lower urinary tract diminish clearance, these conditions must be properly evaluated before low clearance values can be accepted as evidence of primary renal disease.

Glomerular Filtration Rate (GFR)

Inulin, a polysaccharide, is eliminated exclusively through the glomeruli, is neither excreted nor absorbed by the tubules. Inulin clearance is therefore a measure of the glomerular filtration rate. Other radioactive labelled substances can be used. Normal in adults is 100–130 ml/minute per 1.73 sqm of body surface.

Normal values of renal function tests are given in Table 13.6.

Tests of Tubular Function

Concentration Tests

A number of tests have been devised to examine for impairment of the important function of water reabsorption. They are all based on the ability of the kidney (nephron) to concentrate urine. These tests measuring the tubular reabsorption (concentration) function of the nephron have been called, as a group, the specific

Table 13.6: Renal function tests

Determination		*Normal values*	
Phenolsulfon-phthlein (PSP, Phenol red)	1 m I/V	15 min 35% (28–51) 30 min 17% (13–24) 60 min 12% (9–17) 120 min 6% (3–10)	55–60%
Clearance tests	Glome-rular	Corrected to 1.73 sqm SA	
Inulin clearance	filtration rate	Male: 110–150 ml/min	
Iothalamate	–do–	Female:105–132 ml/min	
Endogenous creatinine clearance	–do–		
Iodohippurate ^{131}IPAH clearance	Renal flow	Plasma	Male: 560–830 ml/min Female: 490–700 ml/min
Filtration fraction	FF = GFR/RPF	Male: 17–21% Female: 17–23%	
Urea clearance (C_4)		Standard: 40–65 ml/min Maximal: 60–100 ml/min	
Maximal glucose reabsorptive capacity	TmG	Male: 300–450 mg/min Female: 250–350 mg/min	
Maximal iodopyracet capacity	TmD	Male: 43–59 mg/min Female: 33–51 mg/min	
Maximal PAH excretory capacity	Tm PAH	80–90 mg/min	

gravity tests. They are extremely important, for the ability to concentrate urine is an early kidney activity to show significant impairment in nephritis.

Dilution and Concentration Test

The healthy kidney can excrete variable quantities of fluid or water through the mechanism of reabsorption under the control of the anti-diuretic hormone of the pituitary. This power to do osmotic work can be roughly gauged by measuring the specific gravity of the urine. These tests are a challenge to the physiological function of absorption of water by the tubular epithelium.

Procedure: The patient should be on a diet containing reasonable amounts of water, salt and proteins before the test. At least an interval of 24 hours should elapse between the dilution and the concentration test.

Dilution test: The test is done in the morning after a 12-hour fast. The patient is made to empty the bladder and then he drinks 1,200 ml of water in half an hour. Thereafter the bladder is emptied every hour for 4 hours. The total volume of the urine excreted in 4 hours should be 80 to 120% of the water ingested and in at least one of the four samples the specific gravity should be 1003 or lower. If the amount of albumin in the urine is more than 1 +, the specific gravity figures have to be corrected by subtracting 0.003 for each gram of albumin per 100 ml of urine.

Concentration test: All fluids are restricted after breakfast until the following morning; the usual diet is allowed omitting foods containing free fluid. On retiring the patient empties the bladder, this sample is discarded. The following morning the bladder is emptied and the sample saved. Two additional samples are collected at hourly intervals. At least in one of the three samples the specific gravity should be 1025 or higher. The test is contraindicated in old persons, in patients with heart diseases or those with incipient renal failure.

The dilution and the concentration tests are simple and can be done at the bed side without special equipment. They are sensitive tests, the concentration test being positive even in the case of compensated renal damage. The tests are not reliable in oedematous patients, in pregnancy, in patients with chronic liver disease and in patients with adrenocortical insufficiency. Further, they do not distinguish primary renal dysfunction from that due to external causes.

Tests of Tubular Excretion and Reabsorption

The reserve function of secretion of foreign nonendogenous materials by the tubular epithelium is most conveniently test for by the use of certain dyes and measuring their rate of excretion.

Indigo-Carmine test: The patient is given 100 mg of the dye intravenously. Normally the blue dye appears at the ureteric opening in the bladder 15 minutes after the injection. Late appearance or failure to appear indicates dysfunction on that side.

Phenolsulfonphthalein (PSP) test: PSP is a dye which, when injected intravenously, is excreted mainly by the kidney (both glomerules and tubules); about 15–25% is excreted by the liver, the amount increasing with liver disease. The urinary concentration is determined after alkalinising the urine (when the dye appears red) by colourimetry. By ureteric catheterisation the excretion by each kidney can be estimated separately.

Procedure: The patient empties the bladder. He is given about 600 ml of water to drink to promote the urine flow. After 30 minutes 1 ml of the dye (6 mg) is injected intravenously. The dye should appear in the urine within 10 minutes normally. Beginning after 10 minutes of the injection, samples of the urine are collected at 1 hour and 2 hours. The volume of the urine and the concentration of the dye are measured. If the kidneys are healthy about 40 to 60% of the dye is excreted in the 1st hour and 20 to 25% in the next. A fall in the exeretion of the dye below 50% in 2 hours indicates renal impairment.

Choice of Renal Function Tests

The selection of a renal function test for use in any instance is influenced by three primary considerations—the type of information desired, the nature and severity of the kidney lesion under investigation, and the scope of laboratory facilities available. If a quick, rough estimate of severe functional impairment is desired as in the case of known urinary tract obstruction or in the presence of clinical symptoms suggesting uremia, determination of the blood urea nitrogen, nonprotein nitrogen or serum creatinine is often sufficient. However, it is usually desirable to have a more accurate evaluation of the degree of reduction of renal function. Adequate assessment of kidney function requires consideration of the renal blood flow, glomerular filtration rate and tubular cell activity.

Under conditions where inadequate laboratory facilities prevent the use of tests requiring chemical determinations on blood and urine, entirely satisfactory results may be obtained by employing the specific gravity and the 15-minute phthalein excretion tests. These utilize simple equipment and procedure within the scope of any laboratory or physician's office. They test the reabsorptive and excretory abilities of the renal tubular cell and also the adequacy of renal blood flow. Combined with the examination of the urine they afford a fair appraisal of the functional and structural state of the kidneys. The picture of the functional state will be more complete with some measure of glomerular filtration rate, such as urea or creatinine clearance. Further clarification of the structural state may require needle biopsy of the kidney.

If accurate information of kidney functional is needed for diagnostic or prognostic purposes, the rate of renal blood flow and maximal tubular reabsorptive capacity should be determined.

Renal biopsy: Needle biopsy of the kidneys has been introduced recently. The technique, though safe in experienced hands, is much more difficult than that of liver biopsy. The tissue bit removed is submitted for histological examination. If positive, it gives the exact information of the nature of the lesion.

Chapter 14

Stool Examination

Chapter Outline

- Normal Appearance and Composition
- Importance of stool examination
- Collection of specimens for stool examination
- Physical examination
- Chemical examination
- Microscopic examination
- Concentration techniques

NORMAL APPEARANCE AND COMPOSITION

Stool/faeces is the end product of the digestive system of the body. The faeces are normally composed of food residues, materials secreted through the wall of the intestines and in the bile, leukocytes, desquamated epithelial cells and bacteria.

The contents of jejunum and terminal ileum are liquid and about 400 g in weight per 24 hours. As they pass through caecum and colon, most of the water is absorbed converting the contents to a soft formed mass, about 150–200 g in weight. Normal characteristics of stool are as follows:

Macroscopic

1. No. of evacuations/day	Usually 2 (2–4)
2. Weight in g/day	150–200
3. Form and consistency	Soft but formed
4. Colour	Light to dark brown due to stercobilin
5. Odour	Aromatic
6. Reaction	6.9–7.2
7. Mucous	Scanty, intimately mixed with stool

Microscopic

1. Undigested and indigestible remnants of food—details to be discussed under text.
2. Desquamated epithelial cells.
3. Bacteria—commensals of alimentary tract.
4. Protozoa—commensals in intestines.

IMPORTANCE OF STOOL EXAMINATION

Most clinicians consider examination of faeces as being limited to a search for intestinal parasites or their ova, or for pathogenic bacteria. Much, of clinical value, may be learned, however, by physical, chemical and detailed microscopic examinations of the stool. Examination of stool may therefore be:

1. **Physical**
   a. Amount
   b. Form and consistency
   c. Colour
   d. Odour
   e. Reaction, and
   f. Mucous
2. **Chemical**
   a. Occult blood
   b. Bilirubin
   c. Urobilin (stercobilin)
   d. Urobilinogen
   e. Fats, and
   f. Nitrogen
3. **Microscopic**
   a. Intestinal parasites/ova/cyst
   b. Pathogenic bacteria
   c. Remnants of food
   d. Cellular exudates, and
   e. Erythrocytes

COLLECTION OF SPECIMENS FOR STOOL EXAMINATION

In this section we will mention not only collection of stool specimens for routine examination but also discuss something about the other techniques which improve the chances of finding ova/cyst, etc.

Collection of Faeces

1. The faeces to be examined, should be passed into a clean vessel without admixture of urine and antibiotics.
2. A small portion of stool sample is sufficient for routine examination, collected in a wide mouth glass container, it should be sent to the laboratory within a few hours owing to changes caused by decomposition.

3. The stool should not be sent in a matchbox or wrapped in a paper as it is unhygienic and decomposition takes place quickly.
4. The patient should not usually be given any purgative before the stool is collected, oils should especially be avoided.
5. For benzidine test for occult blood it is advised that patient be given a diet free from meat and green vegetable for 3 days to avoid a false positive test.
6. In case of delay, stool may be collected in a suitable transport medium and may be sent within 4–5 hours or even 24 hours; various transport media in use include:
   i. For vibrios: Alkaline peptone water and Venkat Ramakrishnan (VR) fluid.
   ii. For other enteropathogens: Cary and Blair medium.
   iii. For all parasite/ova/cyst: Stool should be collected in a 30 ml bottle containing 15 ml of 10% formaldehyde solution.
   iv. Hanks solution (salt, 0.4% bovine albumin, pencillin and streptomycin) especially useful for preserving rectal swabs.

Rectal Swab

Sterile swabs are dipped in sterile buffered glycerol. Separate the buttocks before introducing the swab in the rectum to avoid contamination with the perianal skin. The swab is inserted either in a sterile glass container or in a preservative medium like VR fluid or Cary and Blair's medium. Rectal swabs are taken when stool samples are not available.

NIH Swab

This consists of a wooden applicator to which a piece of cellophane tape is attached. Early in the morning without washing, sticky face of the applicator is applied against perianal skin. Immediately transfer to a microslide. Wash away the glue with xylol and examine immediately under microscope. This swan is especially useful for identifying the ova of *Enterobius vermicularis* (pinworms).

Labelling and Registration of Specimens

The technician at the reception bench receives the specimen, check the name of the patient on the container with the name on the request form, provides container and request form with a lab number and register the specimen on the registration sheet. Then the specimen is brought to the parasitology lab and placed on the safety bench.

The technician assigned to the parasitology work writes on the worksheet, if the stool is *formed soft, liquid or watery*, if it contains blood and mucous, and if worm or tapeworm segments are present.

Processing of Stool Specimens

The wet mount is the simplest and most widely used method for diagnosis of intestinal parasites in tropical countries. However, a wet mount contains only 2 mg of faecal matter, and it may not be sufficient to identify all parasitic infections. An adult person produces as an average 125–150 g of stool per day and a child proportionally less. A single female roundworm makes per day about 200,000 eggs, so even a single female roundworm will be identified by examination of one wet mount. However, one female hookworm of whipworm produces about 10,000–30,000 eggs per day, and examination of a wet mount will identify less than half of the infections with a single female worm, and for *Schistosoma mansoni*, which produces only about 300 eggs per day, a single wet mount will identify less than 1% of the infections with a single worm.

There is a direct connection between the number of eggs and the seriousness of the disease which some worms produce. More than 5 hookworm eggs per wet mount indicates a clinically significant infection, while more than 10 whipworm eggs per mount will be needed to produce a significant infection with this worm. This is contrary to infections with Schistosoma and Ascaris where even a single egg may be significant, due to the serious complication these infections may cause.

For protozoa, the percentage of infections identified with a single mount is extremely variable depending on a number of factors in the host and parasite. Besides, there is no relationship between the number of protozoa in stool and the severity of the infection.

The conclusion must be to start with a wet mount, if parasites are not found and a parasitic bowel infection is still suspected on clinical grounds, do a concentration method. Formol-ether sedimentation method is recognised as the best all-round method for both protozoa, helminthis eggs and larvae.

A "standard" wet mount is made directly from a freshly passed stool specimen, preferably not more than 1 hour old. Examine carefully the appearance of the stool and pick out both normal and abnormal looking parts for examination.

Place a drop of saline and a drop of iodine solution on either half of a glass slide. With a wooden applicator stick pick up a very small portion of faeces and emulsify it in the saline and then in the iodine solution. Mix the stool and solution until the preparation are an even mixture. Observe if the smear has the right thickness, which is when newspaper print can just be read through the mount. Cover the two preparations with 22 mm coverslips, and examine the mount under the microscope. One must learn by experience the right proportion of specimen to fluid. Too much fluid will make the preparation to flow over, and too little produce air pockets under the coverslip. Large particles should be avoided.

If there is mucous or blood on part of the stool, make an extra wet mount preparation in a drop of buffered methylene blue (BMB) stain for faecal leucocytes and trophozoites, and let it stand for 10 minutes to allow the cells to take up the stain. BMB will overstain trophozoites in about 30 minutes, so the mount should be examined between 10 and 30 minutes after preparation.

First examine the mount with low power (10x) to detect eggs, larvae, cysts and trophozoites, and use medium (40x) power for identifying the species. Increase the contrast by closing down the aperture diaphragm. Start with the saline mount and then do the iodine mount. If trophozoites of amoebae are observed or suspected, examine the BMB preparation. This will bring out the nuclear structures more clearly. Count the number of eggs seen in the mount. For protozoa, it is sufficient to report "few" = (+). "Intermediary" = (++) or "many" = (+++) cyst or trophozoites of each species observed.

PHYSICAL EXAMINATION

In the complete routine examination of faeces, attention should be paid to the physical characteristics. Much information of clinical value may be derived in relation to amount, form and consistency, colour, odour , mucous, concretions and animal parasites.

Physical examinations are especially indicated in most patients with suspected gastrointestinal diseases and should be rarely omitted in cases of diarrhoea, constipation, jaundice, anaemia or in infants with feeding problem.

Amount: The amount is commonly characteristically increased in states producing:

i. Steatorrhoea—due to an increase in faecal lipids, e.g. obstructive jaundice.
ii. Indigestion of carbohydrate—e.g. sprue when stools are foamy.

Form and consistency

i. Excessively hard faeces, sometimes called scybala are commonly observed in habitual constipation and indicate atony of muscular coat of colon.
ii. In spastic constipation the faeces are characterised by numerous hard, ball-like masses.
iii. Flattened, ribbon-like stools may result from taking mineral oil but otherwise indicate obstruction of rectum, generally a structure from a healed ulcer (most frequently syphillis or LGV).
iv. In dysentry, stools are invariably small, numerous and composed largely of mucus and blood with very small amount of faecal material.

Colour: Colour of faeces may depend a lot on diet, any drugs taken or disease:

i. Diet: Milk diet — Light yellow faeces.
Cocoa chocolate—dark grey faeces
Fruits—reddish black faeces
Spinach and other chlorophyllic Vegetables—green faeces
Beetroot—red coloured faeces
Rhubarb—yellow coloured faeces.

ii. Drugs: Calomet — Green stools due to biliverdin:
Iron—dark brown or black stools
Neoprontasil—red stools
Santonin/senna—yellow stools
$BaSO_4$—clay coloured stools

iii. Diseases: *Obstructive jaundice*—clay coloured stools
Haemorrhage in upper GIT—black tarry stools (melena)
Diarrhoea due to chromogenic bacteria—green coloured stools.

Odour: Variations of odour may occur:

i. Sour rancid odour—increased faecal fat.
ii. Putrid odour—in severe diarrhoeas.
iii. A foul stench—ulcerative/gangrenous lesions.

Blood and mucus: Obvious pus, blood and mucus in faeces indicate the presence of ulcerative lesions or infections of the lower bowel. Blood (bright red) coating surface of stools may be due to haemorrhoids, fissure in and/or ulceration in the rectum.

In the so-called mucous colitis, shreds and ribbons of mucous, sometimes representing complete casts of portions of colon, are passed especially after an enema. This mucous does not contain pus cells.

Reaction: Various methods may be used to test pH of stool:

i. Thoroughly mix the stool and test with red and blue litmus paper, red paper turns blue with alkali.
ii. Test with Congo red paper.
iii. To a watery suspension of faeces, add a few drops of 1% alcoholic solution of phenolphthalein. It turns pink if alkaline.

CHEMICAL EXAMINATION

Blood in Faeces

Quite often blood in the stool is not visible grossly and may be revealed only by specific tests (occult blood).

Principles: Haem compounds catalyze the oxidation of organic substances such as benzidine, orthotolidine by H_2O_2 (hydrogen peroxide). The tests are made specific by boiling the faeces, which destroys true peroxidases, leaving only haem compounds that are thermostable.

Precautions

1. To avoid false positive reactions patients should be on a meat free diet for 72 hours before collection of specimen.
2. Faeces should be mixed thoroughly before testing.
3. Cross check results by 2 methods.

4. Exclude aspirin and related drugs.
5. Exclude lettuce, apples and oranges from diets.

1. **Benzidine test**
   1. Prepare a thin emulsion of faeces with water in a test tube.
   2. Prepare the benzidine reagent by dissolving a knife point of benzidine HCl crystals in 5 ml of glacial acetic acid and adding an equal volume of 10 Vol% H_2O_2. (Alternatively, prepare a saturated solution of benzidine in glacial acetic acid and store away in a brown bottle in a dark place.)
   3. Now add 5 ml of boiled faecal emulsion to the reagent. (Alternatively, haem compounds can be extracted from faeces using 3% v/v acetic acid.)
   4. A deep green colour indicates a positive test for occult blood.
2. **Orthotolidine test**
   1. Prepare the reagent by dissolving 4 g of *O*-tolidine in 100 ml glacial acetic acid. Keep in a brown bottle and prepare at monthly intervals.
   2. To a 1 ml of water suspension of faeces add 1 ml of reagent and 1 ml of 3% H_2O_2.
   3. A positive reaction is indicated by development of a bluish/bluish green colour within 30–60 secs.
3. **Alvarez and Weight's modification of Gregersen test**
   1. Dissolve 225 mg of a mixture of 8 parts barium peroxide (200 mg) and 1 part benzidine (25 mg) in 5 ml of a 50% solution of acetic acid. Prepare a fresh before use.
   2. Rub a small portion of faeces into a few drops of water on a porcelein plate. Add a few drops of the above solution. Interpret results according to Gregersen scale mentioned below:

      Deep blue in 3 seconds –+++

      Distinct blue in 15 secs –++

      Blue green in 30–60 secs: Doubtful positive ±
4. **Guaiac test**
   1. Prepare reagent by dissolving 2 g of powdered guaiac in 10 ml of 95% ethyl alcohol.
   2. Prepare a smear of faeces on a filter paper.
   3. Add 10 drops of reagent followed by 1–2 drops of glacial acetic acid and 1–2 drops of H_2O_2.
   4. Development of blue/dark colour within 30 seconds constitute a positive reaction.

Test for reducing substances: Benedict's qualitative test is used in a way similar to urine except that a faecal suspension is used instead of urine.

Test for bile acids

1. Extract a small amount of faeces with alcohol and filter. Evaporate the filtrate in a dish over a water bath.
2. Dissolve the residue in water made slightly alkaline with KOH solution.
3. Add 0.3 ml of a 5% sucrose solution.
4. Transfer to a test tube and carefully run down the sides about 3 ml of concentrated sulfoxylic acid (H_2SO_2). Cool in running water.

   A red ring at the point of contact is a positive reaction.

Test for urobilin: The test depends on formation of urobilin mercury with production of red colour.

1. Rub a small amount of faeces in a mortar with a saturated solution of $HgCl_2$.
2. Transfer to a shallow white dish and let stand for 24 hours.

Presence of urobilin is indicated by a deep colour imparted to particles of faeces. If unaltered bilirubin is present, a green colour is produced through its oxidation to biliverdin.

Urobilin is absent to greatly reduced in obstructive jaundice and its return to faeces often the first sign of relief.

MICROSCOPIC EXAMINATION

a. Preparation

1. **Saline preparation:** A minute portion of faeces is diluted with normal saline (0.9%) and a drop taken on a clean glass slide. A coverslip is gently put over it so as to spread the emulsion into a thin, uniform and transparent layer.
2. **Iodine preparation:** Lugol's iodine solution is prepared as follows:

Powdered iodine crystals	5 g
Potassium iodine	10 g
Distilled water	100 ml

Potassium iodine is dissolved in distilled water, iodine crystals slowly added while shaking. Filter and store in an amber coloured bottle. One drop of saline emulsion is taken on a glass slide. Add 1 drop of Lugol's iodine and place a coverslip over it.

b. Examination: Both unstained and stained preparations are first examined under low power objective starting from one end of the coverslip, the whole slide is examined. Any suspicious object is focussed under high power objective for detailed diagnosis.

CONCENTRATION TECHNIQUES

1. Cellophane Faecal Thick Smear

With this method 60 mg of faecal matter is examined in a single preparation, which gives a 30 times concentration compared to the standard wet mount. Even light infections of Schistosoma will be identified with this method. However, the technique is not suitable for protozoa, which are difficult to recognise in this preparation.

Cut out pieces of cellophane from the roll into 25 × 30 mm sections and place them in a wide-mouth, flat bottom jar containing:

Glycerol	50 ml
Distilled water	30 ml

Formalin	10 ml
Malachite green	30 mg

A part of the stool specimen is placed on a disposable plastic sheet and with the help of a metal screen and a spatula, the faecal matter is forced through the screen, so the fine faecal material is separated from large debris. Transfer an amount of the screened faecal matter about the size of a pea to a microscopic slide. Place a "cellophane" coverslip soaked in glycerol-malachite green solution over the screened faecal matter.

Invert the slide and press it smoothly against a hard surface, so the faecal matter is spread evenly under the cellophane. To prevent air bubbles to form during storage cover the cellophane with 1–2 drops of glycerol. Roundworm and whipworm eggs are visible at any time. Hookworm eggs are only visible for 30 minutes after preparation of the smear, while Schistosoma eggs are best observed 24–48 hours after preparing the smear. Therefore, the routine should be to examine the thick "cellophane smear" 10–15 minutes after preparation, then add 1–2 drops of glycerol to the cellophane, leave it overnight on the bench and examine it again the next day.

Search the whole film with a low power 10x objective and count the number of helminth eggs of each species present.

2. Formalin Ether Sedimentation Technique

It is equally effective in concentrating protozoan cysts, helminth eggs and larvae. It is more efficient than zinc sulphate floatation method for most parasites, except in detecting *Giardia intestinalis, lodamoeba butchli*, cysts and *Hymenolepis nana* eggs. Add 10 ml of saline to the container with the stool sample, screw on the lid and shake it to get a thin suspension of the stool and saline. Place a folded square of surgical gauze in a small glass funnel. Pour the stool suspension through the gauze into a centrifuge tube. Centrifuge the tube at 1,500 rpm for 5 minutes. Pour away the supernatant fluid into the sink in the safety bench. Add 7–10 ml of 10% formalin, break the sediment with an applicator stick, add 3 ml of ether, and close the tube with a rubber stopper and shake the tube vigorously for 1 minute. Centrifuge the tube at 1,500 rpm for 3 minutes.

After centrifugation four layers would have developed in the centrifuge tube: At the top a clear, yellowish layer of ether, below this a narrow layer of faecal debris, then a liquid layer of formalin and at the botton a little deposit of sediment with the concentrated parasites.

With the applicator stick loosen the second upper layer of faecal debris and tip away the supernatant layers, except for the deposit at the very bottom of the tube.

Add one drop of water to deposit and with the tip of a Pasteur pipette break the deposit and make an even suspension. Transfer the deposit to a microscopic slide, add one drop of iodine, cover with coverslip and examine under the microscope with low 10x and medium 40x power objectives.

3. Zinc Sulphate Floatation Method

It is useful for concentration of cyst, larvae and most helminth eggs, except eggs of Schistosoma and the operculated eggs of liver and intestinal flukes and *Diphylobotrium latum*.

Start by preparing a zinc sulphate solution with a specific gravity of 1.195:

Granular $Z_nSO_47H_2O$	33.6 g
Distilled water	100 ml

Adjust the specific gravity with a hydrometer by adding extra zinc sulphate or water.

Pour 10 ml of saline into the container with the stool sample, screw on the lid and shake it well to get a thin suspension.

Place a folded square of surgical gauze in a small glass funnel and pour the stool suspension through this into a centrifuge tube. Centrifuge the suspension at 2,500 rpm for 2–3 minutes.

Pour off the supernatant fluid and resuspend the deposit in 10% formalin with the help of an applicator stick, close the tube with a rubber stopper, and shake the tube to get an even suspension.

Centrifuge the suspension at 2,500 rpm for 2–3 minutes and pour off the supernatant fluid.

Resuspend the deposit in zinc sulphate solution with a specific gravity of 1.195, mix well with the applicator stick and add extra zinc sulphate solution to fill the tube.

Centrifuge the tube at 3,000 rpm for 2 minutes. Transfer immediately the surface layer with the help of a bacteriological loop to a microscopic slide, add an extra drop of water or iodine, cover with coverslip and examine the preparation under the microscope.

4. Scotch Tape Swab for *Enterobius vermicularis*

The female threadworm rarely lays its eggs inside the bowel, but in the skin folds around anus during the night. The patient should therefore be examined in the morning before visiting the toilet.

Take a strip of Scotch Tape and fold it round the bottom of a test tube or the end of a tongue depressor with the sticky side outwards. Press the sticky surface of the Scotch Tape firmly on the skin round the anus, while flattening the skin folds with your left hand. The eggs on the skin will stick to the Scotch Tape.

Cut off the middle part of the Scotch Tape which has been in contact with the perianal skin.

Put 1–2 drops of immersion oil on the middle part of a microscopic slide and place the sticky side of the tape on top of it. Examine the tape with low power objective for eggs of *Enterobius vermicularis*.

5. Harada-Mori's Test Tube Cultivation of Larvae

The rearing of the infective stage larvae is necessary for the specific identification of the species of Necator,

Anchylostoma, Ternidens, and Trichostrongylus infections, since the eggs of these species are almost identical. The method may also be useful for the diagnosis of Strongyloides infections, if other methods have failed.

The filariform larvae are highly infectious Strongyloides larvae may even migrate upwards on the filter paper. Wash your hand carefully after the examination.

Smear an amount of faeces of the size as an almond on the middle portion of a 10 cm long and 2 cm broad filter paper strip. Fold the filter paper over the faeces and stick the filter paper into a test tube to the bottom.

Add 2–3 ml of water to the test tube and close it with a loosefitted cotton wool stopper. Incubate the test tube at 25–27°C for 7–10 days.

The eggs of hookworm will hatch on the filter paper into rhabditiform larvae and migrate to the water at the bottom of the tube, where he develops into filariform larvae in 1–3 days. Strongyloides' larvae also migrate to the water, where he develops into filariform larvae. Ternidens and Trichostrongylus have only a rhabditiform stage.

Remove the filter paper with a forceps. Aspirate a small portion of the sediment in the bottom of the test tube with a Pasteur pipette and transfer it to a microscopic slide. Add one drop of formalin, cover with coverslip, and examine for larvae under the low power (10 × objective). Identify the larvae.

The bulk of stool consists of granular debris. Among the recognizable microscopic structures encountered in normal and diseased conditions are:

1. **Remnants of food (Fig. 14.1)**
   a. *Vegetable fibres:* Spiral structure, with pits, dots or reticulate marketing.
   b. *Vegetable cells:* Show double contours and sometimes chlorophyll bodies.
   c. *Vegetable hairs:* Are homogenous, elongated, tube like structures with highly refractile wall.
   d. *Starch granules:* Best identified by adding drop of Lugol's iodine which stains them blue.
   e. *Muscle fibres:* Usually appear as short, transversely striated cylinders.
   f. *Fats:* May appear as:
      1. Neutral fats (droplets).
      2. Fatty acids (needle-like crystals).
      3. Soap (yellow masses or coarse crystals).
   g. *Elastic fibres and connective tissue:* Appear as colourless/yellowish threads, rendered more distinct by acetic acid.
2. **PUS cells:** Present in ulcerative conditions of the intestine. In amebic dysentery, their presence indicates superadded infection.
3. **Macrophages:** These are sometimes present and are liable to be mistaken as *E. histolytica*. They are most common in bacillary dysentery.
4. **Epithelial cells:** A few cells are always present. Increase number of epithelial cells occur in catarrhal condition of the colon.
5. **Red blood cells:** Unaltered erythrocytes are seen in diseases of colon, rectum or anus. In amoebic dysentery RBCs are present in clumps and are reddish yellow, while in bacillary dysentery, they are bright, discrete or in rouleaux.
6. **Crystals:** Various crystals may occur:
   i. *Triple phosphates:* More likely in a vegetable diet.
   ii. *Calcium oxalate:* More likely in a vegetable diet.
   iii. *Charcot Leyden crystals:* Particularly common in ulcerative conditions of colon, especially amoebic dysentery. Absent in bacillary dysentery. These crystals are colourless, pointed, often needle like, hexagonal on cross-section and variable size.
   iv. *Haematoidin crystals:* Yellowish brown needle like or rhombic crystals. They may occur after haemorrhages within gastrointestinal tract.
   v. *Bismuth suboxide crystals:* Seen after administration of Bismuth.
   vi. *Cholesterin crystals:* Especially found in cases of cholelithiasis.
   vii. *Calcium bilirubiate:* Same as above.
7. **Bacteria:** A study of bacteria in a saline or iodine preparation of stool is usually unnecessary.
8. **Yeasts and moulds:** Yeast cells are present in large number in cases of intestinal fermentation. The cells show buds and form short chains. Moulds, if present, are commonly contamination from unclean vessels or air.
9. **Protozoa:** Amongst the protozoa, a medical laboratory has to mainly identify *Entamoeba histolytica* and *Giardia intestinalis*. In fresh stool, trophozoites are seen, whereas cysts should be identified in iodine preparations, preferably after concentration. The cyst may be present in carriers. This is the infective form and carriers are public health hazards.
   i. *Giardia intestinalis:* Trophozoites are not usually seen in stool.

      Cysts oval in shape, 12 micron × 7 micron axostyles diagonally split the cyst into two. Four nuclei, clustered at one end or paired at opposite poles. (Fig. 14.2).

      Trophozoite is pear shaped, 12–20 microns in length. Has a depression on one side of the blunt and 3 pairs of flagellae around the depression and one at the pointed end. Two nuclei seen.
   ii. *E. histolytica:* It is to be differentiated from the *Endolimax nana* and *Entamoeba coli* by the under-mentioned characteristics (Fig. 14.3 and Table 14.1).

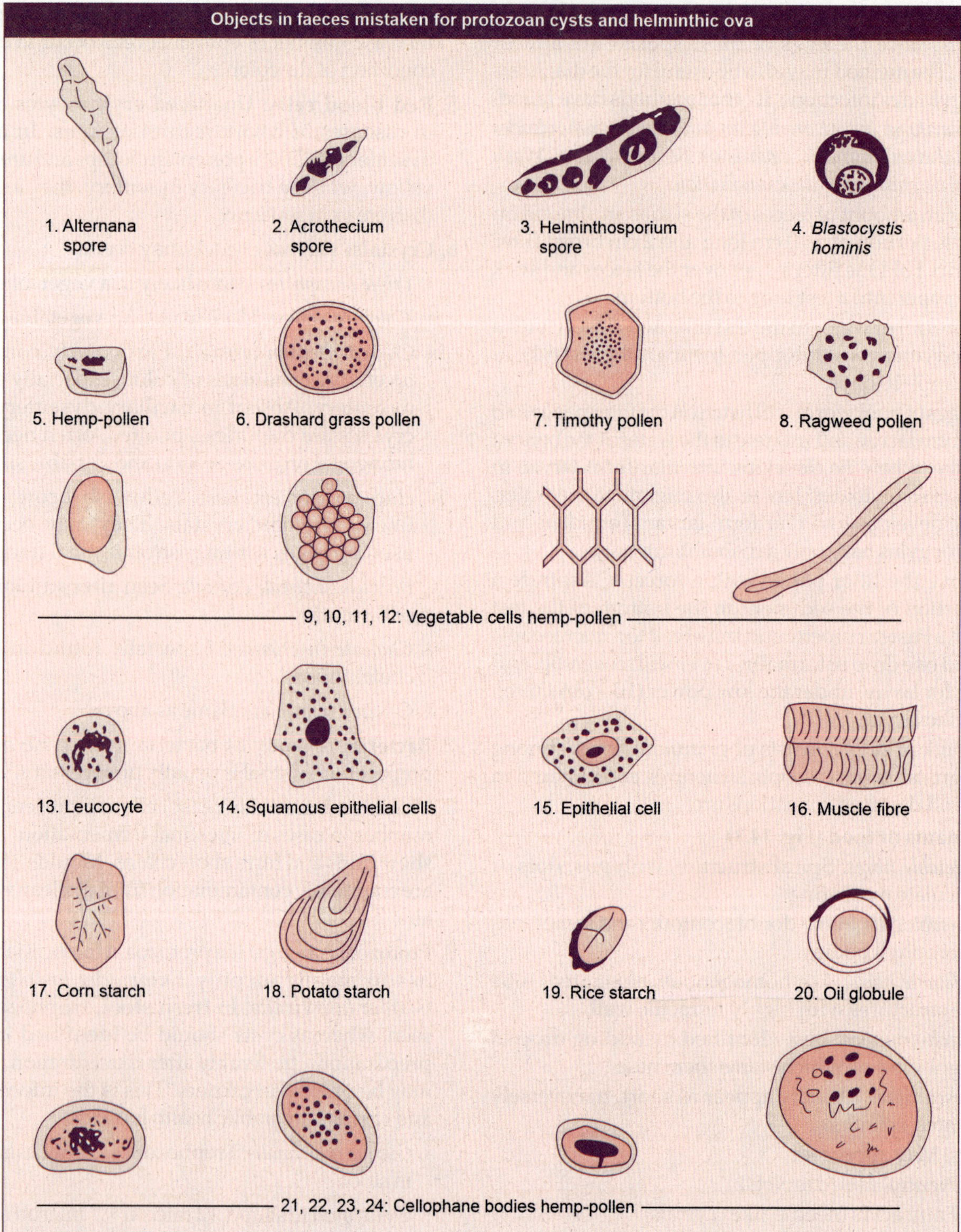

Fig. 14.1: Serial Nos (1–24): Remnants of food labelled diagrams resembling protozoan cysts and helminthic ova

Demonstration of Entamoeba histolytica in fresh stool: The trophozoite of *Entamoeba histolytica* is a shapeless cell 2–4 times as big as a red blood cell. The cytoplasma of the trophozoite is divided into an outer clear ectoplasma and an inner granular endoplasma. In the endoplasma one may find histolytica not detected. Does the cellular exudate look like an amoebic infection, but if *Entamoeba histolytica* not found, the specimen is reported as "*Entamoeba histolytica* not detected. The cellular exudate in accordance with amoebic infection. New specimen is requested. If possible, sample by rectoscopy from ulcerations". If *Entamoeba histolytica* is found, but the cellular exudate is in agreement with bacillary dysentery, the specimen is reported as "*Entamoeba histolytica* detected. Cellular exudate in accordance with bacillary dysentery. The specimen will be send for culture for enteropathogenic bacteria". Is

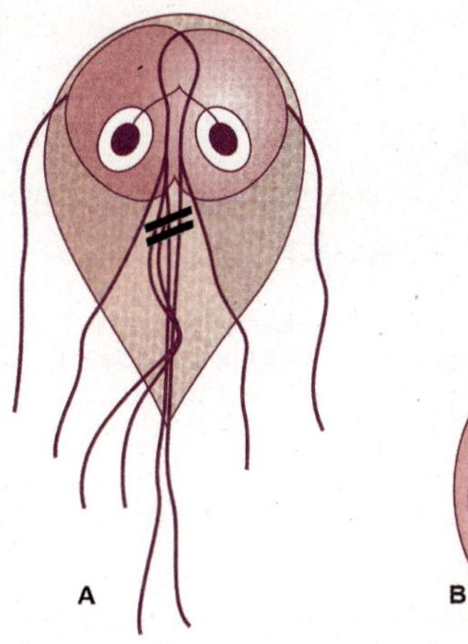

Fig.14.2: Giardia intestinalis: (A) Trophozoite; (B) Cyst

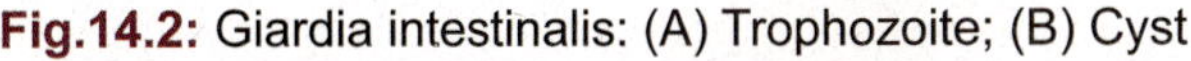

Table 14.1: Differentiation characteristics of *E. histolytica*, *E. coli* and *E. nana*

Morphology	*1. E. histolytica*	*2. E. coli*	*3. E. nana*
Trophozoite			
(Fresh unstained) size	20–30 microns	20–40 microns	8 microns
Motility	Actively motile	Sluggish	Sluggish
Nucleus	Not visible	Visible	Visible
Cytoplasmic inclusions	Red cells, leucocytes tissue debris present, bacteria absent	Bacteria and other materials present	Red cells never found
Cytoplasm	Clearly defined into ectoplasm and endoplasm	No clear division	No clear division
(Iodine stained) nuclear character	Central karyosome, fine chromatin granules line nuclear membrane	Eccentric karyosome coarse, chromatin granules line nuclear membrane	Large, irregular and eccentric karyosome, no chromatin granules
Cyst (stained with iodine)			
1. Size	6–15 microns	15–20 microns	8–9 microns
2. Nucleus	1–4 central karyosome	1–8 eccentric karyosome	1–4 karyosome may be central or eccentric
3. Glycogen mass	Rounded bars Chromatoid bars	Filamentous with square or pointed ends	Not seen

Entamoeba histolytica found and is cellular exudate in accordance with amoebic dysentery, then report "*Entamoeba histolytica* detected".

iii. *Chilomastix mesnili:* Pear shaped, 13–24 microns long with 3 anterior flagella and no undulating membrane. Contains a large round nucleus and a large, elongated cystostome anteriorly. Posterior end is projected into a narrow tail like process (Fig. 14.4).

Cyst is pear shaped to oval 7.5–8.5 microns in length.

iv. *Balantidium coli:* Oval shaped, 60–100 microns long and 50–70 microns wide. It is covered with cilia . It contains a bean-shaped macronucleus, a globular microns nucleus, contractile vocuoles and various sizes granules. At anterior end is a funnel-shaped mouth. It is actively motile (Fig. 14.5).

10. **Helminthic ova:** The ova which may be encountered in faeces of man are:

i. *Ascaris lumbricoides* (Fig. 14.6)

a. *Fertilised egg:* Round or oval in shape (60–75 microns in length by 40 to 50 microns in breadth).

- Always bile stained and brownish (golden brown) in colour.
- Surrounded by a thick smooth translucent shell with an outer albuminous coat which is thrown into rugosities or mamillations, this outer layer is sometimes lost (decortacated egg).
- Contains a very large conspicuous, unsegmented ovum (the nucleus is concealed by a larger amount of coarse yolk granules there is a clean crescentric space at the each pole).
- Floats in saturated solution of common salt.

b. *Unfertilised egg*

- Narrower, longer (80 microns by 55 microns and more elliptical).
- Brownish in colour (bile stained).
- Has a thinner shell with an irregular coating of albumin.
- Contains small atrophied ovum with a mass of unorganised highly refractile granules of various sizes.
- Do not float in salt solution (heaviest of all helminthic eggs).

ii. *Trichuris trichura*

- Size about 50 to 25 microns.
- Colour brown (bile stained). It has a double shell, outer one being bile stained.
- Barrel-shaped with a mucous plug at each pole.
- Contains an unsegmented ovum when the egg leaves the human host.
- Floats in saturated solution of common salt.

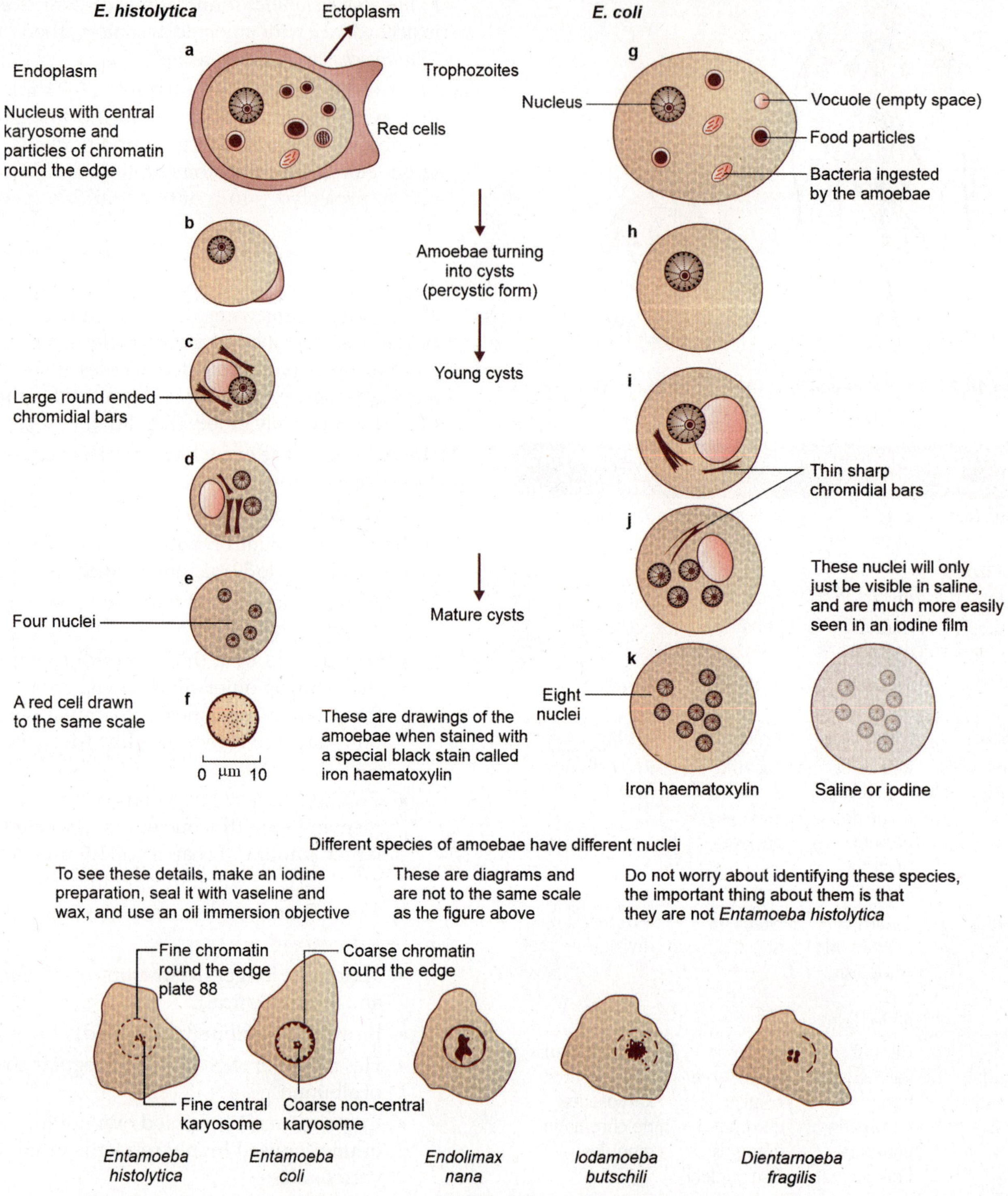

E. histolytica
Ectoplasm
E. coli
a
Endoplasm
Trophozoites
g
Nucleus with central karyosome and particles of chromatin round the edge
Red cells
Nucleus
Vocuole (empty space)
Food particles
Bacteria ingested by the amoebae
b
Amoebae turning into cysts (percystic form)
h
c
Young cysts
Large round ended chromidial bars
i
d
Thin sharp chromidial bars
j
e
These nuclei will only just be visible in saline, and are much more easily seen in an iodine film
Four nuclei
Mature cysts
k
A red cell drawn to the same scale
f
These are drawings of the amoebae when stained with a special black stain called iron haematoxylin
Eight nuclei
0 μm 10
Iron haematoxylin
Saline or iodine
Different species of amoebae have different nuclei
To see these details, make an iodine preparation, seal it with vaseline and wax, and use an oil immersion objective
These are diagrams and are not to the same scale as the figure above
Do not worry about identifying these species, the important thing about them is that they are not Entamoeba histolytica
Fine chromatin round the edge plate 88
Coarse chromatin round the edge
Fine central karyosome
Coarse non-central karyosome
Entamoeba histolytica
Entamoeba coli
Endolimax nana
Iodamoeba butschili
Dientamoeba fragilis

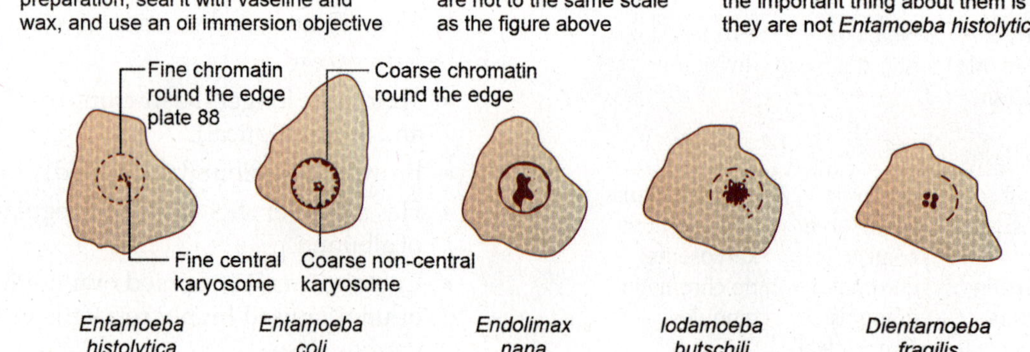

Fig. 14.3: *Entamoeba histolytica* and *Entamoeba coli*

iii. *Ankylostoma duodenale*

- Oval or elliptical in shape 65 microns by 40 microns.
- Colourless (not bile stained).
- Surrounded by a transparent hyaline shell.
- Contains a segmented ovum usually with 4 blastomeres; has a clear space between the egg shell and segmented ovum.
- Floats in saturated solution of common salt.

iv. *Enterobius vermicularis:*

Colourless (not bile stained).

- Asymmetrical in shape being planoconvex, i.e. flattened on one side and convex on the other side.
- Measures 50 to 60 microns by 30 microns.
- Surrounded by a transport shell.
- Contains a coiled tadpole like larva.
- Floats in saturated solution of common salt.

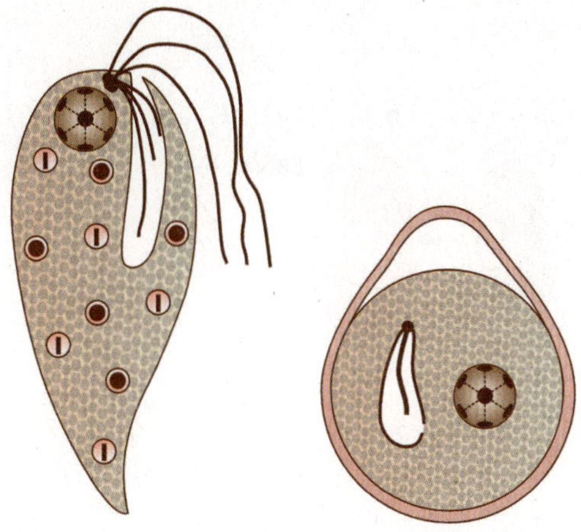

Fig. 14.4: *Chilomastix mesnili*, trophozoite and cyst

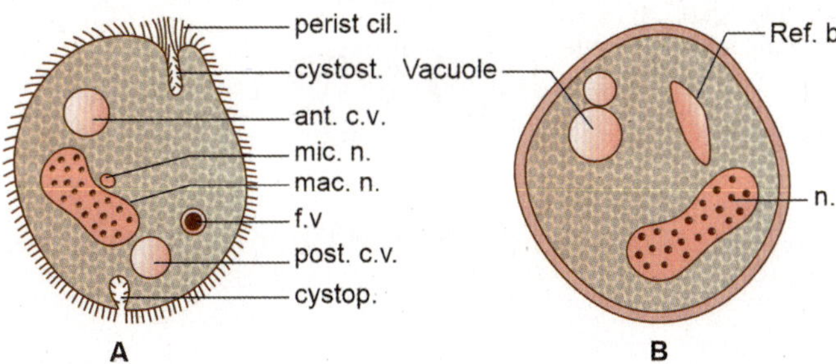

Fig. 14.5: *Balantidium coli:* (A) *Trophozoite;* (B) *Cyst c.v.*: Anterior contractile vacuole, *Cystost.*: Cystostome, *Cystop.* Cytophyge, *f.v.*: Food vacuoles, *mac. n.*: Macronucleus, *perist. cil.*: Peristomel cilia, post *c.v.*: Posterior contractile vacuoles, *mic. n.*: Micronucleus. *ref. b.*: Refractile vacuole, *n.*: Vacuole

v. *Hymenolepis nana*

- Spherical or oval in shape measuring 30 to 45 microns in diameter (not bile stained).
- There are two distinct membranes: (a) The outer membrane is thin and colourless and (b) The inner embryophore enclosed an oncosphere with three pairs of lancet-shaped hooklets.
- The space between the two membranes is filled with yolk granules and polar filaments emanating from little knobs at either end of embryo phore.
- Floats in saturated solution of common salt.

vi. *Taenia soluium/saginata/echinococcus granulosus (Fig. 14.7)*

- Spherical and brown in colour (bile stained).
- Measures 30 to 43 microns in diameter.
- Thin, outer transparent shell, when present, represents the remnant of the yolk mass; it causes the eggs to clump together.
- The inner embryophore is brown, thick walled and radially striated (bile stained).
- Contains an oncosphere (14 to 20 microns in diameter) with 3 pairs of hooklets.
- Does not float in saturated solution of common salt.

vii. *Schistosoma (general):* Eggs are non-operculated and when laid are fully embryonated (containing a ciliated embryo, miracidium).

S. Haematobium	150 microns by 50 microns, terminal spine.
S. Mansoni	150 microns by 60 microns, lateral spine.
S. Japonicum	100 microns by 65 microns, lateral knob.

viii. *Fasciola hepatica/Fasciolopsis buski*

- Large operculated, brownish yellow (bile stained).
- Size 140 microns by 80 microns.
- Contains a large unsegmented ovum in a mass of yolk cells.
- Does not float in saturated salt solution.

ix. *Clonorchis sinensis*

- Large operculated brownish yellow (bile stained) flask-shaped and operculated.
- Possesses a terminal hook-like spine (resembling an electric-bulb).
- Small in size, measuring 35 microns by 20 microns.
- When oviposited, contains a ciliated embryo (miracidium).
- Does not float in saturated salt solution.

x. *Diphyllobothrium latum* (Fig. 14.7)

- Oval and brown in colour (bile stained).
- Measures 70 microns by 45 microns.
- Contains abundant yolk granules and an unsegmented ovum.
- There is an inconspicuous operculum at one end with a small knob at the other end. Does not float in saturated solution of common salt.

xi. *Paragonimus westermani*

- Golden brown in colour (bile stained).
- Oval in shape.
- Flattened operculca.
- Measure 80 microns by 55 microns.
- Contains an unsegmented ovum surrounded by yolk cells.

xii. *Strongyloides stercoralis:* As soon as the eggs of the *Strongyloides sterconalis* are laid, the rhabditiform larvae start hatching and move their way out, into the lumen from where they are passed in the faeces. Hence it is the larvae, not the eggs which are found in the faeces. Two types of larvae are found:

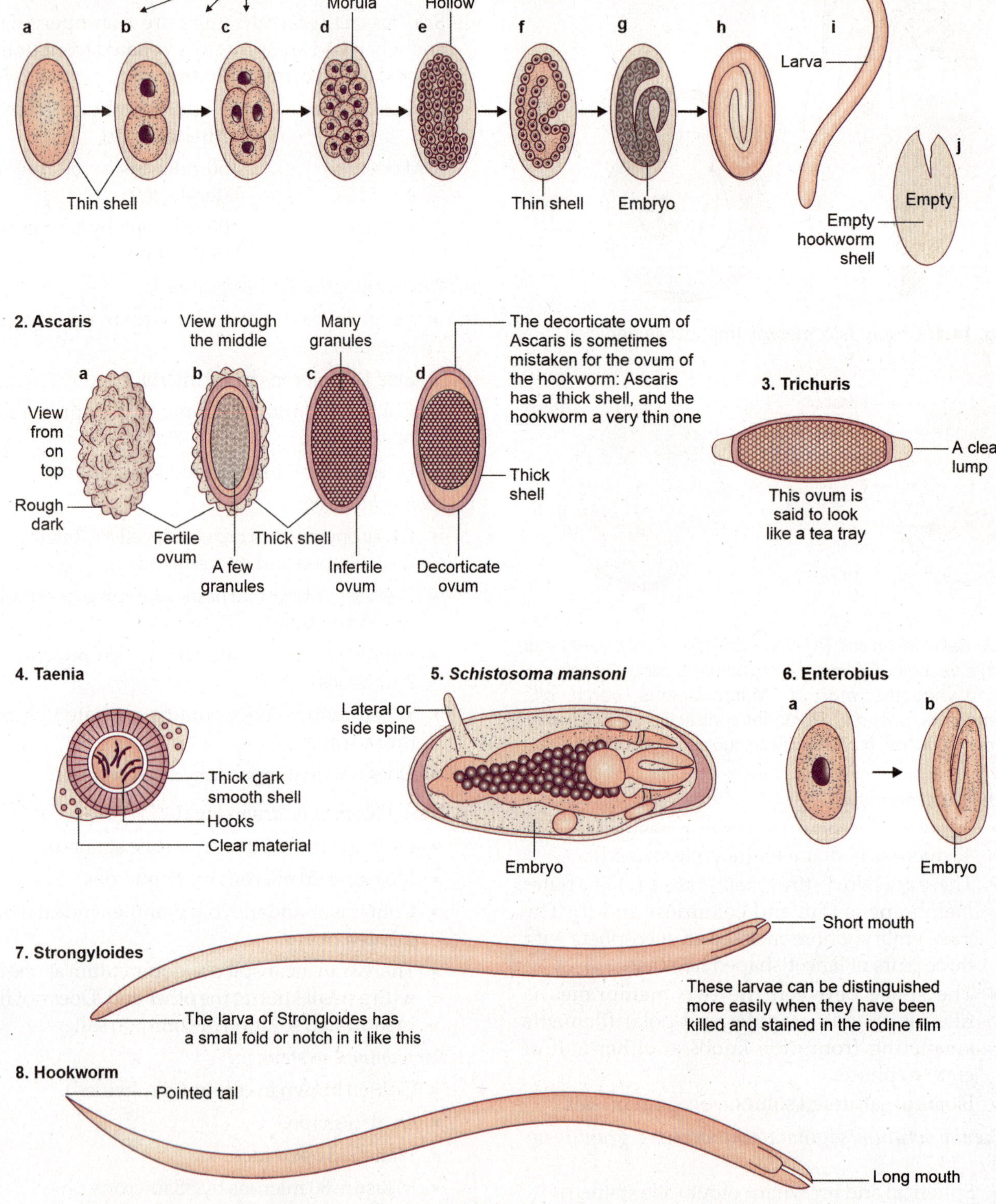

Fig. 14.6: Some common ova and worms in diagram

a. Rhabditiform larvae measure 200 to 250 microns in length by 16 microns in breadth, they have short mouth and double bulb esophagus.

b. Filariform larvae are longer, more slender. They have short mouth and cylindrical esophagus.

An overview of the most common parasitic infections of the intestinal tract are given in Table 14.2.

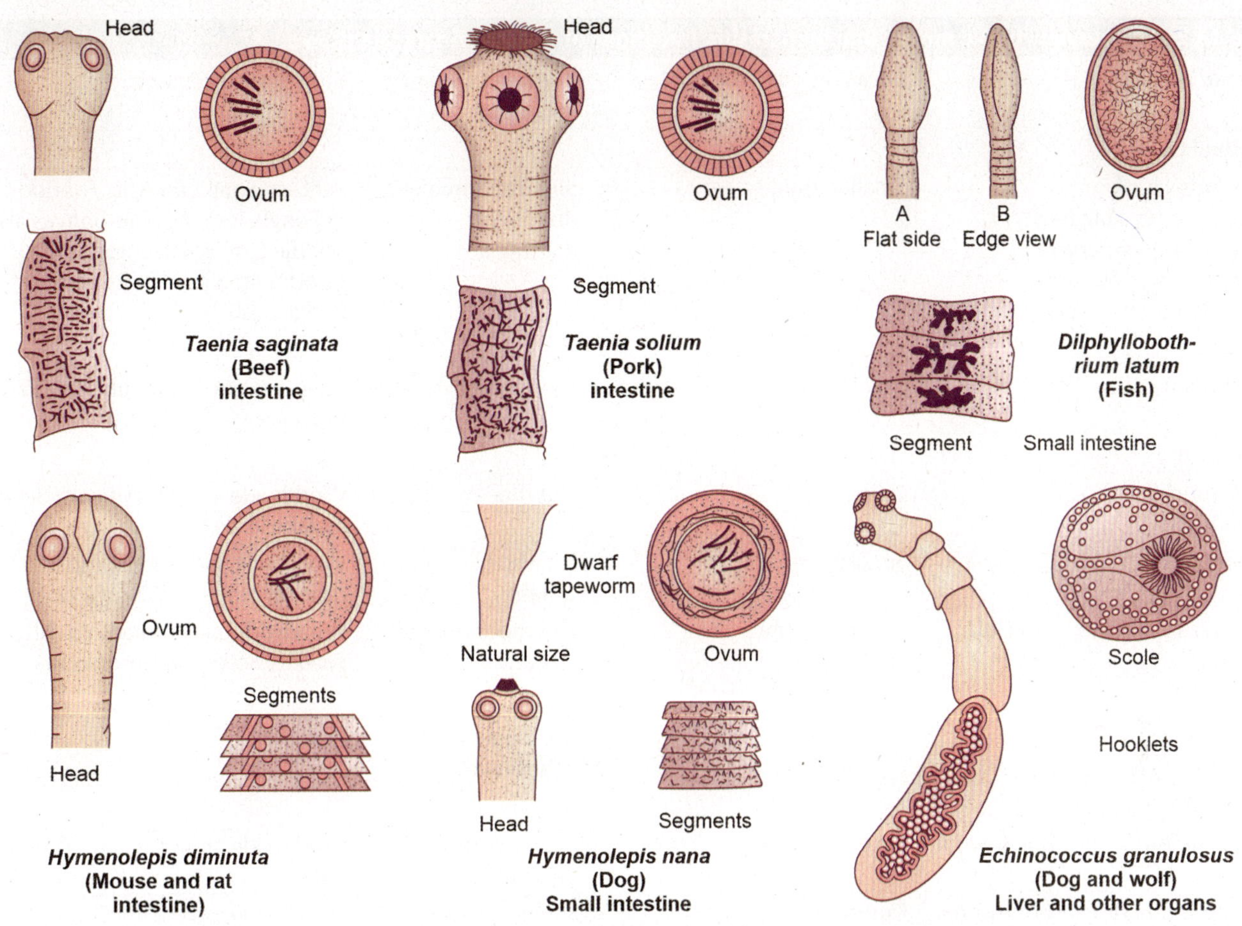

Fig. 14.7: Cystodes—tapeworms

Table 14.2: An overview of the most common parasitic infections of the intestinal tract

Name of parasite	*Localization in the host*	*The most common symptoms*	*Distribution remarks*
Amoeba			
Entamoeba histolytica	Lumen and wall of large intestine, liver	Diarrhoea, dysentery, painful swollen liver (liver abscess)	Worldwide, several races, pathogenic races usually in the tropics and subtropics, many asymptomatic infections
Entamoeba hartmani	Lumen of upper large intestine	Apathogenic	Worldwide
Entamoeba coli	Lumen of upper large intestine	Apathogenic	Worldwide
Entamoeba polecki	Lumen of upper large intestine	Apathogenic	Worldwide
Iodamoeba butschlii	Lumen of upper large intestine	Apathogenic	Worldwide
Endolimax nada	Lumen of upper large intestine	Apathogenic	Worldwide
Dientamoeba fragilis	Lumen of upper large intestine	Apathogenic	Worldwide
Flagellates			
Pentatrichomanas hominis	Lumen of small intestine	Apathogenic	Worldwide
Giardia intestinalis Giardia	Attach to the wall of upper small intestine	Diarrhoea malabsorption	Worldwide asymptomatic infections
Chilomastix mesnili	Coecum	Apathogenic	Worldwide
Enteromonas hominis	Coecum	Apathogenic	Worldwide
Retoramonas intestinalis	Coecum	Apathogenic	Worldwide
Opisthorchis viverini *Opisthorchis felineus*			*F. hepatica* also in South Europe, South and Central America

Contd.

Table 14.2: An overview of the most common parasitic infections of the intestinal tract (Contd.)

Name of parasite		*Localization in the host*	*The most common symptoms*	*Distribution remarks*
Intestinal flukes				
Fasciolopsis buski *Metagonimus yokagawai* *Heterophyes heterophyes* *Gastrodiscoides hominis* Echinostoma and related species		Small intestine	Slight abdominal discomfort, diarrhoea	Far East, Southeast Asia, *F. buski* also in Bangladesh, *H. heterophyes* also in Middle East, South Europe, *G. hominis* also in India and Bangladesh
Ciliates				
Balantidium coli		Colon	Diarrhoea dysentery	Rare, sporatic in the subtropics and tropics
Sporozoae				
Cryptosporidium (parvum?)		Colon	Diarrhoea	Worldwide in AIDS patients: Severe malabsorption
Isospora belli :	Coccidia	Small intestine	Diarrhoea, loss of weight	Worldwide, rare, sporadic in AIDS patients: Severe malabsorption
Sacrocystis sui/bovi : *hominis*	Coccidia	Small intestine	Diarrhoea, loss of weight	Worldwide, rare, sporadic in AIDS patients: Severe malabsorption
Unknown				
Blastocytis hominis		Colon	Apathogenic (diarrhoea?)	Worldwide
Nematodes				
Ascaris lumbri-coides :	Roundworm	Small intestine	Slight abdominal discomfort	Worldwide, may migrate to the bili duct
Trichuris trichiura :	Whipworm	Colon	Slight abdominal discomfort	Worldwide, severe infection: anaemia, dysentery, rectal prolapse
Capillaria philipineses		Small intestine in burrows in the wall	Diarrhoea stomach pain, malabsorption	Philippines, Thailand may be lethal
Capillaria hepatica		Liver	Hepatitis	Worldwide (rare)
Enterobius vermicularis :	Pinworm	Appendix, coecum	Anal itch	Worldwide, whole family usually infected
Ancylostoma duodenale :	Old world hookworm	Small intestine, sucks to the wall	Gastric ulcer-like symptoms	Tropics and subtropics moderate/ severe infections
Necator amricanus :	American hookworm	Small intestine, sucks to the wall	Gastric ulcer-like symptoms	Tropics and subtropics moderate/ severe infections anaemia, diarrhoea
Strongyloides stercoralis		Small intestine in burrows in the wall	Gastric ulcer-like symptoms, diarrhoea	Tropics and subtropics disseminated infections in patients on immunosuppressive therapy
Ternidens deminutus		Small intestine and colon in cystic noduli	Slight abdominal discomfort	Tropical Africa, severe infections: Anaemia
Oesophagostomum apiostomum		Colon in cystic noduli	Slight abdominal discomfort	Nigeria, East Africa, Indonesia
Trichostrongyloides		Small intestine	Slight abdominal discomfort	North Africa, Middle East, India, Far East
Cestopdes				
Hymenolepis nana :	Dwarf tapeworm	Small intestine	Slight abdominal discomfort	Tropics and subtropics
Hymenolepis diminuta :	Rat tapeworm	Small intestine	Slight abdominal discomfort	Tropics and subtropics
Taenia saginata :	Oxe tapeworm	Small intestine	Slight abdominal discomfort	Worldwide segment in stool

Contd.

Table 14.2: An overview of the most common parasitic infections of the intestinal tract (Contd.)				
Name of parasite		***Localization in the host***	***The most common symptoms***	***Distribution remarks***
Taenia solium	Pig tapeworm	Small intestine	Slight abdominal discomfort	Worldwide
Diphylobotriurn latum	Fish tapeworm	Small intestine	Slight abdominal discomfort	Finland, Greenland, Japan
Dipylidium caninum	Dog tapeworm	Small intestine	Slight abdominal discomfort	Worldwide, rare
Bertiella studeri	–	Small intestine	Slight intestinal discomfort	Southeast Asia, India, Yemen, rare
Blood flukes				
Schistosoma mansoni	–	The veins of colon, ova in	Slight intestinal discomfort diarrhoea	Africa, South America, severe infections: Dysentery, hepatosplenomegali, cirrhosis of the liver
Schistosoma haematobium :	Bilharzia	The veins of the urinary bladder	Slight urinary discomfort, dysuria, haematuria	North and Central America, Central and South America, severe infections
Schistosoma japonicum :		The veins of colon	Slight intestinal discomfort, diarrhoea	China, Japan, Philippines, severe infections: Dysentery, hepatosplenomegaly, cirrhosis of the liver
Schistosoma mekongi		The veins of the colon	Slight intestinal discomfort, diarrhoea	Laos, Cambodia, severe infections: Dysentery, hepatosplenomegaly, cirrhosis of the liver
Liver flukes				
Fasciola hepatica	Great liver fluke	Bile duct, gall bladder	Slight intestinal discomfort, diarrhoea	*O. felineus* in Ukraine, Siberia and Polen, the other species in Far East and Southeast Asia
Opisthorchis siniensis	Chinese liver fluke			

Chapter 15

Gastric Analysis

Chapter Outline

INTRODUCTION

Digestion in the stomach consists of the action of pepsin on proteins in the presence of hydrochloric acid and of the curding of milk by rennin. Lipase of the gastric juice has very little activity except on previously emulsified fats, such as those of milk and egg yolk.

Gastric analysis denotes an examination of the gastric contents at various phases of digestion. Yet, the results of such analysis are influenced by many intragastric factors, and need to be interpreted only in the light of the clinical findings.

Although the gastric juice is secreted continuously quantities sufficiently large for examination are better obtained after administration of a suitable food. Different foods stimulate secretion to different degrees, hence for the sake of uniform results certain standard test meals have been adopted.

The highly acidic environment in the stomach lumen degrades proteins (e.g., food). Peptide bonds, which comprise proteins, are labilized. The gastric chief cells of the stomach secrete enzymes for protein breakdown (inactive pepsinogen, and in infancy rennin). The low pH activates pepsinogen into the enzyme pepsin, which then aids digestion by breaking the amino acid bonds, a process called proteolysis. In addition, many microorganisms are inhibited or destroyed in an acidic environment, preventing infection or sickness.

Gastric acid, gastric juice, or stomach acid, is a digestive fluid formed within the stomach lining. With a pH between 1 and 3, gastric acid plays a key role in digestion of proteins by activating digestive enzymes, which together break down the long chains of amino acids of proteins. Gastric acid is regulated in feedback systems to increase production when needed, such as after a meal. Other cells in the stomach produce bicarbonate, a base, to buffer the fluid, ensuring a regulated pH. These cells also produce mucus—a viscous barrier to prevent gastric acid from damaging the stomach. The pancreas further produces large amounts of bicarbonate and secretes bicarbonate through the pancreatic duct to the duodenum to neutralize gastric acid passing into the digestive tract.

Definition: Gastric analysis is a method to measure secretion of hydrochloric acid under basal (baseline) and augmented (stimulated) conditions.

COMPOSITION OF GASTRIC SECRETIONS (Fig. 15.1)

- Gastric juice is a mixture of water, HCl, electrolytes and organic substances.
- The gastric juice is 97–99% water.
- The remainder consists of inorganic salts, and organic components that include mucin, digestive enzymes.

The chief constituents of gastric juice are:

1. Hydrochloric acid, secreted by parietal cells.
2. Pepsinogen secreted by chief cells. (It is activated to pepsin by acid which also provides acid medium in which pepsin acts.
3. Renin which clots milk by converting milk casein into caseinogen.
4. Intrinsic factor which binds vitamin B_{12} and aids its absorption in the intestine.
5. Mucous.

Gastric secretion is secreted in response to varied stimulants, important among which are:

i. Psychic factors such as sight, taste, smell of food, mediated by vagus nerve.
ii. Gastrin (a hormone secreted by gastric mucosa in response to food present in the stomach).
iii. Presence of digested products in the intestine.

Other stimulants include:

1. Insulin
2. Histamine and
3. Alcohol

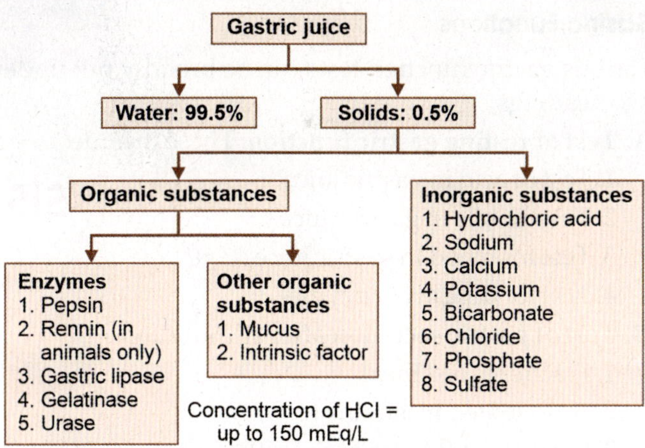

Fig. 15.1: Composition of gastric juice

ORIGIN AND REGULATION OF GASTRIC SECRETIONS

- Secrete hormones that regulate stomach functions, peristalsis, and secretions.
- Initiate digestion of proteins
- Converse hormones
- Chemical digestion
- Provides optimal pH
- Destroys some bacteria
- Stops carbohydrate digestion
- Secrete a mucus protect the epithelium from chemical insults.
- Secrete a mucus that coats and lubricates the gastric surface.

The active components of gastric acid are protons and chloride. Often simplistically described as hydrochloric acid, these species are produced by parietal cells in the gastric glands in the stomach. The secretion is a complex and relatively energetically expensive process. Parietal cells contain an extensive secretory network (called canaliculi) from which the "hydrochloric acid" is secreted into the lumen of the stomach. The pH of gastric acid is 1.5 to 3.5 in the human stomach lumen, a level maintained by the proton pump H^+/K^+ ATPase. The parietal cell releases bicarbonate into the bloodstream in the process, which causes a temporary rise of pH in the blood, known as an alkaline tide.

SECRETION OF GASTRIC JUICE

There is always a small quantity of gastric juice present in the stomach, even when it contains no food. This is known as fasting juice. Secretion reaches its maximum level about 1 hour after a meal, then declines to the fasting level after about 4 hours.

There are three phases of secretion of gastric juice regulated.

- Cephalic phase.
- Gastric phase.
- Intestinal phase.

1. **Reflex phase (cephalic):** A few minutes prior to food entry: Smell/taste.
2. **Gastric phase:** 3–4 hours after food enters the stomach.
3. **Intestinal phase:** Brief stimulatory effect as chyme enters the duodenum, followed by inhibitory effects.
    - Cell types responsible for secreting gastric acid.
    - Mucous neck cells, found in the upper, or "neck," regions of the glands, produce a thin, soluble mucus.
    - Parietal cells: Found mainly in the middle region of the glands, simultaneously secrete hydrochloric acid (HCl) and intrinsic factor. This structure provides a huge surface area for secreting H and Cl into the stomach lumen. HCl makes the stomach contents extremely acidic (pH 1.5–3.5), a condition necessary for activation and optimal activity of pepsin.
    - Chief cells occur mainly in the basal regions of the gastric glands. The chief cells produce pepsinogen, the inactive form of the protein-digesting enzyme pepsin.
    - Enteroendocrine cells ("gut endocrine"): Typically located deep in the gastric glands, release a variety of chemical messengers directly into the interstitial fluid of the lamina propria.

Indications

With the advent of more sophisticated techniques for diagnosis of ulcer disease, indications of gastric analysis are now very much specific and limited. Gastric analysis is mostly done for estimation of acid secretion.

1. To confirm suspected Zollinger-Ellison syndrome.
2. To demonstrate achlorhydria.
3. To estimate or reflect parietal cell mass.

Gastric acidity estimation is influenced by a number of factors, so instead of determining concentration of acid produced, total acid output as a timed volume is determined to reflect a more complete picture of acid secretory capacity.

Zollinger-Ellison Syndrome

A rare condition characterized by severe and recurrent peptic ulcers in the stomach, duodenum, and upper small intestine, caused by a tumor or tumors, usually found in the pancreas. The tumor secretes the hormone gastrin.

The test is also used to evaluate a patient with elevated serum gastrin levels. Hyperchlorhydria in the presence of elevated gastrin usually indicates Zollinger-Ellison syndrome.

Hypochlorhydria in the presence of elevated gastrin indicates impairment of acid output, such as occurs in pernicious anaemia, atrophic gastritis, and Ménétrier disease and after inhibition of gastric acid secretion by potent antisecretory drugs.

Functions of Gastric Juice

1. Digestive function
    - Pepsin
    - Action of pepsin

- Gastric lipase
- Action of other enzymes of gastric juice

2. Hemopoietic function
3. Protective function: Function of mucus
4. Functions of hyorochloric acid
   - Food is stored in the stomach
   - Mixed with acid mucus and pepsin
   - Stomach also adds a significant amount of digestive juices to meal
   - Stomach is ready to receive the food
   - As cephalic phase of gastric secretion start earlier
   - This food is released in steady into the duodenum
   - Water further liquefies the food swallowed.
   - Hydrochloric acid:
     - Acidifies the food and stop the action of salivary amylase.
     - Kills ingested microbes.
     - Provides the acid environment needed for the action of pepsins.
   - Pepsinogens.
   - Intrinsic factor.
   - Mucus.

Functions of HCl

- HCl activates pepsinogen to active enzyme pepsin.
- It provides acid medium in which pepsin acts optimally.
- HCl breaks down connective tissue and muscle fibers reducing large food particle into smaller particle.
- Denatures protein
- It kills micro-organism ingested with food.
- Due to acid and pepsin it can digest proteins.
- Digestion of some lipids and carbohydrates (hydrolysis by acid) is achieved by gastric juice.
- It helps the absorption of extrinsic factor, so, helps in haemopoesis.
- It helps to form the chyme.

Functions of Mucus

- Surface of gastric mucosa is covered by mucus.
- It is derived from surface epithelial cells and mucous cells.
- Mucus works as protective barrier.
- It protects stomach wall from self-digestion by pepsin.
- As mucus is alkaline, pH 7, it protects stomach from HCl [pH 2].

Importance of Detection

- Diagnosis of gastric diseases and assist in the selection of therapy, i.e. peptic ulcer.
- It measures the amount of acid produced by a patient with symptoms of peptic ulcer.
- Diagnosis of Zollinger-Ellison syndrome (adenoma of islet of Langerhans), a condition of gastric hypersecretion produced by a gastrin secreting tumour of the pancreas.

Gastric Functions

Various gastric function tests can be broadly put under two headings.

A. **Test of resting gastric function:** These include:
   1. Test of acid in gastric juice
   2. Test for bile in gastric juice
   3. Test for blood in gastric juice
   4. Test for digestive enzymes

B. **Test of gastric secretion after stimulation**
   1. Fractional test meal
   2. Augmented histamine test
   3. Insulin test (Hollander's test)

Gastric analysis can be of two types

1. Tube gastric analysis: Gastric contents are collected by means of a double lumen tube.
2. Tubeless gastric analysis

Withdrawal of gastric contents: The gastric fluid is obtained by aspiration through a tube. There are many tubes on the market, of which Sawyer tube, Levin tube, Rehfuss tube, or a Ryle's tube may be used (Fig. 15.2).

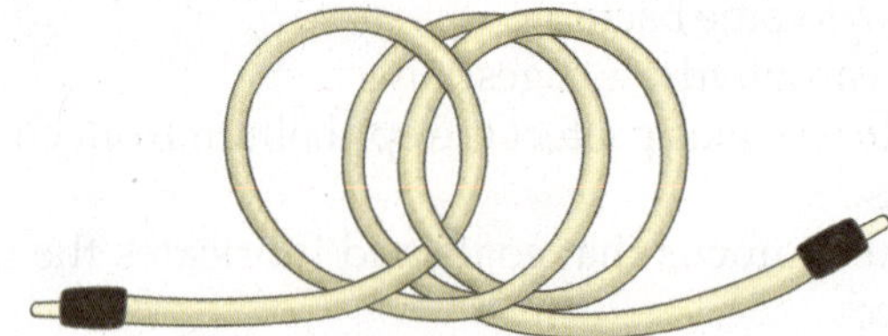

Fig. 15.2: Ryle's stomach tube

Precautions: Because both the basal acid output test and the gastric acid stimulation test require gastric intubation through the mouth or nasal passage, neither test is recommended for patients with esophageal problems, aortic aneurysm, severe gastric hemorrhage, or congestive heart failure.

If the patient is neurotic or has marked pharyngeal hyperaesthesia, spray the fauces and the nostrils with a 2% solution of cocaine hydrochloride. The patient should be seated with the head tilted slightly forward and the clothing protected with towels. Place the tip of the tube on the tongue held well out and pass it back to the throat or introduce the tube along the floor of the nose until it is felt that the top turns down into the pharynx. Then the patient is encouraged to swallow quickly until the tube is passed to the desired length.

Examination of resting contents: The tube is passed after a night's fast (no food or drink) and the stomach contents removed.

Gastric Juice

Following things have to be checked.

1. Colour
2. Volume

3. Any specific odour
4. Detection of acid
5. Presence of mucus (normal or excessive)
6. Detection of blood
7. Detection of bile
8. Detection for digestive enzymes

Each of these will be discussed in detail in the text.

Colour: A colourless to grayish or yellowish watery fluid with a low specific gravity secreted by the surface epithelium, gastric cells and the various glands of the tract.

Volume: In most normal cases after a night fast only a small quantity (20–50 ml) of resting contents is obtained, volumes above 100–200 ml may be considered.

Odour: Fermentation which gives rise to lactic acid and other organic acids may produce a rather characteristic smell with which the dealing persons soon become familiar.

Mucous: Presence of excessive amounts of mucus implies mixture of excessive amounts of saliva in the gastric juice.

Detection of blood: Blood should not normally be present. A small amount of fresh red blood may be present and usually signifies trauma and is easily distinguished macroscopically from that arising due to any pathological condition; since blood which has been in the stomach for some time is usually brown or reddish brown in colour, because of formation of acid haematin (coffee ground), various chemical tests for detection of blood include:

1. Ortho-toluidine test
2. Guaiac test
3. Benzidine test

All these have been discussed in detail under the chapter of stool.

Interpretation: The blood may be

1. Swallowed
2. From stomach itself in various conditions like:
   - Gastritis
   - Gastric ulcer
   - Gastric carcinoma

Detection of bile: Bile may be found occasionally but may not be of any particular significance. A small amount may regurgitate into the stomach during intubation.

Various tests for detection of bile include:

1. Iodine test
2. Gmelin's nitric acid test
3. Fouchet's test
4. Hunter's diazo test
5. Ictotest

(All have been discussed in the chapter on urine)

Some pathophysiologists believe that bile is important in the pathogenesis of gastric ulcers. Therefore, detection of bile may be important and significant in some patients of gastric ulcer.

Detection and estimation of gastric acid: Total acid of gastric juice is divided into two parts:

1. Free hydrochloric acid (free acid)
2. Combined acid, this includes organic acids and HCl found in combinations with proteins or more appropriately acid that is not free for first titration with NaOH.

Testing for Free and Total Acid

Take 1.0 ml of gastric juice in a test tube and to it add 2–4 drops of Topfer's reagent. If there is an initial yellow colour on adding the indicator, no free acid is present, then only titrate for total acid.

If initially red colour appears, titrate with 0.1 N sodium hydroxide (NaOH) until initial red colour becomes yellow.

Note down the volume of NaOH used.

Now add 2–4 drops of phenolphtalein. Again titrate with 0.1N NaOH until pink colour reappears and note down the total NaOH used up for titration.

Vol. of free acid = Vol. of NaOH used for first titration × 10

Total acid = Total vol. of NaOH used for both titrations × 10

(Topfer's reagent-p-dimethylamino azobenzene 1 g in 100 ml of 95% ethyl alcohol. 0.1% methyl orange can be used in its place).

Thymol blue can be used as the only indicator in test for free and total acid because it has 2 colour changes, one at pH 1.2–2.8 and the second at pH 8.0 to 9.5.

Interpretation: There is only a small amount of free HCl, normally present in gastric juice. This is 0–30 mEq/L. Up to 50 mEq/L may be taken to be normal. Concentrations above this point to hyperacidity. Lactic acid is the most important, among the organic acids found. All these are formed by action of microorganisms on food which is favoured by achlorhydria associated with prolonged retention of food.

Tests for Lactic Acid

1. **Ferric chloride test:** 2 ml of filtered gastric contents + 1–3 drops of $FeCl_3$ (10% solution) in a test tube.

   A yellow colour that remains on dilution with water points to presence of lactic acid.

2. **Maclean's test:** (Maclean's solution—100 ml saturated $HgCl_2$ + 1.5 ml HCl in which 5 g $FeCl_3$ is dissolved)

5 ml filtered gastric contents + few drops of Maclean's solution. Reddish colour points to lactic acid.

It can be quantitized colourimetrically with a blank of normal gastric contents.

Tests for HCl

(Gunzberg's reagent—2 g phloroglucinol + 1 g Vanillin in 100 ml of 95% ethanol)

- 1–2 drops gastric contents + 1–2 drops of Gunzberg's reagent in a Petri dish.
- Evaporate to dryness in a waterbath.
- Reddish colour signifies HCl.

(This test is positive for all mineral acids and HCl is the only mineral acid expected in gastric contents).

Fractional Test Meal (Fig. 15.3)

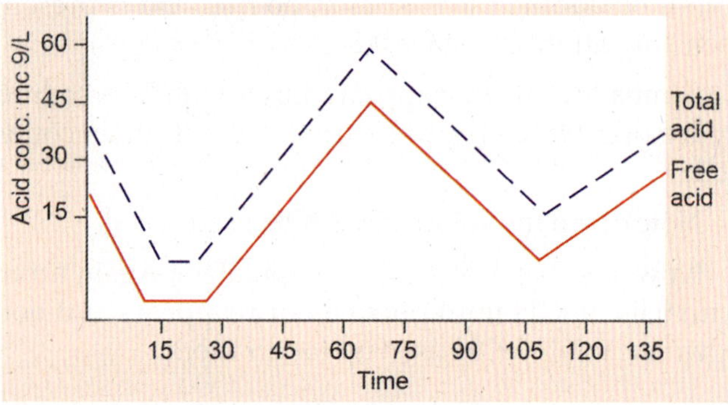

Fig. 15.3: Free and total acid concentration with time relation

This test has now lost its importance and is not of much use in the diagnosis of gastric diseases (Fig. 15.3).

1. Begin the test after overnight fasting. Analyze the fasting contents as discussed earlier.
2. Now give the patient a meal. Various types of meals that have been used include
   (a) 50 ml of 7% ethyl alcohol solution.
   (b) 2 spoonfuls of oat meal to ½ a glass of water.
   (c) Tea/coffee
3. After the meal samples are drawn at interval of 15 minutes for 2 hours. At least 10 ml of sample should be drawn.
4. Analyze for free and total acid as discussed earlier.

Interpretation:

1. *Normal:* After the meal free acid is found after about 45 minutes to 1 hour. It rises steadily to reach maximum at about 1½ hours after which concentration starts decreasing. Maximum level is 15–45 mEq/L of free acid. 25–55 m Eq/L of total acid.
2. *Hyperchlorhydria:* Occurs when maximum free acidity exceeds 45 mEq/L. Combined acidity is same as for normal persons. It is typically seen in
   a. Duodenal ulcer
   b. Zollinger-Ellison syndrome
   c. Gastric ulcer (50% cases).
3. *Achlorhydria:* This term is used when no HCl is secreted by gastric mucosa. Seen in
   a. Tuberculosis
   b. Atrophic gastritis
   c. Late stages of gastric malignancies
   d. Microcytic hypochronic anaemia due to iron deficiency.

Defined as inability of stomach to produce juice with a pH < 7.1 even after maximal stimulation.

Histamine Test (Pentagastrin Test)

Only useful test for diagnostic purposes.

Histamine or pentagastrin is used for stimulating gastric acid secretion.

1. After overnight fasting, collect the resting contents.
2. Collect gastric contents for 1 hour by aspirating at 15 minutes intervals. At 30 minutes point give 1 amp avil intramuscular.
3. At the end of the first hour give the dose of histamine. It is given in doses of 0.25 mg by SC injection (Pentagastrin in doses of 6 mg/kg can be given instead, S/C or I/M: In fact this is now preferred over histamine.)
4. Specimens are again collected for the next 1 hour at 15 minute intervals.
5. Now titrate for presence of acid both free and total.

Interpretation mEq/L/hr

	Basal acid output	*Maximal output*
Normal	3–4	18.5
Gastric ulcer	2	14.6
Duodenal ulcer	0	37.5
Anastomotic ulcer	2.7	31
Zollinger-Ellison syndrome	22	50–100 or even more

Hollander Test (Insulin Test)

It is of value postoperatively to verify completeness of vagal section.

To a fasting patient give 20 unit/10 kg body weight by I/V injection and perform serial 15 min aspirations for 4 hours (blood sugar should fall below 35 mg/dl).

Early response: Rise in concentration of acid 20 mmol/L above basal level within 1st hour suggests incomplete vagotomy.

Delayed response: Rise in concentration of acid between 1 and 4 hours suggests less than complete vagotomy.

Negative response: No increase in gastric acid concentration suggests complete vagotomy.

Tubeless Gastric Analysis

In 1950–53 Segal et al published a series of papers in which a new method for determining the production of free acid by stomach was put forward.

Principle: When a quininium—resin indicator is given by mouth, hydrogen ions from HCl in stomach can liberate quinine ions (the QH cation). At pH values less than 3 quinine HCl is formed, and absorbed in the intestine and begins to be excreted in the urine. The quinine can be extracted from the urine and determined by measuring its fluorescence in U-V light.

Procedure: This test is marketed as a ready made kit in foreign countries.

It is called Gastro test marked by ortho pharmaceuticals Diagnex Test marketed by Squibb Ltd.

It contains the reagent Diagnex Blue (Azure A-3 amino 7-dimethylamino-phenothiazin-5-ium Chloride: Diagnex blue).

Tablets for this test are available. Each test unit contains two 250 mg tablets of caffeine sodium benzoate.

1. Do not breakfast in the morning.
2. Empty the bladder on rising and discard the urine.
3. Take the tablets of caffeine sodium benzoate with a glass of water.
4. Empty the bladder 2 hours later. This is the test urine.
5. Azure A may be excreted in blue form or colourless form which may be converted to blue form by acidification boiling and standing for 2 hours.
6. It is measured by a visual type of coloured comparator.

Cerebrospinal Fluid (CSF) Examination

Chapter Outline

INTRODUCTION

Cerebrospinal fluid is a clear fluid which is formed as an ultrafiltrate of plasma. CSF is present in both the intracranial and spinal compartments. It is continuously being secreted by the choroid plexus at a constant rate inside the ventricles of the brain and circulates in the subarachnoid space of the brain and spinal cord through CSF pathways. The total volume of CSF in the adult is approximately 140 ml. CSF is produced at a rate of 0.2–0. 7 ml per minute or 500–700 ml per day. The main function of the CSF is to reduce buoyancy of the brain. It also supplies nutrients as well as helps in removal of various substances like amino acids, neurotransmitters, metabolic by products and cells.

The composition of the CSF and its pressure is maintained relatively constant by various mechanisms. However, in disease conditions the composition and pressure of CSF can be altered. Hence analysis of CSF by various methods will help in diagnosis as well as prognostication and response to therapy. CSF analysis is particularly useful in various acute neurological conditions and helps in rapid diagnosis of the conditions and initiate therapeutic measures.

Indications

- Diagnostic purpose
  - *Infections:* Meningitis, encephalitis.
  - Inflammatory conditions.
  - *Infiltrative conditions:* Leukaemia, lymphoma, carcinomatous meningitis.
- History of seizures or CNS diseases.
- Relief of abnormally high pressure and drainage of blood or exudate.
- As a prognostic tool for evaluation of CNS diseases.
- To assess the response to treatment.

FORMATION OF CEREBROSPINAL FLUID

- CSF is largely formed by the choroid plexus of the lateral ventricle and remainder in the third and fourth ventricles.
- 30% of the CSF is also formed from the ependymal cells lining the ventricles and other brain capillaries.
- The choroid plexus of the ventricles actively secrete cerebrospinal fluid.
- The choroid plexuses are highly vascular tufts covered by ependyma.

Examination of Cerebrospinal Fluid

Whenever there is clinical evidence of central nervous system disease, examination of CSF is indicated. Removal of spinal fluid is also indicated for relief of abnormal pressure and for the drainage of blood or exudates, for injection of drugs, for spinal anaesthesia, etc. In certain conditions, however, extra caution is required. These are:

1. A brain tumour at the cerebellopontine angle or in the region of the 3rd ventricle associated with papilloedema
2. A recent intracranial haemorrhage
3. A brain abscess
4. Septicaemias and acute exanthemata
5. A state of convulsion, and
6. Advanced diseases of the heart and arteries.

Normal Physiology: The cerebrospinal fluid (CSF) is formed by a process of selective dialysis of plasma by the choroid plexuses of the ventricles of the brain. It then passes through the foramina in the fourth ventricle into sub-arachnoidal systems at the base of the brain and travels over surfaces of the cerebral hemispheres. It is eventually absorbed into the blood in the cerebral veins and dural sinuses through arachnoidal villi and pachionian granulations. Thus it fills ventricles of the brain and subarachnoid spaces of the brain and the spinal cord. The total quantity is about 150–200 ml, but the daily turnover is probably to the tune of about 1000 ml. The normal pressure is 80 to 180 mm of water (Table 16.1).

The functions of the CSF are:

1. To serve as a fluid buffer, as a water jacket for the brain and the spinal cord
2. To act as a reservoir to regulate contents of the cranium; and
3. To serve as a medium for the exchange of substances especially removal of waste-products—between the blood and the brain. The normal composition is shown in Tables 16.2 and 16.3.

The CSF is very poor in colloids so that it does not clot on standing. Compared to the plasma it has less sugar, calcium and non-protein nitrogen; it contains very little cholesterol and no bilirubin at all.

Table 16.1: Normal values for lumbar CSF in adults

Pressure	70–150 mm of water column (patient lying on side)
Volume	90–150 ml
Specific gravity	1.006–1.008
Total solids	0.85–1.70 g%
Cells	0–8 lymphocytes/cu mm Neutrophils and erythrocytes absent
Protein	20–50 mg%
Of this	
⁎ Albumin	50–70%
⁎ α_1 globulin	3–9%
⁎ α_2 globulin	4–10%
⁎ β globulin	10–18%
⁎ γ globulin	3–9%
⁎ Fibrinogen	Absent
Sodium	144–154 mEq/L
Potassium	2.0–3.5 mEq/L
Chloride	118–132 mEq/L
pH	7.30–7.40
Creatinine	0.5–1.2 mg%
Cholesterol	0.2–0.5 mg%
Glucose	50–80 mg%
Glutamine	6–16 mg%
Iron	1–2 mg%
Thyroxine	0.1–0.2 mg%
Urea	6–16 mg%
Uric acid	0.5–4.5 mg%

Table 16.2: Normal CSF characteristics and main pathological alterations

Charac-teristics	*Normal*	*Meningitis*		
		Acute bacterial	*Viral*	*Chronic*
Pressure (mm/H_2O)	100–200	N or ↑	N or ↑	N or ↑
Aspect	Clear	Turbid/ purulent	Clear/ cloudy	Clear/ cloudy
Colour	Clear	White	Clear	Clear/ white
Cytology (mm^3)	Unit 4	>1,000	500–1,000	<500
Cell type	Lympho-cytes	Neutrophils	Lympho-cytes	Lympho-cytes
Protein (mg/dl)	V5–10 SO 10–25 L 15–45	↑↑	Normal or ↑	Normal or ↑
Glucose (mg/dl)	2/3 from serum	↓	Normal	Normal or ↓
Lactic acid (mmol/L)	<3.5	>3.5	<3.5	<3.5

Collection of Cerebrospinal Fluid

The CSF is obtained by puncturing the subarachnoidal space in the interspace between the 3rd and 5th lumbar vertebrae. The puncture is done with all aspetic and under local anaesthesia. A special lumbar puncture needle is used.

Routine examination of CSF includes:

1. Pressure
2. Physical examination
3. Chemical examination
4. Cytological examination
5. Bacteriological examination
6. Serological examination

Values to be filled up in format of reporting form (Table 16.4).

Pressure

CSF under normal pressure flows from the needle at a rate varying from 20 to 60 drops per minute. True evaluation of the pressure is attained by the use of a manometer.

The normal adult pressure in the horizontal position is from 100 to 200 mm of water or 7 to 15 mm of mercury. Pressure above 250 mm or under 50 mm are pathological. In children the pressure is slightly lower.

Physical Examination

1. **Appearance and Colour:** The pathological changes in appearance may consist of cloudiness or opalescence to frank turbidity. Opalescence and turbidity are due

Table 16.3: The CSF in differential diagnosis

Disease	*Initial pressure mm H_2O column*	*Appearance*	*Cells/ cu mm*	*Protein mg%*	*Glucose mg%*	*Remarks*
Normal	70–150	Crystal clear	0–8, lymphocytes	20–50	50–80	In fasting afebrile individuals.
Acute purulent meningitis	↑	Opalescent to purulent clot	500–20,000 mostly polymorphs	50–1000 +	0–45	Organism in sediment or clot
Tuberculous meningitis	↑	Opalescent fibrin web, pellicle	10–500 mostly lymphocytes	45–500 +	0–45	Sugar and chloride values falling
Early, acute syphilitic meningitis	↑	Clear to turbid, occasional clot	25–2000 mostly lymphocytes	45–400 +	15–75	+ ve (often serologic test in CSF and blood)
Late CNS syphilis	↑	Normal	Normal or ↑	Normal or ↑	Normal	Often + ve serologic test in CSF
Aseptic meningeal reaction (brain or extradural abscess, throm-bosis, etc.)	Usually normal	Clear or turbid, often xanthochromic	↑	Normal or ↑	Normal	CSF culture negative.
Acute polio-myelitis	Usually normal	Usually clear and colourless	↑	↑	45–100	
Viral ence-phalitis (arthropod borne)	Normal or ↑	Normal	0–100 mostly lymphocytes	Normal or increased	45–100	Proved by serologic tests.
Viral meningo-encephalitis	Normal or ↑	Normal	0–2000 + mostly	Normal or ↑	Normal	Proved by virus isolation and serologic tests
Post-infectious encephalitis	Usually ↑	Normal	Slightly ↑	Normal or Increased	Increased	
Traumatic (bloody) tap	Normal	Bloody	Many fresh RBCs	↑	Normal	Most blood in Ist tube, least blood in last tube
Cerebral haemorrhage ventricular, subarachnoid	Slightly ↑	Bloody, supernatant yellow	Many RBCs crenated or fresh	↑	Variable	Blood present in all specimens equally
Subdural haematoma	Usually ↑	Clear/yellow	Normal	Normal or ↑	Variable	
Brain tumour	Usually ↑	Clear/ xanthochromic	Normal or increased	Usually ↑	Normal or increased	If papilledema is present, lumbar puncture is contra-indicated.
Spinal cord tumor (subara-chnoid block)	Normal or low	Often xantho-chromic	Normal or ↑	Usually 1	Normal or increased ↑	Little fluid obtained
Multiple sclerosis	Low	Normal	Normal or increased	Normal or increased	Normal	50% cases have normal CSF.
Uremia	Usually ↑	Normal	Normal or ↑	Normal or ↑	Normal or ↑	CSF NPN is high.
Diabetic coma	Low	Normal	Normal or ↑	Normal	Increased	May have spasticity, weakness, convulsions

to the presence of cells in the fluid. In meningitis, therefore, the CSF will show these changes. When the CSF is frankly yellow, the change is described as "xanthochromia", it is caused by:

a. Haemorrhage in the subarachnoid space with conversion of haemoglobin into bilirubin
b. Severe jaundice of the obstructive (regurgitation) type; and
c. In Froin's syndrome in which xanthochromia is associated with a rise in proteins of the fluid (above 500 mg) but not in the cell count.

Froin's syndrome is seen in obstruction in the subarachnoid space produced by a spinal tumour or by chronic meningitis. Another change in colour is reddish discolouration ("erythrochromasia") due to blood in the CSF. If blood has appeared from accidental puncture of vein during the lumbar puncture, it is seen most in the first portion (first tube) of the CSF during collection. If such a sample of the CSF is centrifuged, the upper portion is clear. On the other hand, a spontaneous haemorrhage in the subarachnoid space will produce a uniformly bloody fluid in all the successive tubes and, if it has been of some standing, on centrifugation of supernatant is xanthochromic. Frank blood in the CSF not produced by the puncture of a vein, may be due to a cerebral haemorrhage (intraventricular or elsewhere with rupture into the subarachnoid space), spontaneous subarachnoid haemorrhage or due to a vascular tumour. A third type of discolouration is the greenish discolouration seen in a turbid fluid, this occur in pneumococcal.

2. **Formation of a clot:** This occurs in meningitis. In tuberculous meningitis, on standing for a few hours (especially in a refrigerator), the CSF shows a fine coagulum or pellicle described as a "cobweb". Such a cobweb is used for the demonstration of Myco. Tuberculosis which gets caught in it. In purulent meningitis the clot is formed quickly and is of a coarse type. Cobweb and clot are due to the appearance of fibrinogen in the fluid.

Table 16.4: Routine hospital reporting form on a specimen of cerebrospinal fluid

A. Physical examination	Colour .....
	Transparency ......
	Coagulum or cobweb
B. Chemical examination	Proteins.....
	Tests for globulins, sugar....
	Qualitative—Quantitative.....
	Chlorides......
C. Cytological examination	Total cell count.....
	Predominant cell.....
D. Staining	Ziehl-Neelsen, Gram

Chemical Examination

1. **Estimation of total proteins:** This is done by taking 1 ml of the CSF in a tube and adding 3 ml of 3% sulphosalicylic acid. Mix and allow to stand for 5 minutes, and compare the turbidity with that of the standard protein tubes, or in a photoelectric colourimeter.
2. **Qualitative tests for increase in globulin:**
   a. In Pandy's test 1 ml of the reagent (10% carbolic acid) is taken in a Kahn or Wassermann tube and to it is added one drop of the CSF. Normal fluid does not produce any change. If globulins are increased, a bluish ring or a cloud develops immediately.
   b. In the Nonne-Apelt test 1 ml of saturated ammonium sulphate solution is taken in a small tube and 1 ml of the CSF is layered on it. Allow to stand for 3 minutes and compare with the rest of CSF. Normal fluid produces just a faint opalescence at the junction; if globulins are increased, a distinct ring develops at the junction of the two fluids.

Obviously, if the CSF is contaminated with blood, the tests for proteins and globulins will give false reactions. Heavy bacterial contamination of the CSF (due to improper collection and storage) will also falsify the results. In all the conditions, mentioned in Table 16.3, the rise in the cell count (pleocytosis) is seen. Some entities are characterised by a rise in proteins without pleocytosis; these are cerebral thrombosis, subdural haematoma, brain tumours and polyneuritis.

Quantitative Protein Estimation

Principle: There are 2 types of methods.

1. Protein is precipitated by using 3% sulphosalicyclic acid. The resultant turbidity is proportional to the amount of protein present.
2. Proteins are simultaneously precipitated and dyed by a trichloracetic acid (ponceau S regeant). The protein bound dye is dissolved in alkali, and its absorbance compared with that derived from similarly treated protein standard.

Method I

1. Take 0.5 ml of CSF in a small test tube.
2. Add 1.5 ml of 3% sulphosalicyclic acid, shake and keep the tube for 10 minutes.
3. Compare the tube with the turbidity standard which are marked in mg of protein per 100 ml of fluid.

Method II

1. Determine approximate range of protein level in CSF by albustix.
   Reading 100, use 0.2 ml for assay
   Reading between 100 and 300, use 0.1 ml
   300–1000, use 0.02 ml
2. Set up the following tubes

	Test	*Std.*
a. Std. (80 mg/dl)	–	0.2 ml
b. Test serum	0.2 ml	–

c. Working trichloroacetic acid (centrifuge and decant) 1.0 ml 1.0 ml

d. NaOH (0.2 m) 2.5 ml 2.5 ml

(Read absorbance at 560 nm setting 0 with water)

CSF protein (mg/dl) = T/S × 0.32 × 100/0.2
= T/S × 160 mg/dl

Interpretation: Total protein content of CSF is 10–40 mg/dl. Upon electrophoresis it contains albumin, pre-albumin, β_1, β_2 and globulins with an A:G ratio of 2:1. Total proteins in CSF may increase in:

1. Meningitis (inflammations)
2. Guillain-Barré syndrome (infective polyneuritis)
3. Encephalitis
4. Cerebral malignancies, etc.
5. Froin's syndrome (A block in spinal canal).

Test for Sugar and Quantitative Estimation

a. Qualitative test: In a test tube take 0.5 ml of Benedict's qualitative reagent and add to it 4.5 ml of distilled water. Heat to boil and add 1 ml of the CSF. Boil for 2 minutes and allow to cool. A change of colour to turbid greenish yellow is the normal reaction. Absence of any change in the colour indicates diminished sugar content.

b. The quantitative estimation is done by Folin and Wu technique. Tests for sugar should be always done on fresh samples.

Interpretation: Glucose in CSF is characteristically reduced in pyogenic and tuberculosis meningitis and the reduction is the result of the metabolic requirement of the infecting organisms. CSF glucose is also reduced in disseminated leptomeningeal malignancies. In viral infections glucose may be normal or even raised. Whenever CSF sugar is being estimated, a sample of blood should be taken at the same time for glucose determination because CSF sugar is always judged in relation to blood glucose.

Determination of chloride in CSF: This is an outmoded investigation of no clinical value but only of historical interest.

Cell Counts

A. **Diluting the fluid:**

1. Draw Unna's polychrone methylene blue to the '1' mark in a RBC pipette and fill pipette to '101' mark with spinal fluid. This colours white cells blue and red cells yellow.
2. *Turbid fluid:* When many cells are present (as in turbid or purulent fluid), better counts are obtained with a WBC pipette and WBC diluting fluid.
3. *Bloody fluid:* When significant number of red cell are present in the fluid, the possibility of traumatic bleeding should be considered. Fresh RBCs are intact with a smooth round margin. Older cells have crenated appearance.

B. **Count:** Count 9 large squares in the counting chamber for both RBCs and WBCs. The total multiplied by 1.1 gives the number of cells per cubic mm.

Differential count: Centrifuge the CSF and make smears from the sediment. Stain and count as for a blood smear.

Bacteriologic Examination

Smears and cultures for bacteria should be made of all fluids when indicated.

- **Smears:** Make smears directly if fluid is very turbid, otherwise from sediment of centrifuged CSF. All smears should be stained with Gram's stain. If no characteristic bacteria are found, do an acid-fast stain (Ziehl-Neelsen stain) and search for mycobacteria. AFB stain should also be done if a pellicle forms on standing. An India ink preparation is required for cryptococcus. Immunofluorescent stains can be used for *Haemophilus influenzae* and some other organisms.
- **Cultures:** Cloudy fluid should be streaked on chocolate agar, Sabouraud's agar, and agar plates and inoculated into blood broth and thioglycollate medium. All media are incubated at 37°C, some in candle jars (for CO_2 atmosphere). Sediment of centrifuged fluid should be cultured on special media for tuberculous bacilli and fungi and inoculated into guinea pigs. Mice should be inoculated intraperitoneally if coccidioidomycosis is suspected.
- **Virus isolation:** This is possible only in very sophisticated laboratories and is helpful in aseptic meningitis and arthropod borne encephalitis.
- **Serological examination:** These are undertaken when neurosyphilis (meningovascular syphilis, tabes dorsalis or general paralysis of the insane) is suspected. The Wassermann reaction (complement fixation test) is considered the most dependable of various serlogical tests available. A test on the CSF is warranted because tests on the blood may be negative in neurosyphilis.
- **Lange's colloidal gold test:** About 5 to 7 ml of very fresh fluid collected in scrupulously clean; sterile tubes are required. The fluid must not be contaminated with blood.
- **Lange's test** is an empirical non-specific test depending upon the alterations in the total proteins and the albumin-globulin fractions in the CSF. In some diseases serial dilutions of the fluid when added to colloidal gold chloride solution (brilliant orange-red colour) brings about a somewhat characteristic pattern of colour changes with precipitation, the normal fluid has no effect.

The utility of the test is very limited. Compared to the labour involved, the information given is hardly conclusive. The test is, therefore, falling into background.

One can do—VDRL using CSF in syphilis. Latex agglutination and complement fixation tests in cryptococcal meningitis.

Chapter 17

Semen Analysis (Seminal Fluid Examination)

Chapter Outline

SEMEN ANALYSIS

Semen analysis is a test of a man's sperm and semen. Also known as a sperm count or male fertility test. Semen is the thick fluid that comes from men's penis when they ejaculate during sexual activity. It carries sperm out of a man's body so it can fertilize an egg and create an embryo (the first stage of pregnancy); fertility test, its results show how many sperms are released, as well as how they are shaped and how well they move.

Providing a Semen Sample

A semen sample for a semen analysis. There are four main ways to collect a semen sample:

- Masturbation
- Sex with a condom
- Sex with withdrawal before ejaculation
- Ejaculation stimulated by electricity

Masturbation is considered the preferred way to get a clean sample.

Preparing for the Semen Analysis

Here are a few things to keep in mind before giving the sample:

- Do not have sex or masturbate for 2 to 5 days before your test to make sure your sperm count will be as high as possible.
- Do not avoid ejaculation for more than 2 weeks before your test. That can result in a sample with sperm that are less active.
- It is best not to drink alcohol before your semen analysis.
- Do not use lubricants when you collect your sample because they can affect how easily your sperm can move around.

The semen sample is collected in a clean, dry container preferably in the pathology laboratory. It is recommended that the sample be collected following a three-day period of abstinence. Freshly ejaculated semen is highly viscid, opaque, white or gray-white or grey-white coagulum that may have a distinct musty or acrid odour. After 10–20 minutes it liquifies spontaneously to form a translucent, turbid viscous fluid which is mildly alkaline (pH 7.7). The normal semen volume averages 3.5 ml with a range of 1.5 to 5.0 ml.

Examination of Seminal Fluid

Semen is formed by the testes as well as accessary male reproductive organs. It consists of spermatozoa suspended in seminal plasma. The seminal plasma provides medium for the spermatozoa. Examination of seminal fluid is usually performed as part of infertility investigation involving both partners of a barren marriage. It is a relatively simple examination and hence, is often done before the more complicated and expensive examination of the female partner. The results of the semen analysis must be interpreted in the light of the detailed history and thorough medical examination of the male and female partners. Indeed, it has been suggested that for the purpose of infertility investigation the male and female involved should be considered not as individuals but as a reproductive unit. In case of an abnormal result on first examination it is recommended that the test be repeated one or more times. It is required in forensic studies to examine vaginal secretions or clothing stains for the presence of semen in alleged or suspected rape. Semen examination is also requested to investigate the effectiveness of vasectomy, of recanalization operation and it also supports or disproves a denial of paternity on the grounds of sterility.

A. Macroscopic Examination

i. **Quantity:** Measure the volume of semen in a small graduated cylinder. There is quite a variation in amount in different samples from one donor, depending on the period of continence preceding the examination. The average lies between 3 and 4 ml.

ii. **Viscosity:** Freshly ejaculated semen is highly viscous: Self-liquefaction takes places and should be completed in 15 to 30 minutes. The absence of liquefaction may inhibit the movements of spermatozoa, thereby interfering with fertilization.

iii. **Colour:** The normal semen is whitish with the typical seminal smell. Frank haemorrhage in the vesicles may colour the fluid red, and suppurative infection imparts a yellow colour and a foul smell.

iv. **Reaction:** It is always found to be on the alkaline side (pH 7.2 to 8.0).

B. Microscopic Examination

a. **Motility of spermatozoa:** Make a hanging drop preparation using a well slide. Ring the well with vaseline. Place a large drop of seminal fluid on a cover-glass, invert it over the well and press it down gently to make an airtight seal. Motility can then be observed:

   i. Absence of spermatozoa (*Azoospermia*), which should be confirmed after centrifugation of the specimen.

   ii. Only a few motile spermatozoa found (*Oligozoospermia*).

   iii. Spermatozoa are present but immobile (*Necrozoospermia*).

   iv. When motile spermatozoa are present, the proportion of motile to immobile cells should be noted. The microscopic field is made very small by fitting in the eyepiece of the microscope a disc of black paper with a central slit. Immobile spermatozoa are counted after motile ones.

   v. If the motility is very low, the specimen is incubated at 37°C, which may restore motility. Ten to fifteen per cent of immobile spermatozoa are encountered in fertile samples.

Duration of motility is one essential to fecundation. For studying the duration, a thick smear covered with a coverglass is prepared and the preparation is sealed with vaseline. Hour to hour examination should be made for studying the motility. A normal specimen shows a little cessation of motility at the third hour after emission, and considerable cellular activity is noted at the fifth or sixth hour. Complete or considerable subsidence of motility within this limitation should be regarded as an index of deficiency.

Individual sperm look and swim like tadpoles. Some sperms move less well (asthenozoospermia) than others and so they are less likely to survive and fertilise a waiting egg. The more sperm actively moving are present, the higher the chances of pregnancy.

Active motility is necessary for the sperms to penetrate the cervical mucous and subsequently migrate to fertilize the ovum in the fallopian tube. Motility can be assessed by placing a small drop of liquified semen on a microscopic slide. It is covered by coverslip which is ringed by vaseline to prevent drying. The preparation is scanned under the high dry objective of a microscope until at least a total of 200 sperms are observed. Normally about 80% of the spermatozoa are actively motile and about 20 percent are sluggishly motile or non-motile. Decreased sperm motility is associated with infertility.

Microscopic Examination of Semen

a. It is done as soon as possible after liquefaction of the semen has taken place, i.e. within 15–30 minutes of collection.

b. **Sperm count:** Mix the semen sample thoroughly and draw the sample to the 0.5 mark on a white blood cell pipette (WBC pipette). Dilute to the mark with the semen diluting fluid:

   Semen diluting fluid:

Sodium bicarbonate	5 g
Formalin (neutral) or phenol	1 ml
Distilled water	100 ml

   Charge the improved Neubauer counting chamber. Allow the semen to settle (for 2 minutes) and then count the sperm in the four corner squares as in a WBC count. The formula for calculation is similar to the WBC counting formula except that we report sperm count per cc or ml instead of per cu mm, so an additional multiplication factor of 1000 is added.

   Sperm/ml = $(N \times 10 \times 20 \times 1000)/4$

   The total number of sperms is multiplied by 50,000

   Normal sperm count is between 60 and 150 million/ml. Even if the count is below 60 million/ml (oligospermia), the patient may still be fertile. Total absence of sperm is known as azo-spermia and is associated with sterility.

c. **Morphological examination of spermatozoa:** Stained smears are employed for the purpose.

   A thin smear of semen on a clean glass slide is dried in air, and fixed by heat. Add one per cent chloramine for several minutes to remove excess of mucus. Wash by blotting on filter paper. Stain for 2 to 5 minutes with the following:

Ziehl-Neelsen's carbol fuchsin	2 parts
Conc. alcoholic sol. of eosin	1 part
Alcohol 95%	1 part

   Wash with water and counterstain with Loeffler's methylene blue for a few seconds. Wash, dry and examine under oil immersion. The heads of the spermatozoa are stained purplish, while the tail and middle piece are red.

Count the number of spermatozoa in a microscopic field. The same field is searched for immature forms of spermatozoa. The different developmental stages may be encountered in pathological semen but rare in fertile specimens.

Examine 100 to 500 spermatozoa for the following abnormalities (Figs 17.1 to 17.5):

i. Heads—too small or too large, pointed, ragged edges, atypical distribution of chromatin, presence of acidophilic vacuoles, double heads.
ii. *Middle pieces:* Absent, swollen, bifurcated, etc.
iii. *Tails:* Double, curled, rudimentary or absent.

Semen containing up to 20%, abnormal spermatozoa is still considered fertile.

Morphology of normal sperm is shown in Fig. 17.1.

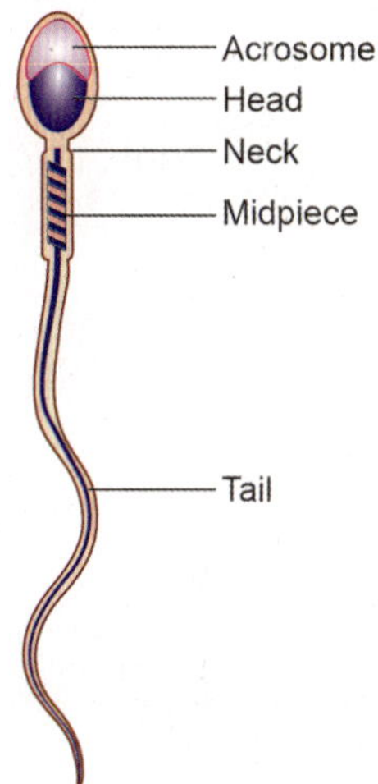

Fig. 17.1: Morphology of normal sperm, diagrammatic parts labelled

Normal sperms have an oval head with a long tail. Abnormal sperms have head or tail defects—such as a large or misshapen head or a crooked or double tail. These defects might affect the ability of the sperm to reach and penetrate an egg. However, having a large percentage of misshapen sperm is not uncommon. Typically, only around 4% to 10% of the sperms in a semen sample are normal, meaning that the vast majority do not look perfect under the microscope.

Sperm morphology is poorly understood, and it can be subjective. Scores can vary on the same semen sample, in the same lab, using the same scoring techniques.

Wet preparation morphology of sperm under microscope is given in Fig. 17.2.

Normal Range

Sperm count: At least 20 million per milliliter (m/ml). Sperm motility, or the ability to move rapidly: 60% to 80% actively moving. Sperm morphology, or the sperm's shape and size: 70% to 90% normally shaped.

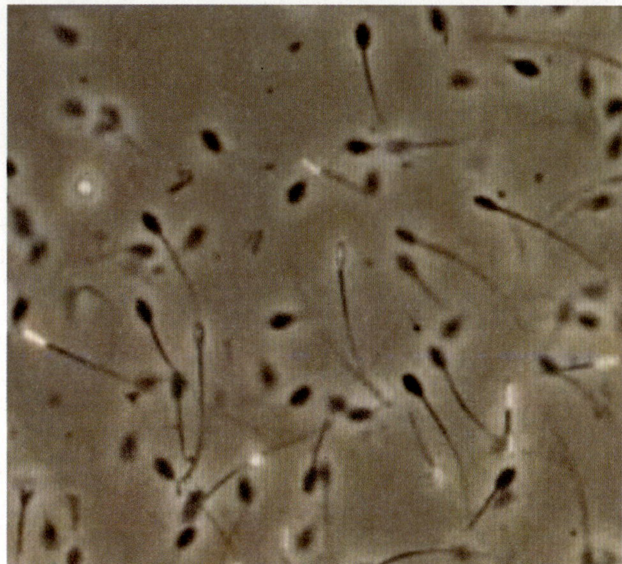

Fig. 17.2: Sperm under microscopy wet film

The detail normal morphology labelled diagram is shown in Fig. 17.3.

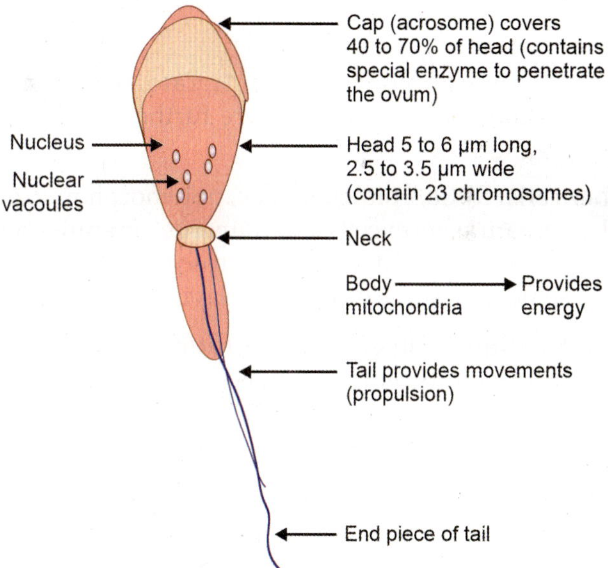

Fig. 17.3: Spermatozoa normal labelled structure

When the shape and size of sperm (this is referred to as sperm 'morphology') are not normal (teratozoospermia), this can reduce the chances for egg fertilisation.

Interpretation: Semen analysis can either be:

- **Normal:** All the elements are satisfactory
- **Abnormal:** Most or all of the elements are unsatisfactory
- **Inbetween:** Some normal and abnormal sperm to different degrees

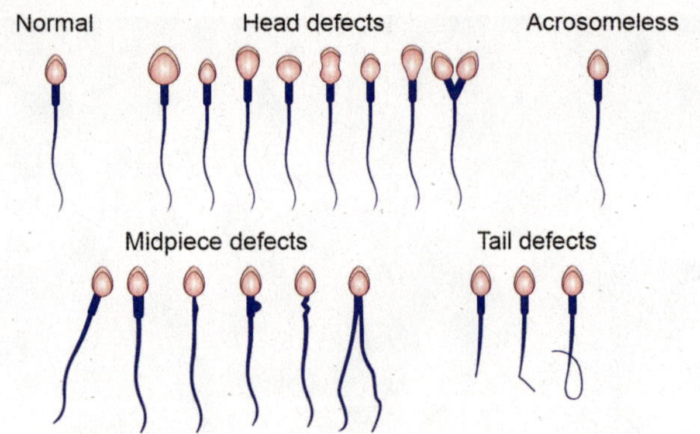

Fig. 17.4: Sperm morphology defects: Teratozoospermia

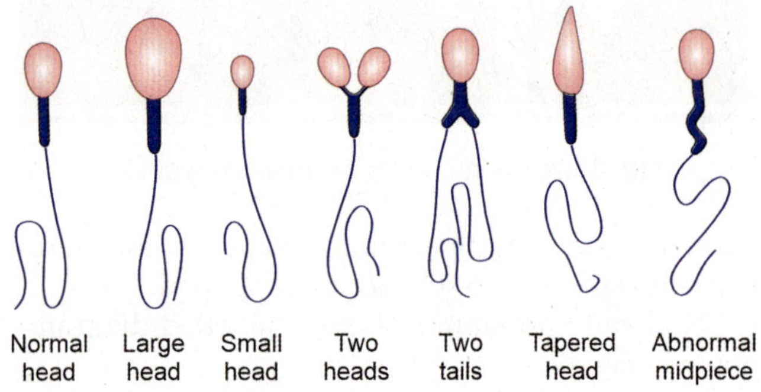

Fig. 17.5: Head abnormalities compared with normal labelled diagram

Sperm morphology defects "teratozoospermia" in males and the head defects are further labelled in Figs 17.4 and 17.5.

Other cells: RBCs, epithelial, cells, polymorphonuclear cells, immature germ cells and numerous granules and globules are observed during the microscopic examination of the semen. Presence of trichomonas is also looked for.

Investigations: Other tests performed on seminal fluid: Post-coital (Sims-Huhner) test, determination of antibodies to spermatozoa, etc. are some additional elaborate tests carried out in the infertility investigations.

Form for reporting routine semen examination:

A. **Microscopic or physical examination:**
   1. Volume
   2. Viscosity
   3. Colour and
   4. Reaction

B. **Microscopic examination:**
   1. Count of sperm
   2. Motility of sperm
   3. Morphology or abnormal forms and
   4. Other cells

Specimen analysis report: Table 17.1 depicts report of patient of 100% motility.

Table 17.1: Semen analysis report

Duration of abstinence:		06 (days)
Liquefaction time (min):		30 min
Interval between start of ejaculation and analysis (before liquefaction):		10 (min)
Gross		
Appearance	Creamy white	
Consistency	Thin	
Volume	3.0 ml	pH: 8.0
Fructose	Present	
Sperm motility (%) (100 spermatozoa)		
a. Rapid progression	05%	
b. Slow progression	25%	
c. Non-progressive motility	05%	
d. Immotile	65%	
Agglutination	–	
Vitality	–	
Count/ml	05 millions	
Morphology (%)		
Normal	30%	
Abnormal	70%	
▪ Head defects	25%	
▪ Tail defects	30%	
▪ Neck and midpiece defects	05%	
▪ Cytoplasmic droplets	08%	
▪ Headless 'pinhead'	02%	
Pus cells	1–2	
Red blood cells	0–1	
Epithelial cells	Nil	
Miscellaneous	Nil	

The morphology revealed 70% abnormal and 30% normal.

WHO 2010 recommended the following parameters with lower limit reference values (Table 17.2) along with range of reference (Table 17.3).

Table 17.2: WHO 2010 (World Health Organization)

Parameter	*Lower reference limit*
Semen volume (ml)	1.5
Sperm concentration (10^6/ml)	15
Total sperm number (10^6/ejaculate)	39
Progressive motility (PR, %)	32
Total motility (PR + NP, %)	40
Vitality (live sperms, %)	58
Sperm morphology (NF, %)	4
pH^+	>/=.72
Leucocyte (10^6/ml)	<1
MAR/Immunobead test (%)	<50

Table 17.3: Parameters with reference limit

Parameter	*Reference limit*
Semen volume (ml)	1.5 (1.4–1.7)
Total sperm number (million/ejaculate)	39 (33–46)
Sperm concentration (millions/ml)	15 (12–16)
Total motility (%)	40 (38–42)
Progressive motility (%)	32 (31–34)
Vitality (live spermatozoa (%))	58 (55–63)
Sperm morphology (normal forms (%))	4 (3.0–4.0)

Diagnosing Male Infertility

Issues like low or no sperm count, abnormal sperm morphology (shape of sperm) and poor sperm motility (ability of sperm to move forward and fertilise the egg) can be detected from a semen analysis.

Further investigations like ultrasound, hormone testing, post-ejaculation urinalysis, genetic tests, testicular biopsy, and specialised sperm function tests may be recommended to explain the anomalies detected in the semen analysis.

While both men and women can have problems, issues with male fertility can play a part in as many as half of all infertility cases. And male infertility is often caused by low sperm production.

Another reason you might need a semen analysis is to make sure a vasectomy (a procedure to prevent pregnancy) was successful. It is usually done 8 to 16 weeks after the surgery to see if you are still making any healthy sperm.

An abnormal semen analysis does not mean that you are infertile. Many men with low semen analysis values can still be father of children—it just might take longer. If you and your partner are not able to conceive through sexual intercourse, assisted reproductive technology such as *in vitro* fertilization might be an option.

Chapter 18

Examination of Sputum

Chapter Outline

- Introduction
- Examination of Sputum
- Collection and Transport of Sputum
- Prerequisites: Cytological Examination
- Gram Stain

INTRODUCTION

Mucus is the fluid secreted by the airways (also known as bronchial and windpipes) and lungs. In the setting of an infection or a longstanding health condition, the term of phlegm is also used. The mixture of saliva and mucus specifically coughed up from the respiratory tract, often either following an infection or an irritation of the mucosa, is precisely labelled "sputum."

EXAMINATION OF SPUTUM

The sputum is the material coughed up from the lungs, the bronchi, the trachea and the larynx, and consists of mucus secreted by the respiratory mucosa, products of tissue disintegration due to disease, exudate from lesions and materials from near-by structures that might have established communication with the respiratory tract. Expectoration of the sputum is the body's attempt to rid itself of material irritating the respiratory mucosa. The amount of mucus secreted in health is so small that normally there is no expectoration. Lesions in the lungs will produce sputum provided they are communicating with the bronchi and provided the material to be coughed out is fluid enough.

Examination of the sputum is a valuable means of investigation diseases of the respiratory tract.

COLLECTION AND TRANSPORT OF SPUTUM

Collection of specimen: The patient is instructed to rinse the mouth with water to avoid contamination by food residues. He is further explained that the material required is expectoration brought out after a fit of coughing and not saliva. The sputum is collected directly into the container. Conveniently the container can be clean, widemouthed bottle (capacity 30 to 60 ml) with a tight-fitting screw-cap.

Caution: When a sputum specimen is being collected, adequate safety precautions must be taken to prevent the spread of infectious organisms and to avoid contaminating the outside of the container. Use a phenol-containing disinfectant to wipe the outside of the container after collecting the specimen.

☞ **Important:** The specimen must be sputum, not saliva. Sputum is best collected in the morning soon after the patient wakes and before any mouthwash is used.

When pulmonary tuberculosis is suspected, up to three specimens may need to be examined to detect AFB.

The most common examination of the sputum is the detection of tubercle bacilli and for this, the early morning specimen (consisting of the material collected overnight in the bronchi) is preferred. If this specimen proves negative, a specimen collected over a period of 24 hours is the next step. When a cultural examination for pyogenic organisms or fungi is to be done, the sputum should be collected in a sterile Petri dish and examined immediately; in the case of the cultural examination for the tubercle bacillus a 24 hours sample in a clean bottle is sufficient. Cultural examination of any kind should, however, be done before antibiotics or chemotherapeutic drugs have been given. After the specimen has been examined, the remnants should be destroyed by heat or a chemical disinfectant (strong lysol).

When a sputum specimen is being collected, adequate safety precautions must be taken to prevent the spread of infectious organisms and to avoid contaminating the outside of the container. Use a phenol containing disinfectant to wipe the outside of the container after collecting the specimen.

☞ **Important:** The specimen must be sputum, not saliva. Sputum is best collected in the morning soon after the patient wakes and before any mouthwash is used.

When pulmonary tuberculosis is suspected, up to three specimens may need to be examined to detect AFB.

Mucopus aspirated from the nasopharynx. When it is not possible to get sputum from children with suspected pneumonia or bronchopneumonia, pathogens can often be isolated from mucopus aspirated from the nasopharynx.

Sample Transport

1. Samples should be, immediately, transported to laboratory as such if nearby.
2. If distant laboratory, transport in 25 ml of the following solution.

N acetyl pyridinium chloride	5 g
Sodium chloride	10 g
Distilled water	1 g

If sputum is allowed to stand without medium:

a. Rapid proliferation of contaminating bacterial flora from oral cavity and throat.
b. *H. influenzae* do not survive for long.

Do not Refrigerate in any Case

The procedure for the routine liquefaction of sputum is as follows:

- The sputum is expectorated into a sterile universal container or other wide mouthed screw-capped bottle.
- Add approximately 5 times the volume of 0.85% saline and agitate to free the sputum from adherent saliva. Remove the saline with a sterile Pasteur pipette.
- To the washed sputum, add an equal volume of Sputasol solution.
- Shake the mixture well, place in a 37°C water bath and incubate, with periodic shaking, until liquifaction is complete.
- Inoculate onto a suitable culture medium. For the total cell count, place a drop of the liquefied sputum in a haemocytometer for enumeration. For a differential cell count, fix a dried smear in methyl alcohol and stain with haematoxylin and eosin or with Lieshmann stain.

The working solution of Sputasol will remain stable for at least 48 hours stored at 2–8°C.

An investigation into the survival of respiratory pathogens in specimens that had been stored for 48 hours at 4°C following homogenisation using Sputasol, showed that the organisms remained viable and, when necessary, treated specimens could be successfully re-cultured.

In a health centre for dispatch to a microbiology laboratory

1. Collect the sputum in a container supplied by the microbiology laboratory. Follow the technique and observe the precautions mentioned under the hospital collection of sputum.
2. To ensure the survival of pathogens such as *S. pneumoniae* and *H. influenzae*, transfer a purulent part of the sputum to a cotton-wool swab, and insert it in a container of Amies transport medium. Label the container using a lead pencil. Amies medium will help the pathogens to survive and avoid the overgrowth of fast-multiplying commensals.
3. Send the sputum specimen and swab with a request form to reach the microbiology laboratory within 6 hours.
   Sputum specimens should be examined in a biological safety cabinet.

Describe the Appearance of the Specimen

Describe whether the sputum is:

- Purulent: Green-looking, mostly pus
- Mucopurulent: Green-looking with pus and mucus
- Mucoid: Mostly mucus
- Mucosalivary: Mucus with a small amount of saliva
- When the sputum contains blood, this must also be reported.
- When the sputum is mostly saliva, report the specimen as 'unsuitable for microbiological investigation' and request another specimen.

☞ **Note:** Before culturing sputum, many laboratories examine a wet preparation or Field's stained smear microscopically for cells. When a large number of squamous epithelial cells (often covered with bacteria) are present and only a few or no pus or macrophage cells, this indicates that the specimen is unsuitable for culturing.

Label the container, and complete a request. When pneumonia or bronchopneumonia is suspected, deliver the sputum to the laboratory with as little delay as possible because organisms such as *S. pneumoniae* and *H. influenzae* require culturing as soon as possible.

☞ **Note:** Specimens for the isolation of *S. pneumoniae* and *H. influenzae* must never be refrigerated.

PREREQUISITES: CYTOLOGICAL EXAMINATION

1. Fresh morning sample.
2. Transport without delay.
3. For suspected lung Ca collect sample for 5 consecutive days.
4. If delay anticipated, prefix with Saccomanno's fixative (50% ethyl alcohol and 2% carbowax).

Procedure for Routine Examination (Table 18.1)

1. Physical Examination

- **Quantity:** A large amount of sputum (over 100 ml per day) are produced in bronchiectasis and lung abscess.
- **Appearance and consistency:** Sputum is described as mucoid, mucopurulent serous (watery) and blood-stained. The characteristic appearance are watery, frothy sputum in pulmonary oedema: Tenacious rusty (blood-stained) sputum in lobar pneumonia; purulent sputum in lung abscess; and thin sputum separating

Table 18.1: Sputum collection and challenges

Processes	*Challenges*
Screening and referral	⁎ Staff awareness and use of TB case finding forms ⁎ Inconsistent use of presumptive TB registers ⁎ Lack of awareness among clinicians regarding which patients should be referred for Xpert testing
Sputum collection	⁎ Shortage of sputum containers (8 of 23, 35% health centers) ⁎ Lack of electricity and/or refrigerator to store sputum samples until transport (10 of 23, 43% health centers). ⁎ Failure of patients to return on anticipated sputum transport day (if sputum could not be stored) at all health centers.
Sputum transport to Xpert testing	⁎ Irregular sputum transport (range 1.3 times/ week) ⁎ Improper packaging of the sputum samples before they are sent to Xperts sites in over half of the health centers. ⁎ A large number of health centers assigned to each hub rider (4–8 sites/day per hub rider). ⁎ Last-minute delays or absence by boda-riders limiting sputum transport at multiple health centers. ⁎ Impassable roads especially during the rainy season.
Diagnostics testing with Xpert	⁎ Malfunctioning modules (5 of 15, 33% testing sites) ⁎ Testing not done for at least 30 days of the year due to lack of power back-up (2 of 15, 13% testing sites) ⁎ Recommended daily maintenance not performed (7 of 15, 47% testing sites) ⁎ Error/invalid rates > 5% (10 of 15, 66% testing sites) ⁎ Ineffective supply-chain logistics, to address gaps in Xpert cartridge inventory at all Xpert referral sites.
Return of results and treatment	⁎ Delayed notification of Xpert results (up to two weeks from sputum collection when notified at all). ⁎ Failure of patients to return to collect Xpert results and initiate treatment. ⁎ Inconsistent recording or Xpert results in lab register. ⁎ Lack of system to notify patients with positive results (21/23, 91% health centers).

into layer on standing in bronchiectasis. Frank blood may be seen in the sputum in pulmonary tuberculosis, pneumonias, congestive cardiac failure from mitral stenosis, pulmonary infarction and malignant tumours of the bronchi and the lungs. Rupture of an amoebic abscess of the liver into the lung produces sputum with the appearance of "anchovy sauce".

- **Odour:** A foul odour is seen in abscess of the lung and in an empyema that has ruptured into the lung. The sputum of bronchiectasis has usually a sweet smell.

2. Microscopic Examination

a. **A wet or coverslip preparation:** Suspicious portions of the sputum, as judged by the physical examination after pouring the sputum in a Petri dish, are selected. A small portion is put on a glass slide; add saline, if necessary to thin and put a coverslip. Examine under the low and the high power.

i. *Elastic fibres:* Appear as slender, curled, highly refrectile fibres; they are seen in any destructive lesion of the lung-tuberculosis, abscess, bronchiectasis or carcinoma. Curschman's spirals are spirally twisted, mucoid strands closing epithelial cells and leucocytes (chiefly eosinophils). Curschman's spirals are seen in bronchial asthma.

ii. *Charcot-Leyden crystals:* These are either colourless, painted hexagons, or needle-like. They are supposed to be derived from disintegration of eosinophils. They are encountered in bronchial asthma or parasitic infection of lung.

iii. *Fungi:* These may take the form of yeast-like cells, non-branching or branching double-contoured filaments or as tangled masses of filaments with "clubbed" ends (ray fungus). Fungi may occur in the sputum as contaminants from the mucous membrance of the upper respiratory tract and have no significance. That they come from bronchi or lungs is proved by demonstrating their presence repeatedly in the sputum raised by deep coughing or in specimens obtained by bronchoscopy. Fungi can also be demonstrated by special staining methods and cultural examinations.

iv. *Animal parasites:* On rare occasions parasites may be found in the sputum. *E. histolytica* may be discovered in the sputum if any amoebic liver abscess has ruptured into the lung. In the case of hydatid disease of the lung the sputum may show the laminar membrane and the germinal layers or scolices containing groups of minute hooklets. Other parasites found are *Trichomonas* hominis, ova of *P. westermani* and larvae of *S. stercoralis* and hookworms.

v. *Cells:* A coverslip preparation may show red cells, pus cells and haemosiderin-containing macrophages ("heart-failure cells"). The last type seen in congestive cardiac failure, must be distinguished from macrophages containing carbon pigment, a common findings in the sputum city-dwellers.

b. **Stained smears:** The suspicious portion is selected and, with a pointed match-stick or a platinum loop, a thin smear is made on a clean glass slide. The smear meant for bacteriological examination is fixed by passing it slowly through the flame three to four times.

Cytological Examination

1. For malignant cells
2. Looking for viral inclusions
3. Asbestosis

The medical professionals will check the amount and gross qualities of the sputum, which should be thick to allow a proper investigation by the laboratory medical staff. In several institutions, clear and runny samples are not acceptable.

Collection of Sputum

1. Early morning deep cough sample is preferred.
2. If unable to cough, induction of sputum can be done by:
   a. 15% NaCl aerosol spray and propylene glycol for 20 min, or
   b. Nebulized hypertonic saline and distilled water.

Spray-cyte or cyto-spray. If this is not available, fix and process for mailing.

A much less satisfactory alternative, to be used only when facilities are not available, is collection and mailing of sputum in one of the following fixatives: 75 to 95% ethanol, Bouin's fluid, Brasil's fixative, or formol-acetic-alcohol. Upon receiving such specimens in the cytology laboratory, attempts (rarely satisfactory) may be made to make smears on albuminized slides, but the buttons of coagulated sputums may be processed and embedded in paraffin wax, and step-serial sections may be cut and examined.

Leishman or Giemsa stained smear for cytological study: This smear is not to be fixed by heat. It is handled exactly like the blood smear. In bacterial infections the sputum will show a large number of polymorphs. Monocytes (macrophages) are seen in chronic infections macrophages with vacuolated cytoplasm (due to fat) may be seen in lipoid pneumonias. However, the only significant finding is the presence of a large number of eosinophils in bronchial asthma and tropical eosinophilia.

Grocott-Gomori's methenamine silver stain (GMS) is a standard staining method used to detect fungal microorganisms. GMS staining is critical in identifying *Pneumocystis jirovecii*. This microorganism first appeared in patients with human immunodeficiency virus (HIV) infection in the 1980s, and it was used to be classified as a protozoan. This microorganism, which is now classified as a fungus, was initially called *Pneumocystis carinii*. Colony morphology is a method that describes the characteristics.

Smears stained by Gram stain: The sputum is always contaminated by organisms contained in the upper respiratory tract and the mouth. A mixture of organisms is the usual findings. None carry a diagnostic significance. The different type of cells, referred to above, can be identified with a little experience in the smears stained by Gram's stain also.

Smear and Culture

Identification of causative organism in a suspected infection, like pneumonia, TB, fungal infection, *P. carinii* in HIV, bronchiectasis, etc.

Gram stain is the first staining technique performed in preliminary bacterial identification, which helps determine if there is an adequate amount of pathogens in the culture and make a definitive diagnosis.

GRAM STAIN

Prerequisites

1. There should not be squamous cells covered with masses of bacteria—indicates sample is mostly from mouth or throat.
2. If PMNs are < 10 per epithelial cell—no need for culture.
3. Knowledge of flora of mouth and pharynx necessary before analysing.

Gram smear: Using a piece of stick, transfer a *purulent part* of the sputum to a glass slide, and make a thin smear.

Allow the smear to air-dry in a safe place. Fix examine the smear for pus cells and *predominant* bacteria. Look especially among the pus cells for (Tables 18.2 and 18.3):

Table 18.2: Normal flora of oral cavity and pharynx
Gram-positive
1. *Staphylococcus aureus* and *epidermidis*
2. *Streptcoccus viridans* and *pneumoniae*
3. Diphtheroids
4. Enterococci
5. Micrococci
6. Lactobacilli
7. Yeasts (Candida)
Gram-negative
1. Neiserria
2. *H. influenzae*
3. Fusobacterim
4. Coliforms
5. *M. catarrhalis*

Table 18.3: Possible pathogens	
Bacteria	
Gram-positive	
• *Streptococcus pneumoniae*	• *Streptococcus pyogenes*
• *Staphylococcus aureus*	• Also *Mycobacterium tuberculosis*
Gram-negative	
• *Haemophilus influenzae*	• *Proteus* species
• *Klebsiella pneumoniae*	• *Yersina pestis*
• *Pseudomonas aeruginosa*	• *Moraxella catarrhalis* and *Legionella pneumophila*

- Gram-positive diplococci (capsulated) that could be *S. pneumoniae*.
- Gram-positive cocci in groups that could be *S. aureus*, but not often seen.
- Gram-negative rods and cocco-bacilli that could be *H. influenzae*, particularly when these are the predominant organisms.
- Gram-negative capsulated rods that could be *K. pneumoniae*, but not often seen.
- Gram-negative diplococci in and between pus cells that could be *M. catarrhalis*.

Finally, sputum antimicrobial susceptibility testing is performed on the bacteria or fungi, leading to lung infection after being identified in a sputum culture sample. The most common approaches consist of the disk diffusion and minimum inhibitory concentration (MIC) methods. These tests are used to detect the effectiveness of the specific antibiotics on the bacteria or to detect whether the bacteria have already developed resistance to certain antibiotics or not.

Smear stained by Ziehl-Neelsen method: This is by far the most important step in the routine examination of the sputum because it shows the presence of *Mycobacterium tuberculosis*. The technique of Ziehl-Neelsen staining is given below.

1. Fix the smears by passing through the flame 3–4 times.
2. Cover the smear with carbol fuchsin.
3. Warm the slide until steam rises from the staining solution; this is done twice. Do not boil the staining solution. Allow the heated stain to act for 5 minutes.
4. Wash the smear with water.
5. Decolourise the smear with 20% (by volume) sulphuric acid.
6. Now counterstain with Lowffler's methylene blue for 1 minute.
7. Wash with water. Dry the smear in air. Examine with the oil-immersion lens (Fig. 18.1).

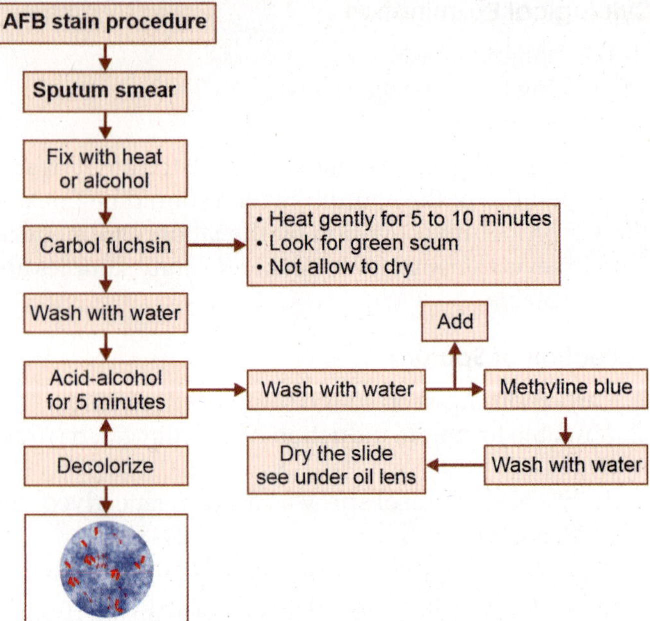

Fig. 18.1: ZN staining process

Mycobacterium tuberculosis is an acid-fast bacillus and appears as a red stained rod with beaded appearance. To detect *Mycobacterim tuberculosis* by this in the sputum-estimated to be about 50,000 per cu mm. A negative result does not, therefore, exclude pulmonary tuberculosis. At least three different specimens of sputum should be examined before the negative report is accepted. When direct microscopy is negative, further procedures are available to detect *Mycobacterim tuberculosis* in the sputum. These are described separately below.

Reporting results of AFB (ZN staining) is given in Table 18.4.

Table 18.4: Grading of slides in AFB microscopy

Examination	*Result*	*Grading*	*No. of fields to be examined*
More than 10 AFB per oil immersion field	Positive	3 +	20
1–10 AFB per oil immersion field	Positive	2 +	50
10–99 AFB per 100 oil immersion fields	Positive	1 +	100
1–9 AFB per 100 oil immersion fields	Positive	Scanty (Record exact number seen)	100
No. AFB per 100 oil immersion fields	Negative	–	100

Special Methods for Detection of *M. tuberculosis*

a. Fluorescence Microscopy

This is a simple and efficient method but requires special equipment. The bacilli in the sputum are stained with a fluorescent dye Auramine O. The stained bacilli when irradiated with ultraviolet light and observed with the fluorescent microscope, appear as brilliant yellow rods against a black background, and can be easily spotted out. The yield of positives by this method in trained hands is better than with smears stained by Ziehl-Neelsen method.

b. Concentration Method for Mycobacterium tuberculosis

Many techniques are available. The principle under all is the same; destroy the extraneous matter like mucus, cells and the contaminating organism by means of chemical digestion so that only live tubercle bacilli are preserved and concentrated in a small amount of the deposit obtained from the original volume of the sputum. The most commonly used method for concentration is that of Petroff. This is as follows:

A 24 hours collection of the sputum is made. The sputum is mixed with an equal volume of 4% NaOH and placed in the incubator at 37°C for 30 minutes; the container is shaken every few minutes. The mixture or digest is now centrifuged at 3000 rpm for 30 minutes and the supernatant discarded. The deposit is neutralised with 8% HCl; the acid is added, drop by drop, using phenol red as an indicator. The neutralised deposit is the concentrated material ready for examination. Three kinds of examinations can be done on the deposit:

1. Smears can be prepared and stained by Ziehl-Neelsen stain.
2. The deposit can be cultured on special media; the most commonly used media are Lowenstein-Jensen medium and Dorsett's egg medium.
3. Guinea pig inoculation. About 1 to 2 ml of the deposit from the concentrated material is injected subcutaneously (in the flank) or intramuscularly (in the thigh). A nodule appears at the site of injection in 7 to 21 days. The neighbouring lymph nodes are also affected and later lymph nodes in other parts of the body; they become enlarged and caseous. The animal loses weight and dies within 6 weeks to 3 months. At the autopsy it will show tubercles in the liver and the spleen in a large number; the lungs may show a few tubercles. In the living animal *Mycobactrim tuberculosis* is demonstrated in smears made from enlarged regional node at the autopsy. The organism is present in smears from different lesions.

In the diagnosis of pulmonary tuberculosis examination of gastric contents or of post-pharyngeal or larynegeal swabs for *M. tuberculosis* are available alternatives, especially in children.

Respiratory viruses have been tested in sputum specimens from patients with cystic fibrosis, asthma, and chronic obstructive pulmonary disease (COPD).

Typically, viral testing is also performed on upper airway samples such as nasopharyngeal swabs or nasal washes. However, some viral pathogens such as severe acute respiratory syndrome (SARS) coronavirus, H1N1 influenza, Middle Eastern respiratory syndrome coronavirus (MERS-CoV), and SARS coronavirus 2 (SARS-CoV-2), the causative agent of coronavirus disease 2019 (COVID-19), may be absent in upper airway secretions.

Sputum samples are also frequently used for viral diagnosis testing by using the clinical real-time polymerase chain reaction (RT-PCR) method or the newly developed next-generation sequencing (NGS) method.

Potentially, face masks, which reduce the aerosol-related risk of transmission in the current era of the COVID-19 pandemic, may also represent a useful source for NGS investigations.

Sputum cytology examination is using a microscope to determine whether abnormal cells are present in sputum samples. The thin layer of sputum placed on a slide before specific staining and diagnosed directly under the microscope helps find out some abnormal cells. Sputum cytology helps detect both lung cancer cells and non-cancer cellular and acellular material useful for the diagnosis of conditions such as pneumonia, tuberculosis, interstitial lung diseases, or pneumoconiosis (e.g., asbestosis). Hematoxylin and eosin stain is the worldwide.

Clinical Diagnostic Sputum Analysis

Lung Cancer and Sputum Cytology

Sputum cytology refers to the examination of sputum (mucus) under a microscope to look for abnormal or cancerous cells.

Sputum, or phlegm, is the fluid that is secreted by cells in the lower respiratory tract such as the bronchi and the trachea.

Sputum cytology, at least at the current time, is not a good test for screening for lung cancer. In one study comparing the effectiveness of sputum cytology with low-dose spiral CT scans for diagnosing lung cancer in asymptomatic people (people who had no symptoms of lung cancer but were at an increased risk for the disease), the test was positive 58% of the time. This meant that sputum cytology alone missed the diagnosis 42% of the time. The test is more accurate in diagnosing squamous cell carcinoma of the lungs than lung adenocarcinoma.

Sputum cytology, however, can be helpful if lung cancer cells are found in the sputum, and the risk of false positive diagnoses (the appearance of lung cancer cells on a sample when lung cancer is not actually present) is very low (less than 1%). Sputum cytology also lacks the ability to determine the location of the cancer or to accurately determine the subtype of lung cancer (histology) present, so further tests will be needed.

Sputum molecular analysis is a new insight and advanced technique used to detect lung cancer-related biomarkers to assist in the early stage of a lung cancer diagnosis. Many DNA mutations, such as *p53*, *KRAS*, *EML4- ALK*, and *GFR* mutations, have been investigated on sputum specimens.

- **Bronchoscopy** is a procedure used to investigate the throat and airway through a thin viewing camera. It is also used to collect the sputum samples in some special situations such as a persistent infection, cough, or something unusual seen on clinical laboratory tests or chest X-rays. The sputum specimen will be examined under a microscope to detect whether abnormal cells are present.
- Flexible bronchoscopy is used more often than rigid bronchoscopy to collect the sputum samples. Before having a flexible bronchoscopy, the doctor may give the patient.
- **Exfoliative cytology on sputum:** This is a useful method for the diagnosis of bronchial and lung carcinomas. Smears of the fresh material are fixed immediately (while wet) in ether-alcohol and stained by Papanicolaou stain. The diagnosis depends upon the identification of cancer cells by their special features (cytological diagnosis of cancer). The bronchial secretion obtained by bronchoscopy gives even better results.

Chapter 19

Synovial Fluid (SF) Analysis–Synovia

Chapter Outline

INTRODUCTION

Normal Synovial Fluid

Synovial or diarthrodial joints are the most sophisticated in the body. Unlike fibrous or cartilaginous joints in which the bone ends are effectively tethered together with bands of motion limiting fibrous tissue or cartilage, in synovial joints each bone end is covered by an independent layer of hyaline cartilage. The two cartilage-covered bone ends are separated by a narrow space containing the lubricant, synovial fluid. This arrangement allows two adjacent bones the freedom to move in multiple directions.

Synovial fluids are joint fluids, they are also termed synovia. It is a viscous, non-newtonian fluid present in the cavity of synovial joints between the bones. This fluid looks like egg white fluid with a transcellular fluid component of extracellular fluid. The primary synovial fluid function is to reduce friction between the articular cartilages during the movement of synovial joints.

The synovial membrane present in the inner membrane of synovial joints will secrete the synovial fluid into the joint cavity. This synovial fluid acts as an ultrafiltration membrane for blood plasma, which contains the protein derivative produced by the cells present inside the joint tissues. Synovial fluid contains hyaluronan, which is secreted by the fibroblast-like cells present in the synovial membrane. Synovial fluid contains proteoglycan 4, the lubricant secreted by the chondrocytes surface present in articular cartilage and interstitial fluid filtered from the blood plasma.

Here, the viscosity of the synovial fluid between bones will decrease with an increase in the speed of the fluid during its motion. On the other hand, the elasticity of the fluid will increase with an increase in the speed of the fluid. Thixotropy features of synovial joints are mainly due to the presence of hyaluronic acid present in the synovia. The main source of the hyaluronic acid present in synovial fluid is the synovial lining cells. Further, the thixotropic properties help to make the elastohydrodynamic lubricant films between the movement and the fixed cone articular surfaces between the bone pairs.

Synovial fluid is produced by the synovium and coats the tendons in the tendon sheaths and the surface of the synovium in normal joints. Synovial fluid is cleared through the subintimal lymphatic vessels which are assisted by joint motion. Synovial fluid is essential for the nutrition and lubrication of articular cartilage and tendons. It is composed of plasma ultrafiltrate, which diffuses in the joint space from the subintimal vasculature, and hyaluronic acid and lubricin secreted by the fibroblast.

The synovium is covered by an incomplete layer of cells—the synoviocytes. There are two main types of synoviocyte: Type A, derived from macrophages that phagocytose any debris that falls into the fluid from the joint lining, and type B, derived from synovial fibroblasts with a synthesising function.

Synovial fluid is a transudate of plasma supplemented with high-molecular-weight saccharide-rich molecules, notably hyaluronans, and a molecule called lubricin, produced by the type B synoviocytes.

Synovial fluid differs from all other body fluids in that the surfaces of synovium and cartilage (the tissues in immediate contact with the synovial fluid) are covered by an incomplete layer of cells. This means that there is no intact basement membrane, which in other tissues is a significant physical and chemical barrier to the movement of molecules and cells. It also means that the matrix or cartilage and synovium are in contact with the synovial fluid, allowing a relatively homogeneous chemical environment to develop within the joint. Because of this unusual arranagement it is perhaps better to regard the synovial fluid as a semi-liquid, avascular, hypocellular connective tissue rather than a true body fluid, such as may form in the pericardial, abdominal or pleural cavity.

Structure of Synovial Fluid

The synovial membrane present in the inner membrane of synovial joints will secrete the synovial fluid into the joint cavity. This synovial lubricates the surface between synovium and cartilage. It also contains phagocytic cells, which remove microbes and debris and helps protect joints from normal wear and tears.

Features of Synovial Joints

The synovial fluids present between the joints of the bone will act as the chemical dialyzer of blood plasma. This means it purifies and filters the portion of the blood plasma through the membrane which contains a larger amount of hyaluronic acid than the other plasma dialyzates. Since the synovial joints have both viscous and elastic characteristics, they are marked as the thixotropic fluid.

Synovial fluid (SF) is the viscous liquid in the synovial cavity and is secreted by the synovial membrane. Its function is to reduce friction between the articular cartilages of the synovial joint during movement. It is a dialysate from plasma to which components produced locally by joint tissue is added. The composition of the SF changes during an individual's lifetime due to changes in mechanical loading.

Arthrocentesis (Figs 19.1 and 19.2)

Arthrocentesis is the process by which synovial fluid collection occurs by penetrating the joint space through aspiration. This procedure should be done under sterile procedural conditions and performed by a physician with intimate knowledge of the involved anatomy. Sterility is essential not only to prevent transmission of infection but also to ensure accurate fluid analysis. Ultrasound technology may be useful in ensuring correct needle placement but is often unnecessary. Fluoroscopy and CT guided arthrocentesis.

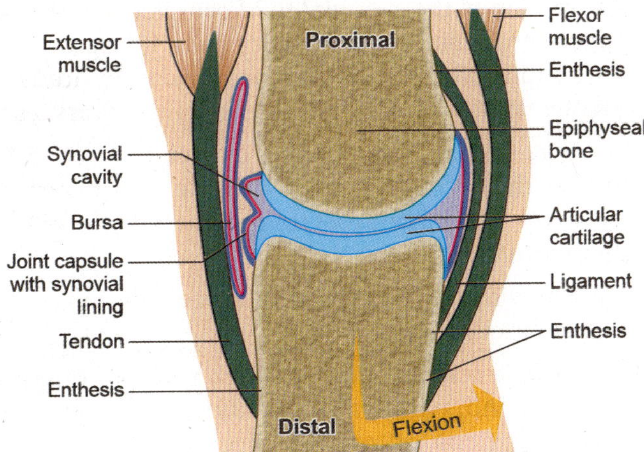

Fig. 19.1: A typical joint

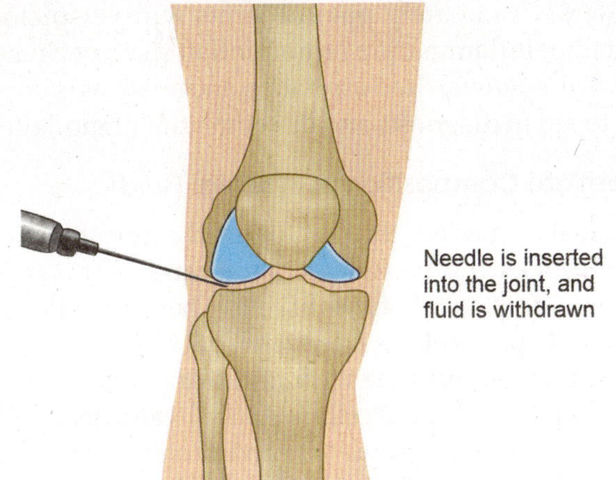

Fig. 19.2: Arthrocentesis

SPECIMEN COLLECTION

Synovial Fluid Collection

Synovial fluid can be aspirated from most joints with a 1-inch, 18- to 20-gauge needle. The skin should be prepared by clipping the hair and performing a surgical scrub to avoid introducing bacteria into the joint. Ethyl chloride spray may be used, if needed, on the overlying skin to lessen the sensation of the needle penetration. Fluid for cytologic evaluation should be placed in an EDTA tube.

Several factors can interfere with aspiration and, therefore, analysis of synovial fluid. Unsuccessful aspiration is common as synovium can clog the needle and interfere with sample collection. Non-sterile technique can contaminate the collected fluid. It is important to remember that multiple etiologies can co-exist, i.e. the presence of gout does not rule out the presence of concomitant infection.

Indications

Indications for synovial fluid aspiration and analysis include the presentation of acute painful joint with surrounding warmth/erythema, suspicion of septic arthritis, suspicion for subacute or chronic periprosthetic joint infection, acute exacerbation of chronic knee pain from osteoarthritis or non-inflammatory arthritis, or acute trauma with painful effusion. In the clinical presentation of acute injury, often arthrocentesis of hemarthrosis can be therapeutic and provide significant pain relief in the acutely traumatic knee.

Effusions from chronic inflammatory arthritis can undergo therapeutic aspiration for pain relief. A definitive diagnosis of gout or pseudogout is also an indication for aspiration. It is important to note that infection and gout can co-exist within a joint space.

Physiologic changes in synovial fluid volume and content occur in response to trauma, inflammation, and bacterial, fungal, or viral penetrance. When patients present with acutely painful joints with suspicion of infection, inflammation or non-inflammatory causes of effusion, synovial fluid aspiration and analysis is imperative to aid in diagnosis and direct treatment modality.

Chemical Composition of Synovial Fluid

Synovial tissues are the vascularized connective tissue, which lacks the basement membrane. The synovial tissues consist of two types of cells. They are Type A and Type B. Type A cells are derived from blood monocytes. Further, it removes the wear and tears debris from the synovial fluid. Type B cells produce hyaluronan, which is made up of hyaluronic acid and proteinases, lubricin, and collagenases. The synovial fluid shows the non-newtonian flow characteristic:

Hyaluronan is synthesized by the synovial membrane, which is secreted into the joint cavity to increase the viscosity and elasticity of articular cartilages, and it lubricates the surface between synovium and cartilage. It also contains phagocytic cells, which remove microbes and debris and helps protect joints from normal wear and tears.

Usually, the synovial fluid contains 3–4 mg/ml of hyaluronic acid. It is a polymer of disaccharides and composed of D-N-acetylglucosamine and D-glucuronic acid combined by alternating beta-1,4 and beta-1,3 glycosidic bonds.

Hyaluronic acid content has been measured directly in synovial fluid, but this test is not performed in most clinical laboratories.

Hyaluronan is the major component of synovial fluid and is important in maintaining synovial fluid viscosity and prevents fluid loss from the articular cavity. Lubricin is present at the articular cartilage interface and is essential for joint lubrication and maintenance of a healthy joint.

The concentrations of small molecules and electrolytes in the synovial fluid mirror those in plasma, while the concentration of large molecules is inversely proportional to their molecular weight.

Total Protein Concentration

Most plasma proteins, especially those with higher molecular weight, are excluded from synovial fluid by the dialyzing properties of the synovial membrane and hyaluronic acid in the perisynovial connective tissue.

Features of Synovial Joints

The synovial fluids present between the joints of the bone will act as the chemical dialyzer of blood plasma. This means it purifies and filters the portion of the blood plasma through the membrane which contains a larger amount of hyaluronic acid than the other plasma dialyzates. Since the synovial joints have both viscous and elastic characteristics, they are marked as the thixotropic fluid.

Here, the viscosity of the synovial fluid between bones will decrease with an increase in the speed of the fluid during its motion. On the other hand, the elasticity of the fluid will increase with an increase in the speed of the fluid. Thixotropy features of synovial joints are mainly due to the presence of hyaluronic acid present in the synovia. The main source of the hyaluronic acid present in synovial fluid is the synovial lining cells. Further, the thixotropic properties help to make the elastohydrodynamic lubricant films between the movement and the fixed conarticular surfaces between the bone pairs.

Main Function of Synovial Fluid

The synovial fluids are produced by the synovium. It is the composition of water, inorganic salts, hyaluronic acid, lubricin, aggrecans, and macromolecules. Synovial fluid is termed joint fluid. This is a thick liquid present between the joints of bones. Synovial fluid between bones acts as cushions for the end of the bones. Further, it reduces the friction between bones, which is caused by the movement of joints.

- As the synovial fluid acts as a dilatant fluid, it possesses rheopectic properties. Synovial fluid has a more vicious capacity when the pressure is applied. The synovial fluid present in diarthrotic joints will become thick the moment shear in order to protect the joint and subsequently. Normal viscosity of the synovial fluid instantaneously resumes its lubricating function between shocks.
- The pressure acts on the joints forces to secrete hyaluronan in the fluid acts on the synovial membrane, which acts as a barrier against cells and helps to migrate into or out through the joint space. The molecular sieving is completely dependent on the molecular weight of the hyaluronan.
- The primary functions of the synovial fluids are two parts. They are nutrition and lubrication. As the synovial fluid acts as a blood-plasma dialyzate, it can nourish the articulating parts of the articular cartilages. The motion of the synovial fluid completely depends on the connections with the fatty pads. It helps for the distribution of nutritions over the articular surfaces and it slowly passes through the interior layer of cartilage.
- Synovial fluid usually supplies oxygen and nutrients, further they remove carbon dioxide and metabolic waste from the chondrocytes present in the surrounding cartilage tissues.
- The synovial fluid lubricates the articulating joints and reduces friction.
- Hyaluronic acid provides the high viscosity of synovial fluid and, with water, its lubricating properties. Concentrations of small molecules (electrolytes, glucose) are similar to those in plasma.

ANALYSIS OF SYNOVIAL FLUID

Gross Analysis

Because synovial fluids from inflamed joints have a tendency to clot, they should be received in the laboratory in anticoagulant. Choosing the most appropriate anticoagulant is problematic. Because one of the key elements of synovial fluid analysis is examination for crystals, crystalline anticoagulants have to be avoided, as do chelating anticoagulants, which destroy crystals by removing core structural metal ions such as Ca^{2+}. We find lithium heparin to be the best anticoagulant.

- Synovial fluid analysis is a group of tests that examine joint (synovial) fluid. The tests help diagnose and treat joint-related problems.
- Removal of joint fluid has a dual purpose—diagnostic and therapeutic. Finding the cause of joint swelling is the diagnostic goal. The removal of fluid is the therapeutic goal, which may help relieve pain and pressure on the joint.

The test may be used to diagnose:

- Gout
- Infection
- Other inflammatory joint conditions
- Joint injury
- Osteoarthritis

Synovial Fluid (SF)

Normally about 1 ml of SF is present in each large joint: knee, ankle, hip, elbow, wrist, and shoulder.

The most important reason for performing joint fluid analysis is to rule out septic arthritis. Synovial fluid analysis can demonstrate local inflammatory response, infection and the presence of crystals.

Synovial fluid effusions are classified into five general etiologic categories: Noninflammatory responses, inflammation, sepsis, crystal induced and haemorrhage. The most common diseases associated with each category are summarized in Table 19.1.

Synovial Fluid in Diseased Joints

Variations in the volume and composition of synovial fluid reflect pathological processing occurring within the joint. Because of the relationship between the tissues within the joint, chemically mediated events such as inflammation or enzyme-mediated degradation occurring within the synovium and cartilage reflected in changes within the synovial fluid. These changes include the production of factors responsible for the accumulation of different cell types within the fluid, and it is this that explains why the complement of cells within the joint varies between diseases.

- **Viscosity:** When normal fluid drips from a syringe, a tenacious 'string' at least 4 cm long forms with each drop. This provides an estimate of whether viscosity is normal, decreased (string less than 4 cm in length), or markedly decreased (string less than 1 cm in length).
  Another method for evaluating viscosity is to see how far a drop of fluid can be stretched between the thumb and index finger before breaking. Fluids with very low viscosity will behave like water. Decreased viscosity reflects decreased hyaluronate in the synovial fluid.
- **Mucin clot test (Ropes' test):** This is done by adding 1 ml of synovial fluid to 20 ml of 5% v/v acetic acid

Table 19.1: Synovial analysis in arthritis

	Appearance	*Viscosity*	*White cells*	*Mucin clot*	*Protein (Avg-gm%)*		*Remarks*
					Total	*Globulin*	
Normal	Straw-coloured clear, cloudy	High	200–600 25% polymorph	Good	1.36	0.05	
Traumatic	Yellow to bloody	High	±2000 30% polymorph	Good	4.27		
Osteoarthritis	Yellow, clear	High	± 1000 20% polymorph	Good	3.08	0.75	Cartilage fibrils
Rheumatic fever	Yellow, slightly cloudy	Low	± 10,000 50% polymorph	Good	3.74	1.07	
Systemic lupus erythematosus	Straw-coloured, slightly cloudy	High	± 5000 10% polymorph	Good			
Gout	Yellow to milky cloudy	Low	± 12,000 60% polymorph	Fragile	4.18	1.54	Urate crystals
Tuberculous arthritis	Yellow, cloudy	Low	± 25,000 50–60% polymorph	Fragile	5.3	2.0	Tubercle bacilli
Septic arthritis	Grayish or bloody, turbid	Low	± 80,000 90% polymorph	Fragile	5.64	2.45	Bacteria
Rheumatoid arthritis	Yellow to greenish, cloudy	Low	± 15 ,000, 65% polymorph	Fragile	4.74	1.79	Rheumatoid factor

in a small beaker. Normally a compact large clot will form, surrounded by clear solution; this is graded as 'good'. If a soft clot forms in a turbid solution, this is graded as fair. A friable clot with cloudy surrounding fluid is graded as 'poor' or 'fragile'. No clot formation, with flakes in a cloudy suspension, is graded as 'very poor'. Good clots do not break up when agitated, while poor clots break up into small shreds. This procedure actually is an estimate of synovial hyaluronate and not mucin, which is absent in joint fluid.

Table 19.2 gives differentiation of various parameters in noninflammatory, inflammatory and septic diseases in comparison to normal SF.

Table 19.3 gives comparison of total WCC and PMNs.

- **Microscopic examination:** Total and differential counts as for CSF. But the usual leucocyte with 1% glacial acetic acid precipitates synovial fluid hyaluronate and is unsatisfactory, instead methylene blue in saline can be used. If the fluid is very turbid, use saline dilution or digestion with hyaluronidase (2 ml SF incubated with 150 IU hyaluronidase for 1 hr at 37°C) may be helpful. Differential count can be done from EDTA sample (sediment) that has been centrifuged, a film made and stained as for peripheral blood.
- LE cells are frequently seen in stained SF from patients with systemic lupus erythematosus. Sometimes they can be seen in cases of rhematoid arthritis. Large phagocytes containing neutrophils may be found in SF and are called 'Reiter cells'; they are non-specific and may be present in effusions of varying etiology. RA cells or 'ragocytes' are neutrophils containing 0.5 to 1.5 μ inclusions better seen with phase microscopy. They are seen in 94% cases of rheumatoid joint fluids but are non-specific for they can also be found in septic arthritis, gout, etc.
- Synovial fluid protein concentration is usually 25% of serum (1–3 g/dl). Synovial fluid glucose is normally within 10 mg/dl of plasma glucose. Neither synovial fluid glucose nor protein provides much useful diagnostic information.

Table 19.2: Various parameters to differentiate non-inflammatory, inflammatory and sepsis

Test	*Normal*	*Non-inflammatory*	*Inflammatory*	*Sepsis*
Clarity	Clear	Slightly turbid	Turbid	Turbid
Colour	Yellow	Yellow	Yellow	Gray-green
Viscosity	High	Reduced	Low	Low
Mucin clot	Firm	Firm to friable	Friable	Friable
Clotted	no	Occasional	Occasional	Often
WBC/uL	0–200	0–2000	2000–100,000	50,000–200,000
% Polys	<25	<30	>50	>90
Glucose difference	0–10	0–10	0–40	20–100
Crystals	Absent	Absent	Absent	Absent
Culture	Sterile	Sterile	Sterile	Positive

Table 19.3: Comparison of total WCC and PMNs

	White cell count (WCC)	*Polymorphonuclear neutrophils (PMNs)*
Non-inflammatory	< 2000	< 25%
Inflammatory	2–50,000	> 50%

Microscopic analysis of synovial fluid is performed to evaluate for cell count and crystals. Crystals include monosodium urate, calcium pyrophosphate, hydroxyapatite and corticosteroid crystals.

Monosodium urate crystals are seen in gout or gouty arthritis and appear as needle-shaped negatively birefringent crystals varying in length from 2 to 20 μm. With negative birefringence, the crystals appear yellow in parallel light and blue with perpendicular light.

Calcium pyrophosphate crystals are seen in pseudogout (also known as calcium pyrophosphate deposition disease, or CPPD). These crystals are rod-shaped or rhomboids varying in length from 2 to 20 μm and with positive birefringence (blue with parallel light, yellow with perpendicular light).

Performing manual white blood cell counts on blood. Saline should be used as the diluent for synovial fluid rather than the dilute acetic acid that is sometimes used as a diluent for blood. Acetic acid causes precipitation of the mucin in synovial fluid. A standard white blood cell pipette may be filled to the 0.5 mark with synovial fluid and then filled to the 11 mark with saline. After the diluted synovial fluid is mixed and the first few drops discarded, a hemacytometer chamber should be charged with fluid.

White cell counts (WBCs) are normally less than 200/ul with fewer than 25% neutrophils A WBC count of 2,000/ul and a neutrophil count of 75% serve as useful cutoff points to distinguish inflammatory from noninflammatory disease. However, there is much overlap in synovial fluid WBCs between the inflammatory, crystal-induced, and sepsis categories, WBC is greater than 50, 000/uL in 70% of patients with septic arthritis, 15% with gout, 10% with pseudogout, and 4% with rheumatoid arthritis (Table 19.3).

Various diseases and type of effusion are shown in Table 19.4.

Table 19.4: Indicates various diseases and types of effusion

Effusion	*Diseases*
Noninflammatory	Osteoarthritis, trauma, osteochondritis, pigmented villonodular synovitis, sickle cell disease, neuropathic.
Inflammation	Rheumatoid arthritis SLE, Reiter's syndrome ankylosing spondylitis, ulcerative colitis, psoriasis.
Infection	Bacteria, fungi, mycobacteria
Crystal	Gout, pseudogout
Haemorrhage	Trauma, haemophilia, haemangioma, pigmented villonodular synovitis, anticoagulant therapy.

Differential Diagnosis

- Cytocentrifuge prepared smears
- Write values of:
  - Neutrophils %
  - Lymphocytes %
  - Monocytes (histocytes) 48%
  - Macrophages %
  - Synovial lining cells %
  - Cytocentrifugation of the specimen provides good smears for Wright staining and observation.

Elevated Monocytes

- Serum sickness associated arthritis
- Viral infections
- Crystal-induced arthritis
- A high number of monocytes may be found in arthritis associated with serum sickness, viral infections, and crystal-induced arthritis.

Elevated Lymphocytes

- Early stages of RA
- A high number of lymphocytes may be seen in early stages of RA.

The mean distribution of nucleated cells is neutrophils 7%, lymphocytes 24%, monocytes 48%, macrophages 10%, and synovial lining cells 4%.

The presence of synovial lining cells is of no significant diagnostic concern. Neutrophils may be vacuolated or contain bacteria or crystals. In addition, cells may exhibit pyknotic nuclei or karyorrhexis.

Septic arthritis exhibits a high number of neutrophils.

- Neutrophils present in later stages of RA may exhibit inclusions that contain immune complexes such as IgG, IgM, complement and RF. These neutrophils will appear to have dark cytoplasmic granules and are sometimes called RA cells or ragocytes. This image is from synovial fluid with acute inflammation demonstrating neutrophilic pleocytosis. Synovial fluid with acute inflammation demonstrating neutrophilic pleocytosis (Wright-Giemsa).
- The current benchmark for identification of the causative microorganism and ascertaining its antimicrobial susceptibility is the conventional culture of aspirated joint fluid. The synovial fluid obtained should be sent for immediate Gram staining, culture, cell counts, and crystal analysis. Measuring erythrocyte sedimentation rates or C-reactive protein levels may be helpful in the following treatment course. A C-reactive protein of more than 10.5 mg/dl is predictive of infection.

Microbiology

- Infectious organisms
- Bacteria
- Fungi
- Mycobacteria
- Viruses
- Route of entry
- Bloodstream
- Penetrating wounds
- Osteomyelitis rupture
- Arthroscopy
- Intra-articular steroid injections prosthetic joint surgery
- Infectious agents that can enter the synovial fluid include: Bacteria, fungi, mycobacteria, and viruses, with bacteria being the most common. Bacteria and other microorganisms enter the synovial capsule through the bloodstream, deep penetrating wounds, and rupture of osteomyelitis into the joint. In addition, bacteria may be introduced during procedures such as arthroscopy, intra-articular steroid injections, and prosthetic joint surgery.
- **Staining:** Smears prepared by centrifugation or cytocentrifugation
  - Saline dilution reduces clustering of cells
  - Gram's stain most common
  - Positive in only 50% of cases
- **Culture:** Set up with positive or negative stain results
  - Aerobic
  - Anaerobic
- Gram stain is performed on synovial fluid smears prepared by centrifugation or cytocentrifugation.

Diluting synovial fluid with saline helps separate cells that tend to cluster. Even if Gram staining does not suggest the presence of infectious agents, both aerobic and anaerobic cultures should be performed. Synovial fluid Gram stains are positive in only 50% of cases with joint sepsis.

- Molecular methods such as polymerase chain reaction (PCR) technique are used to identify bacteria by their genotypes. The advantage of automated multiplex PCR (MPCR) lies in the rapid identification of causative pathogens and their antibiotic sensitivities (5 hours compared with several days in standard tissue culture techniques). Results appear promising for the diagnosis of periprosthetic joint infection in sonication and synovial fluid as well as septic arthritis in synovial fluid of native joints.

Other Test

In addition to direct measurement of hyaluronic acid content, other chemical tests that have been performed on equine synovial fluid include measurement of creatine kinase and lactate dehydrogenase total activity and isoenzyme activity, alkaline phosphatase activity, and glucose content. None of these has been used widely in diagnosis of joint disease.

Dehydrogenase

May be elevated in synovial fluid, while serum levels remain normal. Increased in rheumatoid arthritis (RA), infectious arthritis, gout.

Neutrophils increased during the acute phase of these disorders contribute to this increased LD be elevated in synovial fluid, while serum levels remain normal. Synovial fluid LD levels are usually increased in RA, infectious arthritis, and gout. The neutrophils that are increased during the acute phase of these disorders contribute to this increased LD levels.

Rheumatoid Factor

- RF is an antibody to immunoglobulins.
- Present in rheumatoid arthritis:
  - Serum—most cases
  - Synovial fluid—50%
- Rarely elevated only in synovial fluid and not serum

Clinical Significance

Synovial fluid aspiration and analysis is a necessary therapeutic and diagnostic procedure useful in alleviating pain from a joint effusion and in the diagnosis of potentially serious joint pathologies. It is a low cost, highly effective means of pain reduction and diagnosis, and can be performed quickly, without general anaesthesia, at the bedside. Arthrocentesis does not require a specialized surgeon which increases its utility in prompt therapy and diagnosis.

Potential Diagnosis

Potential diagnosis from synovial fluid aspiration and analysis include:

- Inflammatory arthritis including gout, pseudogout, infection, or spondyloarthritis, or non-inflammatory arthritis which can include effusion from osteoarthritis or meniscal tears.
- Septic arthropathy: Acute septic arthropathy, subacute or chronic septic arthropathy, or periprosthetic joint infection.

False positives in other chronic inflammatory diseases.

Rheumatoid factor (RF) is an antibody to immunoglobulins. RF is present in the serum of most patients with RA, whereas just more than half of these patients will demonstrate RF in synovial fluid.

However, if RF is only being produced by joint tissue, synovial fluid RF may be positive while the serum RF is negative. False-positive RF can result from other chronic inflammatory diseases.

Review of Key Points: Synovial Fluid Analysis

Fluid analysis is a well-established procedure for evaluation of joint disease.

- Determines the presence of arthritis
- Assists in the classification of joint disorders
- Helps guides appropriate treatments.
- Synovial fluid analysis is a well-established procedure in the evaluation of joint disease. The purpose of synovial fluid analysis is to determine the presence of arthritis and to place a fluid into one of several categories.
- Appropriate treatment of joint disease depends on proper identification of disease.

Laboratory form

- Appearance
- WCC
- RBC
- Microscopy + culture
- Protein
- LDH
- Glucose
- Crystals
- Gram stain and culture.

Interpretation Results

Appearance

- Normally clear to light yellow

WCC

Suggests:

- Infection
- Gout
- Pseudogout
- Inflammatory arthritides (RA seronegative)

RCC

Suggests:

- Traumatic tap
- Haemarthrosis (spontaneous or traumatic)

Protein

- > 30 g/L = Exudate
  - Infection and inflammatory arthritides

LDH

> 300 IU/L

- RA
- Gout
- Infection

Glucose

- ½ serum
  - Infection
  - Severe inflammation

Crystals

- Either
  - Gout: Monosodium urate, needle shaped
  - Pseudogout: Calcium pyrophosphate dehydrate, birefringent, rhomboidal crystals
- Calcium urate (gout)
- Negative birefringence
- Needle-shaped crystals, blue crystals

Gram Stain and Culture

Gram stain and bacterial culture: Synovial fluid aspirate is analyzed for Gram stain and both aerobic and anaerobic culture to determine the presence of infection; the presence of any organism indicates abnormal findings.

- Positive in < 25% gonococcal infections
- Positive in 50–75% non-gonococcal

Chapter 20

Pericardial Fluid Analysis

Chapter Outline

INTRODUCTION

The pericardium, also called pericardial sac, is a double-walled sac containing the heart and the roots of the great vessels.

The pericardial sac has two layers, a serous layer and a fibrous layer. It encloses the pericardial cavity which contains pericardial fluid.

The normal pericardial sac contains about 50 ml of fluid, similar to lymph.

Functions

Lubricates the surface of the heart. The pericardium limits distension of the heart, and acts as a barrier to infections.

Inflammation of the pericardium and increased fluid in the pericardial cavity can lead to pericardial effusion (accumulation of excess fluid around the heart). The rate of accumulation and the type of fluid (serous, sanguineous, lymph, or pus) that accumulates vary by the type of pericardial effusion. A major sequela of pericardial effusion occurs when compression of the heart from the fluid buildup interferes with its normal functioning (i.e. compromises the heart's ability to pump blood, leading to decreased cardiac output and stroke volume). This potentially fatal condition, called cardiac tamponade, occurs in up to 15% of patients with idiopathic pericarditis.

Acute pericarditis refers to inflammation of the pericardial sac.

Acute pericarditis is the most common disorder involving the pericardium.

Diseases of the Pericardium

1. **Pericardial effusion**
   A. Hemopericardium
   B. Cardiac tamponade
2. **Pericarditis**
   A. Serous
   B. Fibrinous
   C. Purulent
   D. Haemorrhagic
   E. Constrictive

PERICARDIAL EFFUSION

Definition: Pericardial effusion is defined as an increased amount of pericardial fluid. Pericardial effusion is defined as the collection of fluid in the pericardial sac (typically around 10–50 ml of pericardial fluid within the pericardial sac) that can lead to cardiac tamponade.

Etiology and pathology: The etiology of a pericardial effusion can often be deduced from the clinical presentation patients who present with severe hypothyroidism, end-stage kidney failure, acute myocardial infarction, or who underwent a recent invasive cardiac procedure. The relative frequency of different etiologies of pericardial effusions depends on the geography and the patient population.

- The speed of accumulation determines the physiologic importance of the effusion.
- Because the pericardium stretches, large effusions (>1000 ml) that develop slowly may produce no haemodynamic effects. Conversely, smaller effusions that appear rapidly can cause tamponade.

Complications

Cardiac Tamponade

Tamponade is characterized by elevated intrapericardial pressure (>15 mm Hg), which restricts venous return and ventricular filling. As a result, the stroke volume and pulse pressure fall and the heart rate and venous pressure rise. Shock and death may result.

It is acute heart failure due to compression of heart by a large or rapidly developing effusion.

"Cardiac tamponade, also known as pericardial tamponade, is an acute type of pericardial effusion in which fluid accumulates in the pericardial cavity leads to pressure on the heart muscle which occurs when the pericardial space fills up with fluid faster than the pericardial sac can stretch."

- Cardiac tamponade is a clinical syndrome caused by the accumulation of fluid in the pericardial space, resulting in reduced ventricular filling and subsequent haemodynamic compromise.
- The condition is a medical emergency.

Pericardial effusion is a common complication of acute pericarditis; however, malignancy or autoimmune diseases can cause pericardial effusion with or without acute pericarditis. The clinical presentation of pericardial effusion ranges from dyspnea, orthopnea, chest pain and/or fullness to overt cardiac tamponade.

Pathophysiology: The pericardial sac normally contains up to 50 ml of fluid; it can hold 80 to 200 ml of fluid acutely, and even up to 2 L if the fluid accumulates slowly.

Small effusions are not necessarily dangerous and are commonly caused by infection such as HIV or can occur after cardiac surgery. Large and rapidly accumulating effusions may cause cardiac tamponade, a life-threatening complication, that puts pressure on the heart preventing the ventricles from filling correctly.

Causes (Table 20.1): Pericardial effusion can result from inflammation of the pericardium (pericarditis) after an illness or injury. In some settings, large effusions may be caused by certain cancers. A blockage of pericardial fluids or a collection of blood within the pericardium also can lead to this condition.

Sometimes the cause cannot be determined (idiopathic pericarditis).

Causes of pericardial effusion may include:

- Autoimmune disorders, such as rheumatoid arthritis or lupus
- Cancer of the heart or pericardium
- Spread of cancer (metastasis), particularly lung cancer, breast cancer or Hodgkin's lymphoma
- Radiation therapy for cancer if the heart was in the area of the radiation
- Chest trauma

Type of Pericardial Effusion

1. Transudative
2. Exudative
3. Haemorrhagic
4. Malignant (due to fluid accumulation caused by metastasis)

The two main reasons for fluid accumulation in the pericardial space are:

An imbalance between the pressure within blood vessels—which drives fluid out of blood vessels—and the amount of protein in blood—which keeps fluid in blood vessels. The fluid that accumulates in this case is called a transudate.

Transudates are most often caused by congestive heart failure or cirrhosis.

Transudate (Table 20.2)

Transudates are most often caused by either congestive heart failure or cirrhosis. Typical fluid analysis results include:

Table 20.1: Aetiology of pericardial disease

Infectious causes
Viral: Coxsackieviruses echoviruses, Epstein-Barr virus, cytomegalovirus, parvovirus B19
Bacterial: TB, other bacterial causes are rare, e.g. Staphylococcus
Fungal: Very rare, e.g. *Candida* species in immunocompromised patients
Parasitic: Very rare, e.g. Echinococcus
Non-infectious causes
Autoimmune: Systemic lupus erythematosus, scleroderma, rheumatoid arthritis, Sjögren syndrome, acute rheumatic fever
Neoplastic: Primary tumours are rare; metastases from lung, breast and lymphoma are more common
Metabolic: Renal failure, hypothyroidism
Traumatic: Early—penetrating or non-penetrating traumatic injury; delayed—postmyocardial infarction, post-cardiac surgery
Drug-induced: Rare, e.g. hydralazine, all-trans retinoic acid
Other: Sarcoidosis, aortic dissection (the pericardium includes the proximal 2–3 cm of the great vessels)

Table 20.2: Pericardial effusion: Exudate versus transudate

Parameter	*Exudate*	*Transudate*
Cause	Malignancy	Radiation
	Infectious, parainfectious	Uremia
	Postpericardiotomy syndrome	Hypothyroidism
	Collagen vascular disease	Trauma
Specific gravity (g/ml)	>1.015	<1.015
Total protein (g/dl)	>3.0	<3.0
Fluid-to-serum protein ratio	>0.5	<0.5
Fluid-to-serum LDH ratio	>0.6	<0.6
Fluid-to-serum glucose ratio	<1.0	>1.0

LDH: Lactate dehydrogenase.

- Physical characteristics—fluid appears clear
- Protein or albumin level—low
- Cell count—a few cells are present

Exudate

Exudates can be caused by a variety of conditions and diseases. Initial test results may show:

- **Exudate:** Injury or inflammation of the pericardium may cause abnormal collection of fluid (called an exudate). Exudates are associated with a variety of conditions and diseases.
- **Inflammatory conditions:** Pericarditis may follow a heart attack, radiation treatment, or be part of autoimmune disorders such as rheumatoid arthritis and lupus.
- **Infectious diseases:** Caused by viruses, bacteria, or fungi.
- **Cancer:** Such as mesothelioma that has arisen in the pericardium or metastatic cancer that has spread to it.
- Most pericardial effusions in patients with HIV infection are idiopathic. Culture of pericardial fluid usually is unrevealing; however, opportunistic infections and neoplasms can be diagnosed.

Function: The pericardial fluid reduces friction within the pericardium by lubricating the epicardial surface allowing the membranes to glide over each other with each heart beat.

Composition: Composition of pericardial fluid in patients undergoing open heart surgery. They found that the fluid is made up of a high concentration of lactate dehydrogenase (LDH), protein and lymphocytes. In a healthy adult there is up to 50 ml of clear, straw-coloured fluid. However, there is a little data on the normal composition of pericardial fluid to serve as a reference.

Analysis of Pericardial Fluid (Table 20.3)

Normal pericardial fluid has the features of a plasma ultrafiltrate. Lymphocytes are the predominant cell type.

Table 20.3: Pericardial fluid analysis

pH	7.69
Glucose (mg/dl)	52
Total protein (g/dl)	5.9
Fluid volume (ml)	8.10
Nuc cell Ct (/μl)	1,465
Segs	81
Lymph	10
Monos	7
Eos	2
ANA titer	<80
Rheumatoid factor (unit/ml)	185
C-reactive protein	4.4
CCP (unit)	122

Although routine analysis of fluid does not have a very high yield for disease etiology, analysis is rewarding with bacterial infections and malignant effusions. Measurements should include WBCs and differential, haematocrit, and protein content. Although most effusions are exudates, detection of a transudate reduces diagnostic possibilities.

Analysis of pericardial fluid showing general chemistry, cytology, PCR and microbiology is given in Table 20.4.

Table 20.4: Analysis of pericardial fluid

Analysis	*Test*
General chemistry	Protein level >3 g/dl, protein fluid/serum ratio >0.5, LDH >200 IU/L, fluid/serum ratio >0.6[a], blood cell count
Cytology	Cytology (higher volumes of fluid, centrifugation, and rapid analysis improve diagnostic yield)
Polymerase chain reaction (PCR)	PCR for TB
Microbiology	Mycobacterium cultures, aerobic and anaerobic cultures

LDH—lactate dehydrogenase: TB—tuberculosis.

[a]High values of protein and LDH are commonly interpreted as an exudate, as in pleural fluid, but have not been validated for pericardial fluid.

Increased production of cytokines such as *interleukin-2* and a tumor necrosis factor in patients with end-stage HIV infection has been associated with *capillary leak syndrome*, which also can be seen in patients with AIDS-wasting and malnutrition.

The initial inspection should assess whether the fluid is haemorrhagic, purulent, or chylous. A red blood cell count higher than 100,000/mm^3 is suggestive of trauma, malignancy, or pulmonary embolism (rare). Chylous fluid implies injury to the thoracic duct by trauma or infiltration. The fluid should be sent for a cell count; Gram stain; culture; cytology; acid-fast bacilli; determination of glucose, protein, and lactate dehydrogenase (LDH) levels; and specific gravity.

An elevated protein level higher than 6.0 g/dl often indicates tuberculous, purulent, or parapneumonic effusion.

- Gram stain—for direct observation of bacteria or fungi under a microscope. There should be no organisms present in pericardial fluid.
- Bacterial culture and susceptibility testing—if bacteria are present, susceptibility testing can be performed to guide antimicrobial therapy. If there are no microorganisms present, it does not rule out an infection. Bacteria may be present in small numbers or their growth may be inhibited because of prior antibiotic therapy.
- Adenosine deaminase—a markedly elevated level in pericardial fluid in a person with symptoms that

suggest tuberculosis means it is likely that person has a *Mycobacterium tuberculosis* infection in the pericardium. This is especially true when there is a high prevalence of tuberculosis in the geographic region where a person lives.

ACUTE PERICARDITIS

- **Definition:** Acute pericarditis is an inflammatory process involving the pericardium that results in a clinical syndrome characterized by chest pain, pericardial friction rub, changes in the electrocardiogram (ECG) and occasionally, a pericardial effusion. Generally, the diagnosis requires 2 of these 3 features.
- **Prevalence:** Acute pericarditis is the admitting diagnosis in 0.1% of hospital admissions and 5% of admissions with chest pain. It occurs more commonly in men than in women.
- **Etiology (Table 20.5):** The most common form of acute pericarditis is idiopathic, which accounts for about 90% of cases. Other common causes include infection, renal failure, myocardial infarction (MI).

Table 20.5: Causes of acute pericarditis
Idiopathic
Infectious
- Viral (including HIV)
- Bacterial
- Mycobacterial
- Fungal and protozoal
Post-myocardial infarction (early and late)
Postoperatively after open heart surgery
Chest trauma
- Blunt
- Sharp
Radiation
Malignancy
- Primary: Mesothelioma, angiosarcoma
- Metastatic: Lung, breast, bone, lymphoma, melanoma
Collagen vascular diseases
- Rheumatoid arthritis
- Systemic lupus erythematosus
Inflammatory/infiltrative diseases
- Sarcoidosis
- Amyloidosis
Metabolic
- Hypothyroidism
- Uremia
Pharmacologic
- Cromolyn sodium
- Doxorubicin
- Hydralazine
- Methysergide
- Minoxidil
- Penicillin
- Phenytoin
- Procainamide

Types

I. **Acute pericarditis:**
   1. Serous pericarditis
   2. Fibrinous and serofibrinous pericarditis
   3. Purulent (suppurative) pericarditis
   4. Haemorrhagic pericarditis
   5. Caseous pericarditis

II. **Chronic or healed pericarditis**

Specific Types

Idiopathic pericarditis: The cause of acute pericarditis is often difficult to establish, and idiopathic pericarditis remains the most common diagnosis. Most cases are presumed to have a viral etiology.

Viral pericarditis: Coxsackievirus B and echovirus are the most common viruses, and a fourfold increase in antiviral titers is required for the diagnosis. Patients often experience a prodrome of an upper respiratory tract infection. The prognosis of viral pericarditis is generally good, with a self-limited course, and if uncomplicated, patients may be treated on an outpatient basis.

Purulent pericarditis: Before the antibiotic era, pneumonia was the prime cause of purulent pericarditis. Currently, causes include thoracic surgery, chemotherapy, immunosuppression, and hemodialysis, as well as extension from pneumonia and empyema. Presentation is usually acute with high fevers, chills, night sweats, and dyspnea, but the classic findings of chest pain or friction rub are rare. Cardiac tamponade is common (42 to 77% of patients in selected series), and mortality is high.

If purulent pericarditis is suspected, hospital admission, treatment with intravenous, broad-spectrum antibiotics and urgent drainage is recommended. Findings on pericardial fluid analysis include a high protein level (>6 g/dl), a low glucose level (<35 mg/dl), and a very high leukocyte count (6,000–240,000/mm^3).

Malignancy: Pericarditis associated with malignancy is caused mainly by metastatic disease. Pericarditis is common in metastasized bronchogenic or breast carcinoma, Hodgkin's disease, and lymphoma, it is rare in primary mesothelioma and angiosarcoma. Diagnosis is based on analysis of pericardial fluid cytology, which has a sensitivity ranging from 70 to 90% and a specificity of 95 to 100%.

Radiation pericarditis: Recent or remote mediastinal radiation can cause pericarditis at any time from weeks to months after the exposure.

Traumatic pericarditis: Sharp or blunt trauma and invasive cardiac procedures such as electrophysiological ablation procedures, cardiac diagnostic, or interventional catheterization have been associated with pericardial irritation and inflammation.

Uremic and dialysis-associated pericarditis: Uremic pericarditis occurs in 6 to 10% of patients with advanced renal failure before hemodialysis is initiated; blood urea nitrogen levels usually exceed 60 mg/dl. The typical ST-segment elevation on the ECG usually is absent. A large haemorrhagic effusion facilitated by impaired platelet function may occur, although tamponade is rare. Alternatively, a serous pericardial effusion related to fluid overload may occur. With both forms, initiation or intensification of haemodialysis is indicated, usually leading to improvement in 1 to 2 weeks.

Tuberculous pericarditis occurs in 1 to 2% of cases of pulmonary tuberculosis. It remains the leading cause of pericarditis in some developing countries. Immunocompromised or human immunodeficiency virus (HIV)-positive patients are at increased risk. Nonspecific symptoms such as dyspnoea, fever, chills, and night sweats develop slowly, and a friction rub or chest pain is often absent. A patient with suspected or diagnosed pericardial tuberculosis should be hospitalized and antituberculous therapy started promptly.

Analysis of the pericardial fluid shows high specific gravity, very high protein level (often >6 g/dl), and predominantly lymphocytic cells. A pericardial biopsy with acid-fast bacilli polymerase chain reaction testing is recommended for all patients with suspected tuberculous pericarditis. However, a normal pericardial biopsy does not exclude the diagnosis.

Constrictive Pericarditis

Definition: Constrictive pericarditis refers to an abnormal scarring and loss of elasticity of the pericardium, resulting in impaired ventricular filling and decreased cardiac output.

Etiology: The frequency of different causes of constrictive pericarditis depends on the population and geography in question. In developed countries, cardiac surgery and idiopathic constriction are the leading cause, while in certain developing countries tuberculous remains the number one Etiology.

- Constrictive pericarditis results from an abnormal scarring of the pericardium that causes impairment of diastolic filling.
- A diagnostic challenge often lies in differentiating constriction from restriction. The diagnosis can be made by noting haemodynamic derangements on echocardiography/CMR/right heart catheterization and a thickening of the pericardium on echo/CT/MRI.
- About 20% of patients do not demonstrate thickening of the pericardium by CT.
- For patients that do not respond to medical therapy, the treatment of choice is surgical excision of the pericardium.

Diagnosis: The diagnosis of acute pericarditis remains a clinical one based on history, physical examination, ECG and the echocardiogram. Other imaging studies, including computed tomography (CT) and magnetic resonance imaging (MRI) may be used in selected cases to investigate the pericardium.

Electrocardiography: The ECG does not show specific findings, but low voltage may be seen.

Blood Tests

Testing should include a complete blood count, markers of inflammation including erythrocyte sedimentation rate and/or C-reactive protein, markers of myocardial ischaemia (troponins/CK-MB) to assess for myopericarditis, and assessment of renal function. Depending on presentation and clinical evaluation, additional blood testing may be necessary such as viral titers, blood cultures, thyroid-stimulating hormone, antinuclear antibodies, HIV serology, or QuantiFERON-TB assay.

- **Chemical tests:** In addition to protein or albumin, a glucose test may be performed. Glucose in pericardial fluid samples is typically about the same as blood glucose levels. It may be lower with infection.
- **Microscopic examination:** Normal pericardial fluid has small numbers of white blood cells (WBCs) but no red blood cells (RBCs) or microorganisms. Results of an evaluation of the different kinds of cells present may include:
  - **Total cell counts:** Quantity of WBCs and RBCs in the sample. Increased WBCs may be seen with infections and other causes of pericarditis.
- **Brain natriuretic peptide (BNP)** is a serum biomarker that can help distinguish constrictive pericarditis from restrictive cardiomyopathy. Despite elevated filling pressures in both conditions, levels of BNP are significantly higher in restrictive cardiomyopathy.
- Additional testing on exudate fluid may include:
  - Pericardial fluid glucose
  - Microscopic examination: A laboratory professional may place a sample of the fluid on a slide and examine it under a microscope. Normal pericardial fluid has small numbers of white blood cells (WBCs) but no red blood cells (RBCs) or microorganisms. Laboratories may examine drops of the pericardial fluid and/or use a special centrifuge (cytocentrifuge) to concentrate the fluid's cells at the bottom of a test tube. Samples are placed on a slide, treated with a

special stain, and an evaluation of the different kinds of cells present is performed.

- Cytology: A laboratory professional may use a cytocentrifuge to concentrate the fluid's cells on a slide. The slide is treated with a special stain and evaluated for abnormal cells, such as malignant cells (cancer cells).
- Gram stain: For direct observation of bacteria.

Complications: A potential complication of pericardial effusion is cardiac tamponade (tam-pon-AYD). In this condition, the excess fluid within the pericardium puts pressure on the heart. The strain prevents the heart chambers from filling completely with blood.

Increased in: Condition/test showing increased result

- Bacterial pericarditis (RBC count, WBC count with a predominance of neutrophils)
- Haemorrhagic pericarditis (RBC count, WBC count)
- Malignancy (RBC count, abnormal cytology)
- Post-myocardial infarction syndrome, also called Dressler syndrome (RBC count, WBC count with a predominance of neutrophils)
- Rheumatoid disease or systemic lupus erythematosus (SLE) (RBC count, WBC count)
- Tuberculous or fungal pericarditis (RBC count, WBC count with a predominance of lymphocytes)
- Viral pericarditis (RBC count, WBC count with a predominance of neutrophils)

Decreased in: Condition/test showing decreased result

- Bacterial pericarditis (glucose)
- Malignancy (glucose)
- Rheumatoid disease or SLE (glucose)

Chapter 21

Pleural Fluid Examination

Chapter Outline

INTRODUCTION

Pleural fluid serves a physiologic function in respiration, while also being a useful measure to diagnose and assess disease, trauma, and other abnormalities. A brief review of the anatomy and physiology of normal pleural fluid gives a point of reference for assessing the causes of abnormal pleural fluid collections and pleural effusions.

The light criteria is a useful way to differentiate between transudate and exudate, which can then be further evaluated.

Pleural fluid is a liquid that is located between the layers of the pleura. The pleura is a two layer membrane that covers the lungs and lines the chest cavity. Pleural fluid keeps the pleura moist and reduces friction between the membranes when you breathe.

Pleural fluid is continuously produced by the parietal circulation in the way of bulk flow, while it is also continuously reabsorbed by the lymphatic system via the stomata in the parietal pleura. In a healthy human, the pleural space contains a small amount of fluid (about 10 to 20 ml), with a low protein concentration (less than 1.5 g/dl).

Pleural Effusions

Pleural effusions result from excessive fluid formation and its accumulation in the pleural space. The most common conditions causing pleural effusions are heart failure, malignancy, pneumonia, tuberculosis and pulmonary embolism. In patients presenting with pleural effusions, efforts should be made to find out the cause so that appropriate treatment can be instituted.

The pathological accumulation of serous fluids in the pleural, peritoneal and pericardial space occurs in a variety of conditions. Since patient management depends on right and timely diagnosis, biochemical analysis of extravascular body fluids is considered a valuable tool in the patient management process.

The biochemical evaluation of serous fluids includes the determination of gross appearance, differentiation of transudative from exudative effusions and additional specific biochemical testing to assess the effusion etiology.

The accumulation of fluid in the pleural space is due to the rate of pleural fluid production exceeding the rate of reabsorption. Effusion of exudative type occurs when filtration rate exceeds maximum lymph flow, resulting in an effusion with higher than usual protein content. Exudate forms when protein permeability of the systemic capillaries is increased, causing an increase in pleural liquid protein concentration.

A pleural fluid analysis is used to find the cause of pleural effusion. There are two main types of pleural effusion.

Light's Criteria

Light's criteria are a traditional method of separating transudates and exudates that measures serum and pleural fluid protein and LDH. If at least one of the following three criteria is present, the fluid is defined as an exudate.

1. Ratio of pleural-fluid protein level to serum protein level >0.5
2. Ratio of pleural-fluid LDH level to serum LDH level >0.6
3. Pleural-fluid LDH level > 0.67 or two-thirds of the upper limit of normal for serum LDH level

Transudate—an imbalance between the pressure within blood vessels (which drives fluid out of the blood vessel) and the amount of protein in blood (which keeps fluid in the blood vessel) can result in accumulation of fluid.

- Transudates are most often caused by congestive heart failure or cirrhosis. If the fluid is determined to be a transudate, then usually no more tests on the fluid are necessary.

- Transudate, which happens when there is an imbalance of pressure in certain blood vessels. This causes extra fluid to leak into the pleural space. Transudate pleural effusion is most often caused by heart failure or cirrhosis.

Congestive heart failure (CHF): The most common cause of a pleural effusion, CHF occurs as a result of poor heart function and a decreased ability for the heart to pump blood effectively.

Infections: Some diseases caused by viruses or bacteria such as pneumonia or tuberculosis can also lead to a pleural effusion (Table 21.1).

Table 21.1: Conditions in which transudate is commonly seen
- Transudates
- Congestive heart failure
- Cirrhotic liver disease
- Renal failure
- Nephrotic syndrome
- Hypoalbuminemia
- Atelecttasis
- Hypothyroidism
- Pulmonary embolism (10–20%)
- Malignancy (5%)

Exudate which happens when there is an injury or inflammation of the pleura. This can make excess fluid leak out of certain blood vessels. Exudate pleural effusion has many causes. (Table 21.2)

Exudative (protein-rich fluid) pleural effusions are most commonly caused by:

- Pneumonia
- Cancer
- Pulmonary embolism

Table 21.2: Exudates seen in conditions
- Parapneumonic effusion—empyema
- Malignancy
- Mesothelioma
- Tuberculosis
- Pulmonary embolism
- Connective tissue disorders
- Pancreatitis
- Drug-induced
- Post-coronary artery bypass surgery
- Chylothorax
- Esophageal rupture
- Asbestos-related benign pleuritis
- Sub-diaphragmatic abscess
- Paragonimiasis
- Ovarian hyperstimulation syndrome
- Yellow-nail syndrome

- Kidney disease
- Inflammatory disease

Other less common causes of pleural effusion include:

- Tuberculosis
- Autoimmune disease
- Bleeding (due to chest trauma)
- Chylothorax (due to filariasis)

The details of exudation effusion of simple exudates, pyothorax; haemothorax, and chylothorax and given in Fig. 21.1.

In most cases of pleural effusions, especially if no underlying diagnosis is apparent, biochemical analyses provide important diagnostic information. Various tests can be performed for pleural fluid (PF) analysis, either as sole or additional diagnostic tools to further determine the effusion's etiology.

Most patients who meet the criteria for an exudative effusion by LDH level but not by protein level have either parapneumonic effusions or malignancy. A pleural fluid absolute total protein concentrations >3 mg/dl suggests an exudate, but when taken alone this parameter misclassifies at least 10% of exudates and 15% of transudates.

Pleural-fluid LDH level > 0.67 or two-thirds the upper limit of normal for serum LDH level.

Very high levels of pleura, fluid LDH (>1000 U/L) are found in patients with complicated parapneumonic effusion and in about 40% of those with tuberculous pleurisy.

Very high levels of pleural fluid LDH (>1,000 U/L) are found in patients with complicated parapneumonic effusion and in about 40% of those with tuberculous pleurisy.

Protein gradient: The difference between protein levels in the serum and pleural fluid greater than 3.1 g/dl suggests transudate.

Albumin gradient: The difference between albumin levels in the serum and pleural fluid greater than 1.2 g/dl suggests transudate.

These are supportive tests to Light's criteria and should not be used alone to distinguish transudates from exudates. Fifteen to 20% of patients with congestive heart failure or cirrhosis will meet Light's criteria for exudative effusions. This is particularly likely if the patient has been receiving diuretics before the thoracentesis. The protein gradient is equally effective as the albumin gradient.

PLEURAL FLUID BIOCHEMICAL ANALYSIS

The first question to be stressed is: Is this fluid an exudate? The answer in most cases is given by pleural protein. Exudates have a higher protein concentration (> 30 g/L) due to an increase in capillary permeability and/or impaired lymphatic drainage.

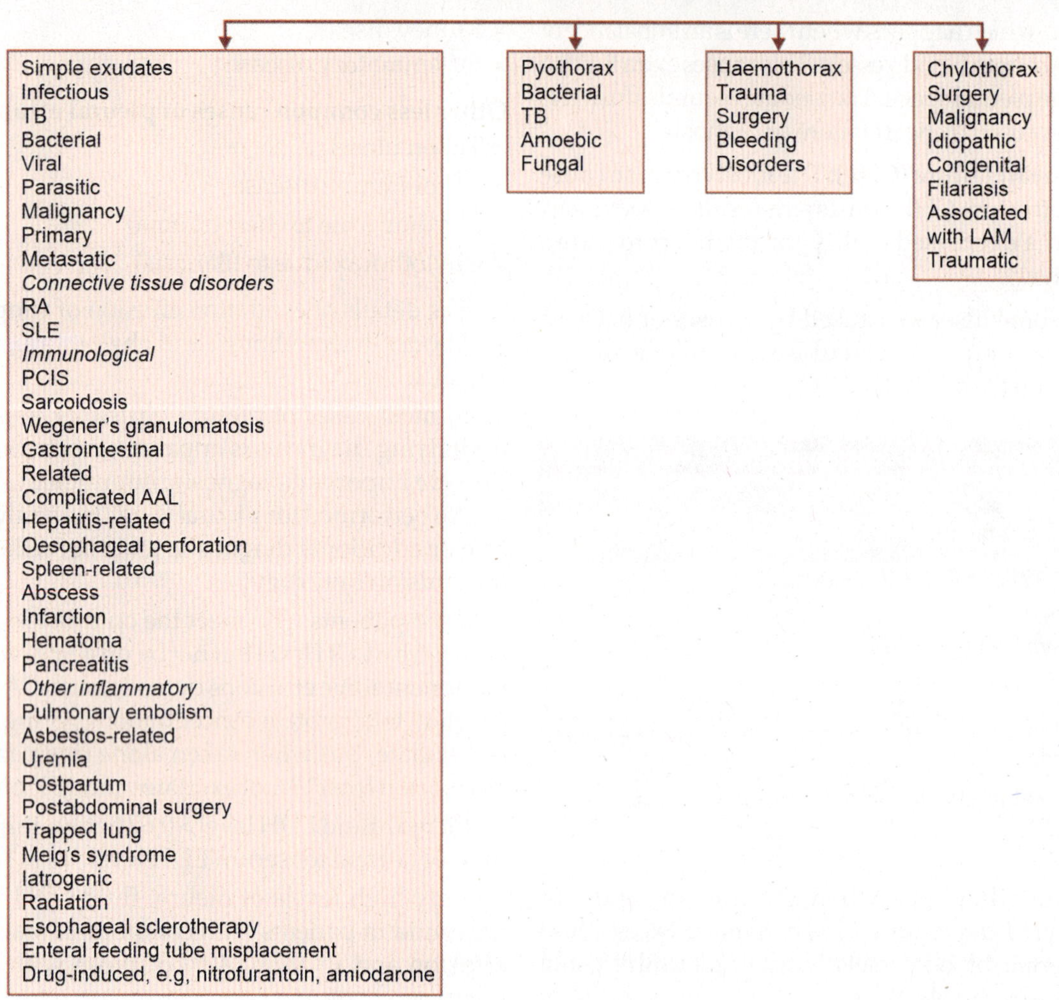

Fig. 21.1: Causes of exudative effusion

Pus is characteristic of pleural empyema and cloudy fluid may be due to parapneumonic pleural effusion and/or to empyema. An underlying disease such as lung carcinoma should be systematically researched. A chocolate or gelatinous pleural fluid may be the consequence of paragonimiasis. A green-coloured fluid may indicate rheumatoid effusion and a 'milky' appearance chylothorax. Classically transudates are limpid, clear yellow-coloured fluids. It is also important to smell the pleural fluid because an unpleasant smell suggests infection by anaerobic bacteria.

Glucose: Pleural glucose can be difficult to interpret in patients with hyperglycemia. Low glucose (< 60 mg/dl) is found in empyema, rheumatoid arthritis, tuberculosis and malignancy. Low glucose levels are found in almost 100% of effusions due to empyema and rheumatoid disease, complicated parapneumonic effusions (30%), tuberculosis (20%), malignancy (< 10%).

Triglyceride: Chylothorax is caused by lymphoma or trauma. Not all chylous pleural effusions appear milky white or whitish.

The fluid is milky if the patient has had laceration of the thoracic duct from recent trauma or thoracic surgery. Triglyceride levels greater than 110 mg/dl are consistent with true chylothorax, whereas levels that are less than 50 mg/dl effectively rule out this entity. For triglyceride levels of 5 to 110 mg/dl, microscopy or electrophoresis revealing chylomicrons supports a diagnosis of chylothorax.

Cholesterol: Optional test for exudative pleural effusion and chylothorax. Cholesterol interpreted alone as a test misclassifies 10% of exudates and 20% of transudates. A level greater than 200 mg/dl suggests a chyliform effusion (pseudochylothorax), which suggests chronic pleural inflammatory state including tuberculosis, solid or hematogenous malignancy, or rheumatoid arthritis. Less common entities include sarcoidosis and amyloidosis.

Adenosine deaminase (ADA): This test may not be routinely required in countries where tuberculosis is rare. Factors such as a positive tuberculin skin test, incarceration, foreign travel, and abnormal chest X-ray should encourage use of this test. Pleural fluid ADA greater than 40 U/L has a sensitivity of 90–100% and a specificity of 85–95% for diagnosing tuberculosis pleurisy.

Appearance: The appearance of the pleural fluid might be useful. Massive and haemorrhagic or sero-haemorrhagic pleural effusions are likely to be malignant. Pus is characteristic of pleural empyema and cloudy fluid may be due to parapneumonic pleural effusion and/or to empyema. An underlying disease such as lung carcinoma should be systematically researched. A chocolate or gelatinous pleural fluid may be the consequence of paragonimiasis.

pH: pH must be measured with an arterial blood gas machine for accurate results. Generally, a pleural fluid pH of less than 7.3 is associated with the same pathologies that cause low pleural fluid glucose levels. In malignant effusions, a pleural fluid pH of less than 7.3 has been associated with more extensive pleural involvement and shorter life expectancies.

A low pleural fluid pH (<7.3) may follow bacterial metabolism and is often associated with a reduced pleural fluid glucose (<3.3 mmol/L) or pleural fluid/serum glucose ratio of <0.5. This combination is relatively specific for parapneumonic pleural effusions and/or empyemas.

Red blood cell count (RBC): Red blood cells are found in most samples of pleural effusion. Fluid for cell counts should be sent in an anticoagulant container to prevent clotting which results in inaccurate results. If fluid appears bloody, obtain haematocrit (Hct). A pleural fluid Hct greater than 50% of the peripheral Hct indicates haemothorax.

White blood cell count and differential: The pleural fluid needs to be sent in an anticoagulant container. If the lymphocyte count is greater than 90%, lymphoma and tuberculosis are the two most likely diagnoses.

- WBC differential—determination of percentages of different types of WBCs. An increased number of neutrophils may be seen with bacterial infections.

Cytology

- Cytology—a cytocentrifuged sample is treated with a special stain and examined under a microscope for abnormal cells. This may be done when a mesothelioma or metastatic cancer is suspected. The presence of certain abnormal cells, such as tumor cells or immature blood cells, can indicate what type of cancer is involved.
- Positive cytology shows low sensitivity (54–73%) and high specificity (97%) for malignancy. Sensitivity will increase on multiple samples: 50%, 66.7% and 73.3% for one, two, and three samples, respectively. Malignancy should not be excluded on the basis of negative pleural cytology results.

INFECTIONS PRODUCING PLEURAL EFFUSIONS

Culture

Pleural effusion should be injected into aerobic blood culture bottles at the bedside. Mycobacterial, fungal and viral cultures should be sent if suspicion of infection.

Bacteria

Bacteria are the pathogens responsible for the majority of pleural effusions from infectious causes. A pleural effusion secondary to a pneumonia is termed a parapneumonic effusion. Parapneumonic effusions progress along a spectrum. In the first stage, termed the exudative phase, the pleural fluid accumulates from increased pulmonary interstitial fluid traversing the visceral pleura as well as increased permeability of the pleural capillaries from inflammation. At this stage the fluid is sterile and the effusion will resolve with proper treatment of the pneumonia. In the second stage, termed the fibropurulent stage, the fluid in the pleural space becomes infected. Gram stain and culture are positive. These effusions may have low pH, low glucose, loculations produced by fibroblasts invading the pleural space, and lactate dehydrogenase greater than three times the upper limit of normal. If a pleural effusion reaches the fibropurulent stage it is termed a complicated parapneumonic effusion. The pleural fluid in all stages of parapneumonic effusions is characterized by having predominantly neutrophils;

The most common bacterial causes of pleural empyema in immunocompetent adults in the community acquired setting include *Streptococcus milleri* group, *Streptococcus pneumoniae*, and *Staphylococcus aureus*. However, gram-negative organisms such as *Escherichia coli, Pseudomonas*.

The diagnosis is confirmed by identification of the acid fast bacteria in sputum, pleural fluid, or pleural fluid biopsy. Often times, however, the pleural fluid will not have the bacteria present. The alternative method of diagnosis is to measure the adenosine deaminase (ADA) level present in the pleural. This test is quite sensitive and specific. When the cut-off of 40 IU/L is used the sensitivity and specificity are 96%. The pleural fluid analysis usually reveals an exudate with a predominance of small lymphocyte. If the effusion is very early, polymorphonuclear cells may dominate but over the next few days the differential of the fluid will invariably turn to lymphocytes.

Other bacteria, Mycoplasma and fungi are also seen in pleural fluid.

- Atypical bacteria: *Mycoplasma pneumoniae*, Actinomycosis, and Nocardiosis are also commonly observed.
- *Mycoplasma pneumoniae* is an obligate intracellular bacteria that produces an illness more resembling a viral pneumonia than a bacterial infection.

VIRUSES

Viruses are less common causes of pleural effusions but may very well account for more effusions than is acknowledged. The effusions are generally smaller than those encountered with bacterial pneumonia. The fluid is an exudate and lymphocytes dominate in the cell differential. The diagnosis of a viral infection is made by observing increasing titers with specific serologic tests or by a positive viral culture.

Adenovirus is the most common viral cause of atypical pneumonia. Pleural effusions occur in anywhere from 15 to 62% of patients. The effusions are often bilateral and are accompanied by a diffuse parenchymal infiltrate typical of a viral pneumonia.

Epstein-Barr virus (EBV) is a common infection and there is evidence of infection in 90% of the world's population. The primary infection is generally acquired in infancy or childhood. Effusions are less commonly seen with EBV.

PATHOPHYSIOLOGY: INTERPRETATIONS

- Pleural effusions develop when changes in fluid and solute homeostasis occur, too much fluid builds up. Pleural fluid is a liquid that is located between the layers of the pleura. The pleura is a two-layer membrane that covers the lungs and lines the chest cavity. Pleural fluid keeps the pleura moist and reduces friction between the membranes when you breathe. The area that contains pleural fluid is known as the pleural space.

Normally, there is a small amount of pleural fluid in the pleural space. This is known as pleural effusion. Pleural effusion prevents the lungs from fully inflating, making it hard to breathe. A pleural fluid analysis is a group of tests that look for the cause of pleural effusion.

- Haemothorax—a build-up of blood in the pleural space; commonly from injury or trauma to the chest.
- Pleurisy—pleura inflammation, causing sharp pain with breathing; most commonly caused by a viral infection.
- Pleural effusion—excess fluid in the pleural space; commonly from congestive heart failure or malignancy.
- Pneumothorax—a build-up of air or gas in the pleural space; commonly from acute lung injury, trauma, or chronic diseases such as a chronic obstructive pulmonary disease or tuberculosis.

An empyema, the third stage of the pleural effusion spectrum, is defined as frank pus in the pleural cavity. It will have the same laboratory characteristics as a complicated parapneumic effusion. Glucose will be less than 60 ml/dl and pH less than 7.20. Loculations can develop very quickly, in a matter of 12 to 24 hours. Quick drainage for complicated parapneumonic effusions and empyema is imperative.

Chapter 22

Peritoneal Fluid Examination

Chapter Outline

- Peritoneal Fluid Production
- Transudate
- Exudate
- Analysate Interpretation
- Peritoneal Fluid Culture
- Risks
- Peritoneal Inclusion Cyst (PIC)

Peritoneal fluid is a serous fluid made by the peritoneum in the abdominal cavity which lubricates the surface of tissue that lines the abdominal wall and pelvic cavity. It covers most of the organs in the abdomen. An increased volume of peritoneal fluid is called ascites.

Ascites is the accumulation of ascitic fluid in the peritoneal cavity. Many diseases can cause ascites, but the most common cause is portal hypertension, which is usually due to liver cirrhosis.

'Ascites'—the abnormal accumulation of fluid within the abdomen.

- The peritoneum is important in osmoregulation
  - Passive diffusion of water and solute (up to a certain size)
  - Maintains osmotic and chemical equilibrium with blood and lymph
- Ascites develops either from:
  - Increased accumulation
    - Increased capillary permeability
    - Increased venous pressure
    - Decreased protein (oncotic pressure)
  - Decreased clearance
    - Increased lymphatic obstruction

Definition: Peritoneal fluid analysis is a lab test. It is done to look at fluid that has built up in the space in the abdomen around the internal organs. This area is called the peritoneal space. The condition is called ascites.

The test is also known as paracentesis or abdominal tap.

Peritoneal fluid production: The amount of fluid is normally small (less than 50 ml in humans) and contains neutrophils, mononuclear cells, eosinophils, macrophages, lymphocytes, desquamated mesothelial cells, and an average of 3.0 g/ml of protein.

Contraindications of peritoneal tap are given in Table 22.1.

Table 22.1: Contraindications to paracentesis

Uncooperative patient
Abdominal skin infection at the proposed puncture sites
Pregnancy
Severe coagulopathy (accelerated fibrinolysis or disseminated intravascular coagulation)
Severe bowel distension

Composition: Contents of peritoneal fluid are shown in Table 22.2.

Table 22.2: Contents of peritoneal fluid

Ascitic fluid	*Results*
Colour	Cloudy
WBC (white blood cell) count	960 cells/mm^3
Segmented neutrophils count	25.0%
Lymphocyte count	75.0%
RBC (red blood cell) count	19,500 Mil cells/mm^3
Mesothelial cells	Many
Macrophage	Many
Albumin	3.2 g/dl
Amylase	46 unit/L
Adenosine deaminase	36.8 U/L
LDH (lactate dehydrogenase)	278 unit/L
Protein	5.2 g/dl
SAAG (serum ascites albumin gradient)	0.7 g/dl

General and specific causes are given in Table 22.3.

Table 22.3: Causes of ascites

General	*Specific*
Liver disease	Cirrhosis Veno-occlusive disease
Heart disease	Congestive cardiac failure Constrictive poricarditis
Malignancy	Liver cancer Ovarion cancer Peritoneal metastasis Pancreatic cancer
Hypoalbuminaemia (low albumin)	Nephrotic syndrome Protein-losing enteropathy Malnutrition
Hepatic vein obstruction	Budd-Chiari syndrome
Chronic inflammation	Pancreatitis Appendicitis Infective peritonitis

Frequency of causes is given in Table 22.4.

Table 22.4: Frequency of causes of ascites

Parenchymal liver disease	78
Cirrhosis	77
Fulminant liver failure	1
Malignancy	12
Cardiovascular disease	5
Congestive heart failure	
Constrictive or restrictive cardiomyopathy	
Thrombosis of inferior vena cava	
Budd-Chiari syndrome	
Veno-occlusive disease	
Infection	2
Tuberculosis	
Fitz-Hugh-Curtis syndrome (chlamydiae, gonococci)	
Coccidioidomycosis	
Whipple's disease (Tropheryma whipplei)	
Renal	1.5
Nephrotic syndrome	
Uremia	
Haemodialysis	
Pancreatic	1
Bacterial peritonitis	0.5
Marked hypothyroidism	
Collagen vascular disease	
Familial Mediterranean fever	
Amyloidosis	
Hereditary angioneurotic edema	
Ménétrier's disease and protein-losing enteropathy	
Starch peritonitis	
Trauma	

Ascitic fluid can accumulate as a transudate or an exudate. Amounts of up to 25 liters are possible. Transudate exudate result of increased pressure in the portal vein (>8 mm Hg, usually around 20 mmHg) exudates are actively secreted fluid due to inflammation.

Non-peritoneal causes of ascites are shown in Table 22.5 with examples.

Table 22.5: Non-peritoneal causes of ascites

Non-peritoneal causes	*Examples*
Intrahepatic portal hypertension	Cirrhosis Fulminant hepatic failure Veno-occlusive disease
Extrahepatic portal hypertension	Hepatic vein obstruction (i.e. Budd-Chiari syndrome) Congestive heart failure
Hypoalbuminemia	Nephrotic syndrome Protein-losing enteropathy Malnutrition
Miscellaneous disorders	Myxedema Ovarian tumours Pancreatic and biliary ascites
Chylous	Secondary to malignancy, trauma

The 3 grades of ascites are shown in Table 22.6.

Table 22.6: Grading of ascites

Grade 1:	Mild ascites: It is only detectable by ultrasound examination
Grade 2:	Moderate ascites: It is manifest by moderate symmetrical distension of abdomen
Grade 3:	Large or gross ascites: It provokes marked abdominal distension

The peritoneum is a tough semi-permeable membrane lining abdominal and visceral cavities. It encloses, supports and lubricates organs within the cavity. Paracentesis is effectively the analysis of 'ascites'—the abnormal accumulation of fluid within the abdomen.

- The peritoneum is important in osmoregulation
  - Passive diffusion of water and solute (up to a certain size)
- Ascites develops either from:
  - Increased accumulation
    - Increased capillary permeability
    - Increased venous pressure
    - Decreased protein (oncotic pressure)
  - Decreased clearance
    - Increased lymphatic obstruction

Peritonitis means that the peritoneum is inflamed. More commonly, infection spreads to the peritoneal space from your biliary or gastrointestinal tract. This is called secondary peritonitis.

Transudate (<30 g/L protein) (systemic disease)
- Liver (cirrhosis)
- Cardiac, e.g. RHF, CCF, SBE right heart valve disease and constrictive pericarditis
- Renal failure
- Hypoalbuminaemia (nephrosis)

Exudate (>30 g/L protein) (local disease)
- Malignancy
- Venous obstruction, e.g. Budd-Chiari, schistosomiasis
- Pancreatitis
- Lymphatic obstruction
- Infection (especially TB)

Analysate interpretation
- Gross appearance: (Table 22.7)

Table 22.7: Gross appearance

Appearance	*Interpretation*
Clear to pale yellow	Normal
Milk-coloured (Chylous)	• Malignant tumour, lymphoma, TB • Parasitic infection, hepatic cirrhosis
Cloudy/turbid	• Peritonitis, primary bacterial infection • Perforated bowel, appendicitis, pancreatitis • Strangulated or infarcted bowel
Bloody tap	• Benign or malignart tumour • Haemorrhagic pancreatitis, perforated ulcer

Ascitic fluid characteristics are given in Table 22.8.

Table 22.8: Ascitic fluid characteristics

Characteristics	*Value*
Colour	Milky and cloudy
Triglyceride level	>200 mg/dl
Cell count	>500 (predominance of lymphocytes)
Total protein	2.5–7.0 g/dl
SAAG	Depends on the underlying aetiology
Cholesterol	Low (ascites/serum ratio <1)
Lactate dehydrogenase	Between 110 and 200 IU/L
Culture	May be positive
Amylase	Elevated in cases of pancreatitis
Cytology	Positive in malignancy
Glucose	<100 mg/dl
Adenosine deaminase	Elevated in cases of tuberculosis

Ascitic fluid biochemistry is given in Table 22.9.

Table 22.9: Ascitic fluid biochemistry

Test	*Levels*	*Interpretation*
Trigiyceride	• Elevated	• Malignant tumour, lymphoma, TB
Protein	• 0.3–4.0 g/dl • >4 g/dl	• Normal • TB, SBP
Glucose	• 7–10 • <6	• Normal • TB and malignancy
Amylase	• 50% of serum level • Increased (up to 5x serum level)	• Normal • Pancreatitis, pancreatic pseudocyst, pancreatic trauma or intestinal strangulation
Alkaline phosphatase	• Increased	• Small bowel perforation and strangulation

Microscopy and analysis are given in Table 22.10

Table 22.10: Microscopy and analysis

Red cell count	*Interpretation*
• None • >100/µl • >100,000/µl	• None • Malignancy, TB • Intra-abdominal trauma (DPL)
White cell count	***Interpretation***
• <300/µl • >300/µl + >25% neutrophils + >25% lymphocytes + Mesothelial cells • Gram +ve cocci • Gram –ve	• Normal • Abnormal + SBP (90%), cirrhosis (50%) + TB or chylous ascites + TB peritonitis • Primary peritonitis • Secondary peritonitis

- The serum-ascites albumin gradient (SAAG) is given in Table 22.11.

Table 22.11: SAAG and albumin gradiant

SAAG >1.1 mg/dl	*SAAG <1.1 mg/dl*
• Cirrhosis • Alcoholic hepatitis • Cardiac ascites • Mixed ascites • Massive liver metastasis • Fulminant hepatic failure • Budd-Chiari syndrome • Portal vein thrombosis • Veno-occlusive disease • Myxoadema • Fatty liver of pregnancy	• Peritoneal carcinomatosis • Tuberculosis peritonitis • Pancreatic ascites • Bowel obstruction • Biliary ascites • Nephrotic syndrome • Postoperative lymphatic leak • Serositis in connective tissue disease

- The SAAG has become more favored in helping to characterize ascites fluid
- The concept surrounds oncotic-hydrostatic balance
- Simple calculation:
  - Serum albumin–ascites albumin = SAAG (Table 22.11)

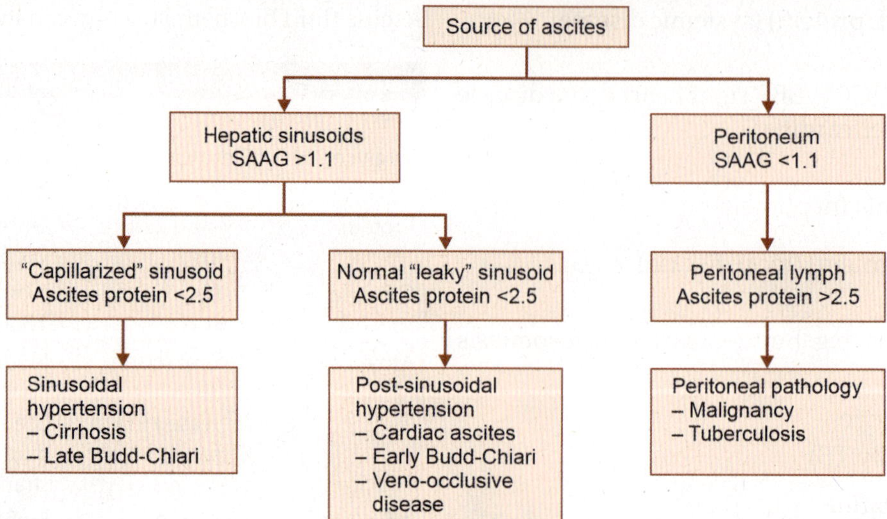

Fig. 22.1: Ascites can be characterised by serum-ascites albumin-gradient (SAAG) and ascites protein

Further characteristics of SAAG and ascitic proteins are given in Fig. 22.1.

Peritoneal fluid culture: The peritoneal space is the area between the abdominal wall and the organs it houses. This space is typically empty, or contains a small amount of fluid. But a buildup of fluid can occur if you have a disease or infection. This fluid is called ascites.

Inflammation of the lining of the abdominal wall, or the peritoneum, can also occur. This can cause pain, nausea, vomiting, and constipation. If left untreated, it can be life-threatening. It can be caused by a variety of diseases.

The growth of any microorganism, such as bacteria or fungi, from peritoneal fluid is abnormal and indicates peritonitis.

The peritoneal fluid culture may be negative, even if you have peritonitis. The diagnosis of peritonitis is based on other factors, in addition to the culture.

Risks: Risks for developing peritonitis include:

- Damage to the bowel, bladder, or a blood vessel in the abdomen from a needle puncture
- Bleeding
- Infection
- Low blood pressure
- Shock
- Scarring of the liver called cirrhosis
- Ulcerative colitis
- Stomach ulcers
- Pelvic inflammatory disease
- A weakened immune system
- Peritoneal dialysis
- Appendicitis
- Diverticulitis
- Pancreatitis

Peritonitis can be dangerous.

Abnormal results

- Bile-stained fluid may mean you have a gallbladder or liver problem.
- Bloody fluid may be a sign of tumor or injury.
- High white blood cell counts may be a sign of peritonitis.
- Milk-coloured peritoneal fluid may be a sign of carcinoma, cirrhosis of the liver, lymphoma, tuberculosis, or infection.

Many diseases can cause ascites, but the most common cause is portal hypertension, which is usually due to liver cirrhosis. Cirrhosis and bacteria is found in peritoneal fluid, may have spontaneous bacterial peritonitis (SBP). This is a life-threatening infection that must be treated with antibiotics. Cirrhosis of the liver causes approximately 85% of peritoneal effusion cases, and cancer causes roughly 10% of cases. While the condition is relatively common among peritoneal mesothelioma patients, this cancer is a rare cause of peritoneal effusion overall.

Regardless of the cause, sequestration of fluid within the abdomen leads to additional fluid retention by the kidneys due to stimulatory effect on blood pressure hormones, notably aldosterone. The sympathetic nervous system is also activated, and renin production is increased due to decreased perfusion of the kidney.

Pathophysiology portal hypertension plays an important role in the production of ascites by raising capillary hydrostatic pressure within the splanchnic bed and a consequent decrease in effective circulating blood volume. This activates the plasma renin, aldosterone, and sympathetic nervous system, resulting in renal sodium and water retention.

Peritoneal inclusion cyst (PIC): Peritoneal fluid in premenopausal women is produced by normally functioning ovaries and is reabsorbed by the mesothelial cells of the peritoneal cavity. A peritoneal inclusion cyst (PIC) represents an abnormal accumulation of pelvic peritoneal fluid that is not resorbed secondary to pelvic adhesions.

Chapter 23

Amniotic Fluid Examination

Chapter Outline

- Amniotic Fluid
- Introduction
- Information
- Definition of Amniotic Fluid
- Objectives of Amniocentesis
- Amniotic Fluid Facts
- Complications of the Amniocentesis Procedure
- Pathophysiology of Amniotic Fluid

AMNIOTIC FLUID

Introduction

Amniotic fluid is a clear, slightly yellowish liquid that surrounds the unborn baby (foetus) during pregnancy. It is contained in the amniotic sac.

Information

While in the womb, the baby floats in the amniotic fluid. The amount of amniotic fluid is greatest at about 34 weeks (gestation) into the pregnancy, when it averages 800 ml. About 600 ml of amniotic fluid surrounds the baby at full term (40 weeks gestation).

The amniotic fluid constantly moves (circulates) as the baby swallows and 'inhales' the fluid, and then releases it.

The amniotic fluid is the protective liquid contained by the amniotic sac of a gravid amniote. This fluid serves as a cushion for the growing foetus, but also serves to facilitate the exchange of nutrients, water, and biochemical products between mother and foetus.

Fluid that looks green or brown usually means that the baby has passed the first bowel movement (meconium) while in the womb. (Usually, the baby has the first bowel movement after birth.)

If the baby passes meconium in the womb, it can get into the lungs through the amniotic fluid. This can cause serious breathing problems, called meconium aspiration syndrome, especially if the fluid is thick.

Some babies who have been in amniotic fluid that has meconium in it may need treatment right away after birth to prevent breathing problems, called meconium aspiration syndrome, especially if the fluid is thick.

Amniotic fluid is present from the formation of the gestational sac. Amniotic fluid is in the amniotic sac. It is generated from maternal plasma, and passes through the foetal membranes by osmotic and hydrostatic forces. When foetal kidneys begin to function around week 16, foetal urine also contributes to the fluid. In earlier times, it was believed that the amniotic fluid was composed entirely of foetal urine.

The fluid is absorbed through the foetal tissue and skin. After 22 to 25 weeks of pregnancy, keratinization of an embryo's skin occurs. When this process completes around the 25th week[2], the fluid is primarily absorbed by the foetal gut for the remainder of gestation.

Definition of Amniotic Fluid

1. Amniotic fluid is the fluid in the amniotic sac that surrounds the foetus.
2. A portion of the amniotic fluid arises from the foetal respiratory system, urine, the amniotic membrane, and the umbilical cord.
3. Amniotic fluid at term is 500 to 1100 ml.

Objectives of Amniocentesis

Following are some of the objectives where examination of amniotic fiuid obtained by amniocentesis is necessary.

1. **RH isoimmunization syndrome:** (Erythroblastosis foetalis). Rh isoimmunization leads to haemolysis in the foetus. This causes an increase in the unconjugated bilirubin in the foetus as well as in the amniotic fiuid. Increase in the amniotic fiuid bilirubin can be estimated by spectrophotometry and accordingly the time for indicated interruption of pregnancy or intrauterine transfusion is selected.
2. Sex determination of the foetus and ABO blood group determination is also done by cytological examination of the amniotic fiuid cells—squamous and red blood cells.
3. Hereditary diseases—chromosomal or genetic (in-born errors of metabolisms) can be diagnosed from the examination of amniotic fiuid. Karyotypic studies of amniotic fluid cells can be used to detect chromosomal abnormalities like Down's syndrome; whereas determination of certain substances like protein bound

iodine can help in diagnosis of genetic abnormality as in hypothyroidism.

4. **Foetal-lung maturity:** Phospholipids (lecithin and sphingomyelin) contents of amniotic fiuid reflect those in the lungs of the growing foetus. The determination of lecithin and sphingomyelin amniotic fiuid predicts foetal lung maturity and is determined by thin-layer chromatography. Lecithin-sphingomyelin ratio increases with foetal lung maturity and thus with duration of pregnancy. This is the single most accurate test for foetal maturity. Immature lung (up to 30th week L/S ratio is less than 1 of gestation)

   Mature lungs (35th week of L/S ratio is more than 2 gestations)

   Postmature lungs — Abundant lecithin with trace or no sphingomyelin

The purpose of the test (indications) for amniotic fluid examination (amniocentesis):

- Around 30 ml of the amniotic fluid is derived from the maternal circulation during the first trimester. Its composition is similar to the mother plasma with the addition of the foetus cells. These cells may provide the basis for cytogenetics analysis.
- After the first trimester, foetal urine is the major contributor to the amniotic fluid volume.
- Now foetal swallowing of arnniotic fluid begins, and it regulates the increase in the fluid from the foetal urine.
- To assess postmature pregnancy >40 weeks.
- To find intrauterine retardation.
- To find congenital infections like:
  1. Toxoplasmosis.
  2. Cytomegalovirus (CMV).
  3. It can do a culture for bacterial infections.
- Amniocentesis help with elective abortion in a defective foetus.
- To diagnose respiratory distress syndrome (RDS). This is a complication in premature newborns.
- To diagnose the genetic disorder (cytogenetics analysis).
- To diagnose chromosomal abnormalities.
- To diagnose inherited metabolic disorders like cystic fibrosis.
- To diagnose neural tube defects like myelomeningocele, anencephaly and spina bifida.
- Measure bilirubin in Rh sensitization for erythroblastosis foetalis.
- To diagnose chorioamnionitis.
- To assess foetal lung maturity, a sample was taken after 32 weeks.
- The lecithin/sphingomyelin ratio is a measure of foetal lung maturity. Phospholipids are measured in amniotic fluids.
- Can diagnose sex-linked disorders like haemophilia.
- Genetic abnormalities like sickle cell anaemia, thalassaemia and Down's syndrome are diagnosed along with supportive diagnostic investigations.
- The determination of foetal maturity is indicated to predict development of the respiratory distress syndrome and to determine when it is safe to interrupt gestation because of threat to foetus.

Amniotic Fluid Facts

1. Amniotic fluid contains protein, hormones, nutrients, and antibodies.
2. There is water transfer between intrauterine compartments:
   a. The placenta
   b. The foetus
   c. Amniotic fluid (Fig. 23.1)

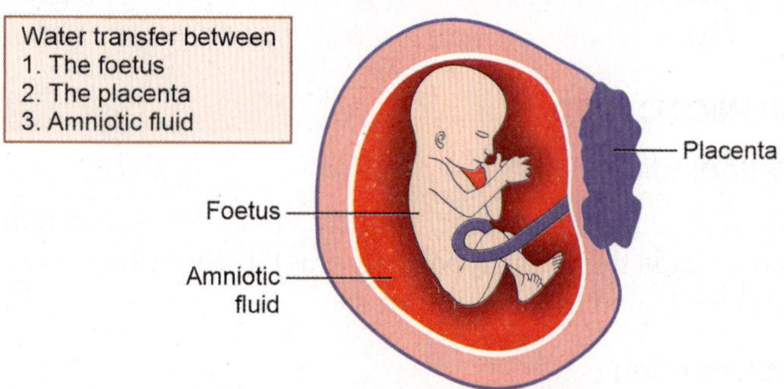

Fig. 23.1: Amniotic fluid circulation

3. As pregnancy (gestation) advances, then there are changes as follows:
   a. After 25 weeks, there is an increase in amylase, alkaline phosphatase, urea, uric acid, creatinine, and phospholipids.
   b. There is a decrease in chloride, bilirubin, protein, glucose, and sodium.
   c. AFP increased level suggests neural tube defect while decreased AFP level is associated with increased risk for trisomy 21.
4. Amniocentesis help with elective abortion in a defective foetus.
5. The sample for foetal lung maturity should be placed on ice for delivery to the laboratory and kept in the fridge
   a. The sample for the cytogenetics may be maintained at room temperature (37°C) before analysis.
   b. The sample for the biochemical testing should be separated immediately from the cellular elements and debris to avoid the effect of cellular metabolism.
6. 30 ml of amniotic fluid is collected in the sterile syringes
   a. The first 2 to 3 ml collected is discarded because this may be contaminated by the maternal blood, tissue fluid, and cells.
   b. In the case of haemolytic disease of the newborn, the sample should be avoided from light. The sample should be kept in an amber-coloured bottle or test tube.

The sample for foetal lung maturity should be placed on ice for delivery to the laboratory and kept in the fridge.

7. Amniocentesis is done during the 14th, 16th, and 18th weeks of gestation.
8. Chorionic villus sampling is better than amniotic fluid for karyotyping and genetic analysis.

Complications of the Amniocentesis Procedure

1. There may be a miscarriage.
2. There are chances for injury to the foetus.
3. There may be a leak of amniotic fluid.
4. There are chances for abortion.
5. There are chances for premature labour.
6. There are chances for infections.
7. There may be amniotic fluid embolism.
8. There are chances for maternal Rh isoimmunization.
9. There may be damage to the urinary bladder or intestine.

Pathophysiology of Amniotic Fluid

i. Amniotic fluid arises from:
   1. Foetal respiratory tract.
   2. Urine.
   3. From amniotic membrane.
   4. From umbilical cord.

ii. Amniotic fluid keeps on increasing throughout the pregnancy and reaches a peak of around one liter (1 L) during the third trimester.

iii. It gradually decreases before delivery.

iv. At first, amniotic fluid consists of water from the mother's body, but gradually, the larger proportion is made up of the baby's urine.

v. It also contains important nutrients, hormones, and antibodies and it helps protect the baby.

vi. It is the fluid contained in the amniotic sac. At term (40 weeks of gestation), the sac contains 5 to 8.5 litres of fluid. The source of the fluid is unknown. The amniotic fluid is in dynamic equilibrium with both foetal and maternal plasma and reflects the physiologic state of the mother and the foetus. Normal amniotic fluid is similar to water in appearance. Its specific gravity and viscocity are slightly greater than water. It consists of 98 to 99% water with 1 to 2% solids. About half of the solids are organic and half of this material is proteins. It also contains foetal cells squamous and RBC.

Amniotic fluid functions: Amniotic fluid has many important functions and is vital for healthy foetal development. However, if the amount of amniotic fluid inside the uterus is too little or too great, complications can occur.

1. A part of the amniotic fluid derived from:
   a. The foetal respiratory system
   b. Amniotic membrane
   c. Urine
   d. Umbilical cord.

   Exchange of the fluid
   A. Water.
   B. Chemicals
   C. Maternal blood and nourishes the foetus during gestation.
2. Allow movements of foetus: The developing baby to move in the womb, which allows for proper bone growth.
3. Prevents pressure on the umbilical cord. A foetus can move freely in the amniotic fluid of the uterus. This will prevent the compression of the umbilical cord.
4. Protective cushion: Protects the baby from outside injury by cushioning sudden blows or movements.
5. Amniotic fluid maintains the temperature. Keep a constant temperature around the baby, protecting from heat loss.
6. The lungs to develop properly.

Amniotic fluid composition: Within days of conception, the amniotic sac will form and fill with fluid. At the beginning of foetal development, the amniotic fluid will mainly consist of water. As the foetus continues to develop, it will pass small amounts of urine into the fluid from around 10 weeks of pregnancy onwards. Amniotic fluid is a clear, pale straw colour.

- It also contains important nutrients, hormones, and antibodies and it helps protect the baby from bumps and injury.
- If the levels of amniotic fluid levels are too low or too high, this can pose a problem.
- It changes when urine formation starts.
  - Creatinine, urea, and uric acid concentrations increase while glucose and protein concentrations decrease.
  - The concentration of urea and creatinine is much lower in the amniotic fluid than in the maternal urine.

Sample	*Creatinine mg/dl*	*Urea mg/dl*
Amniotic fluid	<3.5	<30
Maternal urine	>10	>300

At first, amniotic fluid is mainly water with electrolytes, but by about 12–14th week the liquid also contains proteins, carbohydrates, lipids and phospholipids, and urea, all of which aid in the growth of the foetus.

Mean volume of amniotic fluid during various gestations is shown in Table 23.1.

Table 23.1: Mean volume of amniotic fluid during gestation.	
The mean volume of amniotic fluid during gestation:	
Weeks of gestation	*Quantity of fluid*
10 weeks	30 ml
12 weeks	90 ml
14 weeks	120 ml
16 weeks	230 ml
18 weeks	280 ml
20 weeks	320 ml
40 weeks	1000 ml
Full-term	<1500 ml

Amniotic fluid analysis: Normal amniotic fluid findings are shown in Table 23.2.

Table 23.2: Normal amniotic fluid findings	
General test	*Result*
Appearance	Clear, pale to straw yellow
AFP	14 to 16 weeks ≤5.2 mg/dl 22 weeks ≤3.0 mg/dl
Bilirubin	<0.2 mg/dl
Creatinine	>2.0 mg/dl after 37 weeks
Chromosomal abnormality	Absent
Phosphatidylglycerol	Positive

The lecithin/sphingomyelin (L/S) ratio:

1. It measures foetal lung maturity.
2. Lecithin is the major surfactant required for alveolar ventilation. In the case of deficiency or surfactant, alveoli collapse during expiration and lead to respiratory distress syndrorne (RSD).
3. There is an increased concentration of lecithin between 32 weeks and full-term babies, and there is a slight decrease in the sphingomyelin during the same period.
4. Sphingornyelin is not a surfactant and has no role in lung maturity.
5. This may be a rnajor cause of death in immature babies. As the L/S ratio decreases, the risk of RDS increases.
6. This test is very cumbersome.
7. (a) L/S ratio value 2.0 indicates lung maturity.
   (b) L/S ratio value <2.0, newborns not develop RDS.

Phosphatidylglycerol (PG): This is the minor lung surfactant of about 10%. This is entirely synthesized by the mature lung alveolar cells, which is a good indicator of lung maturity.

Bilirubin level:

1. Analysis of the amniotic fluid for bilirubin level (or absorbance at 450) in the Rh-negative mothers in later weeks of the gestation gives the severity of anaemia due to Rh incompatibility.
2. Lilly plotted the graph to give the severity of the haemolytic anaemia.

Volume

- The volume of amniotic fluid changes with the growth of foetus. From the 10th to the 20th week, it increases from 25 ml to 400 ml approximately.
- Approximately in the 10th–11th week, the breathing and swallowing of the foetus slightly decrease the amount of fluid. Neither urination nor swallowing contributes significantly to fluid quantity changes until the 25th week when keratinization of skin is complete; then the relationship between fluid and foetal growth stops. It reaches a plateau of 800 ml by the 28-week gestational age. The amount of fluid declines to roughly 400 ml at 42 weeks. Some sources indicate about 500 ml to 1000 ml of amniotic fluid is present at birth.
- Too much amniotic fluid is called polyhydramnios. This condition can occur with multiple pregnancies (twins or triplets), congenital anomalies (problems that exist when the baby is born), or gestational diabetes.
- Too little amniotic fluid is known as oligohydramnios. This condition may occur with late pregnancies, ruptured membranes, placental dysfunction, or foetal abnormalities.

Table 23.3: Abnormal amniotic fluid findings	
Lab findings	*Findings*
Appearance	Yellow
	Red-brown (dark red-brown)
	Amber colour
	Green colour
	Pink-red (blood-streaked)
Volume	Increased
	Decreased
Presence of cells	Long bipolar cells, multiple filamentous pseudopodia, large vacuolated cells with inclusions
Bilirubin	At 28 weeks >0.075 At 40 weeks
Saturated phosphatidylcholine	>500 pg/L
AFP	Increased >2.3 MoM
Creatinine	>2.0 mg/dl
Microscopic examination	• There are amniotic epithelial cells from the lining of the sac. • Foetal squamous cells originate from foetal skin, oral mucosa, and vagina.
Chromosomal abnormality	Absent
Phosphatidylglycerol	Positive (negative in immature)
Lecithin/sphingomyelin rafio	Mature > 2.0, immature <2.0, Diabetic mother >3.5

- Abnormal amounts of amniotic fluid may cause the healthcare provider to watch the pregnancy more carefully.
- Polyhydramnios (>2000 ml) seen in diabetic patients increases the chances of congenital abnormality.
- Oligohydramnios when the amniotic fluid is less than 300 ml at 25 weeks of gestation. This is associated with foetal renal disease.

Abnormal amniotic findings are given in Table 23.3.

Interpretation of the amniotic fluid analysis:

1. Haemolytic anaemia shows increased bilirubin.
   a. Rh immunization also shows increased bilirubin.
2. Raised AFP shows a neural tube defect. Acetylcholinesterase can confirm the diagnosis.
3. AFP may also be raised in sacrococcygeal teratoma.
4. Foetal distress: The presence of meconium gives greenish colour to amniotic fluid indicating foetal distress.
5. Can diagnose immature foetal lung.
6. Can diagnose hereditary metabolic disorders like cystic fibrosis, Tay-Sachs disease, and galactosemia.
7. Genetic disorder identified by the amniotic fluid analysis.

Chromosomal anomalies diagnosis is:

Trisomy 21	Down's syndrome
Trisomy 13	Patau's syndrome
XO 45	Turner's syndrome
XXY 47	Klinefelter's syndrome
Trisomy 18	Edward's syndrome

Overview : Significance

Diagnosis of erythroblastosis foetal is:

1. Guidance for foetal rnaturity
2. Genetic counseling

Amniotic fluid embolism: Amniotic fluid embolism is a rare but serious condition that occurs when amniotic fluid—the fluid that surrounds a baby in the uterus during pregnancy—or foetal material, such as foetal cells, enters the mother's bloodstream. Amniotic fluid embolism is most likely to occur during delivery or in the immediate postpartum period.

Section

3A

Microbiology

Chapter 24

General Bacteriology I

Chapter Outline

- Introduction to Microbiology
- Microscope
- Micrometry
- Examination of Specimens for Microbiological Investigation
- Sterilization and Disinfection
- Identification of Bacteria and Preparation of Culture Media
- Containers for Media and Cultures
- Principles of Microbiological Diagnosis

INTRODUCTION TO MICROBIOLOGY

Compared to the wide spectrum of diseases to which mankind is exposed, we have knowledge about the etiopathogenesis is of very few, of which one group is diseases caused by microbes.

The study of microbes is very important because diseases caused by microbes are potentially curable and preventable.

Microbiology has very close link with curative medicine in regard to the precise diagnosis and the rational treatment of disease which are:

A. Microbial—caused by
   1. Bacteria
   2. Spirochaetes
   3. Rickettsiae
   4. Fungi
   5. Viruses
   6. Mycoplasma [Pleuropneumonia-like organisms (PPLO)]
   7. Chlamydiae

B. Parasitic—caused by
   1. Protozoa
   2. Helminths

Before discussing further, certain terms in common use need to be classified.

1. **Saprophytes:** Organisms that grow on decaying matter.
2. **Parasites:** Microbes or larger species that live in or on and obtains nourishment from a living host. Parasites may be:
   i. *Commensals:* Constitute normal flora of body.
   ii. *Pathogens:* Microbes invading the tissues producing diseases.
3. **Opportunistic pathogens:** Commensals which, as and when body defences are impaired, may invade and cause disease.
4. **Toxins:** Poisonous substances, produced by microbes that cause manifestations of diseases.
5. **Infection:** The process of microbial invasion of the body is called infection.
6. **Infectious/contagious disease:** Infective diseases that are readily communicable from person to person.
7. **Sources of infection:** Habitats in which the pathogens ordinarily grow and from which they are disseminated to susceptible hosts.
8. **Vehicles of infection:** Inanimate objects responsible for transfer of pathogens also called fomites, e.g. towels and linen.
9. **Vectors:** Living organisms which transmit disease. Microbes are able to grow in the vectors.
10. **Zoonoses:** Infections prevalent primarily in animals, which accidentally are transmitted from animal to man but not back.
11. **Exogenous infection:** Infections from external sources.
12. **Endogenous infection:** Infection due to opportunistic invasion of tissues by a commensal.

Nosocomial infection: Hospital infection.

Infectivity: Ability of pathogenic microbes to initiate infection.

Virulence: A measure of the infectivity.

Invasiveness: Capacity of microbes to invade and multiply in healthy tissues.

Sources of Infection (Table 24.1)

Modes of Spread

1. **Respiratory infection**
   i. Direct contact with infected secretion, e.g. kissing/hugging.
   ii. Indirect contact involving fomites
   iii. Dustborne
   iv. Droplet spray

Table 24.1: Sources of infection

Exogenous	*Endogenous*
1. Patients	1. Bowel, e.g. *E. coli*
2. Carriers a. Healthy carriers b. Convalescent carriers c. Contact carriers d. Paradoxical carriers	2. Nasopharynx, e.g. pneumococci
3. Infected animals	3. Skin, e.g. *Staphylococcus albus*
4. Soil	4. Nostrils, e.g. *Staphylococcus aureus*

2. **Skin, wound and burn infection**
   i. Contact—direct, indirect.
   ii. Dustborne
   iii. Contamination with droplets
3. **Venereal infection**
   i. Sexual intercourse
   ii. Communal use of bathing facilities and towels
4. **GIT infections:** Transmission is by faecal–oral routes, may be:
   i. Water-borne
   ii. Hand infection
   iii. Food-borne
   iv. Vectors, e.g. housefly (*Musca domestica*)
5. **Arthropod-borne blood infection**
   i. Mosquitoes (malaria, yellow fever)
   ii. Flea (plague)
   iii. Louse (epidemic typhus, European relapsing fever)
   iv. Tsetse fly (trypanosomiasis).
6. **Laboratory infections**
   i. Artificial curtures.
   ii. Diagnostic/necropsy materials (Brucellae, Rickettsiae and *Francisella tularensis* are especially liable to cause laboratory infections).
   iii. Used syringes.
   iv. Blood and blood products.

MICROSCOPE (Fig. 24.1)

Magnification by a Microscope (Table 24.2)

Magnification at 105 mm. Initial magnification of the objective multiplied by the magnification of the eyepiece.

Table 24.2: Magnification

Objective (focal length)	*Magnification of the objective*	*eyepiece*	*Total magnification*
2/3 or 16 mm	10	10x	100
1/6 or 4 mm	45	10x	450
1/12 or 1.8 mm	100	10x	1000

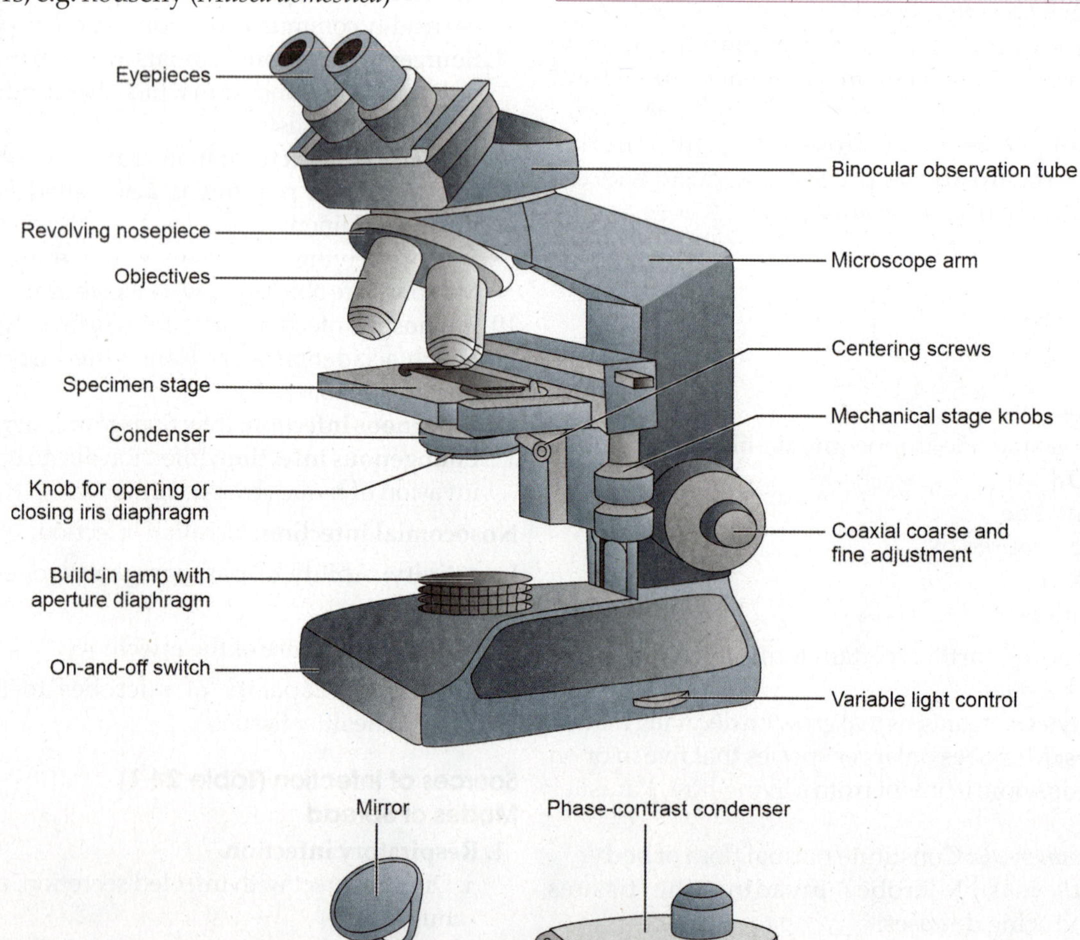

Fig. 24.1: A binocular microscope

Use of Microscope

Put the slide on the stage and focus under low power and then under high power or oil immersion as the case may be.

Focussing: At first use, do the coarse adjustment and then the fine (micrometer) adjustment. When examining a slide under low or high power, lower the condenser and work with concave mirror. In case of an unstained specimen, close the diaphragm for better definition of the object. Diaphragm and condenser should be manipulated each time for critical illumination of the object to be examined.

Use of Oil Immersion Lens

A suitable field is found under low power. A drop of oil is placed, objective lowered until it is in contact with the oil and almost touches the slides. This is observed with the eye on the level with the stage. Then looking through the microscope, the objective is raised by course adjustment until the object is in focus, final focussing is done by fine adjustment, immersion oil should always be removed after work is over with a little xylol. On no account use alcohol.

Causes of failures to focus under the oil immersion:
1. Quick movement of the coarse adjustment.
2. Viewing the wrong side of the slide.
3. Too thick a coverslip.

After working, immersion oil is removed with a little xylol. Never use alcohol.

Dark Ground Illumination

The light which illuminates the object must not enter the objective directly. The only light admitted must be that which has been reflected by the object itself. A special condenser is used which allows a wide cone of light and then stops that portion which normally enters the front of the objective. The oblique rays which normally miss objective when scattered by the object, enter the objective to illuminate image of the specimen against an entirely dark background. It is used to examine organisms in living state without staining. It increases visibility without increase in resolving power.

Care of Microscope

1. Keep it free from dust
2. Handle the microscope by the handle supporting the base with hand in an erect position
3. Avoid jerks
4. Draw tube may be used by a spiral motion
5. Systems should never be separated
6. Lens should be cleaned by xylol
7. Oil immersion lens must be cleaned after using.

Problem while Using Microscope

1. Light	Lower condenser
too strong	1. Use condenser of higher aperture
too faint (dim)	2. Adjust mirror.

2. Under oil immersion, the field appears dark with moving shadows of bubble of air in oil. Oil has left the space between the slide and lens.
3. **Definition is poor:** Objectives have been insufficiently cleaned. If specks appear in field and float about, they are usually in your eyes. If stationery but revolving with the eyepiece, clean the eyepiece. If they do not move, they are due to dust on the back of objectives.

Special Types of Microscope

1. **Phase contrast microscope:** It is a method of illumination which enables observation of entirely transparent objects without staining.
   - **Principle:** Ordinary specimens are visible because they have an amplitude or intensity contrast. Many specimens do not change the amplitude of light but change the phase of light waves. These phase changes are converted into amplitude changes which are visible to the eye. Special phase contrast apparatus in place of condenser and phase contrast objectives are required.
2. **Electron microscope:** In principle, it works by using light of shorter wavelength to increase resolving power. A powerful electron beam is passed in vacuum through magnetic fields which replaces the usual optical system of the microscope and image of the material under examination is photographed. The lenses are circular electromagnets whose focus varies as the strength of applied magnetic field. A magnification of 10,000 to 50,000 can be obtained in practice and objects as small as 1–2 micron photographed.
3. **Fluorescent microscope:** Some substances emit light when stimulated. The source of light is UV lamp or a carbon arc. The filter used in the system permits only short wave blue rays to fall on the object, if the object is autofluorescent, it emits colour. Alternatively, the object can be stained by fluorescent dyes; rhodamine, auramine or fluorescein isothiocyanate; making them visible under fluorescent microscope. The method is widely used for many immunological investigations.

MICROMETRY

Measurement of objects is important in microscopic work. Measurement methods are comparative methods so that degree of magnification is immaterial and need not be known.

Measurement by means of mechanical stage is used for objects not less than 100–200 microns.

Safety Precautions in the Laboratory

Over 4000 laboratory-associated infections have been reported and many more still go unreported. Laboratory acquired infections may be different from natural infections in pathogenesis and clinical presentation.

Biosafety in a microbiological laboratory is very essential and basically depends on three components:

a. Basic standard of laboratory design, operation and equipment.
b. Selection and use of essential biosafety equipment.
c. Safe laboratory procedures

Some practical and easily safe laboratory rules are:

i. Avoid mouth pipetting.
ii. Avoid smoking and eating in the laboratory.
iii. Decontaminate working is at least once a day.
iv. Wash hands with soap and water after handling infectious material.
v. Always wear laboratory coats in the laboratory only.
vi. Decontaminate all waste materials before disposal.
vii. Perform all technical procedures in a way to minimise aerosol formation.
viii. Provide adequate safety training to the laboratory staff.
ix. Actively immunize the workers against specific diseases handled.

EXAMINATION OF SPECIMENS FOR MICROBIOLOGICAL INVESTIGATION

Examination of specimens for this purpose is divided into three topics:

A. Examination of materials from sites normally sterile
B. Examination of materials from sites possessing normal flora
C. Examination of pus from abscesses and swabs from wounds.

A. Examination of Materials from Sites Normally Sterile

1. Blood Culture

i. Incubate the blood culture bottle containing blood sample at 37°C in an incubator till growth appears for a maximum of 7 days.
ii. After 24 hours incubation, a loopful of material is cultured on blood agar and MacConkey's agar plate.
iii. Incubate the plates at 37°C overnight.
iv. Examine next day for growth. If growth is positive, proceed accordingly.
v. If no growth is obtained, incubate culture plate for a further 24 hours.
vi. If still no growth, inoculation of sample may be repeated after 7, 14 and 21 days of incubation of original sample.
vii. If still no growth, sample should be reported as sterile.

2. Examination of Cerebral Fluid (CSF)

i. **Macroscopic examination:** Examine and record appearance and volume of the fluid.
ii. **Microscopic examination:** If the clot is present transfer small pieces of clot on slide, tease it and let it dry. Then perform staining. If no clot is observed, centrifuge a part of specimen under sterile conditions and make three smears from deposit, one each for Gram staining, Leishman staining and Ziehl-Neelsen staining.
iii. **Cell count:** Performed on an uncentrifuged specimen in Neubauer's chamber.

Culture: Culture should be done immediately on its arrival in the laboratory. Deposit is seeded on blood agar and chocolate agar, incubated in presence of 5–10% CO_2 achieved by keeping a lighted candle and closing the lid. The uncentrifuged fluid should be incubated overnight. When the primary culture is sterile, it may be possible to recover pathogen by repeating culture from incubated fluid.

3. Examination of Serous Fluids

Various fluids include pleural, pericardial, ascitic, synovial and hydrocele fluids.

i. Describe volume, colour and appearance. Look for sulphur granules.
ii. Centrifuge, deposit is used for staining.
iii. Culture on MacConkey plate, two blood agar plates and a tube of Robertson's meat medium. Incubate one blood agar plate anaerobically.
iv. Examine culture plates and proceed accordingly.

4. Examination of Urine

For diagnosis of urinary tract infection, the presence of pus cells in the urine is important but more than half the patients of UTI may not show a state of pyuria. A count of over 10^5 bacteria per ml is significant and indicates urinary tract infection. A count of less than 10^5 ml is considered to be due to contamination.

Culture of urine sample should be done within one hour of collection, otherwise refrigerate at 4°C.

Use bacteriological loop with 4 mm internal diameter. Inoculate one loopful, each on blood agar and MacConkey plates. Incubate at 37°C overnight. Examine for bacterial growth. Count number of colonies and give the count as:

No. of colonies × 100 = No. of bacteria/ml. If the growth is confluent, it is always significant. If no growth occurs in 24 hours and if still no growth is observed, report as sterile after 48 hours. If repeated cultures are sterile, isolate for *Mycobacterium tuberculosis*.

B. Examination of Materials from Sites Possessing Normal Flora

The processing of specimen from sites which are normally not sterile differs in the following ways:

a. Direct microscopic examination of the material is not very conclusive except *Mycobacterium tuberculosis* in sputum or Corynebacterium in throat swab.
b. Isolation of the pathogens which are less in number becomes difficult so invariably enrichment media have to be used.
c. The skill to distinguish normal flora from the pathogens on the basis of colony characterisitics needs to be developed.

1. Gastrointestinal Tract

a. **Macroscopic examination:** Make gross examination of stool, noting colour, consistency and presence of blood or excess mucus.
b. **Microscopic examination:** Make a light emulsion of stool in saline. Look for blood, pus, ova and cysts. Gram staining is of a little value.
c. **Culture procedure:** Inoculate a sample of faeces onto several types of solid media and into fluid enrichment medium. On the third day, suspicious colonies can be inoculated alternatively into this system and confirmed by serology.

First Day

a. Plate on bile—lactose media (MacConkey and blood agar)
b. Inoculate small piece into selenite F broth or GN broth.

Second Day

c. After overnight incubation at 37°C, examine blood agar plate for staphylococci and Candida. Transfer non-lactose fermenting colonies from bile-lactose media to a set of five tubes, one tube each of SIM (Sulfide Indole Motility) medium, Koser's citrate, urea agar and Russell's double sugar agar and small tube with charcoal gelatin disc in 1 ml of peptone water.
d. Subculture selenite F broth or GN broth to bile lactose medium.

Third Day

e. Note the pattern of reaction in five tubes. If reactions are suggestive of Salmonella or Shigella, perform slide agglutination test.
f. Inoculate non-lactose fermenters from step (d) into sets of five tubes.

Fourth Day

g. Read reactions from procedure (e). Complete identification may be made at this stage.
h. Read the five tubes from step (f) and if indicated, inoculate as in (e) and continue as in (g). If there is possibility of staphylococci or clostridial food poisoning, stool should be treated accordingly.

2. Female Genital Tract

It can be studied under 3 topics

a. **Acute cervicitis and vaginitis:** If clinically gonorrhoea is suspected, a swab is obtained and inoculated into Thayer-Martin medium.
b. **Chronic vaginitis:** A saline soaked swab should be taken. Make a hanging drop preparation. Look for *Trichomonas vaginalis*. Examine Gram stained film. If positive for *T. vaginalis*, culture in special media for this. For bacterial and fungal causes, plate the swabs onto blood agar, MacConkey and Transgrow media. Examine after 24 hours of incubation at 37°C.
c. **Puerperal sepsis and septic abortion:** A high vaginal swab is taken, smear is made, examined for streptococci, Gram-positive rods and pus cells. Plating is made onto 2 blood agar plates (one for anaerobic culture), a MacConkey plate and Robertson meat medium. Incubate blood agar and MacConkey agar plates at 37°C. Look for growth the next day. Normal flora is excluded.

3. Sputum

The objective of culturing the sputum is to diagnose bacterial infection of lung. Open case of pulmonary tuberculosis can be diagnosed by direct microscopy.

Select purulent or bloody flecks and transfer a loopful to a clean slide, press another slide over it. Press the slide together and then pull them apart. Flame both slides after drying. Stain by Gram stain and look for bacteria. Inoculate a blood agar and MacConkey agar plate with a small loopful of sputum specimen. Put blood agar plate in a candle jar. If incubated, plates show no acceptable pathogens, subculture meat medium both aerobically and anaerobically. If no growth, re-examine meat medium by gram stain and re-culture if necessary.

Processing of sputum for acid-fast bacilli (AFB): A biological safety cabinet (UV sterilized) is used. Small portion of the material is transferred to a clean slide. Prepare the smear with a bacteriological loop or by pressing glass slide on it. Label the slides, air dry and flame immediately.

Stain by Ziehl-Neelsen's stain:

Examine under oil immersion.

Culture: Mix equal volumes of sputum and 3–4% sodium hydroxide containing 0.004% phenol red in a centrifuge tube. Centrifuge at 3000 rpm for 20–30 minutes. Discard supernatant. Add 2N HCl dropwise from a pipette to achieve yellow end-point. Add 4% NaOH to get faint pink end-point. Inoculate two slants of LJ medium. Observe culture every week. If there is growth around 3–4 weeks, stain by ZN stain. Discard the tube after 10 weeks, if there is no growth.

4. Throat Swab/Nasal Swab

Inoculate blood agar and MacConkey agar by rolling the swab over small portion of agar surface and by streaking a sterile wire loop to develop isolate colonies. Incubate at 37°C aerobically overnight. Examine plates next morning for the presence of pathogens.

5. Nasopharyngeal Swab

It is especially useful in study of meningococcal carriers where throat swab is not satisfactory.

Seed blood agar and chocolate agar preferably on bedside. Incubate these plates in air plus 10% CO_2 at 37°C. If growth is obtained, proceed for further identification.

6. Skin

General procedure of skin culture involves inoculating skin onto a portion of blood agar, MacConkey and colistin–nalidixic acid agar plate. Make incisions into surfaces of plates for demonstration of haemolysis. Incubate at 37°C for 24 to 48 hours. If positive growth, perform subculture for identification.

7. Conjunctiva Culture

These are best taken with a sterile bacteriologic loop and plated directly on chocolate and blood agar plates incubated in 10% CO_2. Viral inclusions are shown by Giemsa stain in inclusion conjunctivitis.

8. Male Urethral Discharge

Urethral discharge from patients with urethritis is used for making smears directly on slide. After heat fixation, stain by Gram method. Presence of Gram-negative diplococci is strongly suggestive of gonorrhoea. Culture on chocolate agar and incubate in 10% CO_2 .

C. Examination of Pus from Abscesses and Swabs from Wounds

Procedure: A gross examination is made for volume, colour and consistency. A Gram film preparation is made. Examine for pus cells and bacteria. A ZN preparation should also be made. A drop of pus should be mixed with 10% potassium hydroxide for fungi. Plate out on blood agar and MacConkey plate and inoculate meat medium. Incubate one blood agar plate anaerobically.

The plates are examined after 24–48 hours of incubation at 37°C. If positive growth, then identification is carried out by subcultures and Gram staining.

If plates are found to be sterile, further aerobic and anaerobic subcultures are made from meat medium.

STERILIZATION AND DISINFECTION

Definitions

1. **Sterilization:** Sterilization is the freeing of an article from all living organisms including bacteria and their spores .
2. **Disinfection:** Disinfection is a process having a narrow spectrum of activity, effective principally on non-acid fast vegetative organisms and with an uncertain action on bacterial endospores.

Methods of Sterilization and Disinfection

Physical Methods

1. Heat:
   A. Dry heat
      a. Flaming
      b. Hot air oven
      c. Red heat
   B. Wet heat
2. Radiation:
   A. Ionizing
   B. Non-ionizing
3. Filteration

Chemical Methods

1. Bactericidal
2. Bacteriostatic

☞ **Note:** Sterilization in the strict sense is effected only by physical means. Chemical means are effective only in certain cases in which physical means cannot be employed.

1. Sterilization by Heat

Heat is the most certain method of sterilization. Sterilization by heat can be effected in 2 ways:

A. Dry heat
B. Wet heat

A. Sterilization by Dry Heat

It is suitable for glassware, syringes, metal instruments, paper-wrapped goods which are not spoiled by high temperature and water impermeable oils, waxes and powders. It can be done in 5 ways:

i. **Red heat:** This is done by holding articles, in the flame of burner until hot.
ii. **Flaming:** Here sterilization is effected by passing the article through the Bunsen flame without allowing it to become red hot.
iii. **Burning of spirit:** It is not an effective method.
iv. **Hot air oven:** This allows controlled application of dry heat.

   It is the best method for sterilizing dry glassware such as test tubes, Petri dishes, flask, pipettes and instruments, such as forceps, scalpels, throat swabs and assembled all glass syringes; dry materials sealed in containers and powders, fats, oils and greases that are impermeable to moisture.

   Glassware should be perfectly dry. Before sterilization plug test tubes and flasks with cotton wool stoppers. Other glasswares may be wrapped in kraft paper or sterilized metal cans. Time the holding period of 1 hour at 160ºC when the thermometer first shows that oven air is at 160°C.

v. **Infra-red radiation:** Infra-red radiation generates high temperatures and can be employed in central sterile supply departments only.

B. Sterilization by Moist Heat

Moist heat can be employed in three ways.

i. At temperatures below 100°C.
ii. At temperatures of 100°C.
iii. At temperatures above 100°C.

i. **At temperatures below 100°C:** These are not reliable. Best known is pasteurization of milk. Vaccines prepared from cultures may be sterilized in a special bath (vaccine bath) at a comparatively low temperature, 1 hour at 60°C being usually sufficient.

ii. **Moist heat at a temperature of 100°C:** It can be done in 2 ways:
   a. *Boiling at 100°C:* Boiling at 100°C for a minimum of 10 minutes is sufficient to kill all non-sporing and many, but not all sporing organisms.
   b. *Steaming at 100°C:* Pure steam in equilibrium with water boiling at normal atmosphere pressure has normally a temperature of 100°C. Steaming at 100°C is employed commonly for culture. There are 2 ways:
      1. *By a single exposure at 100°C for 90 minutes:* The spores of some thermophilic and rare mesophilic bacteria survive this treatment.
      2. *Tyndallization:* Intermittent exposure at 100°C for 20–45 minutes on 3 successive days. First exposure kills the vegetative forms. Between heating, the spores become vegetative forms which are killed during subsequent heating.

iii. **Moist heat above 100°C or sterilization in autoclave:** Water boils when its vapour pressure equals the pressure of atmosphere. Thus, when pressure is increased water boils at a higher temperature, thereby raising the temperature of steam above 100°C. It is especially suitable for culture media, aqueous solutions, the steam preventing evaporation during heating. In the autoclave, all parts of the load must be permeated by steam. Once heated up, there is a minimum holding time, given in Table 24.3:

Table 24.3: Holding time

Pressure lb/in²	*Temperature in °C*	*Holding time in minutes*
0	100	—
10	115	45
15	121	18
30	134	3

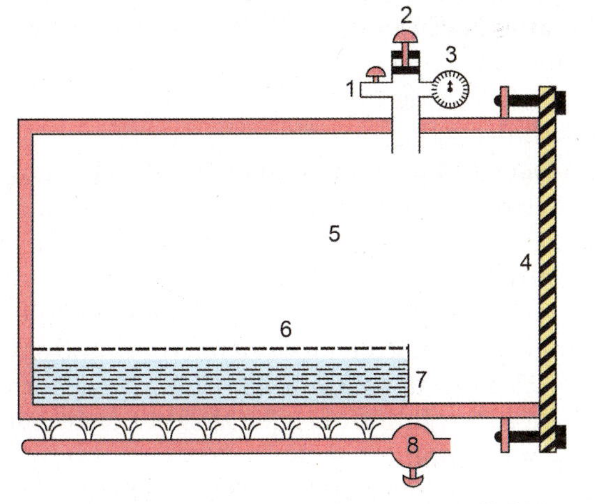

1. Chamber discharge tap
2. Adjustable safety valve
3. Pressure guage
4. Chamber door
5. Chamber
6. Perforated tray
7. Water
8. Gas burner

Fig. 24.2: Simple non-jacketed autoclave

   a. Simple non-jacketed laboratory autoclave. It is of two types (Fig. 24.2):
      1. Horizontal type.
      2. Vertical type.

      Both are pressure cooker types and have a similar basic structure.

      Deficiencies of simple autoclave. The method of air discharge is inefficient. It also lacks means for drying the load after sterilization.
   b. Steam-jacketed autoclave with automatic air and condense discharge. Most are horizontal cylinders or rectangles (20″ × 50″) of rustless metal, e.g. Monel metal. Rectangular chambers are more conveniently loaded. At the front is a swing door, fastened by a capstan head which operates radial bolts and automatically remains locked while the chamber pressure is raised (Fig. 24.3).

C. High Prevacuum Sterilizers

They are the most advanced surgical sterilizers. They are equipped with electrically driven pumps capable of exhausting the chamber almost to a perfect vacuum, thus removing about 98% of the air. The absence of air enables the steam to penetrate very rapidly and heat up all parts of the load.

1. Autoclave Control and Sterilization Indicators

1. *Automatic process control:* It carries out the whole sterilization cycle.
2. *Recording thermometer:* It makes a graphic timed record of temperature changes.
3. *Thermocouple:* It discovers the heating up time required for a given kind of load.
4. *Chemical indicators:* Browne's sterilizer control tubes contain a red solution which turns green when heated at 115°C for 25 minutes (Type I), for 15 min (Type II) or at 160°C for 60 minutes (Type III).

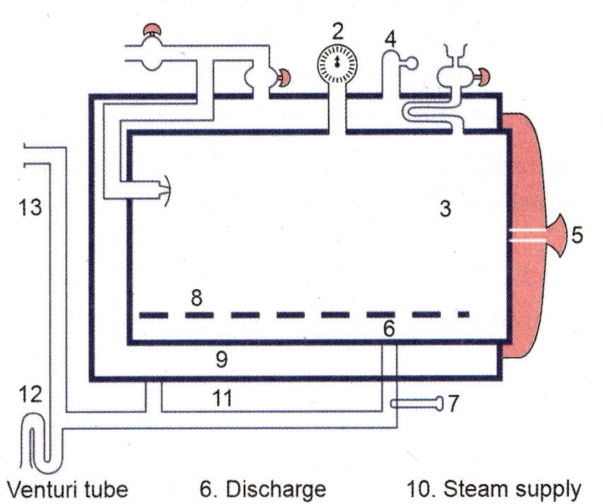

1. Venturi tube
2. Pressure guage
3. Air filter intake
4. Safety valve
5. Chamber door
6. Discharge
7. Thermometer
8. Perforated tray
9. Jacket
10. Steam supply
11. Jacket steam trap
12. Drain
13. Discharge to atmosphere

Fig. 24.3: Steam-jacketed autoclave

5. *Adhesive tape:* Brown Bowie Dick autoclave tape test for steam penetration is used extensively.
6. *Spore indicators:* A preparation of dried bacterial spores is placed within the load in the autoclave and after autoclaving is tested for viability, e.g. *Bacillus stearothermophilus* spores are killed at 121°C in about 12 mins. The indicators are placed in the centre of the largest and most densely packed items of the load and some in the coolest part.

Types of Filters

i. **Earthenware candles:** They are of three types:
   a. Berkefeld filters
   b. Mandler filter
   c. Chamberland filters

   These filters may be used for the removal of organisms from fluid cultures to obtain the bacterial toxin.
ii. **Asbestos or seitz filter:** These consist of a disc of an asbestos composition through which fluid is passed. The discs are available in three grades, namely:
   a. K or clarifying
   b. N or normal
   c. EK or special.
iii. **Sinfered glass filters:** They are made of finely ground glass fused sufficiently to make the small particles adhere.
iv. **Cellulose membrane filters:** Three types are available:
   a. Gradocol membranes
   b. Modern membrane filters
   c. Oxoid membrane filters made of cellulose acetate. They are much less adsorptive and rate filtration is much greater. Also bacteria retained on the surface of a membrane filter can be grown by placing in a culture media.

2. Sterilization by Radiation

Ultraviolet radiation: Effectiveness of UV light increases with decrease in wavelength.

UV radiation is equally effective against Gram-positive and Gram-negative bacteria, spores are 10 times and viruses are 200 times more resistant.

But UV radiation has a low to nil penetrating power.

Ionizing radiation: They are not used because they cause mutations and are not safe for workers.

3. Sterilization by Filtration

Filtration is the only means of sterilizing heat labile fluids, e.g.:

i. Serum
ii. Antibiotic solution
iii. Some culture media

The British Pharmaceutical codex test for bacteria proof filters requires that efficient filters should be able to return *Serratia marcescens*. This indicates a diameter of 0.75 m or less.

However, sterilizing filters render a liquid bacteria free but not virus-free (Fig. 24.4).

Technique of filtration: As fluids do not readily pass through filters by gravity, it is necessary to use positive or negative pressure. Suction is the most convenient method of filtration, the fluid being drained into a sterile filtering flask, which is a conical flask of thick glass with a side-arm.

A negative pressure of about 100–200 mm of mercury is applied.

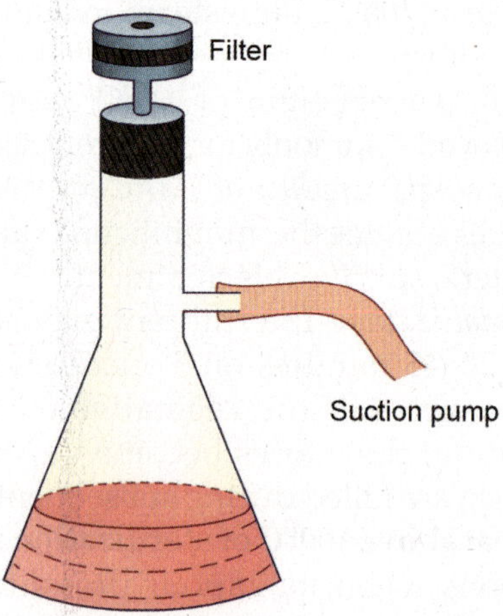

Fig. 24.4: Sterilization by filter

Chemical Methods

1. **Acids**
   i. Inorganic acids
      a. Boric acid: 2–3% aq. soln.
         Dusting powder and borax glycerine.
         Bacteriocidal and antifungal.
      b. Chromic acid: Powerful germicide.
   ii. Organic acids:
      a. Benzoic acid (antifungal and bacteriocidal plus keratolytic action)
      b. Salicylic acid
      c. Mandelic acid
      d. Nalidixic acid
2. **Alkalies NaOH and KOH:** Potent germicides used to disinfect excreta samples, sputum samples, effective against all forms of life.
3. **Alcohols**
   i. *Ethanol:* Maximum activity at 70% concentration. Ineffective against spore forms.
   ii. *Isopropyl alcohol:* More potent than ethanol.
4. **Aldehydes**
   i. *Formaldehyde:* This irritant water soluble gas is highly lethal to all kinds of microbes and spores:
      a. *Disinfection with formalin:* Commercial formalin is a 40% solution of HCHO in H_2O, containing 10% methanol.
      b. *Disinfection by HCHO gas:* Atmosphere must have a relative humidity of 60%, a temperature of 18°C. Concentration should be 2 mg/litre of air. It is used to disinfect blankets, mattresses, rooms,

operation theatres and smaller articles like hair brushes.

ii. Glutaraldehyde: Less irritant than HCHO.

iii. Methenamine.

5. **Phenols and derivatives**

i. *Phenol:* Oldest antiseptic, introduced by Joseph Lister. It is outdated.

ii. *Cresol:* Ortho-para-methyl derivative of phenol. Used as 0.1 % solution.

iii. *Lysol:* Cresol on saponification gives lysol. Used as 3% solution.

iv. *Chlorzylenol (Dettol):* 1–1.5% skin antiseptic prior to surgery. 6% sterilization of surgical instruments.

v. *Picric acid:* Trichlorophenol.

vi. *Hexylresorcinol:* Weak antiseptic.

vii. *Thymol.*

viii. *Bithinol.*

ix. *Hexachlorophane:* It is a chlorinated phenol.

x. *Chlorhexidine:* Contains cetrimide as well.

xi. *Hycolin:* 2% hycolin is suitable as a disinfectant in hospitals.

IDENTIFICATION OF BACTERIA AND PREPARATION OF CULTURE MEDIA

Identification of Bacteria

There are numerous methods on the basis of which bacteria can be differentiated and identified. They together form a complete system of identification.

i. **Morphology and staining reactions:** A Gram-stained smear shows the
   i. Gram reaction;
   ii. Size;
   iii. Shape and
   iv. Grouping

   A hanging drop preparation may be used to demonstrate motility.

ii. **Cultural characters:** Including growth requirements and appearance of cultures to the naked eye. Attention is paid to;
   a. Size of colonies;
   b. outline of colonies;
   c. elevation;
   d. translucency;
   e. Colour and
   f. Haemolysis on blood agar.

iii. **Biochemical reactions**
   a. *Fermentation reactions:* It depends on whether or not a bacterial growth in a liquid medium will ferment particular ugar. There may be production of acid or of acid plus gas.
   b. *Tests dependent on particular end-products:* Indole, H_2S and nitrities, in certain bacteria .
   c. *Certain enzymatic activities:* Such as oxidase, catalae, urease, gelatinase, collagenase, lecithinase or lipase.
   d. *Specialised techniques:* Thin layer chromatography (TLC) and gas liquid chromatography.

iv. **Antigenic characters:** Species can be identified by specific antibody reactions observed in serological tests.

v. **Fluorescence microscopy and fluorescent antibody procedures:** When certain dyes are exposed to UV light, they absorb energy and emit visible light. Such a dye is said to fluoresce. When tissue cells or organisms are stained with such a dye and examined with UV light they are seen as fluorescent.

   Antibody molecules can be labelled by conjugation with such a dye. When fluorescent antibody is allowed to react with homologous antigen on a cell surface, this direct immunofluorescence procedure affords a highly sensitive method for identification.

vi. **Typing of bacteria:** The typing of strains may depend upon special biochemical or serological tests or highly specialized bacteriophage and bacteriocin typing.

vii. **Animal pathogenicity and toxigenicity:** In case of certain organisms the inoculation test provides a reliable method of identification. In case of involved toxins, by use of specific neutralising antisera identification is highly specific.

viii. **Antibiotic specificity:** The organism is tested for its ability to grow on artificial nutrient media containing different concentrations of antibiotics, thereby determining the minimum inhibitory concentration.

General Types of Media

1. **Defined synthetic media:** They are prepared exclusively from pure chemical substances and their exact composition is known. It is of two types:
   a. Simple synthetic media: They contain a carbon and energy source, an inorganic source of NPS and various inorganic salts in a buffered aqueous solution.
   b. Complex synthetic media: Incorporate in addition to basic necessities, certain amino acids, purines, pyrimidines and other growth factors.

2. Routine Laboratory Media

a. **Basal media:** For example, nutrient broth and peptone water are simple routine media and are called basal media.

b. **Enriched media:** Prepared to maintain the nutritional requirements of more exacting.

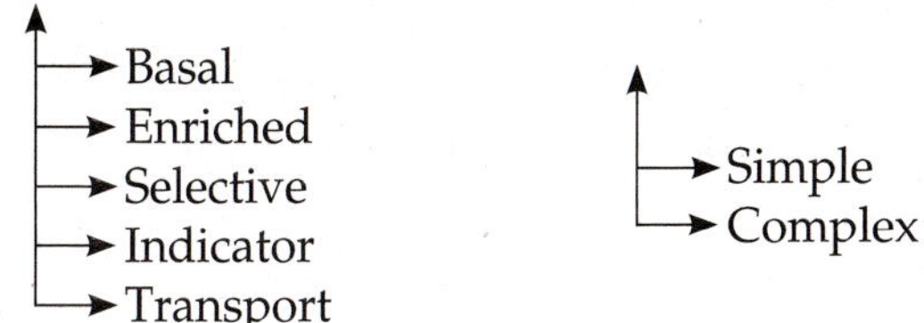

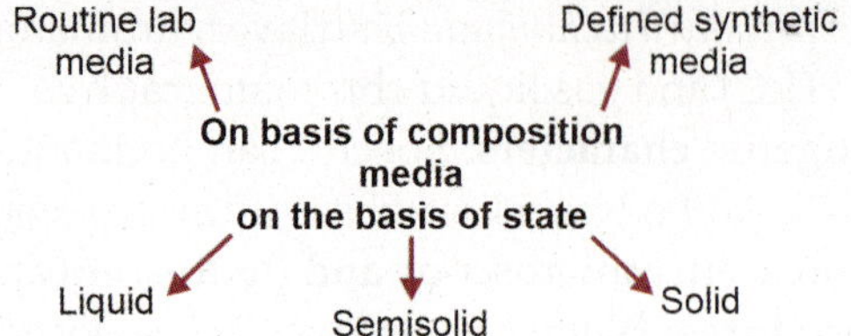

Liquid media are disadvantageous because growth exhibit no specificity and organisms cannot be separated.

Substances used to solidify media

i. Gelatin
ii. Pieces of potato impregnated with nutrient solutions.
iii. Coagulated serum
iv. Inspissated egg
v. Agar

c. **Selective media:** Contain substances that inhibit all but a few bacteria. An enrichment medium is liquid selective medium.

d. **Indicator media:** Incorporate substances that change visibly as a result of metabolic activities of particular organisms.

e. **Transport media:** Used to sustain sensitive organisms for a short period.

CONTAINERS FOR MEDIA AND CULTURES

Flasks stoppered with cotton wool, test tubes stoppered with cotton wool or with slip-on metal caps, and screw capped bottles of different capacity and shape can be used as containers of media and cultures. Glassware must be thoroughly cleaned before use for culture media and new glassware requires special treatment to remove free alkali. Sterilization of glassware is brought about by dry heat in a hot air oven.

The use of sterile disposable Petri dishes supplied by the manufacturer are now freely available in the market at cheaper rates.

Common ingredients of culture media

i. **Water:** Tap water is suitable if low in mineral content. But otherwise glass distilled water may be used.

ii. **Agar:** It is prepared from a variety of sea-weeds. The product is available as dried strands or powder. At concentrations normally used most bacteriological agars melt at about 95°C and solidify only when cooled to about 42°C. Main agars used are: Japanese agar in conc. of 2% and New Zealand agar in conc. of 1.2%.

Peptones
- → Peptones
- → Proteoses
- → Amino acids
- → Inorganic salts (PO_4, K^+, Mg^{+2})
- → Accessory growth factors
  - Nicotinic acid
  - Riboflavin

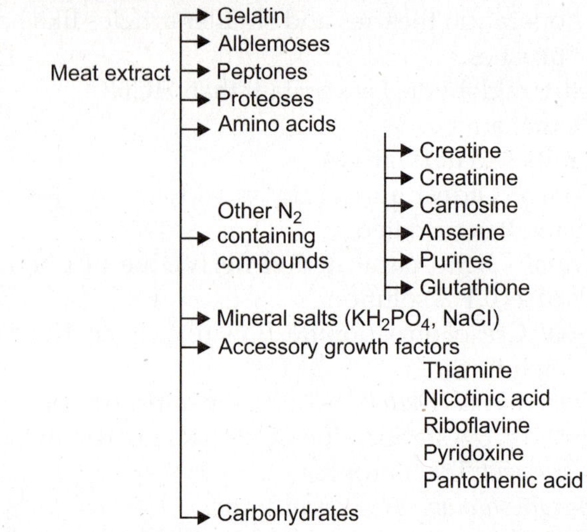

iii. **Peptone:** It consists of water-soluble products obtained from lean meat or other protein material, such as heart muscle, by digestion with proteolytic enzymes.

iv. **Casein hydrolysate:** It consists largely of amino-acids obtained by hydrolysis of milk protein casein.

v. **Meat extract:** Finely divided lean beef is held in boiling water for a short time. After removal of extra fat, it is concentrated by evaporation to a dark viscid paste containing 70–80% solids.

vi. **Yeast extract:** Commercial yeast extract is prepared from washed cells of brewers or bakers yeast.

vii. **Blood:** Blood for use must be collected with aseptic precautions, from man, horse, rabbits or sheep.

viii. **Fildes peptic digest of blood:** It is better because peptic digestion of blood liberates nutrients from red cells. Saline 0.85% + HCl + Defibrinated sheep blood + Pepsin

ix. **Serum:** Serum obtained is sterilized by filtration through a Seitz filter.

Common Media used in Laboratories

1. **Nutrient broth:** It is of three types:
   i. Meat infusion broth consisting of a watery extract of lean meat to which peptone is added.
   ii. Meat extract broth prepared as a mixture of commercial peptone and meat extract.
   iii. Digest broth consisting of a watery extract of lean meat that has been digested with a proteolytic enzyme so that additional peptone is not required.
2. **Nutrient agar:** Nutrient agar is nutrient broth solidified by the addition of agar.
3. **Semi-solid agar:** Agar is added to media concentrations too low to solidify them.
4. **Peptone water:** It is used as basal medium for carbohydrate fermentation tests and formation of indole.

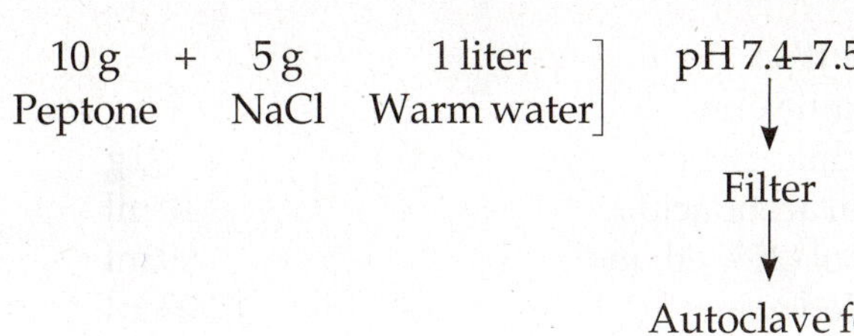

5. **Blood agar:** It is especially suitable for gonnococcus and other delicate pathogens. It is also an indicator medium showing haemolysis. The medium is prepared by adding sterile blood to sterile nutrient agar that has been melted and cooled to 50°C. Blood is used at a conc. of 10%.
6. **Chocolate agar:** It is suitable for *H. influenzae*. During heating, red cells are ruptured and nutrients are liberated. It is prepared by heating 10% of sterile blood in sterile nutrient agar at 75°C .
7. **Serum agar:** It is prepared by adding 10% of sterile serum to sterile nutrient agar that has been melted and cooled to 50°C. It is generally used as slopes.

Staining Procedures

As bacteria consist of clear protoplasmic matter, it is difficult with ordinary microscope to see them in the unstained condition. Staining, is therefore, of primary importance for the recognition of bacteria.

Methods of Making Film or Smear Preparation

Film preparations are made either on cover slips or on 3 × 1″ glass slides, usually the latter. It is essential that the coverslips or slides should be perfectly clean or free from grease, otherwise, films will be uneven.

For ordinary use, wipe the slide with a clean dry cotton cloth and then, holding its end with forceps, roast it free from grease by passing it 6–12 times through a Bunsen's flame.

Alternatively moisten the finger with water, rub on the surface of a fine sand soap and then smear the surface of the slide. After removing the soapy film with a clean cloth, the surface is clean and free from grease.

The slides should not be cleaned and used again since it is difficult to ensure that all organisms are removed.

Coverslips should be 3/4 or 7/8 inches square and 0.1 mm thick. They are cleaned by the dichromate sulphuric acid solution. They are then well-washed, first in tap water and then in distilled water and stored in stoppered jar in 50% alcohol.

Preparation of Films

In the case of fluid material, loopful is taken up, spread thinly on the slide. The slide is then dried by keeping it high on a Bunsen flame. The film is then dried by heating through the glass slide.

Solid material: Cultures on agar. A loopful clean water is placed on the slide. The loop is then sterilized and a minute quantity of material is transferred to the drop, thoroughly emulsified and mixture is spread evenly on the slide. The film is then fixed and dried as above.

A. Simple Stains

These show not only the presence of organisms but also the nature of cellular content in exudates. Commonly used are as follows:

i. **Methylene blue:** Saturated solution of Loffler's methylene blue in alcohol.

   Procedure
   1. Stain for 3 minutes with methylene blue stain.
   2. Wash with water.
   3. Examine directly or after mounting in glycerine.

ii. **Dilute carbol fuchsin:** Ziehl-Neelsen's stain diluted with water, 10–15 times its volume.

   Procedure
   1. Stain for 10–15 seconds.
   2. Wash well with water.
   3. Air dry and examine directly.

B. Gram Staining Method

i.	Methyl violet	0.5 g
	Distilled water	100 ml
ii.	Iodine	1.0 g
	Potassium iodide	2.0 g
	Distilled water	100 ml

Grind potassium iodide and iodine in a mortar and dissolve in not more than 20 ml of distilled water. Make up to 100 ml with distilled water. Store in coloured glass bottles.

iii.	Basic fuchsin	0.1%
	Or safranin	0.5%

Basic fuchsin: Dissolve 0.1 g basic fuchsin in 10 ml alcohol, allow to stand over night and make volume to 100 ml with distilled water.

Safranin: Grind 0.5 g safranin in 10 ml alchol and make up the volume to 100 ml with distilled water.

Procedure

i. Cover the slide with methyl violet solution and allow to act for about 10 seconds.
ii. Pour off stain and wash with Gram's iodine solution thoroughly.
iii. Cover the whole slide with Gram's iodine solution and leave it for about 2 minutes.
iv. Decolorize with acetone (100%). Decolorization is very rapid and complete in 2–3 seconds. After this period of contact, wash thoroughly with water under a running tap, which should be running before the acetone is applied to the slide,
v. Wash with water.
vi. Apply counterstain for 20–30 seconds.
vii. Wash with water and dry between blotting paper.
viii. Examine under oil immersion without mounting.

Results: Gram-positive bacteria are stained violet while Gram-negative bacteria are reddish pink.

C. Ziehl–Neelsen Method

Used for staining acid-fast bacilli.

Preparation of solutions

1. Ziehl–Neelsen's (strong) carbol fuchsin

Basic fuchsin	10 g
Absolute ethanol	100 ml
5% Solution of phenol (in water)	1000 ml

Dissolve the dye in alcohol and add to the phenol solution.

2. Sulphuric acid—20% solution
Place 800 ml water in a large flask. Add 200 ml conc. sulphuric acid—about 50 ml at a time, gently pouring down the side 10% and 5% are also used in special situations mentioned elsewhere in the text.
3. Alcohol—95%
Counterstain Loffler's methylne blue or Malachite green.

Procedure

1. Cover slide with carbol fuchsin and heat until steam rises. Allow to stain for 5 min., heat being applied at intervals to keep stain hot. The stain must not be allowed to evaporate dry.
2. Wash with water.
3. Cover with 20% sulphuric acid. Red colour of the preparation is changed to yellowish brown. After about a minute in acid, wash with water and pour more acid—repeat till the film is very faintly pink.
4. Treat with 95% alcohol for 2 minutes.
5. Wash well with water.
6. Counterstain with Loffler's methylene blue or dilute malchite green for 15–20 seconds.
7. Wash, blot, dry and mount as mentioned.

Results: Acid-fast bacilli stain bright-red and the background issue, cells and other organisms are stained blue or green.

Modification of Ziehl–Neelsen method

1. Leprosy bacilli are also acid fast, but usually to a less degree so that 5% sulphuric acid is used for decolorization.
2. Actinomcyes and Nocardia can be treated with 1% H_2SO_4 to demonstrate the acid fastness.
3. Cultures of some Nocardia are acid fast with 0.5% H_2SO_4.
4. Brucella differential stain: Dilute (1 in 10) carbol fuchsin, allow to stain without heat for 15 min. Decolorize with 0.5% acetic acid solution for 15 seconds, wash and counterstain with Loffler's methylene blue for 1 min.

D. Albert Staining

For *Corynebacterium diphtheriae*.

i. **Albert's I**

Toluidine blue	1.5 g
Malachite green	2.0 g
Glacial acetic acid	10 ml
Alcohol (25% ethanol)	90 ml
Distilled water	1000 ml

Dissolve the dyes in alcohol and add to the water and acetic acid. Allow to stand for one day and then filter.

ii. **Albert's iodine (Albert's II)**

Iodine	6 g
Potassium iodide	9 g
Distilled water	900 ml

Procedure

1. Cover the slide with Albert's stain I and allow to act for 3–5 min.
2. Wash in water and blot dry.
3. Cover the slide with Albert's iodine and allow to act for 1 min.
4. Wash and blot dry

Result: By this method volutin granules within bacilli stain bluish black, the protoplasm green and other organisms mostly light green.

E. Staining of Spores

Spore bearing organisms, when stained with grams, are deeply coloured, whereas the spore is unstained and appears as a clear area in the organism. For the staining of spore, acid-fast stain is used in the following manner:

1. Stain with Ziehl–Neelsen's carbol fuchsin for 3–5 min, heating until steam rises.
2. Wah with water.
3. Treat with 0.5% sulphuric acid for 1–5 minutes. Wash with water. Counterstain with 1% methylene blue for 3 min. Wash in water, blot and dry.

Result: Spores are stained bright red and protoplasm blue.

F. Staining of Capsules

Capsules: The capsules of bacteria present in body fluids and pus are often clearly stained when treated by common stains like methylene blue. Artificial cultures, do not stain for capsule by the common stains. For this purpose, special methods are employed known as relief staining. The methods adopted for staining of capsules are:

1. Wet film India ink method
2. Dry film India ink method
3. Relief staining with eosin

Wet Film India Ink Method

This is the method of choice.

Procedure

1. Clean a slide, put a loopful of India ink on it.
2. Place a small portion of bacterial culture on India ink and emulsify.

3. Place a clean coverslip and press through the sheet of blotting paper so that the ink film becomes very thin and pale in colour.
4. Examine under oil immersion.

Results: Bacteria is seen as a highly refractile outline against dark background of ink particle. The capsular zone is visualized as a clear space between the refractile portion and the dark background of India ink.

Demonstration of flagella by modified Leifson's method: The stain, basic fuchsin with tannic acid is deposited on the bacteria and flagella from an evaporating alcoholic solution. The degree of staining is controlled by an exact determination of duration of exposure.

Procedure

1. Clean the glass slide with absolute alcohol and then with conc. H_2SO_4 saturated with potassium dichromate by immersing for several days. Rinse with water, dry in air and flame.
2. Fix broth culture by 1–2% formalin (W/V).
3. Sediment the bacilli by centrifuging at 2000–3000 rpm.
4. Decant supernatant and suspend bacteria in distilled water.
5. Centrifuge again and gently resuspend in distilled water to obtain a final slightly cloudy suspension.
6. With a flamed platinum loop inoculation, place a loopful of suspension on prepared slide and gently spread over as 2 cm^2 area.
7. Allow to air dry at room temperature.
8. Place slide horizontally on a staining rack and put exactly 1 ml of stain on slide to cover whole of the surface. Stain is prepared as follows:

Tannic acid	10 g
Sodium chloride	5 g
Basic fuchsin	4 g

Prepare the solution by adding 1.9 g of powdered mixture to 33 ml of 95% ethyl alcohol and add distilled water to make volume of 100 ml. Adjust pH to 5.0.

9. Leave at room temperature for exactly required time.
10. Rinse off excess stain through slowly running tap water.
11. Counterstain with methylene blue for 30 min.
12. Wash with water, drain, dry and examine under oil immersion.

Romanowsky stains: Romanowsky stains impart a reddish-purple colour to chromatin of malaria and other parasites due to a substance which forms when methyline blue is ripened either by age or by heating. Various Romanowsky stains are Leishman's, Wright's, Jenner's and Giemsa stains.

Leishman's stain (for protozoa in blood films):

Reagents

Leishman dye	3.8 g
Methyl alcohol	250 ml
Glycerol	250 ml

Preparation of stock solution

1. Grind 3.8 g of Leishman stain and add glycerol in a mortar slowly.
2. Add half of methyl alcohol and continue grinding.
3. Transfer to a glass stoppered bottle.
4. Pour remainder methyl alcohol into mortar and grind the residue. Transfer this to the bottle.

Preparation of buffer solution

Potassium dihydrogen phosphate	0.7 g	Adjust pH to 7.2
Disodium hydrogen phosphate	1.0 g	
Distilled water	1000 ml	

Preparation of working solution

1. Filter the stock solution
2. Add 3 drops of stain for 1 ml of buffer solution.

Procedure

1. Fix thin films with methyl alcohol.
2. Pour off alcohol.
3. Pour 3 ml of diluted stain for 30 min.
4. Differentiate by holding under a stream of water for approx. 15 seconds.
5. Allow slides to drain and dry before examination.

Results: Malarial parasite will to be seen as per stage and species.

Giemsa stain (for protozoa and spirochaetes): This consists of a number of compounds made by mixing different proportions of methylene blue and eosin. These have designated as Azure I, Azure II and Azure II eosin: The following method by Lillie is recommended for preparation:

Azure A eosinate	0.5 g
Azure B eosinate	2.5 g
Methylene blue eosinate	2.0 g
Methylene blue chloride	1.0 g
Glycerol	375.0 ml
Methyl alcohol	375.0 ml

Procedure

Rapid Method

1. Fix films in methyl alcohol for 3 min.
2. Stain in a mixture of 1 part stain and 10 parts of phosphate buffer pH 7.0 for 1 hour.
3. Wash with buffer solution, allowing the preparation to differentiate for about 30 seconds.
4. Blot and allow to dry in air.

Slow Method

Valuable for demonstrating spirochaetes:

1. Fix films in methyl alcohol for 3 min.
2. Make a mixture of 20 ml of buffer (pH 7.0) and 1 ml of stain in Petri dish.
3. Place a thin glass rod in Petri dish.
4. Place slides in Petri dish with one end on the glass rod.
5. Stain for 16–24 hours.
6. Wash in buffer solution.
7. Allow to air dry, mount and examine under oil.

Field's stain (for staining thick blood films for malarial parasite):

Reagents

Solution A (methylene blue)

Methylene blue	1.3 g
Na_2HPO_4 anhydrous	5 g

- Dissolve in 50 ml distilled water.
- Bring to boil and evaporate to dryness
- Add KH_2PO_4 6.25 g
- Add 500 ml of boiled, warmed, distilled water.
- Keep for 24 hours
- Filter

Solution B (Eosin)

Eosin	1.3 g
Na_2HPO_4 (anhydrous)	5.0 g
KH_2PO_4 (anhydrous)	6.25 g
Distilled water (filter before use)	500 ml

Procedure

1. Dip the slide in solution A for 1–2 sec.
2. Rinse in distilled/tap water until the stain ceases to flow from the film.
3. Dip the slide in solution B for 1–2 sec.
4. Rinse in clean water for 2–3 sec.
5. Place vertically on rack to drain and dry.

JSB stain (for malarial parasite) devised by Jaswant Singh and Bhattacharji:

Reagents

Solution I

Methylene blue	0.5 g
Sulphuric acid 1%	3 ml
Potassium hydroxide 1%	10 ml
Distilled water	500 ml

Solution II

Eosin	1 g
Tap water	500 ml

Procedure (for thick film):

1. Put the slide in solution I for 10 seconds.
2. Wash for 2 seconds in a jar containing acidulated water (pH 6–6.6).
3. Stain with solution II for 1 second.
4. Wash in jar (2) for 5 seconds.
5. Immerse in solution I again for 10 seconds.
6. Wash as above for 10 sec. or till the smear gives a pink background.
7. Dry and examine.

Staining of spirochaetes: Fontana's method.

Reagents

a. **Fixative**

Acetic acid	1 ml
Formalin	2 ml
Distilled water	100 ml

b. **Mordant**

Phenol	1 g
Tannic acid	100 ml
Distilled water	100 ml

c. **Ammoniated silver nitrate**

10% Ammonia dissolved to 0.5% sol. of $AgNO_3$ in distilled water till the precipitate formed just dissolves, add $AgNO_3$ drop by drop, till precipitate reappears, and does not dissolve.

Procedure

1. Treat the film three times for 30 sec. each with fixative.
2. Wash off the fixative with alcohol and allow to act for 3 min. Drain excess alcohol.
3. Pour on mordant heating till steam rises and allow to act for 30 sec.
4. Wash well in distilled water and dry the slide.
5. Treat with ammoniated silver nitrate, heating till steam rises for 30 sec., when film becomes brown in colour.
6. Wash well in distilled water, dry and mount in Canada balsam.

Results: Spirochaetes are stained brownish black, background is brownish yellow.

Levaditi's method (for staining spirochaetes in tissues)

Procedure (pyridine modification):

1. Fix the tissue in 10% formalin.
2. Wash the tissue for 1 hour in water.
3. Place in 96–98% alcohol for 24 hours.
4. Place in 1% solution of silver nitrate (to which 1/10th volume of pure pyridine is added) for 2 hours at room temperature and thereafter at 50°C for 4–6 hours.
5. Rapidly wash in 10% pyridine solution.
6. Transfer to reduce fluid, which consists of 4% formalin—100 parts.

Add just before	Acetone	10 parts
use	pyridine	15 parts

   Keep the tissue in fluid for 2 days at room temp. in dark.
7. Wash well with water, dehydrate in increasing strength of alcohol and embedded in paraffin.
8. Cut the section, mount in usual way with Canada balsam.

Staining of Fungi in Wet Mounts with Lacto-Phenol Blue

Reagents

Phenol crystals	20 g
Lactic acid	20 ml
Distilled water	20 ml
Cotton blue/Methyl blue	0.075 g

Phenol crystals dissolved by gentle warming.

Procedure

1. Place a drop of 95% alcohol on slide.
2. Gently tease out a fragment of culture in alcohol and allow alcohol to evaporate.
3. Add a drop of strain.

4. Apply a coverslip and gently press.
5. Remove excess stain around the edges of coverslip.
6. Examine after a few minutes.

Result: Fungal hyphae stain blue black.

Staining of virus inclusion and elementary bodies

Inclusion bodies

Basophilic inclusion bodies	Giemsa stain
Acidophilic inclusion bodies	Manus methyl blue eosin stain

Elementary bodies

- Geimsa stain (useful for vaccinia and psittacosis)
- Brucella differential stain (useful for Chlamydia)
- Gutstein's method (useful for variola–vaccinia group).

PRINCIPLES OF MICROBIOLOGICAL DIAGNOSIS

Best way of diagnosing any infectious disease is to directly demonstrate the causative organism either in direct microscopy or in culture. But this is not always possible due to a variety of reasons.

Diagnosis of a Disease

Direct evidence

1. Demonstration by naked eye, e.g. various intestinal worms.
2. By microscopic evidence, e.g. stained smear showing gonococci in urethral pus and AFB in sputum.
3. Culture is the best way of diagnosis specially for bacteria and fungi.

Indirect evidence

1. Demonstration by naked eye, e.g. by latex agglutination, ELISA, etc.
2. Specific, e.g. serological tests.
3. Non-specific, e.g. ESR, TLC, DLC.

In routine practice, both types of evidences should be attempted, and the two should act as complementary to each other for making a final diagnosis.

Morphological classification of bacteria

A. True bacteria

I. Cocci

i. Gram-positive

1. Streptococci (arranged in chains)
2. Staphylococci (grape-like clusters)
3. Micrococci (irregular clusters)
4. Sarcina (cubical packets of 8)
5. Pneumococci, diplococci

ii. Gram-negative

1. Neisseria—intracellular diplococci
2. Veillonella—irregular clusters.

II. Bacilli

i. Gram-positive

a. Sporing
   1. Bacillus
   2. Clostridia

b. Nonsporing
   1. Corynebacterium
   2. Erysipelothrix
   3. Lactobacillus
   4. Listeria

ii. Gram-negative

a. Polar flagella
   Pseudomonacae

b. Peritrichous flagella
   1. Enterobacteriacae
   2. Achromobacteriacae
   3. Brucellaceae
   4. Bacterioidaceae

iii. Acid fast

a. Mycobacterium

III. Vibrios and Spirilla
   i. Vibrios
   ii. Spirillium

IV. Spirochaetes
   i. Borrelia
   ii. Treponema
   iii. Leptospira

B. Higher bacteria (Filamentous)

1. Actinomycetes
2. Nocardia
3. Streptomyces

Isolation of bacteria: In this chapter, the identification points of most commonly isolated bacterial pathogens in routine hospital practice shall be discussed.

Antibiotic sensitivity tests: Antimicrobial agents include basically 2 groups of drugs:

1. Disinfectants
2. Chemotherapeutic agents.

Assessment of the range of sensitivity of pathogenic bacteria isolated from patients to different antimicrobial agents, performed *in vitro* is of importance to the physician for prescribing the chemotherapeutic agents. However, it has to be kept in mind that *in vitro* result may not be 100% applicable *in vivo* (in the human body).

Principles

A wide range of tests is available, each of which is appropriate for a different purpose. Tests most commonly used are:

1. **Minimal inhibitory concentration:** It measures the lowest concentration of antimicrobial agent that will inhibit the growth of a known strain of bacterium.

   In this test, we use different concentrations of a drug to prevent the growth of an indicator bacterium in solid or liquid media.

   These tests are of importance mainly in pharmacology, especially for determining dosage of drugs.
2. **Rideal-Walker test:** This tests the potency of disinfectants to kill bacteria in reference to a standard (phenol in this case).

Phenol coefficient: It expresses the bactericidal power of a particular disinfectant as compared with pure phenol.

Rideal-Walker test measures the phenol coefficient of disinfectant under standard conditions.

3. **Chick-Martin and Garrod tests:** They also determine the phenol coefficient of the disinfectant in presence of a standard amount of organic matter.
4. Tests for disinfecting actions on surfaces.
5. **Capacity use-dilution test:** Measures effect of repeated challenge by bacteria.
6. **Stability test:** Measures stability and long time effectiveness of a diluted disinfectant.
7. **The in-use test:** Determines the presence/absence of bacteria in-use disinfectants.

What we will discuss in detail here are the antibiotic sensitivity tests as carried out in routine in a microbiology laboratory. These are the disk diffusion tests of sensitivity to antibiotics, which are simple, reliable and specially applicable in routine clinical bacteriology.

Disk Diffusion Tests

Principle: Disk diffusion method consists of impregnating small disks of a standard filter paper with given amounts of chosen range of antibiotics. These are placed on plates of culture medium previously spread uniformly with an inoculum of bacterial isolate. After incubation, degree of sensitivity is determined by measuring visible areas of inhibition of growth produced by diffusion of antibiotic into the surrounding medium.

Preparation of disks: It is the most convenient to use commercially available dry disks. These are 6 mm in diameter and consist of absorbent paper, impregnated with antibiotic. They are marked with letters showing name of antibiotic.

Preparation of wet disks: Punch disks 6.25 mm in diameter from no. 1 Whatman filter paper, dispense in batches of 100 in screw-capped bottles and sterilize by dry heat at 140°C for 2 hours. Prepare solutions of antibiotics so that 1 ml solution contains 100 times the amount of antibiotic required for 1 disk. Add 1 ml solution to each bottle and store in wet conditions. They retain their potency for several months at 40°C (in contrast, dry disks expire very quickly).

Disks: Containing different antibiotics can be recognised by:

1. Typed/printed letters
2. Colour applied to plain paper.
3. Paper on which black spots/lines have been stencilled.

Colouring is done with cotton dyes which are fast and do not interfere with action of antimicrobial agents.

Choice of drugs for disk test: When a large number of sensitivity tests have to be done on isolates from clinical specimens, it is convenient to restrict the routine tests to the number of first line antibiotics that can be conveniently tested on a single culture plate. Preferably 6 and at most 8 disks are used on one plate. Different appropriate first-line sets of 6 or 8 drugs may be selected for use with different types of clinical specimen, e.g. exudates/sputurn/urine/blood selection is also guided by the nature of isolates obtained. The set should depend on frequency of usage by clinicians.

1. **For cultures other than urine:** Sets of antibiotics include ampicillin, cotrimoxazole (Septran), erythromycin, benzylpenicillin, tetracycline, cephalexin and streptomycin.
2. **Cultures from urine:** High content disks are used. Set includes ampicillin, cotrimoxazole (Septran), nalidixic acid, nitrofurantoin, gentamicin, kanamycin, cephalexin and tetracycline.

Culture medium used: A nutrient agar medium should be used which is as far as possible free from substances inhibitory to action of antibiotics. Suitable sensitivity test agars are available from commercial suppliers. pH should be 7.2–7.5. Blood should be added when testing *Streptococcus pyogenes* or pneumococci. Chocolated blood should be used with Haemophilus. A volume of 20 ml medium is poured in 8.5 cm Petri dishes with flat bottoms to obtain a 3–4 mm deep layer.

Identification of Gram-positive cocci from colonies in blood agar (Fig. 24.5) and Gram-negative diplococci (Neissarie) are shown in Fig. 24.6 along with biochemical reactions (Fig. 24.7). Identification of Gram-negative bacilli oxidase positive is shown in Fig. 24.8 and Albert staining reaction from throat swabs and cullture is given in Fig. 24.9.

Test procedure

1. Dry culture plate in incubator, until surface is free from moisture. Inoculate test bacteria by any of the disc diffusion test as mentioned in Fig. 24.7.
2. After plate is dried after inoculation, apply the chosen disks with proper disk spacing, with sterile fine pointed forceps (Fig. 24.10 and Table 24.4) and drug concentration used is shown in Table 24.5.
3. Incubate for 18–24 hours at 37°C.
4. Measure the diameters of zones of inhibition of growth including 6 mm diameter of disk by calipers or viewing against a ruler.
5. Simultaneously a control of known sensitivity is run.
   a. Oxford strain of *Staphylococcus aureus* (Type 6571)
   b. *Escherichia coli* (NCTC 10418)
   c. *Pseudomonas aeruginosa* (NCTC 10662)

Reading interpretation

1. Report the test stain as sensitive if diameter of its zone of inhibition by a drug is greater than, equal to or ≤4 mm less than that on control culture.
2. Report as follows:
   >12 mm — sensitive
   >10 mm — <12 mm — moderately sensitive
   < 10 mm — resistant

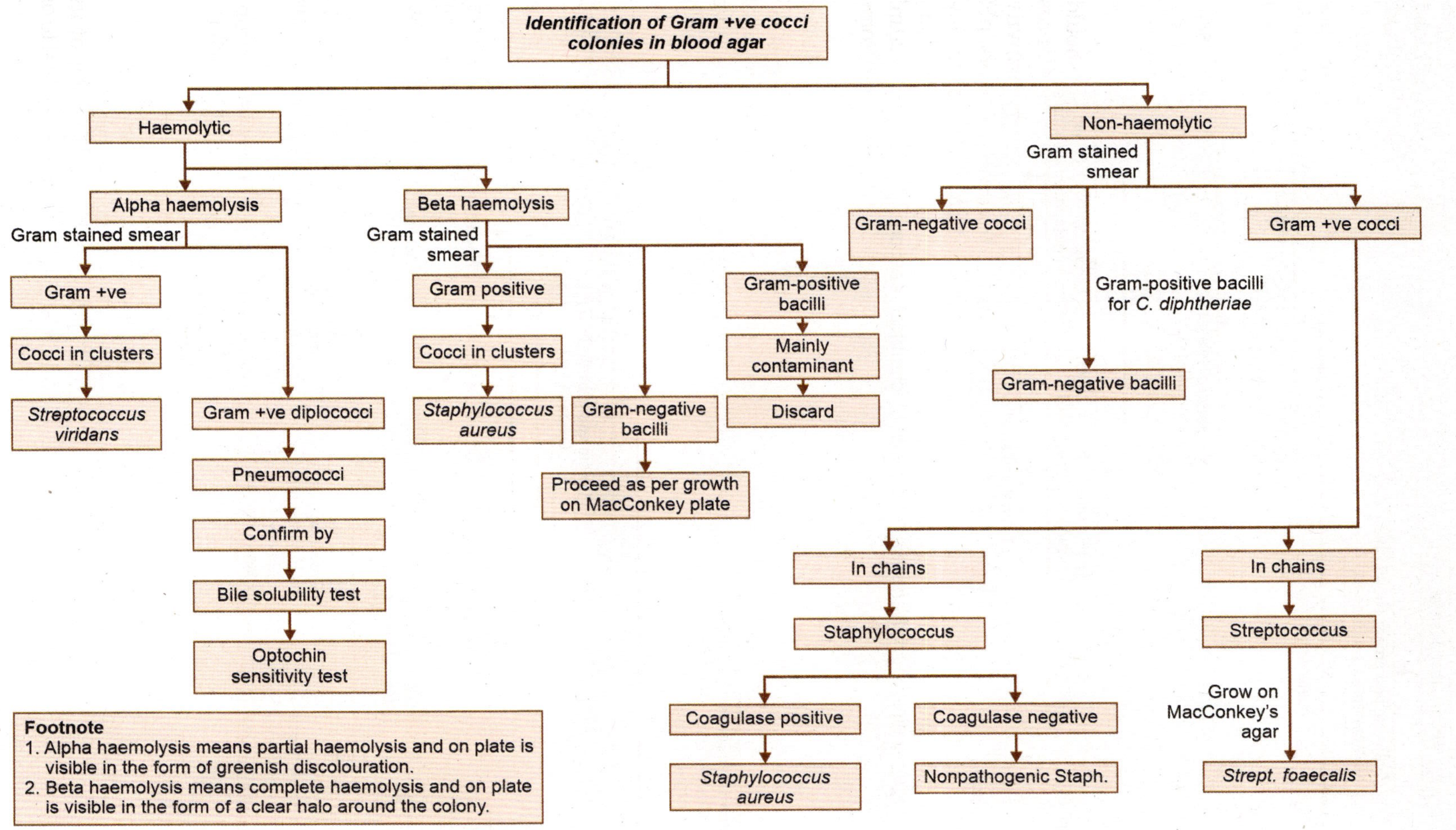

Fig. 24.5: Identification of Gram-positive cocci colonies in blood agar

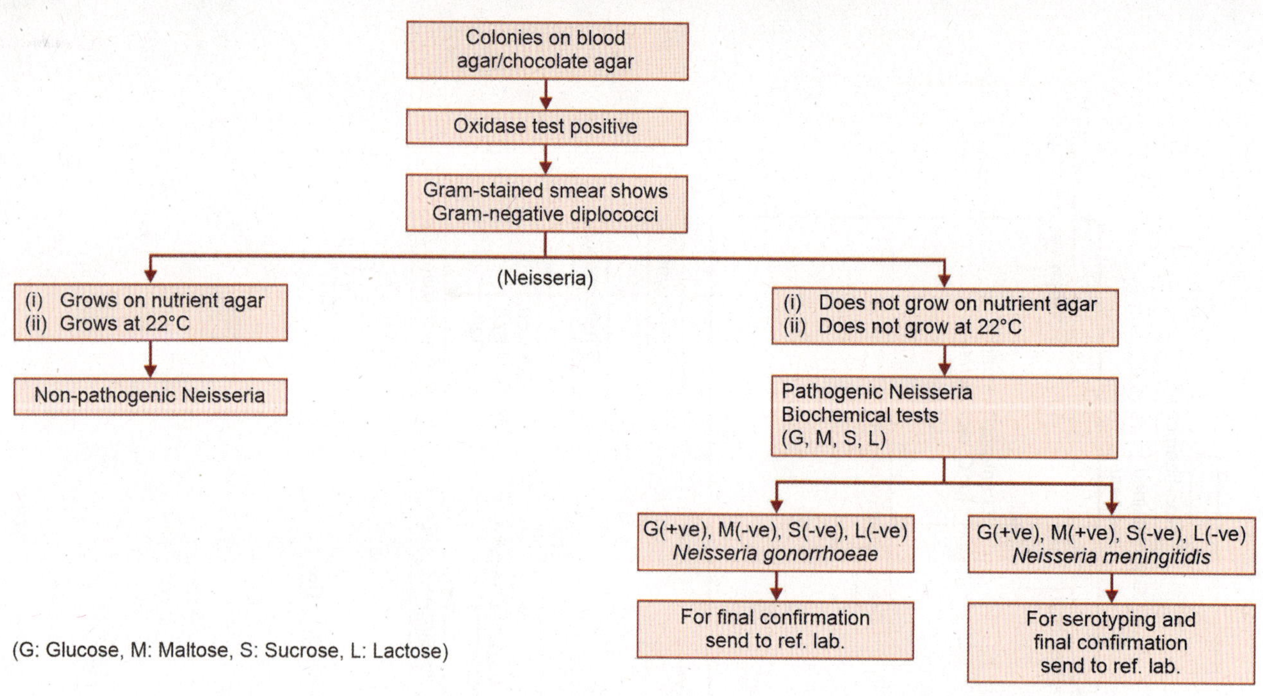

Fig. 24.6: Gram-negative diplococci (*Neisseria*) along with biochemical reactions

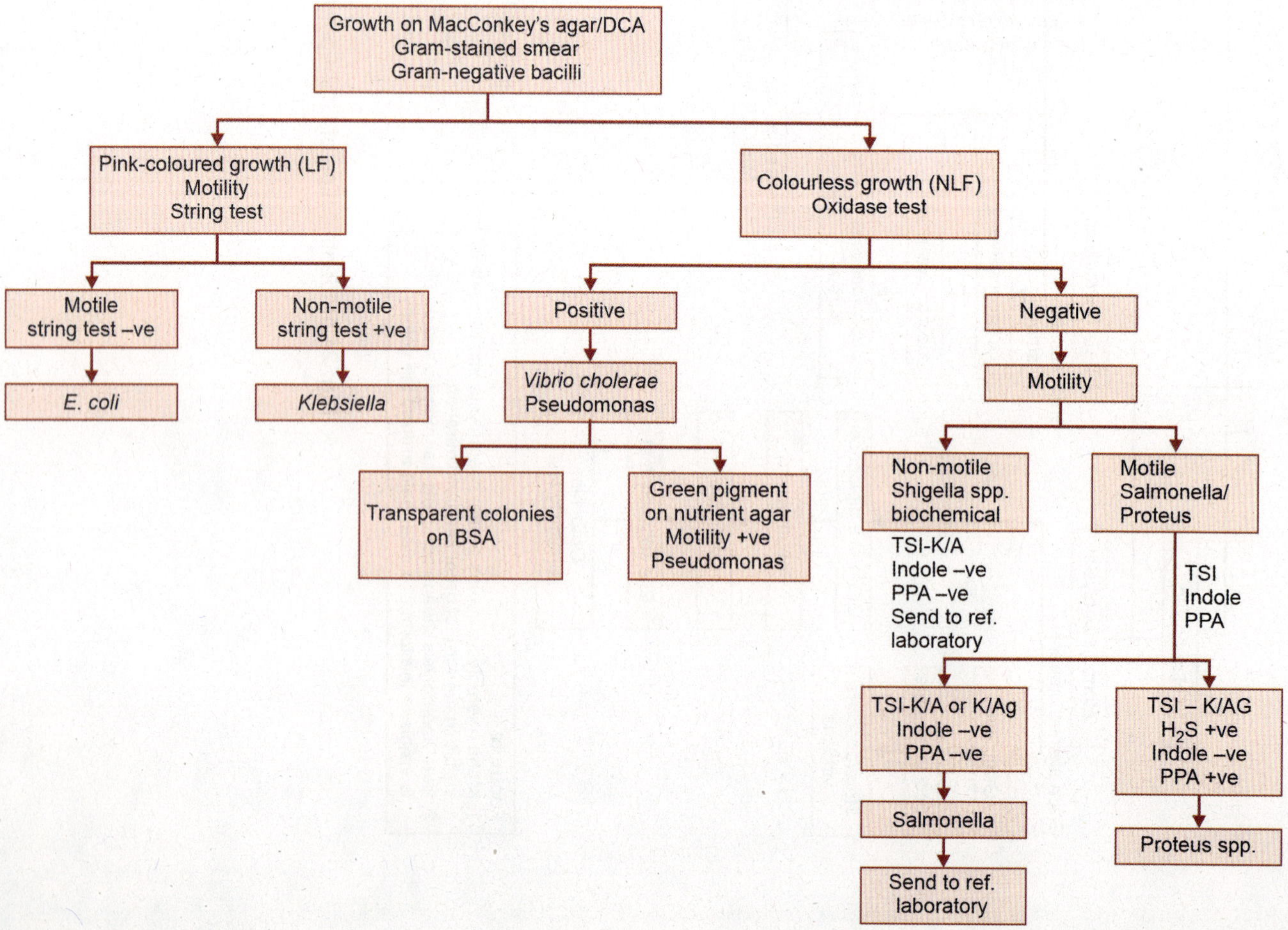

- Growth on MacConkey's agar/DCA, Gram-stained smear, Gram-negative bacilli
  - Pink-coloured growth (LF), Motility, String test
    - Motile, string test –ve → *E. coli*
    - Non-motile, string test +ve → *Klebsiella*
  - Colourless growth (NLF), Oxidase test
    - Positive → *Vibrio cholerae*, Pseudomonas
      - Transparent colonies on BSA
      - Green pigment on nutrient agar, Motility +ve, Pseudomonas
    - Negative → Motility
      - Non-motile, Shigella spp. biochemical: TSI-K/A, Indole –ve, PPA –ve, Send to ref. laboratory
      - Motile, Salmonella/Proteus: TSI, Indole, PPA
        - TSI-K/A or K/Ag, Indole –ve, PPA –ve → Salmonella → Send to ref. laboratory
        - TSI – K/AG, H_2S +ve, Indole –ve, PPA +ve → Proteus spp.

Fig. 24.7: Growth on MacConkey's media as Gram-negative bacilli, lactose fermenting (LF) and non-lactose fermenting (NLF)

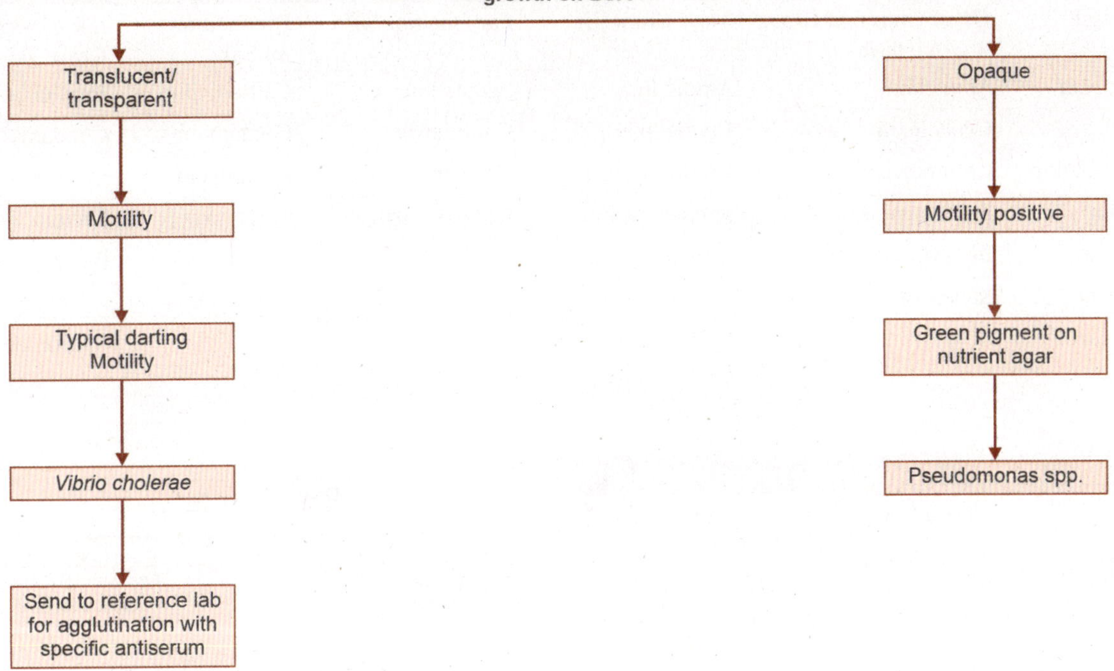

Fig. 24.8: Identification of Gram-negative bacilli—oxidase positive growth on BSA

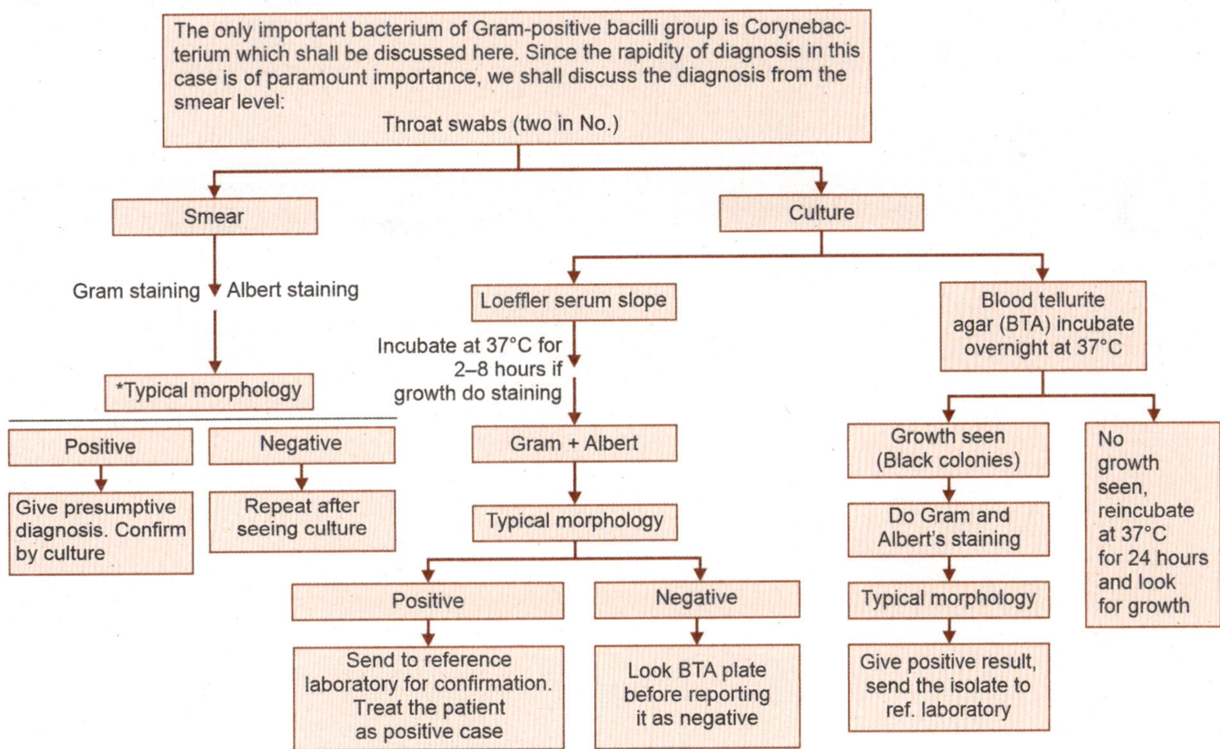

* Thin slender bacilli, pleomorphic, with one and clubbed, weakly Gram-positive and with metachromatic granules. Diphtheroids are thick, short mostly of uniform size and usually without metachromatic granules.

Note: If the Gram-positive bacilli isolated on blood agar not confirmed as *C. diphtheriae*, then do not attach much importance, discard them.

Fig. 24.9: The Albert staining reactions from throat swabs and culture

Table 24.4: Depending on isolate type of antibiotic used

Staphylococci	*Other cocci and Gram +ve bacteria*	*Most Gram –ve*	*For Haemophilus*	*For Pseudo-monas*	*For Clostridia and Gram –ve anaerobes*
1. Erythromycin	Ampicillin	Ampicillin	Ampicillin	Carbenicillin	Ampicillin
2. Fucidin	Cephalexin	Cephalexin	Cephalexin	Gentamicin	Clindamycin
3. Benzylpenicillin	Cotrimoxazole	Cotrimoxazole	Chloramphenicol	Kanamycin	
4. Ampicillin	Erythromycin	Streptomycin	Cotrimoxazole	Polymyxin B	Fucidin
5. Lincomycin	Benzylpenicillin	Gentamicin	Tetracycline		Benzylpenicillin
6. Tetracycline	Kanamycin			Tetracycline	
7. Cotrimoxazole		Chloramphenicol			Metronidazole
8. Gentamicin		Chloramphenicol			

Table 24.5: Drug concentrations used for common antibiotic

Drug	*Normal conc. (pg)*	*High content (pg) for urine*
1. Ampicillin	2	30
2. Benzylpenicillin	1	30
3. Carbenicillin	100	100
4. Cephalexin	5	30
5. Erythromycin	10	—
6. Gentamicin	10	30
7. Kanamycin	10	30
8. Nalidixic acid (Gramoneg)	—	30
9. Nitrofurantoin	—	200
10. Septran (cotrimoxazole)	Trimethoprim 1.25 Sulfamethoxazole 23.75	1.25 23.5
11. Streptomycin	10	30
12. Tetracycline	10	30

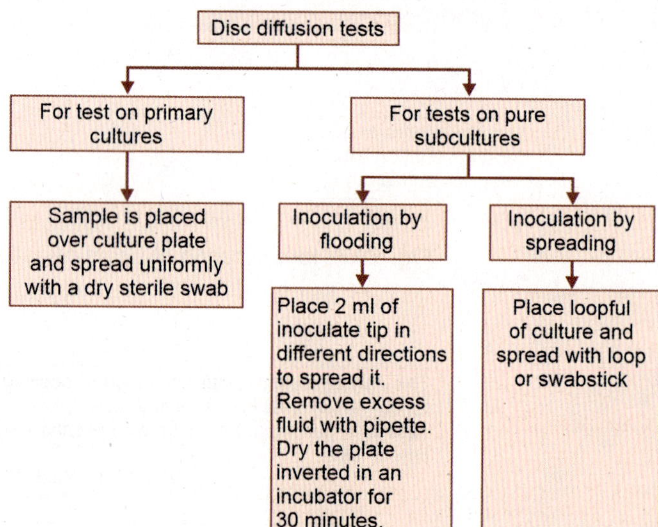

Fig. 24.10: Procedure disc diffusion tests

Chapter 25

General Bacteriology II

(Structure, Metabolism, Stains, Method of Staining, Classification, Culture, Chemotherapy Mechanisms)

Chapter Outline

- Structure of Bacteria
- Typical Shapes and Arrangements of Bacterial Cells
- Staining Methods
- Bacteria and Chemotherapy
- Universal Safety Precautions for Microbiology Laboratories

STRUCTURE OF BACTERIA (Fig. 25.1)

All bacteria, both pathogenic and saprophytic, are unicellular organisms that reproduce by binary fission. Most bacteria are capable of independent metabolic existence and growth, but species of Chlamydia and Rickettsia are obligatory intracellular organisms. Bacterial cells are extremely small and are most conveniently measured in microns (10^{-6} µm). They range in size from large cells such as *Bacillus anthracis* (1.0 to 1.3 pm × 3 to 10 pm) to very small cells such as *Pasteurella tularensis* 2 × 0.2 to 0.7 pm). Mycoplasma (atypical pneumonia group) are even smaller, measuring 0.1 to 0.2 pm in diameter.

Bacteria have characteristic shapes. The common microscopic morphologies are cocci (round or ellipsoidal cells, such as *Staphylococcus aureus* or Streptococcus, respectively); rods, such as Bacillus and Clostridium species; long, filamentous branched cells, such as *Actinomyces* species; and comma-shaped and spiral cells, such as *Vibrio cholerae* and *Treponema pallidum*, respectively. The arrangement of cells is also typical of various species or groups of bacteria. Bacteria have characteristic shapes (cocci, rods, spirals, etc.) and often occur in characteristic aggregates (pairs, chains, tetrads, cluster, etc.). These traits are usually typical for a genus and are useful diagnostically.

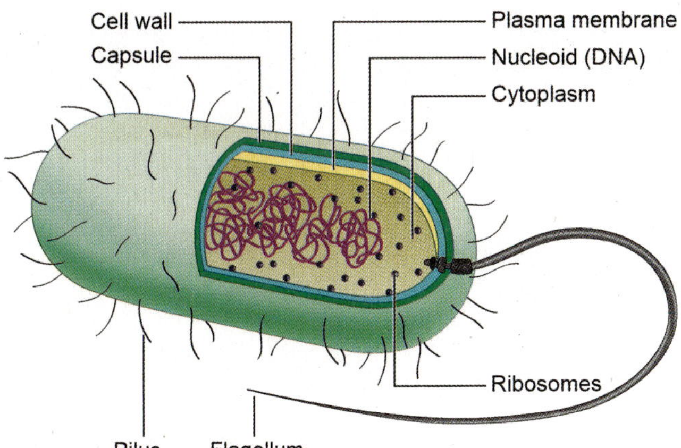

Fig. 25.1: Typical structure and parts of bacterial cell

TYPICAL SHAPES AND ARRANGEMENTS OF BACTERIAL CELLS (Table 25.1)

Surface Structures

The surface structures include the surface appendages (flagella, pili) and the surfae layers (capsule and cell wall).

Surface Appendages

Two types of surface appendage can be recognized on certain bacterial species—the flagella, which are organs of locomotion, and *pili* (Latin hairs), which are also known as *fimbriae* (Latin fringes). Flagella occur on both Gram-positive and Gram-negative bacteria, and their presence can be useful in identification. For example, they are found on many species of bacilli but rarely on cocci. In contrast, pili occur almost exclusively on Gram-negative bacteria. Some bacteria have both flagella and pili (Fig. 25.2).

Structurally, bacterial flagella are long (3 to 12 mm), filamentous surface appendages about 12 to 30 mm in diameter. The protein subunits of a flagellum are assembled to form a cylindrical structure with a hollow core. A flagellum consists of three parts:

1. The long filament, which lies external to the cell surface;
2. The hook structure at the end of the filament; and
3. The basal body, to which the hook is anchored and which imparts motion to the flagellum.

The basal body traverses the outer wall and membrane structures. The thrust that propels the bacterial cell is provided by counterclockwise rotation of the basal body, which causes the helically twisted filament to whirl. The ability of bacteria to swim by means of the propeller-like action of the flagella provides them with the mechanical means to perform chemotaxis (movement in response to attractant and repellent substances in the environment).

Table 25.1: Morphology of bacteria

Bacteria feature	Gram reaction	Morphology	Genus
	Gram-positive	Cocci in clusters	Staphylococci
	Gram-positive	Cocci in chain	Streptococci
	Gram-positive	Ovoid diplococci with/ without capsule	Pneumococci
	Gram-negative	Diplococci	Neisseria
	Gram-positive	Diphtheroids	Corynebacterium
	Gram-positive	Branching chains	Lactobacillus
	Gram-positive	Rods with non-protruding, subterminal spores	Bacillus
	Gram-positive	Rods with protruding subterminal spores	Clostridium
	Gram-positive	Rods with terminal spores	Clostridium
	Gram-positive	(True) branching rods	Actinomyces
	Gram-negative	Rods	Enterobacteria
	Gram-negative	Spindle-shaped rods	Fusobacterium
	Gram-negative	Comma-shaped rods	Vibrio
	Gram-positive	Budding yeasts	

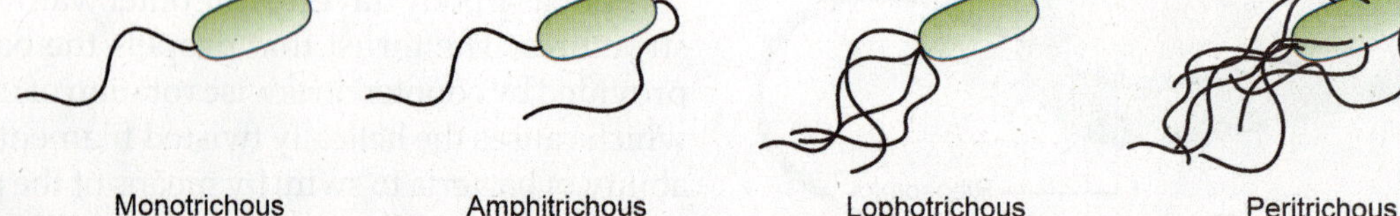

Fig. 25.2: Typical arrangements of bacterial flagella. Monotrichous: Single flagella which is polar in attachment. Lophotrichous: Polar flagella in tufts (multiple flagella attached together). Amphitrichous: Flagella at both poles. Peritrichous: Flagella present all over the cell.

Metabolism of Bacteria

Metabolism refers to all the biochemical reactions that occur in a cell or organism. The study of bacterial metabolism focuses on the chemical diversity of substrate oxidations and dissimilation reactions (reactions by which substrate molecules are broken down), which normally function in bacteria to generate energy. These respective exergonic (energy-yielding) and endergonic (energy-requiring) reactions catalyzed within the living bacterial cell by integrated enzyme systems, the end result being self-replication of the cell.

The bacterial cell is a highly specialized energy transformer. Chemical energy generated by substrate oxidations is conserved by formation of high-energy compounds such as adenosine diphosphate (ADP) and adenosine triphosphate (ATP) or compounds containing the thioester bond (acetyl-CoA or succinyl-CoA). ADP and ATP represent adenosine monophosphate (AMP) plus one and high-energy phosphates (AMPP and AMP ~ P ~ P, respectively); the energy is stored in these compounds as high-energy phosphate bonds. In the presence of proper enzyme systems, these compounds can be used as energy sources to synthesize the new complex organic compounds needed by the cell. All living cells must maintain steady-state biochemical reactions for the formation and use of such high-energy compounds.

Bacteria, like mammalian and plant cells, use ATP or the high-energy phosphate bond (~P) as the primary chemical energy source. Bacteria also require the B-complex vitamins as functional coenzymes for many oxidation–reduction reactions needed for growth and energy transformation.

From a nutritional, or metabolic viewpoint, three major physiologic types of bacteria exist: The heterotrophs (or chemoorganotrophs), the autotrophs (or chemolithotrophs), and the photosynthetic bacteria (or phototrophs).

Cell Wall and Gram-negative Cell Envelope

The Gram stain broadly differentiates bacteria into Gram-positive and Gram-negative groups; a few organisms are consistently Gram-variable. Gram-positive and Gram-negative organisms differ drastically in the organization of the structures outside the plasma membrane but below the capsule. In Gram-negative organisms these structures constitute the cell envelope, whereas in Gram-positive organisms they are called a cell wall (Fig. 25.3).

Note the complexity of the Gram-negative cell envelope (outer membrane, its hydrophobic lipoprotein anchor, periplasmic space).

Most Gram-positive bacteria have a relatively thick (about 20 to 80 nm), continuous cell wall (often called the sacculus), which is composed largely of peptidoglycan (also known as mucopeptide or murein). In contrast, the peptidoglycan layer in Gram-negative bacteria is thin (about 5 to 10 nm thick); *E. coli*, the peptidoglycan is probably only a monolayer thick.

Outside the peptidoglycan layer in the Gram-negative envelope is an outer membrane structure (about 7.5 to 10 nm thick). In most Gram-negative bacteria, this membrane structure is anchored noncovalently to lipoprotein molecules (Braun's lipoprotein which, in turn, are covalently linked to the peptidoglycan. The lipopolysaccharides of the Gram-negative cell envelope form part of the outer leaflet of the outer membrane structure.

STAINING METHODS

Methods of Staining

Mechanism of staining of bacteria is not fully understood. It is probable that both physical and chemical factors are involved. Physical process consists in dye being absorbed on the surface and chemical process in chemical combination between bacterial protoplasm and the dye. The following stains are commonly used in laboratory.

1. **Ordinary aniline stain:** These are derivatives of coal-tar product aniline. Those most frequently employed are basic fuchsin, methylene blue, gentian violet, saffranin and methyl violet. Dilute aqueous solutions are applied for 1/2 to 1 minute to the fixed smear, stains are washed. The smear is dried and examined under oil immersion lense. These tire employed for quick diagnosis of morphology of bacteria.
2. **Differential stains:** Two common examples are: Gram stain
   i. A thin uniform smear is prepared which is dried fixed.
   ii. Smear is covered with gentian violet and is allowed to act for 1 minute.
   iii. Stain is poured off then hold the slide at an angle, the remaining stain is washed away by Gram iodine. Smear is covered with Gram iodine which is allowed to act for 2–3 minutes (this acts as mordant. A mordant is a substance which facilitates a particular staining reaction).
   iv. Wash off iodine with alcohol and continue adding drop-by-drop of fresh alcohol till no more violet colour comes off the smear (this is called decolorisation).
   v. Wash with tap water.
   vi. Counterstain with saffranin for 1 minute.
   vii. Wash with tap water, dry the smear between blotting paper and examine.

Principle of the stain: Organism is stained with gentian violet and is subsequently with Gram iodine the letter acts as mordant under such conditions, certain organism resists subsequent decolourisation with alcohol, whereas others cannot. The organism which resists subsequent decolourisation and therefore retain violet stain are

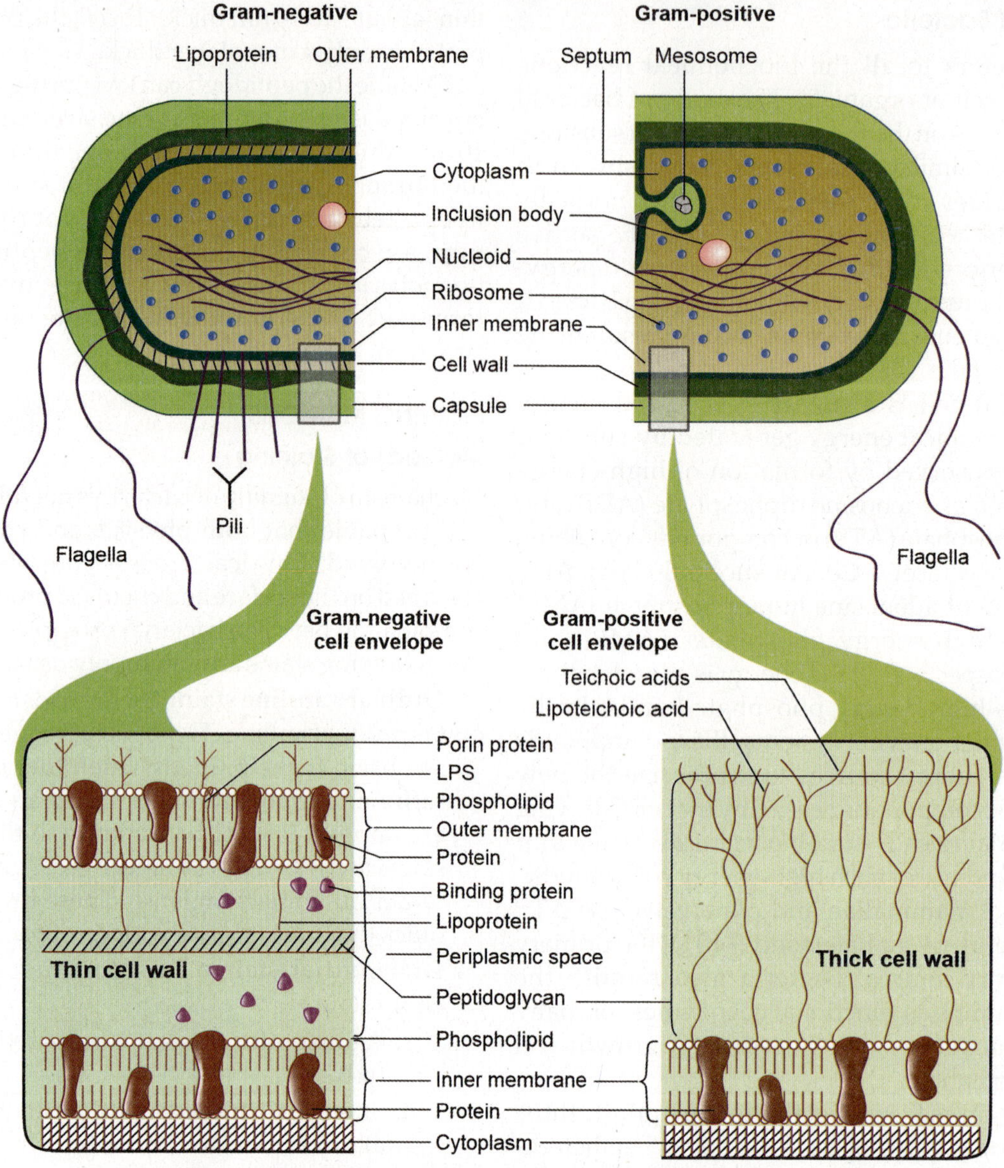

Fig. 25.3: Comparison of the thick cell wall of Gram-positive bacteria with the comparatively thin cell wall of Gram-negative bacteria

termed Gram-positive. As regards reason for Gram positive, it is believed that ribonuclease acid content of cell plays a major role. Some ascribe it to peculiarities in the permeability of cell membrane. The organisms which are decolorised with alcohol and so do not retain violet stain, but are stained red by suffranin, are termed Gram-negative.

1. Gram Staining Method (Rapid)

Procedure:

1. Make a thin film on a slide of the organism or specimen to be tested, air dry and fix shortly over the flame.
2. Flood the smear with crystal violet stain.
3. Wash off the stain with Gram's iodine and allow it to remain on the slide for 10 seconds.
4. Decolourise the smear with 97% alcohol, until no further colours flow from the slide. This usually takes 15–30 seconds, depending on the thickness of the smear. Care should be taken not to overdecolourise the smear.
5. Immediately wash off the alcohol with the back of the slide against a gentle jet of water.
6. Cover the smear with carbol fuchsin for 10 seconds.
7. Wash off the stain and leave it to dry in a staining rack.

Results:

Gram-positive bacteria	Dark purple
Gram-negative bacteria	Pale to dark red
Pus cells	Nuclei and cytoplasm red
Epithelial cells	Cytoplasm
Yeasts	Dark purple

Report:

The number of bacteria	Few, scanty, moderarte, many
The Gram reaction	Gram-positive/Gram-negative

Quality control:

Gram-negetive	*Streptococcus faecalis*
Gram-negetive	*Haemophilus influenzae*

2. Ziehl-Neelsen Stain

Principle: Some organisms retain carbol fuchsin when decolourised with acid. Such organisms ure called acid-fast organism. Mycolic acid is thought to be responsible for acid fastness. Acid-fast organisms take red stain. Acid-fast organisms are mycobacteria (tubercle bacilli, Lepra bacilli), bacterial spores. Nocardia, ascospore of certain yeast, Actinomyces.

Method

i. Cover the smear with hot carbol fuchsin and allow it to act for 5 to 7 minutes (carbol fuchsin is first heated in a test tube and then procedure on the smear (do not boil)
ii. Wash the smear well with tap water.
iii. Decolourise, with dilute sulphuric acid 95% in case of Lepra bacilli and 20% in case of tubercle bacilli. Acid should not be changed two or three times.
iv. Wash well with tap water.
v. Counterstain with methylene blue for 1 minute.
vi. Wash with tap water, blot it dry and examine.

Ziehl-Neelsen stain—cold method:

Formula:	
Basic fuchsin	25 g
Phenol	50 g
Ethanol, absolute	25 ml
Distilled water	500 ml
Triton X-100	5 ml

i. After heat fixation, place a strip of filter paper slightly smaller than the slide over the smear.
ii. Flood the slide with cold method of Ziehl-Neelsen stain and leave it for 3 minutes.
iii. Remove the filter paper and wash off the free stain with the back of the slide against a gentle jet of water.
iv. Decolourise the smear to a faint pink with acid alcohol while continuously rocking the slide until no more stain comes off. This takes approximately 1 min for an average thickness smear. Thoroughness wash off the acid-alcohol with the back of the slide against a gentle jet of water.
v. Counterstain with malachite green for 1 minute.
vi. Rinse off the stain with a gentle water jet, wipe the back of the slide dry with blotting paper and leave it to dry in a draining back.

Results:

Acid-fast bacilli	Bright red
Non-acid bacilli	Dark green

3. Other Stains

Albert stain: Some bacteria may have metachromatic black granules, e.g. *Corynebacterium diphtheriae* which stain dark bluish or black with methylene blue or a mixture of toluidine blue and malachite green.

Spore stain: Spores do not get stained by ordinary method of staining. In Gram stain, spores appear as clear areas in deeply stained body of bacilli. Methods of spore staining are modified acid-fast stain and Moller method.

Capsular stain: They are not stained with ordinary aniline dyes. In Gram stain, they are shown as area of halo around bacterium. India ink method and Hiss method are used for capsular stain.

Factors Influencing Growth of Bacteria

1. **Nutrition:** All bacteria have the following major nutritional needs for growth.
   a. A source of carbon
   b. A source of nitrogen
   c. A source of energy
   d. A variety of metals and ions.
2. **Moisture:** It is very essential for the growth of bacteria because 80% of the body of bacteria is made up of water.
3. **Temperature:** The temperature range at which an organism grows best is called optimum temperature. In human parasitic organisms, optimum temperature ranges between 30°C and 37°C. There are three groups of bacteria as regards the temperature of growth.
   a. *Psychrophilic:* These organisms grow between 0°C to 25°C.
   b. *Mesophilic:* These organisms grow between 20°C and 44°C.
   c. *Thermophilic:* These organisms grow between 50°C and 60°C, e.g. bacillus algae.
4. **pH:** Some bacteria grow in neutral media, some grow in alkaline media and some grow in acidic media.
5. **Oxygen:** On the basis of oxygen requirement, bacteria are classified as:
   a. *Aerobes:* The aerobe organisms grow only in the presence of oxygen, e.g. Pseudomonas.
   b. *Facultative anaerobes:* They are the organisms that can live with or without oxygen, e.g. Vibrio, *Escherichia coli*, Salmonella, Shigella.
   c. *Obligate anaerobes:* The strict anaerobes multiply only in the absence of oxygen, e.g. Bacteroides, Clostridium.
   d. *Micro-aerophilic:* These are aerobic bacteria that require low oxygen tension to grow, e.g. *Campylobacter* species.
   e. *Carboxyphilic (capnophilic):* These bacteria require an atmosphere composed of oxygen and raised level of carbon dioxide, e.g. *Neisseria gonorrhoeae*. This organism grows best in an atmosphere enriched with 5–10% carbon dioxide.
6. **Carbon dioxide:** The metabolic activities of some organisms like *Neisseria gonorrhoeae*, *Brucella abortus* are greatly enhanced by the presence of extra amount of carbon dioxide in atmospheric air.

7. **Light and other radiation**
8. **Osmotic effect**
9. **Mechanical and sonic stresses**

Growth of Bacteria

Following phases are observed in growth and multiplication of bacteria.

- **Lag phase:** It has a short duration. During this phase, there is adaptation of bacteria to new environment and increase in size and metabolic activity of cell.
- **Log phase:** It has also short duration. In this phase, bacteria multiply and their multiplication is like logarithm ratio. Numbers of bacteria increase in large amount in this phase. In this phase, bacteria have high rate of metabolism and are more sensitive to antibiotics.
- **Stationary phase:** In this stage, the death rate and multiplication rate is almost equal. It may be due to depletion of nutrients and collection of toxic products.
- **Decline phase:** In this phase, the population of bacteria is decreased due to death of cells.
- **Generation time:** Time required for bacterium, to give rise to two daughter cells under optimum condition is called generation time or generation gap. Generation time of Coliform bacilli is 20 minutes, *Mycobacterium tuberculosis* is 20 hours, and Lepra bacilli is 20 days. Culture: Growing of bacteria colonies in artificial medium containing all suitable nutrients and favourable condition is called culturing of bacteria.
- **Culture media:** It is the artificial media necessary for the growth of culture of bacteria.

Classification of Culture Media

On the Basis of Consistency

i. **Liquid media:** As the name suggests, it is liquid in state and it is used for putting up biochemical test and antibiotic sensitivity motility. Its types are infusion broth, meat extract broth and bile broth.

ii. **Semi-solid media:** These are used to demonstrate the motility of bacteria.

iii. **Solid media:** Liquid media are incorporated agar to solidify them. It is used to study colonies of individual bacteria. It is essential for isolation of organism in pure form. The constituents of solid media are:
   a. *Gelatin:* It is in liquid form at 37°C and form transparent gel below 25°C.
   b. *Agar:* It melts at 80°C to 100°C and solidifies at 35–42°C.
   c. Serum
   d. Egg

On the Basis of Different Constituent Properties

i. **Simple or basal media:** These media contain basic ingredients of all media such as peptone water, nutrient broth, nutrient agar.

ii. **Complex media:** In this, ingredients are added to bring out certain characteristics of bacteria or for providing specific nutrients for growth of bacteria.

iii. **Synthetic media:** They are prepared from pure chemical substances.

iv. **Special media:** They are further divided as under:
   a. *Enriched media*, e.g. blood agar, chocolate agar, egg yolk.
   b. *Enrichment media*, e.g. selenite F broth, tetrathionate broth.
   c. *Selective media*, e.g. potassium tellurite blood agar, deoxycholate citrate agar, Lowenstein-Jensen (LJ media)
   d. *Indicator media*, e.g. Wilson and Blair medium.
   e. *Differential media*, e.g. MacConkey media, blood agar.
   f. Sugar media
   g. Hiss serum
   h. Transport media.

On the basis of Aeration

i. **Aerobic culture media:** These used for growing aerobic bacteria, e.g. nutrient agar, nutrient broth and blood agar.

ii. **Anaerobic culture media:** For growing anaerobic bacteria, e.g. Robertson's cooked meat broth.

Culture Methods

I. Aerobic Culture Methods

1. **Streak culture:** It is also called surface plating. It is used for isolation of bacteria in pure culture from clinical specimen.
2. **Lawn or carpet culture:** It is prepared by flooding the surface of culture plate with a liquid suspension of bacteria by pipette.
3. **Stroke culture:** It is made in tubes containing agar slope. It is used for producing pure growth of bacteria for slide agglutination.
4. **Stab culture:** It is prepared by puncturing with charged loop, straight wire.
5. **Pour-plate culture:** This method is used for counting the number of living bacteria or groups of bacteria in a liquid culture or suspension.
6. **Liquid culture:** Liquid culture in tubes, bottles or flasks is inoculated by touching with charged loop or by pipetting or by syringes.

II. Anaerobic Culture Methods

Anaerobiasis is created by:

1. Cultivation in vacuum
2. Displacement of oxygen
3. Chemical or biological method
4. Anaerobic jar
5. Anaerobic chamber
6. Gaspak
7. Anaerobic bags.

BACTERIA AND CHEMOTHERAPY

Antibacterial drugs can be bacteriostatic or bactericidal. Bacteria may develop resistance to drugs.

General Concepts of Chemotherapy

Basis of Antimicrobial Action (Fig. 25.4)

Various antimicrobial agents act by interfering with

1. Cell wall synthesis
2. Plasma membrane integrity
3. Nucleic acid synthesis
4. Ribosomal function, and
5. Folate synthesis.

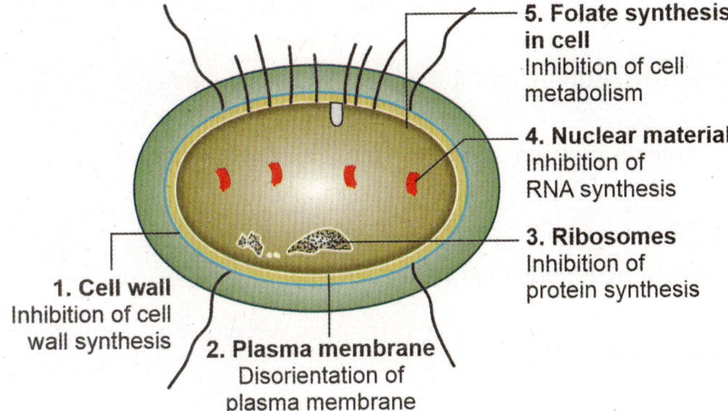

Fig. 25.4: Principles of action of antibiotics

Action of Specific Agents

Cell wall synthesis is inhibited by β-lactams, such as penicillins and cephalosporins, which inhibit peptidoglycan polymerization, and by vancomycin, which combines with cell wall substrates. Polymyxins disrupt the plasma membrane, causing leakage. The plasma membrane sterols of fungi are attacked by polyenes (amphotericin) and imidazoles. Quinolones bind to a bacterial complex of DNA and DNA gyrase, blocking DNA replication. Nitroimidazoles damage DNA. Rifampin blocks RNA synthesis by binding to DNA-directed RNA polymerase. Aminoglycosides, tetracycline, chloramphenicol, erythromycin, and clindamycin all interfere with ribosome function. Sulfonamides and trimethoprim block the synthesis of the folate needed for DNA replication.

Bacterial Resistance

Bacteria can evolve resistance to antibiotics. Resistance factors can be encoded on plasmids or on the chromosome. Resistance may involve decreased entry of the drug, changes in the receptor (target) of the drug, or metabolic inactivation of the drug.

Effects of Combination Therapy

Combinations of antibiotics may act synergistically-producing an effect stronger than the sum of the effects of the two drugs alone or antagonistically, if one agent inhibits the effect of the other.

Adverse Effects of Antimicrobial Agents

Many antibiotics are toxic to the host. Alterations of the normal intestinal flora caused by antibiotics may result in diarrhoea or in superinfection with opportunistic pathogens.

Antimicrobial Sensitivity Testing

Antibiotic effectiveness can be estimated through the determination of the minimal inhibitory concentration and the minimal lethal concentration with dilution susceptibility tests. Disk diffusion tests like the Kirby-Bauer test are often used to estimate a pathogen's susceptibility to drugs quickly.

Mechanisms of Antibacterial Drug Action

Drugs and its mechanism of action are shown in Table 25.2.

UNIVERSAL SAFETY PRECAUTIONS FOR MICROBIOLOGY LABORATORIES

Blood and other body fluids from all patients should be considered as potential source of infection for staff and community.

1. All specimens of blood and body fluids should be put in a well-constructed container with a secure lid to prevent leaking during transport. Care should be taken while collecting specimen to avoid contamination of the outside of the container and of the laboratory form accompanying the specimen.
2. All persons processing blood and body fluid specimens should wear gloves. Masks and protective eyewear should be worn if mucous membrane contact with blood or body fluids is anticipated. Gloves should be changed and hands washed after completion of specimen processing.
3. For routine procedures, such as histologic and pathological studies or microbiologic culturing, a biological safety cabinet is not must. However, biological safety cabinets must be used whenever conducting procedures that have a high potential for generating droplets. These include activities such as blending and vigorous mixing.
4. Mechanical pipetting devices should be used for manipulating all liquids in the laboratory. Mouth pipetting must not be done.
5. Use of needles and syringes should be limited to situations in which there is no alternative, and the recommendations for preventing injuries with needles outlined under universal precautions should be followed.
6. Laboratory work surfaces should be decontaminated with an appropriate chemical germicide after a spill of blood or other body fluids and when work activities are completed.
7. Apparatus, equipement and materials used in laboratory tests should be decontaminated before reprocessing or be placed in bags and disposed of in

Table 25.2: Factors and drugs mechanism of action

Drug	*Mechanism of action*
1. Call wall synthesis inhibitors	
Penicillin, ampicillin carbenicillin, cephalosporins	Inhibit transpeptidation enzymes involved in the cross-linking of the polysaccharide chains of the bacterial cell wall peptidoglycan and activate cell wall lytic enzymes
Vancomycin	Binds directly to the D-Ala-D-Ala terminus and inhibits transpeptidation
Bacitracin	Inhibits cell wall synthesis by interfering with action of the lipid carrier that transports wall precursors across the plasma membrane
2. Protein synthesis inhibitors	
Streptomycin, gentamicin	Binds with the 30S subunit of the bacterial ribosome to inhibit protein synthesis and causes misreading of mRNA
Chloramphenicol	Binds to the 50S ribosomal subunit and blocks peptide bond formation through inhibition of peptidyl transferase
Tetracyclines	Binds to the 30S ribosomal subunit and interfere with aminoacyl-tRNA binding.
Erythromycin and clindamycin	Binds to the 50S ribosomal subunit and inhibit peptide chain elongation
Fusidic acid	Binds to EF-G and blocks translocation
3. Nucleic acid synthesis inhibitors	
Ciprofloxacin and other quinolones	Inhibit bacterial DNA gyrase and thus interfere with DNA replication, transcription, and other activities involving DNA
Rifampin	Blocks RNA synthesis by binding to and inhibiting the DNA-dependent RNA polymerase
4. Cell membrane disruption	
Polymyxin B	Binds to the plasma membrane and disrupts its structure and permeability properties
5. Metabolic antagonism	
Sulfonamides, trimethoprim	Inhibit folic acid synthesis by competition with *p*-aminobenzoic acid. Blocks tetrahydrofolate synthesis through inhibition of the enzyme dihydrofolate reductase
Dapsone	Interferes with folic acid synthesis
Isoniazid	May disrupt pyridoxal or NAD metabolism and functioning. Inhibits the synthesis of the mycolic acid "cord factor"

accordance with institutional policies for disposal of infective waste.

8. Scientific equipment that has been contaminated with blood or other body fluids should be decontaminated and cleaned before being repaired in the laboratory or transported to the manufacturer.
9. All working staff should wash their hands before and after completing laboratory activities and should remove protective clothing before leaving the laboratory.
10. There should be no eating, drinking or smoking in the work areas.

General Bacteriology III
(Various Common Biochemical Tests and Reactions)

Chapter Outline

TESTS FOR METABOLISM OF CARBOHYDRATES AND RELATED COMPOUNDS

These tests are as follows:

1. Tests to distinguish between aerobic and anaerobic breakdown of a carbohydrate.
2. Fermentation reactions (to show the range of carbohydrates and related compounds that can be attacked).
3. Tests for specific breakdown products
4. Tests for ability to use a specific substrate
5. Tests for metabolism of proteins and amino acids
6. Tests for production of enzymes
7. Miscellaneous tests

1. Tests to Distinguish between Aerobic and Anaerobic Breakdown of a Carbohydrate

For this, Hugh and Leifson medium is used. It is a semisolid tube medium containing

1. Peptone 2 g
2. NaCl 5 g
3. K_2HPO 300 mg
4. Agar gel 3 g
5. 1% aqueous bromothynol blue 3 ml.

Make to 1 litre with distilled water (adjust pH to 7.1 before adding indicator). Autoclave at 121°C for 30 min. Carbohydrate to be added is sterilized separately and added to give a final concentration of 1%. The medium is then tubed to a depth of 4 cm using a Durham's tube.

Method: Duplicate tubes of medium are inoculated by stabbing.

One tube is promptly covered with a layer of sterile melted petroleum jelly to a depth of 5–8 mm. Incubate for up to 30 days. Fermenting organisms produce a colour change throughout the medium while oxidising (aerobic organisms) produce colour change only on the surface of uncovered tube.

2. Fermentation Reactions

Majority of these tests are simply for the production of acid and gas or acid alone when a pure culture grows in the presence of test compound.

Carbohydrate or Related Compounds under Test

1. Monosaccharides
   - Pentoses (arabinose, xylose)
   - Hexoses —Glucose —Fructose —Mannose —Galactose
2. Disaccharides —Sucrose —Maltose —Lactose —Trehalose
3. Polysaccharides —Starch —Inulin —Dextrin —Glycogen
4. Polyhydric alcohols —Glycerol —Mannitol —Dulcitol —Sorbitol —Inositol
5. Organic acids —Citrate —Tartrate —Gluconate —Malanate

Media Used for Test

1. Peptone water (most commonly used) 950 ml + 50 ml 10% test solution + indicator

Indicators are:
 i. Andrade's indicator 10 ml or
 ii. Bromocresol purple 25 ml.
2. Broth media (bromothymol blue as indicator).
3. Serum bases (phenol red as indicator).
 i. Serum peptone water.
 ii. Hiss serum water
 (25% serum in distilled water).

Indicators Used with End Points

1. Andrade's indicator (yellow to reddish pink)—1 N NaOH + 0.5%, acid fuchsin till light yellow colour develops.
2. 0.005% Bromocresol purple (violet to yellow).
3. 0.01% Phenol (red-pink-purple to yellow).
4. 0.0025% Bromothymol blue (blue to yellow).

A small inverted tube (Durham tube). Completely filled with liquid and containing no air bubbles is usually included in each culture tube to detect gas.

Method: Inoculate each culture tube with a speck of pure solid culture or a loopful of liquid culture. Incubate for 24 hours or (48 hours) for slow growers. Late fermentation may take up to 40 days.

Colour Codes for Common Fermentation Reactions

Glucose — Green
Lactose — Red
Maltose — Blue/white
Sucrose — Blue
Mannitol — Mauve
Sorbitol — Black/blue
Dulcitol — Pink

3. Tests for Specific Breakdown Products

i. Methyl Red Test (MR Reaction)

It is employed to detect the production of sufficient acid during fermentation of glucose and maintenance of conditions such that pH of old cultures is maintained at 4.5 (Fig. 26.1).

ii. Voges Proskauer (VP) Test (Figs 26.2 and 26.3)

Principle and method

Gluconate Test (Fig. 26.4)

This tests the ability of an organism to oxidize gluconates to 2-keto-gluconate. (Gluconate is non-reducing while 2-K-gluconate is reducing.)

4. Tests to Show Ability to use a Specific Substrate

Citrate Utilization Test

This tests the ability of an organism to use citrate as the sole source of carbohydrate and energy (Fig. 26.5).

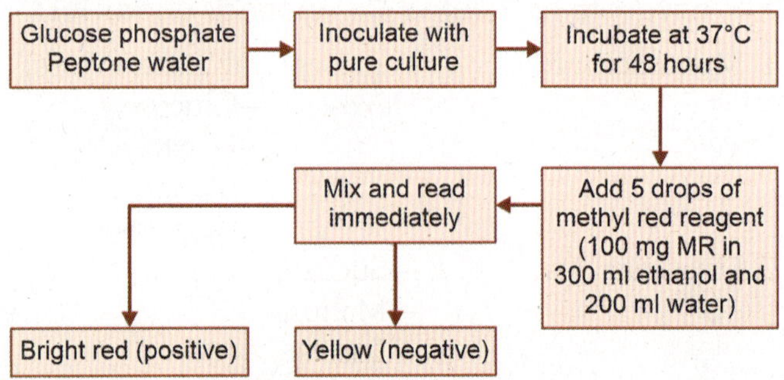

Fig. 26.1: Methyl red reaction

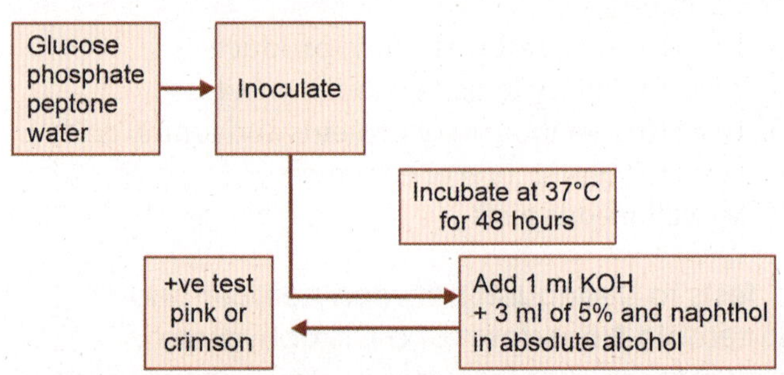

Fig. 26.3: Method of VP test

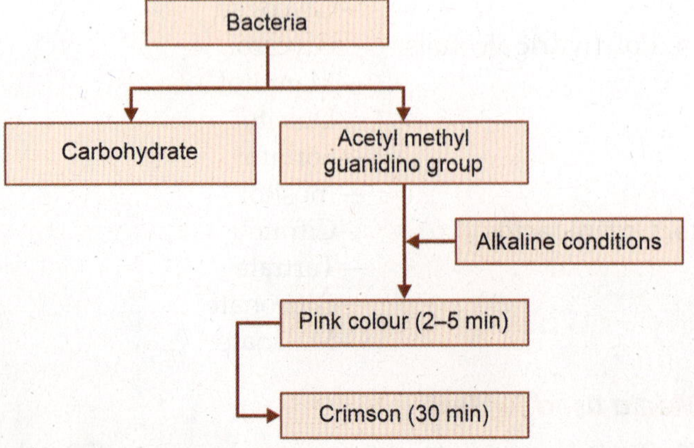

Fig. 26.2: Voges Proskauer (VP) test

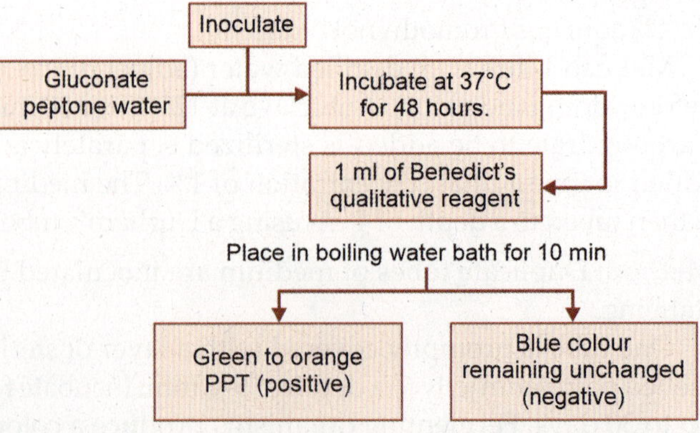

Fig. 26.4: Gluconate test

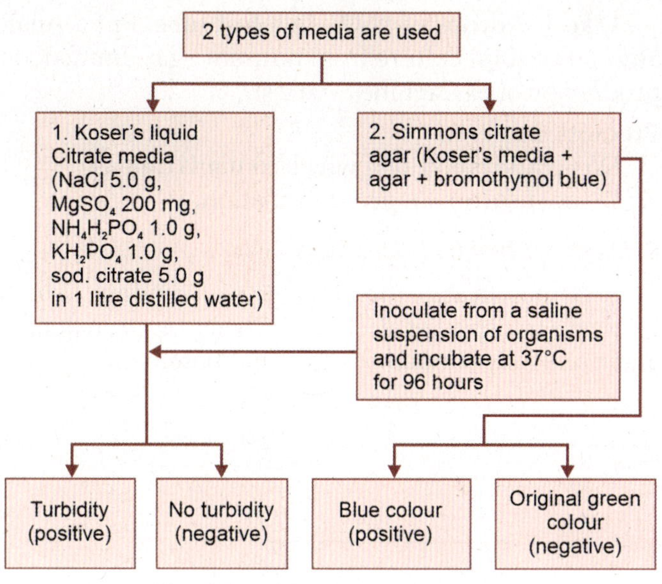

Fig. 26.5: Citrate utilization test

5. Tests for Metabolism of Proteins and Amino Acids

i. Gelatin Liquefaction (Fig. 26.6)

Two methods of demonstrating:

1. Using nutrient broth + Gelatin
2. Using gelatin agar (Fig. 26.7)
   a. Gelatin broth [nutrient broth (1 litre) + Gelatin (120 g) + Egg albumin (2 egg whites)]
   b. Gelatin agar (nutrient agar 11, KH_2PO_4 500 mg, K_2HPO_4 1.5 g, gelatin 4.0 g, glucose 50 mg]

ii. Indole Test

Principle and method (Figs 26.8 and 26.9)

iii. Nitrate Reduction Test (Fig. 26.10)

Peptone water

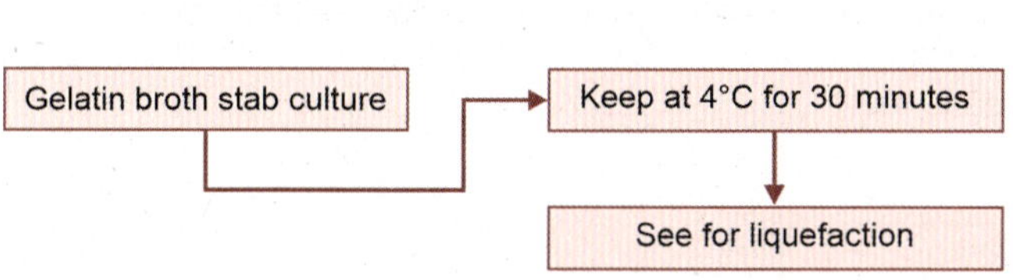

Fig. 26.6: Gelatin liquefaction test

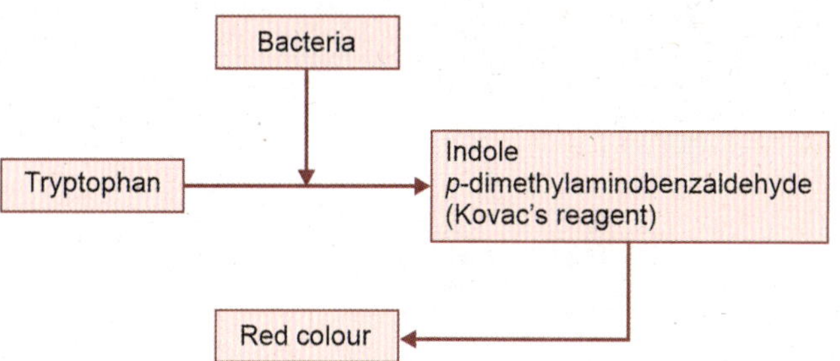

Fig. 26.8: Principle of indole test

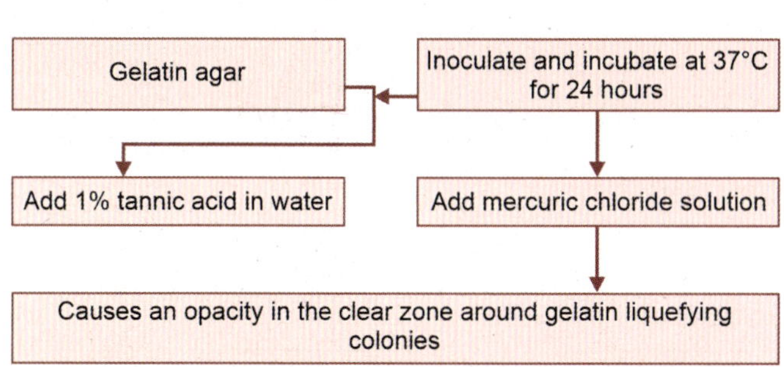

Fig. 26.7: Gelatin agar method

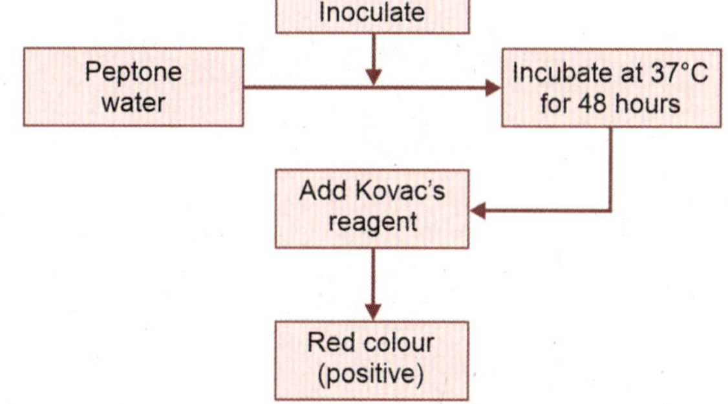

Fig. 26.9: Method of indole test

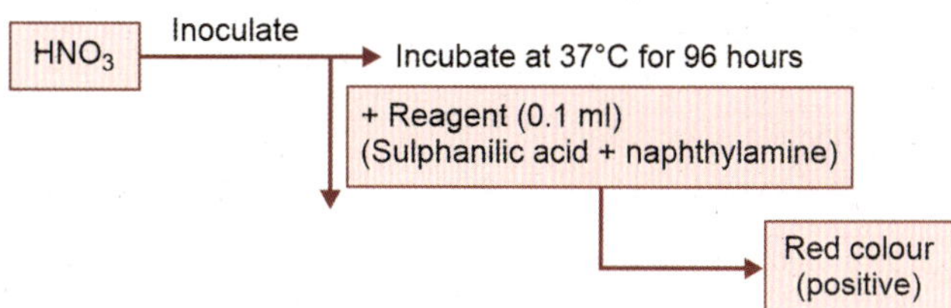

Fig. 26.10: Nitrate reduction test

iv. Urease Test (Fig. 26.11)

v. DNAse Test (Fig. 26.12)

vi. Coagulase Test (Fig. 26.13)

vii. Phenylalanine Deaminase (PPA) Test (Fig. 26.14)

6. Tests for Production of Enzymes

i. Catalase Test

It demonstrates the presence of catalase that releases O_2 from H_2O_2.

Take 1–2 drops of H_2O_2, in a test tube. Put a small amount of solid culture from nutrient agar. Immediate production of gas signifies +ve test.

Precautions

1. Do not use blood agar which contains catalase
2. Do not use iron loop for inoculation.

ii. Oxidase Test (Fig. 26.15)

This demonstrates the presence of oxidase which catalyzes transport of electrons between electron donors and a redox dye (tetramethyl phenyldiamine)

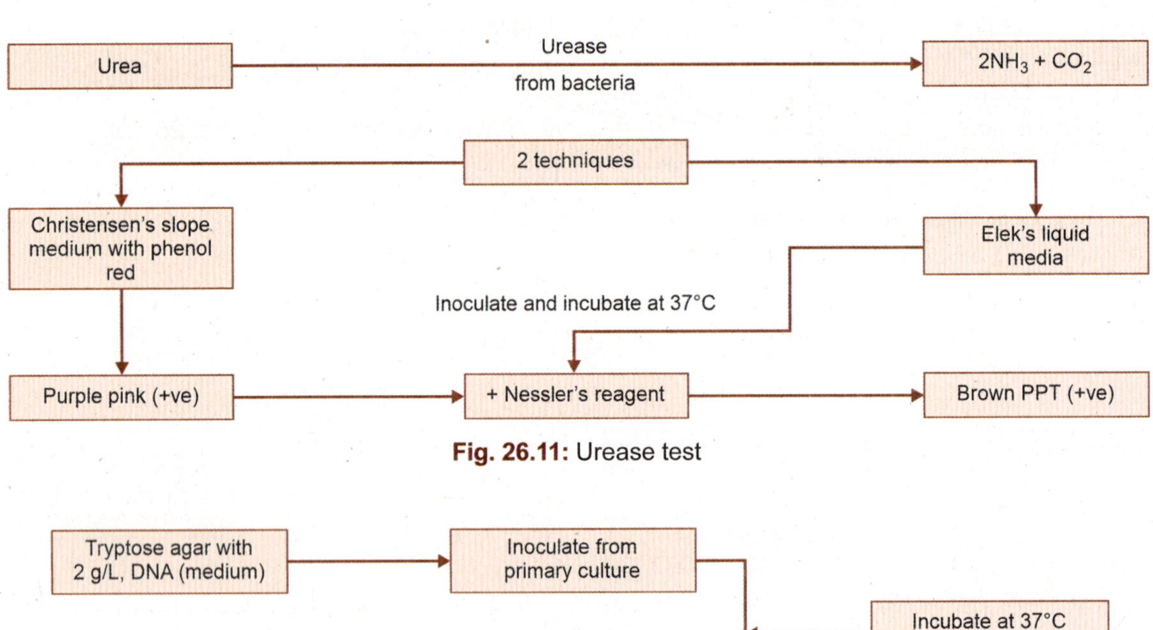

Fig. 26.11: Urease test

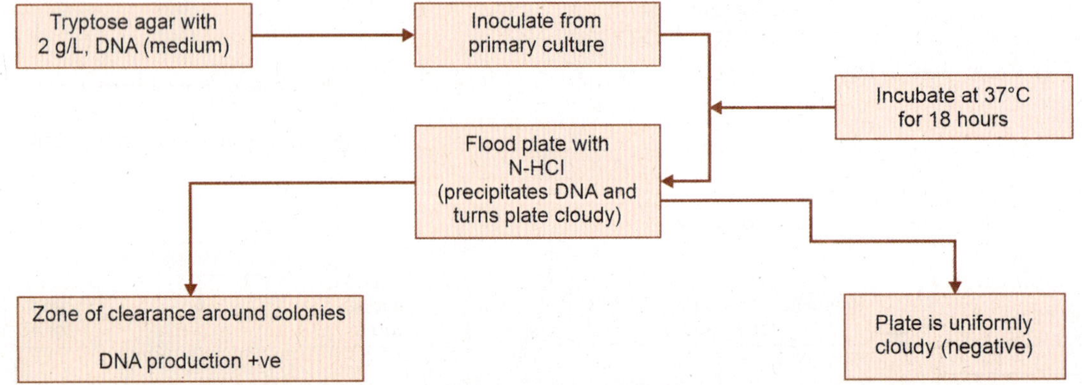

Fig. 26.12: DNAse test

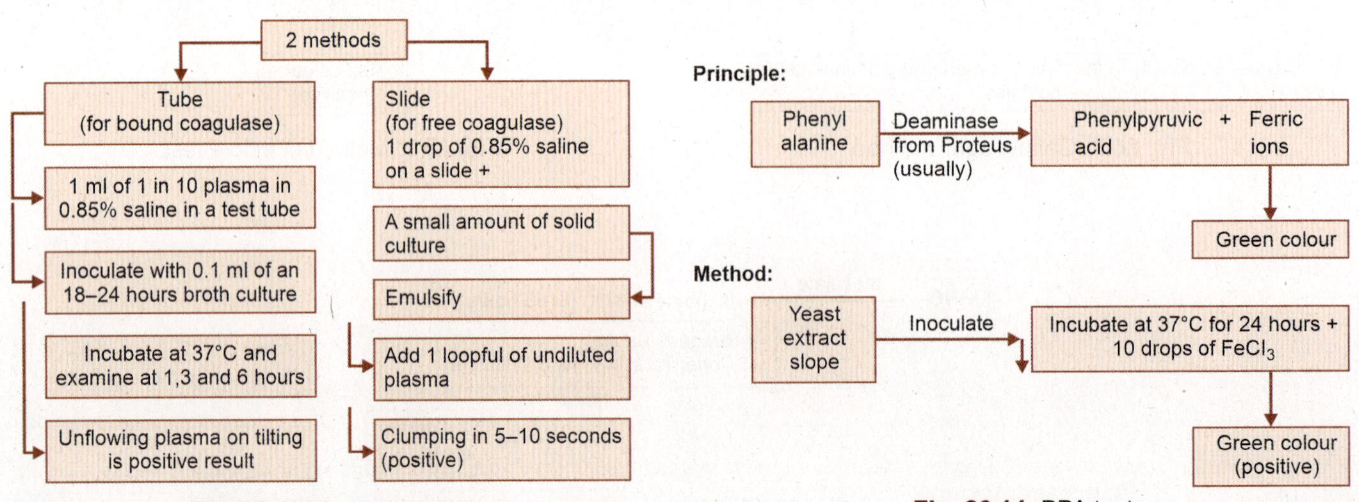

Fig. 26.13: Coagulase test

Fig. 26.14: PPA test

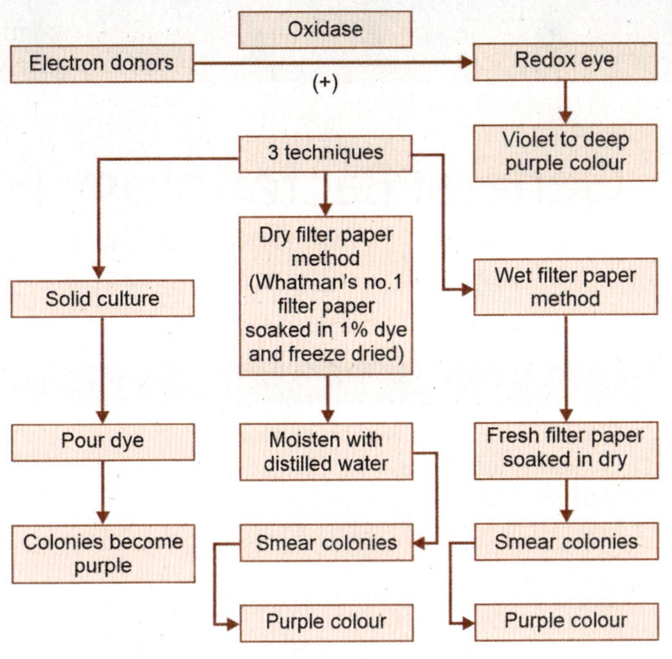

Fig. 26.15: Oxidase test

iii. Lecithinase Test (Naegler's Test)

Some bacteria produce lecithinase or phospholipase that spilt lipoprotein complexes in human serum and hen egg yolk and produce opalescence or turbidity when grown in media containing these substrates.

Medium used: Nutrient broth with human serum or egg yolk suspension.

Test and control media are inoculated with a drop of liquid culture or a colony picked up from plate culture. A known lecithinase producing bacteria is placed in a control tube. Incubate under suitable conditions (aerobic/anaerobic) for 24–48 hours, and lecithinase production is indicated by a pronounced turbidity with a yellowish curd on the surface of the test mixer.

Plate test: Use a medium containing nutrient agar and sterile human serum with 5% Fildes extract. Inoculate and incubate under suitable conditions (anaerobic for Clostridia). Lecithinase producing colonies are surrounded by zones of opalescénc (Naegler reaction).

In some cases an additional test is included by spreading a few drops of antitoxin to a specific lecithinase over half the plate before inoculation. Opalescence should be inhibited around colonies on antitoxin half, if the antitoxin is really specific.

7. Miscellaneous Tests

i. Potassium Cyanide Test

It tests the ability of an organism to grow in the presence of KCN. Basic peptone water is utilized. Add 5% KCN solution to cold medium. Inoculate with the one loopful from a 24-hour nutrient broth culture and incubate at 37°C. Observe after inoculate Dubos and Davis slope medium.

ii. Niacin Test

Tubercle bacilli (hominis) produce niacin (nicotinic acid) and this is detected with cyanogen bromide and aniline. Inoculate Dubos and Davis slope medium. Incubate at 37°C for 72–96 hours.

At regular intervals take a slope in a test tube

+

- 1 ml of 10% cyanogen bromide
- 5 min later add 1 ml of 4% aniline in 96% ethanol.
- Yellow colour (positive)
- Keep testing for 10 weeks.
- Then discard the culture

Chapter 27

General Bacteriology IV
(Bacterial Genetics)

Chapter Outline

Definition

Genetics is the study of heredity and variation. All here dietary characteristics are encoded in DNA. The chromosomal DNA plays a major role in the maintenance of characters constant from generation to generation.

I. BASIC PRINCIPLES

The DNA molecule is composed of two strands of complementary nucleotides wound together in the form of a double helix as deduced by Watson and Crick.

The bacterial nucleus contains a circular chromosome of a double-stranded DNA molecule of approximately 1000 µm (1 mm) long when straightened (Fig. 27.1).

Each strand has a backbone of deoxyribose (sugar) and phosphate groups. There are four nitrogenous bases, two purines: Adenine (A) and guanine (G) and two pyrimidines: Thymine (T) and cytosine (C). One of these four nitrogenous base pairs is attached to each deoxyribose. The two strands are held together by hydrogen bonds between the nitrogenous base pairs on the opposite strands. This bonding is in such a specific manner that hydrogen bonds can only be formed between adenine and thymine (A-T) and between guanine and cytosine (G-C). Adenine and thymine thus form one complementary base pair, and guanine and cytosine form another.

During replication of the DNA molecule, the two strands separate at one end, and each strand then acts as a template for the synthesis of a complementary strand, with which it then forms a double helix.

RNA is structurally similar to DNA, except for two differences, sugar ribose is present instead of deoxyribose and the nitrogenous base uracil replaces thymine. There are three different types of RNA in a cell—messenger RNA (mRNA), ribosomal RNA (rRNA) and transfer RNA (tRNA).

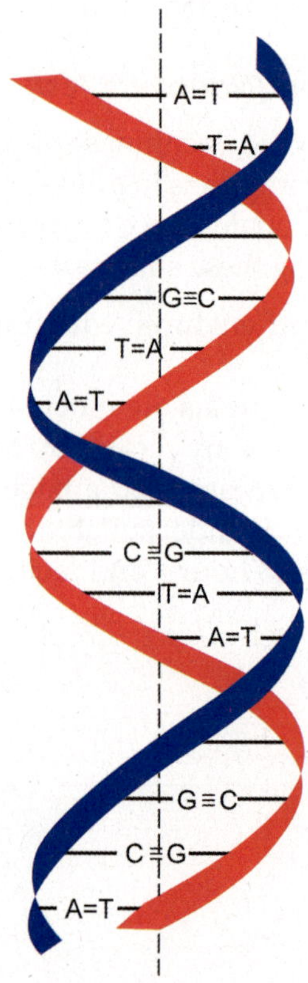

Fig. 27.1: DNA double helix (Watson-Crick model)

Important Definitions in Genetics

- **Gene:** A segment of DNA that specifies for a particular polypeptide is called a gene.
- **Codon:** Genetic information is stored in the DNA as a code. Codon consists of a sequence of three nucleotide base pairs, i.e. the code is triplet. Each codon specifies for production of a single amino acid.
- **Non-sense codons:** Three codons (UAA, UGA and UAG) do not code for any amino acid and act as 'stop

codons for terminating the message for the synthesis of a polypeptide. These are called non-sense codons.

II. SYNTHESIS OF POLYPEPTIDE

Genetic information in DNA is transcribed on to RNA and then translated as the particular polypeptide (Fig. 27.2).

A. Transcription

RNA polymerase attaches itself to the beginning of a gene on DNA and synthesises m-RNA, using one of the strands in DNA as a template. This process is known as *transcription*.

B. Translation

The m-RNA passes into cytoplasm and then m-RNA and t-RNA come together on the surface of ribosome containing r-RNA. The triplet base sequence on m-RNA is known as *codon*. The base sequences on m-RNA are recognised by the anti-codon (corresponding complementary) sequences of t-RNA. The t-RNA molecule contains a triplet at one end and amino acid at the other end. The ribosome moves along the m-RNA until the entire m-RNA molecule has been translated into corresponding sequences of amino acids. This process is called *translation*.

III. EXTRACHROMOSOMAL GENETIC ELEMENTS

Besides the chromosomal DNA, some bacteria may also possess extrachromosomal DNA which may be plasmids (when these are situated in the cytoplasm as free state) or episomes (when integrated with chromosomal DNA of bacteria). Plasmids are circular DNA molecules and can replicate autonomously (independent replicons). Plasmids and *episomes* are not essential for function of the host bacterium but they may carry properties of drug resistance, toxigenicity, conjugation and others.

IV. BACTERIAL VARIATION

There are two types of variation
A. Phenotypic variation
B. Genotypic variation

The *phenotype* (*phaeno*; display) is the expression of various characters by bacterial cells in a given environment.

The *genotype* is the sum total of the genes. It is the genetic constitution of an organism.

A. Phenotypic Variation

A bacterial cell may exhibit different phenotypic appearances in different environmental conditions. Phenotypic variations are reversible. Some examples of environmental influence on bacteria are:

1. **Synthesis of flagella:** *Salmonella typhi* (typhoid bacillus) is generally flagellated, but when grown in phenol agar, the flagella are not formed. This effect is reversed when subcultured from phenol agar into broth.
2. **Synthesis of enzyme:** *E. coli* possesses the genetic information for the synthesis of the enzyme, beta-galactosidase, but the actual synthesis takes place

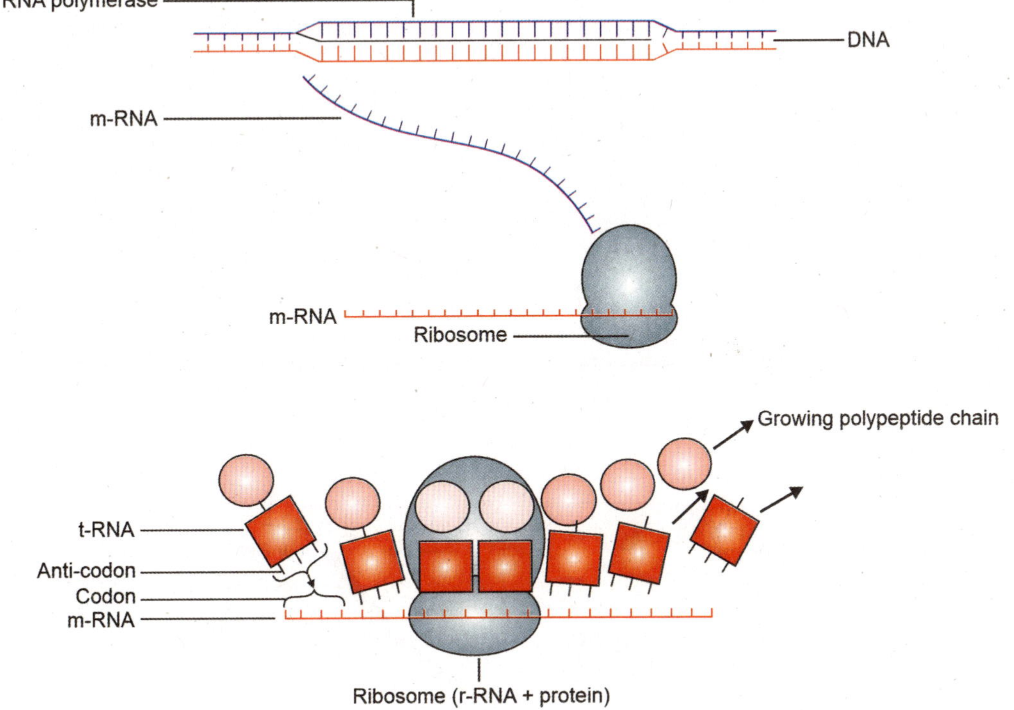

Fig. 27.2: Synthesis of polypeptide

only when grown in a medium containing lactose. This enzyme is necessary for lactose fermentation.

Gene Regulation ('Operon' Concept by Jacob and Monod)

Lactose fermentation of *E. coli* requires three enzymes, beta-galactosidase, galactoside permease and transacetylase. These enzymes are coded by the structural genes *lac* Z, *lac* Y and *lac* A, respectively. These genes are arranged in sequence, forming a functional unit, *lac operon* (Fig. 27.3). The regulator gene is *lac* I, which codes for a 'repressor, which is an allosteric protein molecule. This repressor can combine either with the operator region or with the inducer (lactose in this case). The promoter and operator regions lie between *lac* I and the structural *lac* genes.

B. Genotypic Variation

These variations occur in the genetic material. These are stable, heritable and not influenced by the environment. Genotypic variations may occur in bacteria by mutation or gene transfer.

Mutation

Mutation is a random, undirected heritable variation caused by change in nucleotide sequence of the DNA of the cell. It can involve any of the numerous genes present in bacterial chromosome. The frequency of mutation ranges from 10^{-2} to 100^{-10} per bacterium per division. Mutation occurs spontaneously but its frequency may be enhanced by mutagens such as UV rays, alkylating agents, 5-bromouracil and acridine dyes.

Mutation can affect any gene and hence may modify any characteristic of the bacterium, e.g. sensitivity to bacteriophages, loss of ability to produce capsule or flagella, loss of virulence, alteration in colony morphology, pigment production, drug susceptibility, biochemical reactions, antigenic structure. The practical importance of bacterial mutation is mainly in the field of drug resistance and the development of live vaccines.

Transition

This happens by replacement of one pyrimidine by another pyrimidine, and one purine by another purine, e.g. AT is replaced by GC. Transition is the most frequently occurring mutation.

Transversion

When a purine is replaced by pyrimidine and vice versa, it is named transversion, e.g. GC changes to CG.

Non-sense Mutation

When a non-sense codon (UAG, UAA or UGA) is formed within a gene by mutation, the protein synthesis is terminated prematurely and a partial polypeptide is produced during translation. This is called a nonsense mutation.

Missense Mutation

Both substitution and frame shift mutation give rise to an altered codon which specifies a different amino acid from that is normally located at a particular position in the protein. This is called missense mutation.

V. GENE TRANSFER

Various methods of gene transfer are as follows:

A. Transformation (uptake of naked DNA)

B. Transduction (through bacteriophage)

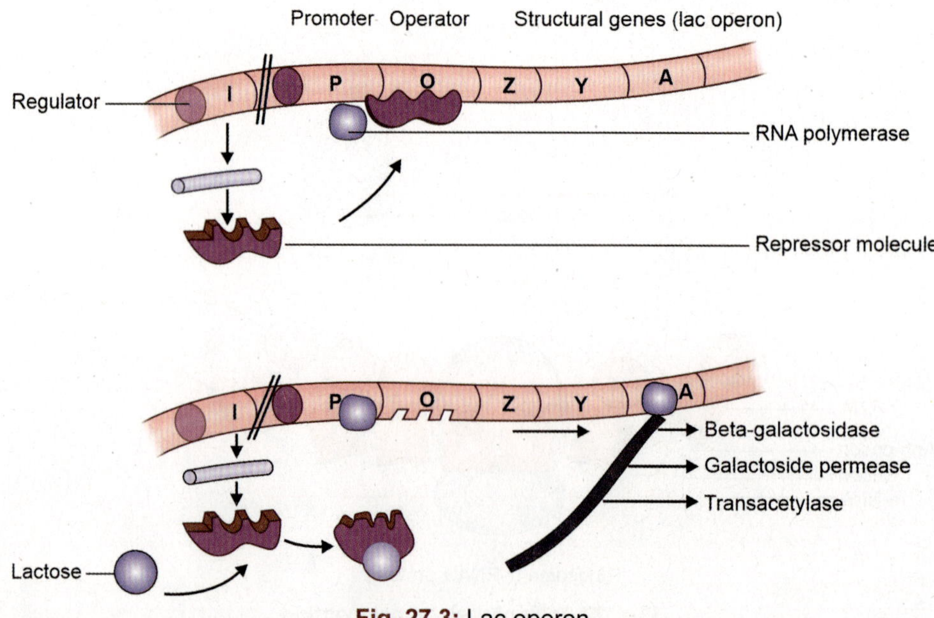

Fig. 27.3: Lac operon

C. Lysogenic conversion
D. Conjugation (plasmid-mediated)

A. Transformation

Transformation is the transfer of genetic information through free or naked DNA. In 1928, Griffith found that mice died when injected a mixture of live noncapsulated (rough: No capsule) pneumococci derived from capsular type II and heat killed (smooth: Capsulated) strain from type I, neither of which separately proved fatal. The live type I capsulated pneumococcus could be isolated from mice that died. It showed that rough forms (noncapsulated) were transformed into the smooth forms (Fig. 27.4).

B. Transduction

Transmission of a portion of DNA from one bacterium to another by a bacteriophage is transduction. During the assembly of bacteriophage progeny inside infected bacteria, errors may happen occasionally. Besides its own nucleic acid, host DNA may accidentally be incorporated into the bacteriophage. This is known as 'packaging error. Hence, when this bacteriophage infects another bacterium, host DNA is transferred and the recipient cell acquires new characters coded by donor DNA.

Types of transduction: 1. Generalised, 2. Restricted

1. Generalised transduction: Transduction may be 'generalised', when it involves any segment of donor DNA at random.

2. Restricted transduction: Transduction may be 'restricted', when a specific bacteriophage transduces only a particular genetic trait.

Role of Transduction

Transduction is not only confined to transfer of chromosomal DNA but episomes and plasmids may also be transduced. Penicillin resistance in staphylococci is due to the plasmids transferred from one bacterium to another by transduction.

C. Lysogenic Conversion

Bacteriophages have two types of life cycles inside the host bacterium.

i. Virulent or lytic cycle
ii. Temperate or non-lytic cycle

i. **Virulent or lytic cycle:** Large number of progeny phages are formed and subsequently, these progeny phages are released causing death and lysis of the host cell.
ii. **Temperate or non-lytic cycle:** In contrast to virulent cycle, the host bacterium is unharmed. The phage DNA remains integrated with the bacterial chromosome as the prophage, which multiplies synchronously with bacterial DNA. The prophage acts as an additional chromosomal element which encodes for new characters and is transferred to the daughter cells. This process is known as lysogeny or lysogenic conversion and bacteria harbouring prophages are known as lysogenic bacteria.

Example of lysogenic conversion: Diphtheria bacillus produces toxin only when lysogenisation with the phage beta occurs.

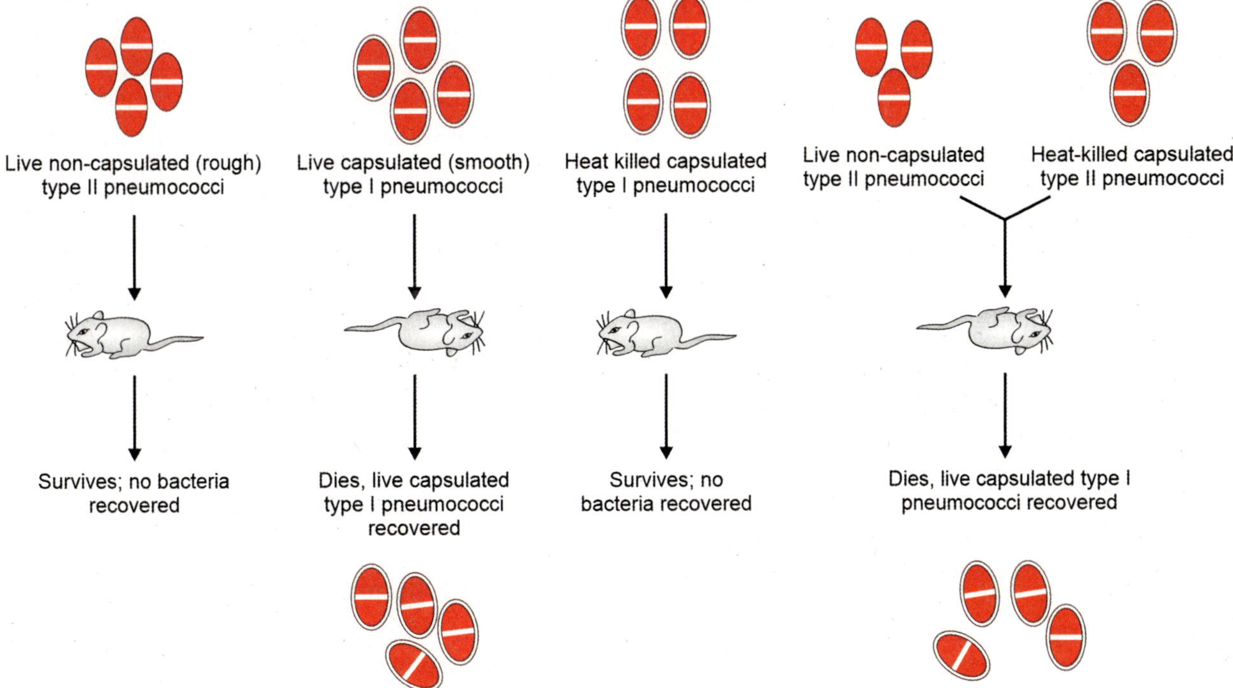

Fig. 27.4: Transformation experiment of Griffith

D. Conjugation

The transfer of genetic material from one bacterium (donor or male) to another (recipient or female) by mating or contact is called conjugation (Fig. 27.5.). Donors are those bacteria that contain F plasmid (F^+ or male cells) while cells lacking F plasmid (F^- or female cells) act as recipients. F plasmid is conjugative plasmid which encodes for sex pilus (in P^+ cells) necessary for conjugation. This plasmid is also named 'sex factor' or 'fertility' (F) factor. When other similar plasmids were also discovered, a name of 'transfer factor' was given to all such plasmids which conferred on their host cells the ability to act as donors or male cells in conjugation.

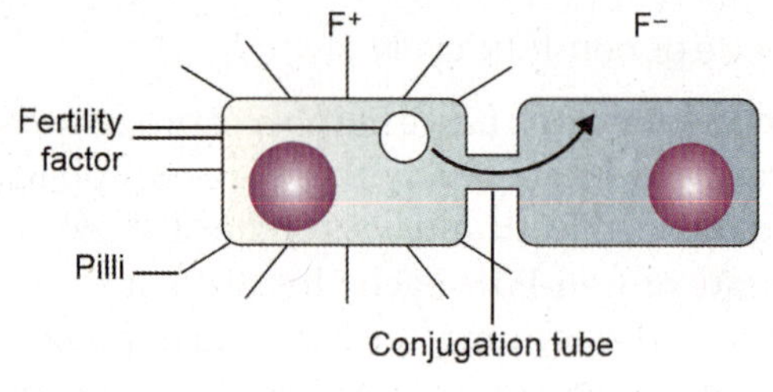

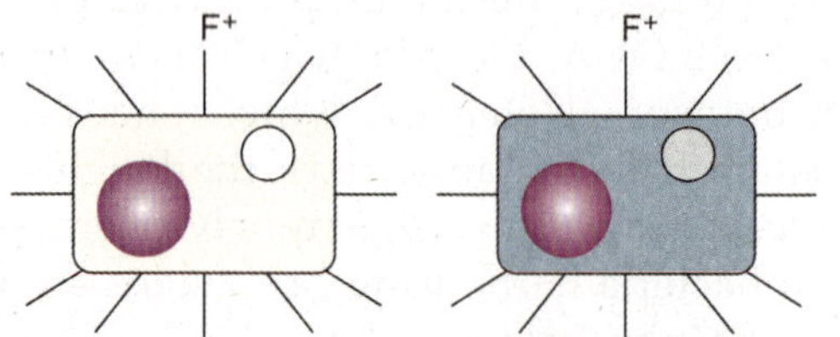

Fig. 27.5: The process of conjugation

During conjugation, the plasmid DNA replicates and copy of it passes from donor to the recipient cell probably along the sex pilus (conjugation tube). As a result, recipient (F^-) becomes donor (F^+) and can in turn conjugate with other female cells (F^-). This character of maleness (F^+) in bacteria is transmissible or infectious.

Resistance Transfer Factor (RTF)

Resistance transfer factor (RTF) and resistance determinant (r) are two components of the plasmid known as an R factor (RTF + r determinants). The RTF is responsible for conjugational transfer while each r determinant carries resistance for one of the several drugs. An R factor can have several r determinants and resistance to many drugs can be transferred simultaneously (Fig. 27.6) The RTF can also attach to its determinants other than those for drug resistance. Enterotoxin and haemolysin production in some enteropathogenic *E. coli* are shown to be transmitted by this transfer factor (RTF). Transferable drug resistance is seen in various pathogenic and commensal bacteria of man and animals such as *E. coli*, Klebsiella, Proteus, Vibrio, Pseudomonas.

Bacteria carrying R factors can be transmitted from animals to man. Hence, indiscriminate use of antibiotics in animals or in animal feeds can lead to an increase of multiple drug resistance in the community.

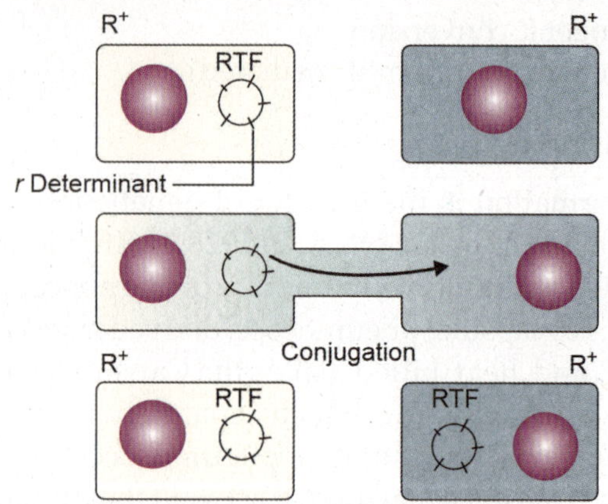

Fig. 27.6: Resistance transfer factor and drug resistance

VI. GENETIC MECHANISMS OF DRUG RESISTANCE

Bacteria may acquire drug resistance by mutation or by one of the methods of gene transfer. In clinical practice, mutational resistance is very important in tuberculosis. If a patient is treated with streptomycin alone, initially organisms die in large numbers but soon resistant mutants appear and multiply unchecked. By use of two or more drugs, a mutant resistant to one drug will be killed by the other drug. The possibility of a mutant developing resistance to more than one drug at one time is remote. This is the rationale of combined treatment in tuberculosis.

Transferable drug resistance mediated by the R factor is an important method of drug resistance. Acquisition of an R factor simultaneously confers resistance to several drugs, therefore, there is no use of combined drug therapy. Table 27.1 shows differences of mutational and transferable drug resistance.

Table 27.1: Differences of mutational and transferable drug resistance

Mutational drug resistance	*Transferable drug resistance*
1. Mutational resistance	1. Transferable resistance
2. Resistance to one drug at a time	2. Multiple drug resistance
3. Low degree resistance	3. High degree resistance
4. Resistance is not transferable to other organisms	4. Resistance is transferable to other organisms
5. Mutants may be defective	5. Not defective
6. Virulence of resistance mutants may be lowered	6. Virulence not decreased
7. Resistance can be prevented by treatment with combination of drugs	7. Cannot be prevented by treatment with combination of drugs

Transposable Genetic Elements

Transposable genetic elements are specific sequences of DNA segments that have the ability to move from one plasmid to another plasmid or from plasmid to chromosome and vice versa and also within the chromosome. Because of their ability to insert into many sites both on plasmid and chromosome, they have assumed the popular name of *jumping genes*.

The transfer of genetic material from one DNA molecule to another is called *transposition*.

Transposons are larger (4–25 kb) transposable genetic elements and contain additional genes that encode for at least one function (often conferment of antibiotic resistance).

Small transposons (1–2 kb) are known as 'insertion sequences' or IS elements. Bacteria acquire new characters by the insertion of transposable elements.

VII. GENETIC ENGINEERING

By genetic engineering or recombinant DNA technology, it is now possible to isolate the genes coding for any desired protein from microorganisms or from cells of higher form of life including man, and to insert them into suitable microorganisms in such a way so that it can be expressed in the formation of specific (desired) protein. Such cloning of genes in microorganisms enables the preparation of the desired protein in pure form and in large quantities at a reasonable cost.

The DNA can be cleaved by enzymes called restriction endonucleases and the fragments containing the desired genes are isolated. These desired DNA fragments are covalently bound to vectors or carriers, such as plasmids or temperate bacteriophages. The recombinant DNA molecule is then introduced into a bacterial host, usually *E. coli*. Many other bacteria and yeasts have also been employed for introduction of recombinant DNA molecule. *E. coli* containing recombinant molecule is grown on a suitable medium and bacterial colonies carrying specified genes are produced. Thus, desired protein is obtained in large quantities by growing these *E. coli* (Fig. 27.7).

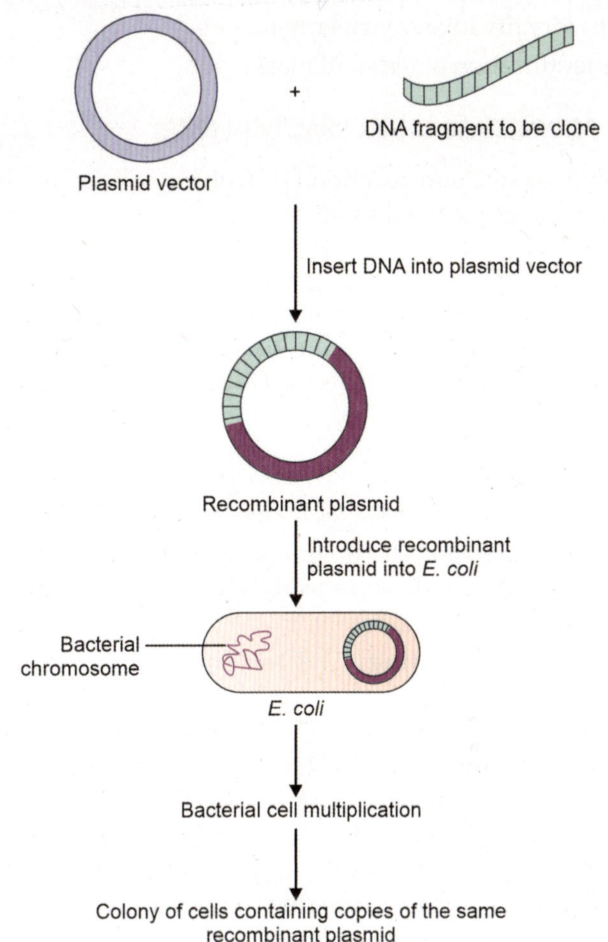

Fig. 27.7: Genetic engineering

Application of Genetic Engineering

1. **Production of vaccines:** Preparation of certain vaccines is done by producing specific antigen against which antibody is required, e.g. hepatitis B, rabies and *B. pertusis* vaccines.
2. **Production of proteins:** Genetic engineering has also been used for the production of proteins of therapeutic interest. These include human growth hormone, insulin, interferons and interleukin-2.

VIII. DNA PROBES

DNA probes are radiolabelled or chromogenically labelled pieces of single-stranded DNA which can be used for the detection of homologous DNA by hybridisation. Hybridisation is the technique in which two single strands of nucleic acid come together to form a stable double-stranded molecule.

All microorganisms contain some unique sequences of nucleic acid within their genome that distinguish them from all other organisms. This unique sequence of nucleic acid can be recognised by hybridisation with a DNA probe.

Various diagnostic DNA probes have been developed for identification of different microorganisms. The advantages of DNA probes are their high degree of specificity and ability to detect minute quantities of DNA. They are also very useful in diagnosis of microbes that are either difficult or impossible to culture.

Application of DNA Probes

Diagnostic DNA probes to recognise *Legionella pneumophila*, *Campylobacter jejuni*, *M. tuberculosis*, *Helicobacter pylori*, *E. coli* (LT and ST toxins), hepatitis B virus, *Plasmodium falciparum*, rotavirus and human immunodeficiency virus have been developed.

Applications of DNA Probe Technology

- In clinical microbiology:
  - Direct detection of microbes in specimens.
  - To detect microbes which are either difficult or impossible to culture.
- Identification of culture isolates
- Strain identification

- To identify toxins, virulence factors
- Identification of resistant markers

IX. POLYMERASE CHAIN REACTION (PCR)

Polymerase chain reaction (PCR) has made a revolutionary impact in molecular biology.

A. Principle

It is a DNA amplification system that produces a large amount of DNA *in vitro* from small amounts of starting material. It amplifies a specific DNA sequence (or gene) of interest.

B. Procedure

It involves four main stages which are as follows:

i. **Denaturation:** The double-stranded DNA is dissociated to a single-stranded DNA at 94°C (denaturing temperature).

ii. **Primer annealing:** The temperature is reduced to 50–60°C, then oligonucleotide primers attach to target DNA. This temperature is called annealing temperature and the process is known as annealing of primers.

iii. **DNA synthesis:** Polymerase enzyme derived from *Thermus aquaticus* (Taq) triggers the formation of new DNA strand from the free nucleotides. Taq polymerase and nucleotides are added in the tube for formation of new strands of DNA.

These three steps are repeated again and again, a process that is automated by the thermocycler or PCR machine. The products of first cycle become the template for the next cycle. After 20–30 cycles or more, an exponential increase in the amount of DNA occurs (Fig. 27.8).

iv. **Detection of amplified product:** Amplified DNA can be detected by gel electrophoresis.

C. Application of PCR

The PCR provides extremely rapid analysis (one day). PCR is a versatile tool useful in infectious, genetic or neoplastic diseases, in forensic investigations and in the examination of phylogenetic relationships in evolution. It has been applied in clinical laboratory for diagnosis of various infectious agents (Table 27.2).

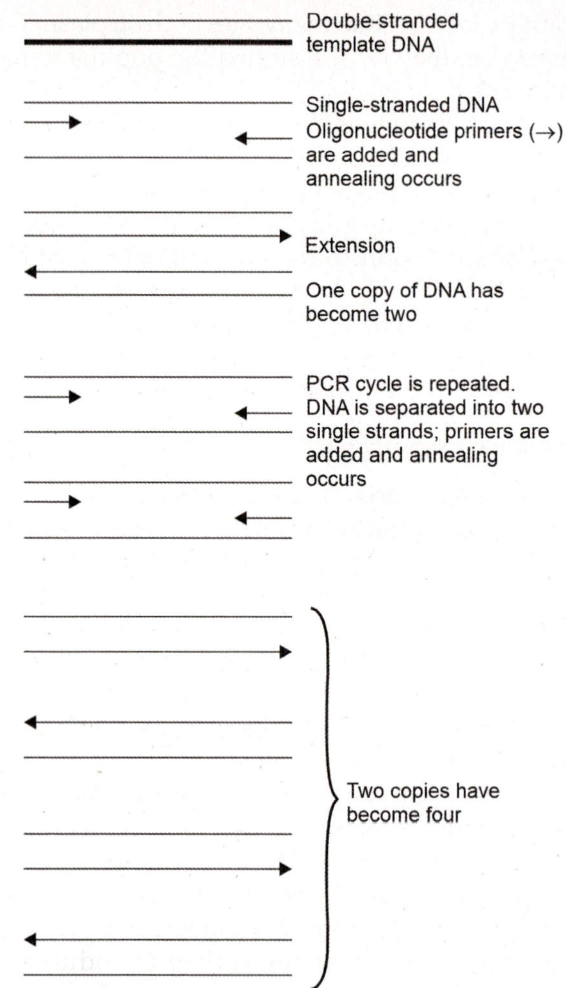

Fig. 27.8: Polymerase chain reaction

Table 27.2: Application of PCR in diagnosis of infectious agents
Bacteria: M. tuberculosis, Legionella pneumophila, Helicobacter pylori, Chlamydia trachomatis, Mycoplasma pneumoniae
Viruses: Cytomegalovirus, herpes simplex virus, hepatitis B virus, hepatitis C virus, coxsackie virus, measles virus, human immunodeficiency virus (HIV-1 and HIV-2), human papillomavirus, rotavirus, rubella virus, human herpes virus-6 (HHV-6), rhinovirus, parvovirus, adenovirus.
Fungi: Candida albicans, Cryptococcus neoformans, Pneumocystis carinii.
Protozoa: Toxoplasma gondii, Trypanosoma cruzi, Plasmodium spp.

Chapter 28

General Bacteriology V
(Microbial Pathogenicity)

Chapter Outline

- Microbes and Related Terms
- Infection
- Types of Infectious Diseases

The host–parasite relationship is determined by the interaction between host factors and the infecting microorganism. Health or disease depends on the equilibrium between the two.

I. MICROBES AND RELATED TERMS

A. Microbes

Microbes can be divided into saprophytes and parasites, based on their relationship to their hosts.

1. **Saprophytes:** These are free-living microbes that live on dead or decaying organic matter. They are generally unable to invade the living body. However, when host resistance is lowered, may cause infection.
2. **Parasite:** A parasite is microorganism which lives on a living host and derives nutrition from the host, without any benefit to the host.

B. Related Terms

1. **Commensals:** Commensals live in complete harmony with the host without causing any harm to it.
2. **Pathogen:** Microorganism capable of producing disease in the host is called pathogen.
3. **Opportunistic pathogens:** Some commensals or saprophytes can produce disease when host resistance is lowered.
4. **Pathogenicity:** It refers to the ability of a class of microbes to produce disease.
5. **Virulence:** It is the degree of pathogenicity of a microbe.

II. INFECTION

Infection: The lodgement and multiplication of a parasite in the body is known as infection. All infections do not invariably result in disease.

A. Types of Infection

1. **Primary infection:** Initial infection with a parasite in a host is termed primary infection.
2. **Reinfection:** Subsequent infection with the same parasite in the same host is called reinfection.
3. **Secondary infection:** When the body resistance is lowered by a pre-existing infectious disease, a new parasite sets up an infection, this is termed secondary infection.
4. **Cross infection:** When a patient already suffering from a disease acquires a new infection from another host or another external source, it is known as cross infection.
5. **Nosocomial infection:** Cross infection acquired in hospitals is called hospital-acquired or hospital associated or nosocomial infection.
6. **Iatrogenic infection:** An iatrogenic infection is defined as physician-induced infection resulting from drug therapy or investigative procedures.
7. **Subclinical infection:** When clinical symptoms of an infection are not apparent, it is known as subclinical infection.
8. **Latent infection:** Following infection, some parasites may remain in a latent or hidden form in host tissues and they proliferate and produce clinical disease when the host resistance is lowered. It is known as latent infection.

B. Transmission of Infection

There are three links in the chain of transmission of communicable diseases. These links include the reservoir, mode of transmission and the susceptible host.

1. Reservoir

It refers to any human being, animal, plant, soil or inanimate matter in which parasite normally lives, multiplies and depends primarily for its survival.

Sources of infection

These may be endogenous sources or exogenous sources.

i. Endogenous sources: Organisms of normal flora are usually non-pathogenic but occasionally they behave as pathogens outside their habitat. Viridans streptococci which are the normal flora of the mouth may cause infective endocarditis.

ii. Exogenous sources: Most of the infections are exogenous in origin. Exogenous sources include:

a. Human cases and carriers
b. Animals
c. Insects
d. Soil and water
e. Food.

a. **Human cases and carriers:** The commonest source of human infection is man himself. The parasite may originate from a patient or a carrier.
   - *Carrier:* A carrier is a person who harbours the pathogenic microorganism without suffering from its ill effects. Several types of carriers are known.
   - *Healthy carrier:* One who harbours the pathogen but has never suffered from the disease caused by that particular pathogen.
   - *Convalescent carrier:* One who has recovered from the disease but continues to harbour the pathogen in his body.

b. **Animals:** Many pathogens are capable of causing infection in both man and animal. Animals may, therefore, act as source of human infection. The infection in animals may be asymptomatic and these animals act as the reservoir of human infections. These are called reservoir hosts. Infectious diseases transmitted from animals to man are called zoonoses. Zoonotic diseases may be
   - *Bacterial:* Bovine tuberculosis, *Salmonella* food poisoning.
   - *Viral:* Rabies from dogs.
   - *Protozoal:* Leishmaniasis.
   - *Helminthic:* Hydatid disease from dogs.
   - *Fungal:* Dermatophytes from cats and dogs.

c. **Insects:** Blood sucking insects such as mosquitoes, ticks, mites, flies, fleas and lice may transmit a number of pathogens to man. The diseases so caused are called *arthropod-borne diseases*. Insects transmitting these pathogens are known as vectors.
   Besides acting as vectors, some insects may also act as reservoir hosts (e.g., ticks in relapsing fever).

d. **Soil and water:** Some pathogens may survive in the soil for very long periods. Spores of tetanus and gas gangrene bacilli remain viable in the soil for several decades and serve as the source of infection.
   Contamination of water with pathogenic microorganisms (e.g. *Vibrio cholerae*, hepatitis virus) may act as the source of infection.

e. **Food:** Contaminated food acts as a source of infection in cases of food poisoning, gastroenteritis, diarrhoea and dysentery.

2. Modes of Transmission

Pathogenic organisms can spread from one host to another by a variety of mechanisms.

i. **Contact:** Contact transmission may be direct or indirect.
   a. *Direct contact:* Sexually transmitted diseases (STD) such as syphilis, gonorrhoea and AIDS are acquired by direct contact.
   b. *Indirect contact:* It may be through the agency of fomites, which are inanimate objects such as clothing, toys, etc. which may be contaminated by a pathogen and act as a vehicle for its transmission.
   - *Contagious disease* is term used for the disease acquired by direct contact.
   - *Infectious disease* is the disease acquired by other modes such as inanimate objects. The distinction between contagious and infectious disease is now not generally employed.

ii. **Inhalation:** Respiratory infections such as common cold, influenza, whooping cough and tuberculosis are acquired by inhalation. These organisms are shed into the environment by patients in secretions from the nose or throat during sneezing, coughing or speaking.

iii. **Ingestion:** Intestinal infections like cholera, dysentery, food poisoning and most of the parasitic infections are acquired by ingestion of food or drink contaminated by pathogens. Food-borne infections occur mostly through carriers engaged in handling or preparation of food and contaminating the foodstuffs. The water supply may get contaminated with the faeces of the patients or carriers.

iv. **Inoculation:** Pathogens, in some instances, may be inoculated directly into the tissues of the host, for example, rabies virus is inoculated directly by bite of a rabid animal.

v. **Vectors:** Vectors are arthropods or other invertebrate hosts, e.g. mosquitoes, flies, fleas, ticks, mites and lice. Transmission by vector may be either mechanical or biological.

vi. **Transplacental:** Some pathogens can cross the placental barrier and infect the foetus *in utero*. This is known as vertical transmission. This may lead to abortion, miscarriage or stillbirth. Infection with rubella virus, especially in the first trimester of pregnancy, may lead to congenital malformations. Such infections are known as teratogenic infections.

vii. **Iatrogenic and laboratory infections:** If meticulous care in asepsis is lacking, certain infections like AIDS and hepatitis B may sometimes be transmitted during procedures such as injections, lumbar puncture, blood transfusion, dialysis and surgery. These are known as iatrogenic infections.

3. Susceptible Host

The infectious agent enters the body by one of the following routes: *Oral, respiratory, genitourinary, conjunctival* or *cutaneous*. This is known as portal of entry.

Incubation period: It is the time interval between the entry of infective agent and the onset of clinical features of the disease.

The outcome of an infection depends on interaction between microbial factors which predispose to pathogenicity and various host factors which contribute to resistance.

C. Factors Predisposing to Microbial Pathogenicity

Determinants of Virulence

i. **Adhesin:** The initial event in the pathogenesis is the attachment of the bacteria to body surfaces. The attachment is a specific reaction between surface receptors on the epithelial cells and adhesive structures on the surface of bacteria. These adhesive structures are named adhesins. Adhesins usually occur as fimbriae or fibrillae and pili or as colonisation factors.

ii. **Invasiveness:** This refers to the ability of an organism to spread within the host tissues after establishing infection. Highly invasive pathogens produce, spreading or generalised lesions (e.g. streptococcal infections), while less invasive pathogens cause localised lesions (e.g. staphylococcal abscess).

iii. **Antiphagocytic factors:** Macrophages and polymorphs play role in phagocytosis of microbes. There are certain factors which oppose phagocytosis for survival of bacteria. These factors are as follows:

a. *Capsule:* Capsule contributes to the virulence of bacteria by preventing phagocytosis. Non-capsulated variants usually exhibit low virulence.

b. *Streptococcal M protein:* The M protein present on the surface of group A streptococci binds both fibrinogen and fibrin to the bacterial cell wall, thus masking the bacterial receptors from complement.

c. *Cytotoxin:* Cytotoxins produced by certain bacteria interfere with chemotaxis or kill the phagocyte. *Staphylococcus aureus* produces haemolysins (can damage both RBCs and WBCs) and leukocidin (only WBCs are damaged).

d. *Bacterial surface antigens:* Vi antigen of *S. typhi* and K antigen of *E. coli* enable these bacteria to resist phagocytosis and lytic activity of complement.

iv. **Survival within the phagocyte:** Ingestion of a microbe by a phagocyte results in the formation of a phagolysosome by the fusion of phagosome with the lysosome. Any organism which interferes with the formation of phagolysosome can survive intracellularly.

v. **Bacterial toxins:** Bacteria produce two types of toxins, endotoxins and exotoxins (Table 28.1).

a. *Endotoxins:* They are lipopolysaccharide (LPS) in nature and form an integral part of the cell wall of Gram-negative bacteria. They are released from the bacterial surface by natural lysis of the bacteria or by the disintegration of the cell wall. They are heat stable. The toxicity of endotoxin depends on the lipid component (lipid A).

Table 28.1: Differences between exotoxins and endotoxins

Exotoxins	*Endotoxins*
1. Protein (polypeptides) MW 10,000 to 900,000	1. Lipopolysaccharide in nature
2. Heat labile (>60°C)	2. Heat stable
3. Actively secreted by living cells into medium	3. Form integral part of the cell wall; released only on disruption of bacterial cell
4. Highly antigenic; stimulates formation of antitoxin which neutralises toxin	4. Weakly antigenic; antitoxin is not formed but antibodies against polysaccharide are raised
5. Converted into toxoid by formaldehyde	5. Cannot be toxoided
6. Enzymic in action	6. No enzymic action.
7. Specific pharmacological effect for each exotoxin	7. Non-specific action of all endotoxins
8. Very high potency	8. Low potency
9. Highly specific for particular tissue, e.g. tetanus toxin for CNS	9. Non-specific in action
10. Do not produce fever in host	10. Usually produce fever
11. Produced mainly by Gram-positive bacteria and also by some Gram-negative bacteria	11. Produced by Gram-negative bacteria

They cannot be toxoided. They are poor antigens and the toxicity is not completely neutralised by the homologous antibodies. Massive Gram-negative septicaemias may cause the syndrome of endotoxic shock characterised by fever, leucopenia, thrombocytopenia, profound fall of blood pressure and circulatory collapse leading to death.

b. *Exotoxins:* They are heat labile proteins which are secreted by certain species of bacteria. They diffuse readily into the surrounding medium. They are highly potent even in minute amounts. Exotoxins can be converted into toxoids by treatment with formaldehyde. Toxoids lack toxicity but retain antigenicity and thus induce protective immunity when used as vaccines.

Exotoxins are highly antigenic and stimulate formation of antitoxin which neutralises toxin. They are highly specific for a particular tissue, e.g. tetanus toxin for CNS. They have specific pharmacological activities and do not produce fever in host. They are mainly produced by Gram-positive bacteria but may also be produced by certain Gram-negative bacteria such as *Vibrio cholerae* and enterotoxigenic *E. coli*.

vi. **Enzymes:** Some bacteria produce enzymes which directly damage host tissue.

a. *Proteases:* These enzymes cleave immunoglobulin IgA which protects at mucosal surfaces.

b. *Hyaluronidase:* It breaks down hyaluronic acid and helps in spread of infection, e.g. Streptococcus.

c. *Coagulase:* It causes deposition of fibrin around the bacteria and thus prevents phagocytosis, e.g. Staphylococcus.

III. TYPES OF INFECTIOUS DISEASES

Infectious diseases may be localised or generalised.

A. Localised

There is an acute inflammatory reaction at the site of invasion to arrest infection. When this process fails, the organisms spread via the lymph channels (lymphangitis) to regional lymph nodes (lymphadenitis) and then to bloodstream (bacteraemia) which leads to dissemination of organisms

B. Generalised

1. **Bacteraemia:** It is the circulation of bacteria in blood.
2. **Septicaemia:** It is the condition where bacteria circulate and multiply in the blood, form toxic products and cause high fever.
3. **Pyaemia:** It is the condition where three pyogenic bacteria produce septicaemia with multiple abscesses in internal organs, e.g. liver, spleen and kidney.

Chapter 29

Systemic Bacteriology I
(Staphylococci, Streptococci, *Diplococcus pneumoniae*, Neisseria)

Chapter Outline

STAPHYLOCOCCI

Morphology: Structure

Staphylococci are Gram-positive spherical cells of about 0.8–1.0 micron in diameter, and are arranged in irregular clusters, which is most evident when super is made form solid media.

Cultural Characteristics

They grow readily on most of the media under aerobic and micro-aerophilic conditions. The optimum temperature is 37°C but pigment is formed best at 20°C. Colonies on nutrient agar are found smooth, glasening with pigment varying with the type of staphylococci.

Staphylococci are widely distributed in nature. They are present in air, water, milk, sewage and exist as members of normal flora of human skin, respiratory and gastrointestinal tract. Some of them are non-pathogenic while others produce a variety of suppurative conditions.

Classification

S. aureus and *S. intermedius* are coagulase positive. All other staphylococci are coagulase negative. They are salt tolerant and often haemolytic. Identification requires biotype analysis. Depending upon the pigment production they are classified as follows:

Staphylococcus aureus—Golden yellow pigment
Citreous—Lemon yellow pigment
Albus—Porcelain white

Pigment is not produced anaerobically or in broth. The ability to ferment sugars varies greatly according to strain employed. Mannitol is usually fermented by aureus and some strains of albus which are pathogenic.

Toxins and Enzymes

Under suitable conditions, pathogenic strains produce a number of toxins.

1. **Exotoxins:** A filtrate substance which is lethal on injection to animals, causes necrosis of skin and demonstrated presence of haemolysins (alpha, beta or gamma type). These haemolysins are antigenically distinct in types and produce lysis of RBCs of sheep and rabbit whereas beta lysis only sheep cells.
2. **Leucotoxins:** Acts on WBCs causes agglutination or kills them on exposure.
3. **Enterotoxin:** It is thermostable in presence of carbohydrates and high concentration of CO_2.
4. **Coagulase:** An enzayme, which clots citrated or oxalated human or rabbit plasma, it is not antigenic. Opacity in medium containing egg yolk—many coagulase—positive staphylococci when grown in glucose egg yolk broth give a dense opacity due to lipolytic (lecithinse) activity. This effect can be neutralised by staphylococcal antiserum. The reaction is given by a high proportion of human stains out only by a few animal strains.

Common lesions: Resulting from staphylococcal infection include abscesses, furuncle, osteomyelitis, empyemema, sinusitis, otitis media, bronchopneumonia, meningitis and in extreme cases bacteraemia and disseminated abscess in most of the organs.

Laboratory Procedure

- **Specimens:** May vary depending on lesions surface swabs, pus, blood, sputum and cerebrospinal fluid. Stain smear—typical morphological appearance, but cannot distinguish between saprophytic and pathogenic organisms.
- **Cultures:** Are studied on nutrient agar for pigment production and blood agar for haemolysis.
- **Biochemical reaction:** For fermentation of mannitol.
- **Coagulase test:** A broth culture of staphylococci is mixed with citrated human or rabbit plasma (1.10 dilution) and incubated at 37°C. A tube with

sterile broth added to plasma is kept as a control clotting occur within three hours in experimental tube.

- **Slide method:** Put a drop of human plasma on the slide on a drop of thick suspension of the organism—agglutination occurs in 1 minute.
- **Drug sensitivity:** Exhibits great variability in respect with sensitivity sulfonamides and antibiotics. Penicillin resistant strains are due to production of enzyme penicillinase.

A pathogenic strain produces golden yellow pigments, gives positive phosphatase test, ferments mannitol, haemolyses RBCs or produces coagulase out at all these tests generally coagulase test is applied for differentiating pathogenic from non-pathogenic staphylococci.

STREPTOCOCCI

Streptococci are arranged in long or short chains and are widely distributed in nature, some are members of normal human flora, others are associated with pathogenic disease.

Morphology

The individual cocci are spherical or oval 0.7 to 1.0 μm in diameter forming chains of varying length depending on environmental factor. They are Gram-positive. Virulent strains may show capsule, if examined within 2–3 hours of growth in serum broth.

Cultural Characteristics

The growth tends to be poor on solid media unless enriched with blood or tissue fluids. Most of the strains are aerobic and facultatively anaerobic, but some strains are obligate anaerobes. Optimum temperature of culture is 37°C. But enterococci grow well between 51° and 45°C. In broth, they give rise to granule deposit. The colonies on blood agar are small, round, semi-transparent and give rise to varying zone of haemolysis favours development of haemolysis.

1. **Beta-haemolysis:** Colonies are surrounded by sharply defined clear, colourless zone of haemolysis, 2–4 mm in diameter, well-developed after 18–24 hours of incubation (*Streptococcus pyogenes*).
2. **Alpha haemolysis:** Colonies are surrounded by greenish discolouration 1–2 mm in size and partial zone of haemolysis. It is well-developed after 24–28 hours of incubation (*Streptococcus viridans*).
3. **Gamma haemolysis:** The colonies develop in blood agar without any change in surrounding medium (*Streptococcus faecalis*).

Resistance and biochemical properties: With the exception of group D (enterococci) which may resist heating at 60°C for 30 minutes, the other varieties are readily by exposure for ½ hour to 55°C, addition of bile does not lyse the growth of streptococci in broth. They ferment most of the sugars with production of acid only. Group A streptococci are more sensitive to bacitracin than other haemolytic streptococci.

Antigenic structures: They possess a complex antigenic structure and have been divided in 15 serological groups and sub-groups (A–Q no. group designated I or J).

Group antigens: Group specific "C" carbohydrate is immunologically distinct for each group. This carbohydrate substance forms the basis of serologic grouping (precipitation reaction) of Lancefield classification.

Typing antigens: M and T antigens (proteins) have been isolated M antigen is associated with virulence and organism producing mucoid colonies, it is present in group A streptococci, and is type specific.

T antigens: It is heat labile, is prepared by proteolytic digestion, is type specific, but not related with virulence.

TOXINS AND ENZYMES

1. **Streptokinase (fibrinolysin):** An active proteolytic enzyme which digests fibrin.
2. **Streptodornase:** An enzyme which depolymerizes deoxyribonucleoprotein and thus lowers viscosity.
3. **Hyaluronidase (spreading factors):** An enzyme. which splits hyalurenic acid, an important constituent of ground substance.
4. **Erythrogenic toxin:** A soluble toxin, heat resistant at 60°C, but destroyed 100°C is responsible for rash that occurs in scarlet fever. The toxin is antigenic and forms the basis of Dick's test and Schultz Charlton reactions.
5. Haemolysins of two types, O and S haemolysins have been described, responsible for giving characteristic haemolysis on blood agar O—is oxygen labile, but reactivated by reduction S—is oxygen stable and soluble in serum and it responsible for β-haemolysis.

Pathogenesis: In addition to causing disease directly which in general is the nature of suppurative inflammation streptococci, also produce disease indirectly by setting up the state of hypersensitivity. Acute rheumatic fever and glomerulonephritis are well-established examples of this and are known as post-streptococci diseases or post-streptococcal infection syndromes.

Group A: Haemolytic strains give rise to a numerous pyogenic and septicaemic infection in man, like erysipelas, puerperal fever and septic infection of wounds. They also produce:

a. *Local infections* like sore throat and other upper respiratory tract infections, impetigo and may act as secondary invaders in viral infections.
b. *Bacterial endocarditis:* Streptococcus haemolytic produces acute and streptoviridans produce sub-acute

type. Genitourinary tract infection may be produced, especially by anaerobic streptococci.

Laboratory Diagnosis

Direct smear: Direct smear is prepared from pus or throat swab and Gram staining is done and we look for Gram +ve cocci in chains.

Culture: Culture is done on blood agar. We get pinpoint colonies producing β-haemolysis on blood agar. Gram staining should be done with culture.

Bile solubility: Inulin fermentation (+); catalase and oxidase (negative).

Drug sensitivity: Optochin sensitivity (+); (*Streptococcus pneumoniae*).

Other tests

1. **ASO test:** ASO titer can raise due to previous infection.
2. **Dick test:** This is a skin test which is used for the diagnosis of scarlet fever. Redness or swelling after 24 hours at injection site indicates Dick test is +ve for scarlet fever.

DIPLOCOCCUS PNEUMONIAE (PNEUMOCOCCI)

Diplococcus pneumoniae is also called *Streptococcus pneumoniae*. These bacteria are found in mouth, nose, upper respiratory tract. Virulent form of these bacteria produces disease.

Morphology: This is oval-shaped, gram +ve cocci arranged in pairs. Capsulated, non-motile, non-sporing.

Culture: Pneumococcus is aerobe and facultative anaerobes. Optimum temperature for its growth is 37°C and optimum pH is 7.4–7.6. They cannot grow on ordinary media. Enriched media, i.e. blood agar and chocolate agar is used for its growth. Growth can be enhanced with 5–10% CO_2. On blood agar a haemolysis is produced by bacteria. Capsule is not developed in artificial culture, it develops only in human being and animals.

Bio-chemical reaction: Bile soluble, catalase –ve, oxidase –ve, ferment inulin.

Toxins and virulent factor: Haemolysin and leucocidin and capsular polysaccharides.

Optochin sensitivity: Pneumococci are sensitive to optochin.

Antigenic structure: The capsular polysaccharide (SSS specific soluble substance) is immunologically distinct for different types of pneumococci and forms the basis of serological typing.

Quellung reaction: When pneumococci are fixed with specific antiserum capsule swells markedly, the reaction is useful for quick identification and typing of the organism.

Pathogenicity: Lobar pneumonia, bronchopneumonia and meningitis and other infections.

Lab diagnosis: Sputum, throat swab, CSF are collected aseptically. Smear is prepared from morbid material with cotton wrapped stick. Gram staining is done after drying and Gram +ve capsulated pneumococci are looked for.

NEISSERIA

These are arranged in pairs. Meningococcus and Gonococcus are pathogenic.

Neisseria meningitidis

Morphology: These are Gram –ve diplococci arranged in pairs. Its size is 0.6–0.8 p. There is a thick capsule in each pair. These are non-sporing and non-flagellated. In human body, this is present intracellular and extracellular. Sometimes, microcapsule may be demonstrated by Quellung reaction.

Culture: These bacteria do not grow on simple culture media. So, enriched media (Chocolate agar) is used for this bacteria. Optimum temperature is 36°C and optimum pH is 7.4–7.6. These are aerobes and grow better in presence of mild carbondioxide. After 24 hours bacterial colonies are pinhead size and transparent and produce a haemolysis around the colonies.

Biochemical reaction: Meningococcus ferments glucose and maltose with the production of acid only, oxidase +ve, catalase +ve.

Pathogenicity: Infection occurs in nasal cavity and bacteria through cribriform plate enter in brain with the help of olfactory nerves. Fever, headache, neck stiffness and, vomiting occurs in patient. Sometimes, infection enters in blood and cause *Meningococcus septicaemia*.

Laboratory diagnosis: Direct examination of CSF: Direct smear is prepared from CSF and Gram staining is done. Gram –ve diplococci seen extracellular and intracellular.

Neisseria gonorrhoeae

Morphology: Gram –ve diplococcus and is bean-shaped. This is non-capsulated, non-motile and non-sporing. In human body, this is present extracellular and intracellular.

Culture: These bacteria do not grow on ordinary media. Enriched media like chocolate agar is used for its growth. Thayer Martin selective media is used for its growth. Chocolate agar is present in this medium. This is an aerobe. In the presence of 5–10% carbon dioxide, this grows better. Optimum temperature for its growth is 36°C and optimum pH is 7.4–7.6.

Biochemical reaction: Oxidase +ve, catalase +ve, ferment maltose, glucose with production of acid only.

Pathogenicity: Gonococcus produces gonorrhoea disease which is sexually transmitted disease. In male, these bacteria produce uretheritis, prostatitis and epididymo-orchitis. In female, these bacteria produce uretheritis, vaginitis and cervicitis. In newborn child these bacteria produce ophthalmia neonatorum disease. Infection is transferred to child from infected mother. In young girls, vulvovaginitis can occur.

Laboratory diagnosis: For the laboratory diagnosis, uretheral discharge is collected. In female, cervical swab is also collected. Direct smear is prepared from discharge and Gram straining is done. We look for Gram –ve diplococci which can be extracellular and intracellular and typical colonies are confirmed by biochemical reaction.

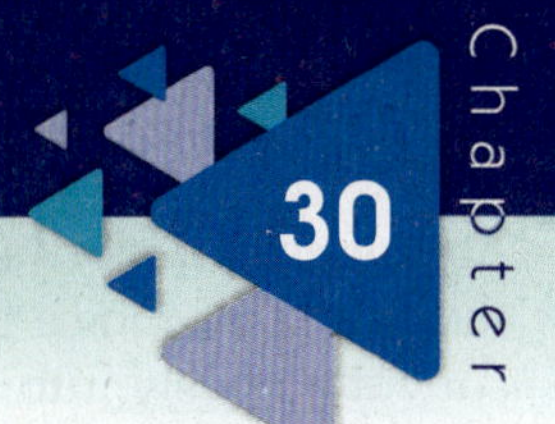

Systemic Bacteriology II
(*Corynebacterium diphtheriae*; Clostridia, *Bacillus anthracis*—Anthrax)

Chapter Outline

- Corynebacteria
- Clostridia
- *Clostridium botulinum*
- Genus Bacillus
- Anthrax

CORYNEBACTERIA

The genus Corynebacterium comprises species which are pathogenic to man and animals as well as others occurring saprophytes which are also known as diphtheroids.

Examples: Pathogenic to man and animal—*C. diphtheriae, C. ovis, C. murium, C. pyogenes.*

Non-pathogenic (diptheroids): C. erosis, C. acnes, C. hofmanni.

Corynebacterium diphtheriae

Morphology and staining reaction: Typical form is evident in a film prepared from 24 hours culture on Loeffler's serum or in a smear from a case of diphtheriae. The organism is long, slender, slightly curved with rounded, some what swollen ends. It stains uniformally with methylene blue, when stained by Albert's or Neisser's method metachromatic granules are demonstrated. Arrangement of bacilli in a film is characteristic. The organisms tend to be arranged at angles to each other like V or letters. Combination of these resembles Chinese letters. This is due to mode of division (one and remaining attached). Pleomorphism which is a characteristic feature of the species diphtheriae bacilli are Gram-positive, but running reaction is variable (Table 30.1).

Cultural characteristic: Loeffler's serum is the medium of choice showing abundant growth within 18–24 hours. Colonies are discrete, circular, convex, slightly raised, opaque and cream coloured. The organisms are classified by morphological appearances of colonies on blood tellurite agar medium (chocolate tellurite agar). Colonies acquire a greyish, black appearance on this media.

Biochemical reactions: Dextrose, maltose and sucrose are commonly used for differentiating species of corynebacterium. *C. diphtheriae* ferments first two, *C. xerosis* ferments all and *C. hofmanni* none, no species produces gas. Within diphtheriae bacilli, gravis ferments, starch, glycogen and dextrin; mitis and intermedius have no action on starch and glycogen and irregular action on dextrin (Hiss serum water is employed for study of these tests).

Toxin production: *C. diphtheriae* produces a powerful exotoxin, which is heat labile and antigenic. This can be inverted by suitable treatment with formalin into toxoid.

Table 30.1: Differentiating characteristics of diphtheriae

	Gravis	*Intermedius*	*Mitis*
Morphology	Short rods, staining uniformly with a few or on granules show some degree of pleomorphism	Long, irregular IP barred rods with poor granulation pleomorphism present	Long, curved, pleomorphic rods with prominent metachromatic granules
Colony on blood tellurite agar	Within 2–3 days, colonies are 2–3 mm in diameter, greyish black colour, raised, darker centre and paler periphery, edges crenated with radial striation (daisy head)	Colonies small uniform, 1–2 mm, a little increase in size with incubation, centre greyish black and raised	Colonies variable size 2–4 mm, circular, convex, darker than gravis
Biochemical reaction	Ferments starch and glycogen	Does not ferment starch and glycogen.	Some as in intermedius
Haemolysis pathogenicity	Occasionally Invariably virulent	No invariable virulent	Usually virulent, but avirulent strains are oncounteral.

In this state, it is no longer toxic, but retains its antigenic character.

Pathogenicity for laboratory animals: Guinea pig is the animal of choice for virulence, test when inoculated subcutaneously into the flank with virulent culture or toxin filtrate a soft oedematous swelling appears at the site within 12–18 hours and animal usually dies within 18–96 hours. Postmortem shows enlarged, congested dark red adrenals effusion to pleural and pericardial cavities congested kidneys, and edematous lungs.

Pathogenicity: Diphtheria disease is produced by *C. diphtheriae*. Sometimes, patient becomes symptomatic. Diphtheria involves tonsils, pharynx, fauces, larynx, nose, uvula. It destroys tissue and create a membrane at the infection site. Cardiovascular system and central nervous system is effected by this membrane.

Laboratory diagnosis: For diagnosis throat swab is collected. From throat swab and Gram stain, Neisser's stain and Albert stain is done. Culture is done on Leoffler's serum slope, blood tellurite agar and blood agar.

Schick test: A skin test based on the fact that diphtheria toxin when injected produces inflammatory reaction unless neutralized by antitoxin. A marked local reaction indicates susceptibility of individual (Schick positive) and should be immunized. Absence of reaction indicates adequate amount of antitoxin present (Schick negative), such individuals do not require immunization.

Active immunization: Formal toxoid, alum precipitated toxoid (APT) or toxoid antitoxin floccules are used.

Laboratory diagnosis: Swabs from suspected lesions are examined by (1) smear, (2) cultural methods: These serve to confirm the clinical findings, however, treatment must never be delayed till diagnosis is established if clinical picture is strongly suggestive for diphtheriae.

Toxigenicity test: *In vitro* (Elek's gel precipitation) test. Loopful of organism is inoculated on half of agar gel plate. The other half is inoculated with known toxigenic strain which acts as a control.

A rectangular filter paper strip dipped in diphtheria antitoxin is placed at right angle to lines of stroke and the plate is incubated for 48 hours.

Antitoxin diffusing from the paper reacts with the toxin diffusing from the organisms and develops lines of precipitates radiating from the margin of the paper to periphery.

CLOSTRIDIA

Morphology: These bacteria are Gram +ve bacilli. They are spore bearers and obligate anaerobes. On the basis of disease production, this is classified as follows:

- *Clostridium tetani* (tetanus),
- *Clostridium botulinum* (food poisoning),
- *Clostridium welchii* (*Clostridium perfringens*): It produces gas gangrene.

Clostridium tetani

Cl. tetani is the causative agent of tetanus. It is widely distributed in soil and intestine of man and animals.

Morphology: It is a Gram-positive, slender bacillus (measuring 4–8 µm × 0.5 µm) with spherical, terminal spores giving the bacillus the characteristic drumstick appearance. It is non-capsulated and motile (except *Cl. tetani* type VI) with peritrichate flagella.

Classification: Ten serological types (types I to X) of *Cl. tetani* have been recognised based on type specific flagellar (H) antigens. Type VI strains are non-flagellated.

Toxins Produced by Clostridia

i. *Clostridium tetani* produce hemolysin and neurotoxin toxins.
ii. *Clostridium perfringens* produces at least 12 distinct toxins besides many other enzymes. The 4 major toxins—alpha, beta, epsilon and iota are responsible for pathogenicity.
iii. *Clostridium botulinum* produces powerful exotoxins responsible for pathogenicity.

Pathogenicity: *Clostridium tetani* produce a serious disease tetanus. *Clostridium botulinum* produces botulism which is a type of food poisoning. *Clostridium welchi* produces gas gangrene and food poisoning.

Biochemical reactions: *Clostridium welchii* ferment glucose, maltose, lactose and sucrose with the production of acid and gas. Indole is negative. MR^{+ve}, VP^{-ve}, H_2S^{+ve}, gelatin-liquified. Non-motile, capsulted in animal body. Special media is Ellner's broth is used for sporulation for *Clostridium perfringens*.

Clostridium botulinum ferment glucose, maltose with acid and gas. $Indole^{-ve}$, $Gelatinase^{+ve}$.

Laboratory diagnosis: Laboratory diagnosis of *Clostridium tetani* is clinical. Laboratory helps to confirm the diagnosis. For laboratory diagnosis, swab is collected from infected wound. Diagnosis is based on demonstration of bacillus or toxin in food or faeces. In early stages, toxin may be detected from patient's blood. Gram staining and culture is done. Colonies are identified by Gram staining and biochemical reaction. For laboratory diagnosis of *Clostridium botulinum* stool sample, part of vomitus and part of remaining food is collected. These bacteria are demonstrated after doing Gram staining and culture. For *Clostridium welchii* swab is collected from local area, pus swab is also collected and necrosed tissue piece is collected. Cooked meat broth, blood agar and lactose egg yolk medium is used for culture. Negler's reaction is useful test for *C. welchii* (Fig. 30.1).

CLOSTRIDIUM BOTULINUM

Clostridium botulinum causes a severe form of food poisoning named botulism. It is a widely distributed

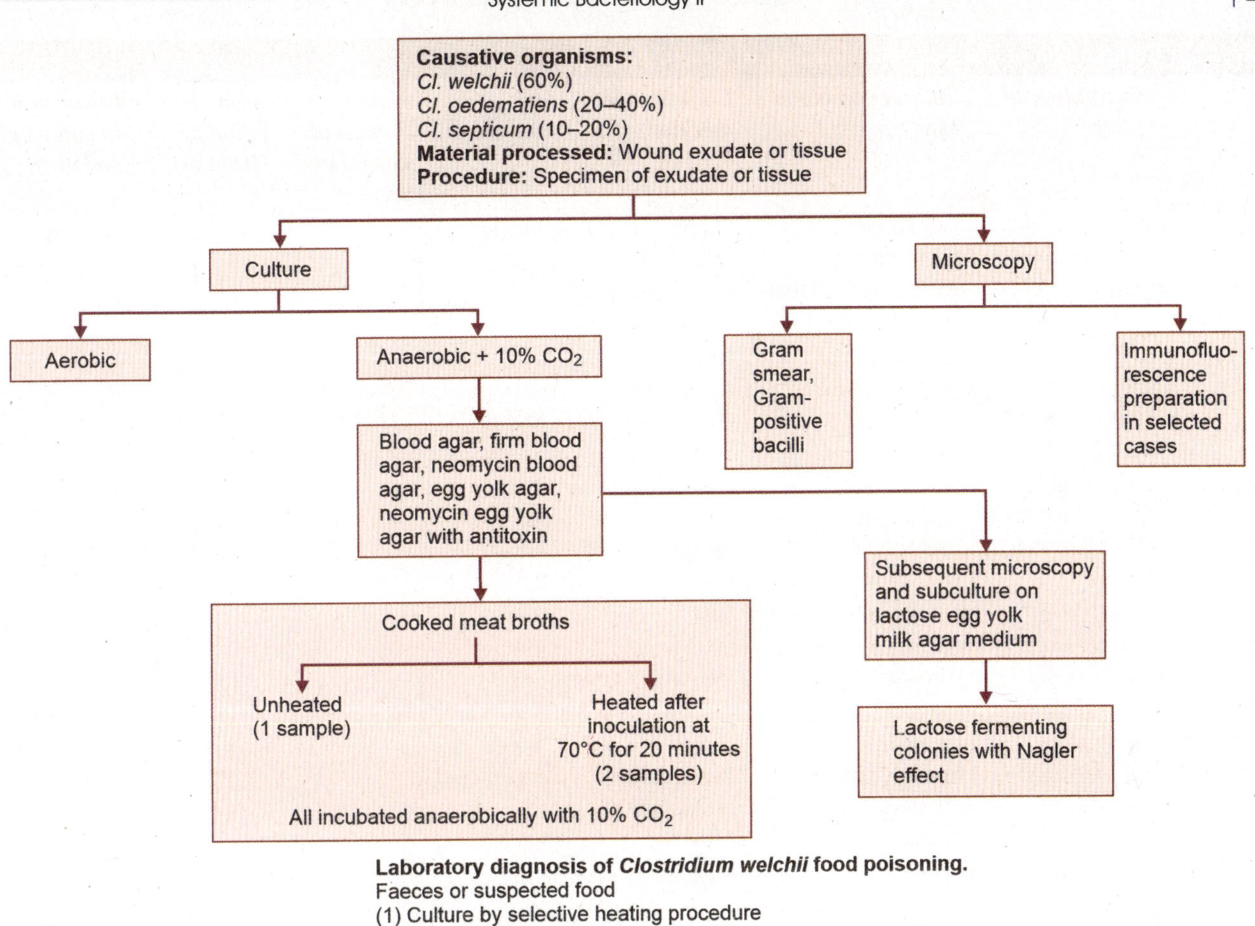

Fig. 30.1: Laboratory diagnosis of gas gangrene

saprophyte and is found in soil, animal manure, vegetables and sea mud.

Morphology: It is a Gram-positive, non-capsulated bacillus about 5 μm × 1 μm, motile by peritrichate flagella and produces subterminal, oval, bulging spores.

Culture: It is a strict anaerobe and can grow on ordinary media. Optimum temperature is 35°C. Commonly used media are blood agar and Robertson cooked meat broth. Colonies are large, irregular, semitransparent, with fimbriate border. On blood agar, haemolysis around the colonies is observed.

Resistance: The spores are highly resistant, and can withstand heat for several hours at 100°C and for up to 10 minutes at 120°C. They are also resistant to radiation.

Classification: Eight types—A, B, C1, C2, D, E, F and G have been identified on the basis of their antigenically distinct toxins.

Toxin: *Cl. botulinum* forms a powerful exotoxin. The toxin differs from other exotoxins in that it is not released during the life of the bacterium. It is produced intracellularly and appears in the medium on autolysis of the cell. The toxin has been isolated as a pure crystalline protein with a MW 70,000. It has a lethal dose for mice 0.000,000,033 mg and a lethal dose for humans is probably one microgram. It is a neurotoxin and acts slowly, therefore, takes several hours to kill. Botulinum toxin is the most toxic substance known so far.

Preformed toxin in food is destroyed by boiling for 20 minutes. It is a good antigen and can be neutralised specifically by its antitoxin.

The toxin acts by blocking the production or release of acetylcholine at synapses and neuromuscular junctions. Death occurs due to respiratory failure.

The comparison of various characteristic features of *Clostridium* species are shown in Table 30.2.

GENUS BACILLUS

It consists of number of spore bearing, Gram-positive rods often occurring in long chains. They are widely distributed; found in water, air, soil milk, and dust. Most of the organisms are non-pathogenic; the important ones being—*B. subtilis*., *B. mesentericus*, *B. mycoides*, *B. megaterfum*, *B. anthracis* is the only pathogenic member which may give rise to disease (anthrax) in man, cattles, sheep and other animals.

Table 30.2: Comparison of characteristic features of *Clostridium* sp.

	Morphology in culture	*Colonies on blood agar*	*Cooked meat medium (CRCM)*	*Milk medium*	*Lique-faction of coagulated serum*	*Fermen-tation of GLSMSa*	*Pathogenicity to guinea pigs and mice*
Tetani	Slender bacilli with round terminal spores	Transparent, haemolytic, swarming with feathery projection	Slight digestion, blackening and pungent odour	Unaltered	–	– – – – –	Tetanus produced +
Welchii	Large, thick stubby bacilli, Spores usually absent	Large, circular, regular outline, haemolytic	Gas, no digestion, meat reddened	Acid, gas, rapid clotting	–	+ + + + –	+
Septicum	Pleomorphic short with central or subterminal spores	Transparent, projection, haemolytic, swarming	Gas, no digestion meat reddened	Acid, gas, slow clotting	–	+ + – + +	+
Oede-matiens	Large, Gram-positive rods, central or sub-terminal spores	Translucent convex, haemolytic, spreading	Gas, no digestion, meat reddened	Slow clotting	–	+ – – + –	+
Botulinum	Large, pleo-morphic bacilli, oval spores, subterminal	Large, irregular, feathery projections opaque, pseudo-haemolytic	Gas, Types vary in proteolytic activity	Casein precipitated No digestion	±	+ – – + –	+

GLSMSa—G = Glucose, L = Lactose, S = Sucrose, M = Maltose, Sa = Salioin

Bacillus Anthracis

Bacillus anthrax are Gram-positive bacilli from family Bacillaceae, causing anthrax.

Structure and classification: Bacillus species are rod-shaped, endospore-forming aerobic or facultatively anaerobic, Gram-positive bacteria; in some species cultures may turn Gram-negative with age. The spores are resistant to heat, cold, radiation, desiccation, and disinfectants. *Bacillus anthracis* needs oxygen to sporulate; this constraint has important consequences for epidemiology and control. *In vivo*, *B. anthracis* produces a polypeptide (polyglutamic acid) capsule that protects it from phagocytosis.

It is an aerobe and grows profusely on ordinary media curved (Medusa-head) hair-locked appearance of colonies on nutrient agar, and inverted for three growth in gelatin stab are important characteristic. It is non-haemolytic, in contrast to other member of this group which are haemolytic, fermentation reaction are not characteristic.

In the vegetative from bacilli are killed at the usual temperature, however, spores are very resistant. They can withstand a temperature of 100°C for 15 minutes. They are killed by dry heat at 150°C or 1 hour and in autoclave at 120°C for 15 minutes.

They appear to be two main antigens: (a) Protein-like substance present in capsule, (b) polysaccharide substance present in the body of the organisms. Specific precipitin for both anitigens are present in serum of animals injected with capsulated organisms, Ascoli's thermo-precipitation test is based on this (extracts of infected tissue show precipitate formation when layered over with immune serum).

ANTHRAX

Anthrax is a primary disease of sheep, cattle and horses, the spores entering the body through the mouth infection of man is uncommon in man and spores enter through a wound in the skin or are inhaled, in the former case a malignant pustule" results, and in the latter a "pneumonia". The inflammation is haemorrhagic and oedema is marked feature.

Pathogenesis: The virulence factors of *B. anthracis* are its capsule and three-component toxin, both encoded on plasmids. *Bacillus cereus* produces numerous enzymes and aggressins. The principal virulence factors are a necrotizing enterotoxin and a potent haemolysin (cereolysin). Emetic food poisoning probably results from the release of emetic factors from specific foods by bacterial enzymes.

Clinical manifestations: Anthrax is caused by *Bacillus anthracis*. Humans acquire the disease directly from contact with infected herbivores or indirectly via their products. The clinical forms include:

1. Cutaneous anthrax (eschar with oedema), from handling infected, material (this accounts for more than 95% of cases);

2. intestinal anthrax, from eating infected meat; and
3. pulmonary anthrax, from inhaling spore-laden dust.

***Bacillus cereus* causes two distinct food poisoning syndromes:** A rapid-onset emetic syndrome characterised by nausea and vomiting, and a slower-onset diarrhoeal syndrome.

Diagnosis: Cutaneous anthrax is diagnosed on the basis of the characteristic papule (early) or eschar (later) with extensive surrounding edema, backed by a history of exposure to animals or their products. Diagnosis is confirmed by observation of characteristic encapsulated bacilli in polychrome methylene blue-stained smears of blood, exudate, lymph, cerebrospinal fluid, etc. and/or by culture. Other bacillus infections are diagnosed by culture of the bacteria.

Laboratory diagnosis: Material consists of fluid from lesions, pus, sputum, blood, infected tissues or other materials like brushes, wool and hair.

Control: Control in animals is essential for control in humans. In endemic areas, animals that die suddenly should be handled cautiously and livestock should be vaccinated annually. A human vaccine is available for individuals in high-risk occupations.

Anthrax: Anthrax is readily treated with antibiotics (e.g. penicillin, tetracycline, chloramphenicol, gentamicin, or erythromycin).

Systemic Bacteriology III

(Salmonella, Shigella, *Escherichia coli*, Vibrio, Klebsiella)

Chapter Outline

- Salmonella
- Shigella (Dysentery Group of Bacilli)
- *Escherichia coli*
- Vibrio
- Klebsiella

1. SALMONELLA

Members of Salmonella group are essentially pathogenic to man and animals. Two main types of Salmonella infection may be produced in man: (a) Continuous fever of the type of typhoid (predominance of septicaemic over intestinal symptoms and (b) acute gastroenteritis of food poisoning type (predominance of intestinal over septicaemic symptoms). Sometime localised manifestations of disease in meninges, bones, joints or other situations may also be encountered. *Salmonella typhi* causes typhoid fever. *Salm. paratyphoid* A, B and C cause paratyphoid fever, *Salm. enteritis*, *Salm. typhimurium*, *Salm. cholera* suis and a large number of other organisms may cause acute gastroenteritis (Salmonella food poisoning).

Morphology and staining reactions: The shapes, size, structure, arrangements and staining reactions of the organisms do not differ from one another and with the other members of Enterobacteriae. The usual length is 2–3 µm and width 0.6 µm. They are Gram-negative and motile.

Cultural characteristics: The members of this group grow readily on ordinary nutrient media. In broth, smooth organisms to uniform turbidity. Resistance of Salmonella group of organisms to different chemicals is utilised for preparation of selective media.

Brilliant green and malachite green: In suitable concentration inhibits growth of *Bacterium coli* and dysentery group of organisms.

Sodium tetrathionate favours growth of Salmonella. Sodium deoxycholate in presence of certain other substances inhibits growth of coliform, but not dysentery and salmonella organisms.

Culture: This is an aerobe. Optimum temperature for its growth is 37°C. This can grow on ordinary media. These bacteria produce rounded, convex and whitish colonies on nutrient agar. These bacteria produce non-lactose fermenting colonies on MacConkey agar. These bacteria produce pale colonies on DCA. DCA and Wilson and Blayer are selective media. Bile broth, selenite F broth and Tetrathionate broth liquid media is also used for its growth.

Biochemical reaction

i. *Salmonella typhi* ferment glucose and mannitol with the production of acid only no gas.
ii Indole –ve, MR +ve. VP –ve.

Antigenic structure of Salmonella: Three antigens:

1. **"O" antigen (somatic antigen):** It is body antigen.
2. **"H" antigen:** It is flagellar antigen.
3. **Vi antigen (virulent):** It is on covering layer on the outside cell wall.

Various serological tests for identifications of organisms and the classification of Salmonella group is based on antigenic structure. As these organisms are motile both flagellar (H) and somatic (O) antigens are present. A formalized suspension of motile organisms demonstrates. H and alcoholic suspension O antigens only. H antigen in many organisms is diphasic, and exists in phase 1; phase 2; phase 1 shows more specific and phase 2 shows less specific antigens. In addition to H and O, some strains of typhoid bacilli may contain a heat-labile somatic antigen called Vi antigen. However, a considerable antigenic variation may be met within this group further, sharing of antigenic structure is a common feature.

Pathogenicity: Salmonella produce various diseases. Enteric fever is important. Food poisoning and gastroenteritis are also produced by these bacteria.

Laboratory diagnosis: For laboratory diagnosis following methods are used:

- *Blood culture:* For typhoid and septicaemia, blood culture is an important method (to be done in first week of onset). In suspected cases of typhoid, 5% bile broth can be used. Smear is prepared from culture and gram staining is done.

- *Stool culture:* In first week of illness, stool culture method is used for diagnosis of Salmonella. Stool sample is collected in Petri dishes and enrichment media like tetrathionate broth is inoculated.

From this, subculture is done on DCA, MacConkey agar and Wilson and Blayer medium.

Widal test: Widal test is positive, preferably after 6–7 days of illness. In this test, we detect antibodies against antigen O and H, Widal test is done by two methods: (i) Slide method, (ii) tube method.

Diagnosis of typhoid fever:

1. **Blood culture in bile broth:** Best results are obtained in the first week of injection. The blood clot (after obtaining the serum aseptically for widal reaction) can be cultivated in bile of glucose broth.
2. **Widal test:** It is generally positive after 10th day.
   a. *O agglutinins:* A titre less than 1:50 is present in normal persons. A titre above 1:100 is considered significant. It rarely goes above 1:250. A rising titre is always diagnostic of typhoid fever.
   b. *H agglutinins:* Diagnosis by H titre is only useful in non-inoculated persons or in those who show rising titre on a subsequent examination.
   c. *Viagglutinins:* A positive even 1:10 titre is diagnostic of typhoid fever provided the person is not a carrier.
3. **Stool and urine culture:** They give best results in third week. Stool gives much better results than the urine culture.

2. SHIGELLA (DYSENTERY GROUP OF BACILLI)

Dysentery may be defined as diarrhoea accompanied by passage of blood and mucous in the stool. It is usually classified into amoebic and bacillary type. Shigella are the cuasative agents of bacillary dysentery. There are several strains of dysentery bacilli which are pathogenic to man. Inspite of much work no satisfactory basis of classification is available. A combination of biochemical and antigenic structure is utilised. The important pathogenic members of this group are *Sh. shiga, Sh. flexneri, Sh. sonnei, Sh. boydii, Sh. schmitzi*. The dysentery produced by *Shigella shiga* tends to be most severe and that by sonnei the least severe. The organisms tend to remain localised in the large intestine and may sometimes reach mesenteric lymph nodes, but bacteriaemia is not produced. The organisms produce potent endotoxin, but *Sh. shiga* and some strains of *Sh. schmitzi* produce powerful exotoxins (neuro-enteric-toxin). The exotoxin is heat labile and antigenic.

Morphological and cultural characteristics: Dysentery bacilli are non-motile and Gram-negative, measuring about 2–3 μm by 0.5 μm. They grow readily on ordinary media. These are aerobes and facultatively anaerobes. For primary isolation from faeces selective medium like desoxycholate citrate agar is used. Growth on nutrient agar shows small, translucent colonies with regular edges and on MacConkeys and desoxycholate citrate agar colourless colonies. Broth culture shows uniform turbidity.

Biochemical reaction: Biochemical reactions are fairly constant. They ferment sugars with the production of acid. The organisms of this group are broadly classified by their action on mannite, into mannite and non-mannite fermenters. With the exception of *Sh. sonnei* (late lactose ferments) non-ferments lactose (Table 31.1).

Table 31.1: Biochemical reactions of *Shigella* species

	Glucose	*Mannite*	*Lactose*	*Indole*
Sh. shiga/ Sh. boydii	A	–	–	–
Sh. schmitzi	A	–	–	–
Sh. flexneri	A	A	–	–
Sh. boydii	A	A	–	–
Sh. sonnei	A	A	A (late)	–

A: Fermentation of sugars with acid production only

Pathogenicity: Shigella cause bacillary dysentery. Patient passes stool mixed with mucus and blood.

Antigenic structure: The serologicial behaviour and hence antigenic structure of dysentery bacilli are complex. As the organisms are non-motile only, somatic antigens are present. Agglutination is the serological test usually employed.

Laboratory diagnosis of dysentery: It is carried out by microscopic and cultural studies on faeces from suspected cases. Blood culture does not help as there is no bacteraemia in this disease. Agglutination reaction for demonstration of specific antibodies in serum is only helpful to certain extent in subacute, chronic dysentery and in carriers.

Stools should be fresh and examined within one hour after passing. If this is impossible, the faeces should be collected in Sach's glycerine buffered saline in faeces tubes. The stools have red currant jelly appearance, odourless, alkaline and microscopically show plenty of polymorphs and RBCs. Cultures should be made from flakes of mucous in desoxycholate citrate agar.

3. *ESCHERICHIA COLI*

Morphology and staining reaction: The typical organism is rod-shaped 2–3 micron in length, 0.6 micron in breadth, with parallel sides and rounded ends. It stains uniformally and is Gram-negative. Most of the organisms are motile by peritrichous flagellas.

Cultural characteristics: They grow on ordinary nutrient media and also in presence of bile salts. They are aerobic and facultatively anaerobic, optimum temperature is 37°C. The colonies are large, circular and raised with smooth surface. Certain chemical substances exert a selective bactericidal or inhibitory action and are used in selective media brilliant green, malachite green, sodium desoxycholate in suitable concentrations inhibit growth of *Escherichia coli* but not Salmonella group of organisms.

Culture is done on MacConkey agar. Colonies produced are identified by colony character and biochemical reaction. Pink, non-mucoid, flat to raised colonies.

Biochemical reactions form one of the important methods of identification of these organisms, their reaction on different types of sugars with the production of acid and gas is highly characteristic. The common sugars used in laboratory are—lactose, glucose and mannitol. *E. coli, Klebsiella aerogenes* (often present in soil and grass) when Gram-negative organisms are isolated from drinking water. Presence of *E. coli* is an indication of faecal pollution of drinking water, whereas the presence of *K. aerogenes* indicate presence of bacteria from soil or grass.

***E. coli* produces indole,** gives a positive methyl red (MR) reaction and negative Voges-Proskauer (VP) test, whereas *K. aerogenes* does not produce indole, gives a negative MR and positive VP test.

Toxin produced: Enterotoxin, haemolysin.

Pathogenicity: Though *E. coli* forms normal flora of intestine, yet they lead to many diseases like diarrhoea, urinary tract infection, pyogenic infection like meningitis, wound infection, peritonitis, cholecystitis and septicaemia.

4. VIBRIO

Vibrios are short comma-shaped organisms. They are widely distributed in nature, mostly as saprophytes in water and sometimes in faeces of man and animals only a few of them are pathogenic. *Vibrio cholerae* in man only. Organisms assembling *V. cholerae*, but not pathogenic are called para-cholera and cholera like vibrios. *El-Tor vibrios* were previously thought to be non-pathogenic, but recently cholera epidemics due to *El-Tor vibrios* have been reported.

Morphology and cultural characteristics: The vibrios are short, curved rods looking like commas. They vary considerably in size about 1–5 μm × 0.3 to 0.6 μm. They may be arranged singly, in 5-shape or in short chains. The organisms or actively motile and show darting or scintillating movement by a single polar flagellum. They stain best with dilute carbol fuchsin (1:10 for 1 minute). They are Gram-negative. Growth occurs readily on most of the common media. Vibrios are strongly aerobic and grow best in the presence of abundant oxygen. The organisms have a high alkali, but a very low acid tolerance. Most of the selective media make use of such properties as alkali tolerance, reduction of bismuth salts and growth in the presence and bile salts. Optimum pH for its growth is 8.2.

Specimens which cannot be cultured immediately should preserved in a solution containing 0.3% boric acid and 0.3% potassium chloride at pH 9.2. Such preserved specimens should be transferred to the suitable laboratory for diagnosis from the epidemic areas.

It grows within a temperature, range of 16–40°C (opt. temp. 3/°C). Nutrient agar—MacConkey agar and blood agar is used for its growth. VR fluid and Carry Blair's transport medium is also used for its growth.

Biochemical reaction: Indole +ve, oxidase +ve, convert nitrate to nitrite, cholera red test is used to show its reaction.

Cholera-red reaction elicited by adding a few drops of H_2SO_4 to a growth on peptone water; a pink colour results when reaction is positive.

Haemolysis test: *Vibrio cholerae* is non-haemolytic (technique—to a 3% suspension of goat's RBCs, add equal quantity of 24 hours broth culture. Incubate for 2 hours at 37°C and keep it at 40°C overnight and observe for haemolysis).

The organisms have a marked proteolytic and saccharolytic activities. Acid without gas is generally produced in most of sugar media late like glucose, maltose, sucrose and mannite. Lactose is fermented (usually after 5 to 14 days). Rapid production of indole from tryptophan in alkali peptone water is well-marked property of cholera Vibrio. It also reduces nitrates to nitrites; and if to such culture medium H_2SO_4, is added, nitrate indole is formed which is red in colour and forms the basis of cholera red reaction.

Pathogenesis: Cholera disease is produced by *Vibrio cholerae*. This generally occurs in the form of epidemics. Patient gets severe diarrhoea. The faecal matter is present in stool. Sometimes, patient passes flakes of mucus and water. This stool is called rice water stools. Patient losses large quantity of water in stool and vomiting leading to severe dehydration that could be fatal. Other symptoms are vomiting, abdominal pain and mild fever.

Antigenic structure: The Vibrio has a somatic and flagellar antigens. The former is heat stable and specific and latter heat labile and non-specific. On the basis of somatic antigen cholera and cholera-like vibrios are divided into six groups. *Vibrio cholerae* belongs to group 1 and is further subdivided into true cholera and *El-Tor* on the basis of haemolysis of sheep cells. True cholera vibrios are non-haemolytic; whereas *El-Tor* are haemolytic. True cholera and *El-Tor* are further subdivided into three types each—Inaba, Ogawa and Hikojima.

Laboratory diagnosis: Stool sample is collected for its diagnosis. Sample is collected in clean container and immediately transferred to laboratory.

It is based on isolation and identification of causative organisms. A smear of mucous flakes from stool of case of a cholera stained with dilute carbol fuchsin shows characteristic morphology and arrangement like "fish in stream". For isolation of organisms, selective media peptone water (pH 8.6) and Dicudoune's medium (blood alkali agar) are used. Identification is based on biochemical characters and agglutination by specific antiserum. When *V. cholerae* are injected intraperitoneally in immunised animals lysis and disintegration of organisms occur as a result of specific antibodies acting on organisms in the presence of complement. This is called Pfeiffer's phenomenon.

5. KLEBSIELLA

These bacteria are widely distributed in nature. They may be found in the intestine or in sewage water. There are three species of Klebsiella.

1. *Klebsiella pneumoniae*
2. *Klebsiella ozaenae*
3. *Klebsiella rhinoscleromatis*.

Morphology: This is Gram –ve bacillus. Its size is 1–2 µm × 0.5–0.2 µm. Capsulated, non-sporing, non-motile bacteria.

Culture: It is an aerobe. Optimum temperature for its growth is 37°C. This can grow on ordinary media. Nutrient agar and MacConkey agar are usually used for these bacteria. On MacConkey agar, these produce pink colonies. Colonies are large, mucoid because of the production of huge amount of capsular material. These mucoid colonies are not identified separately. These colonies are string test +ve.

Pathogenicity of Klebsiella: Klebsiella produces various diseases, i.e. UTI, pneumonia, wound infection. Sometime it causes diarrhoea.

Laboratory diagnosis: Morbid material is collected aseptically. Colonies are identified by biochemical reaction. *Klebsiella ozaenae* is found in atrophic rhinitis or ozaenae patient. *Klebsiella rhinoscleromatis* is found in rhinoscleroma disease.

Chapter 32

Systemic Bacteriology IV

(*Pseudomonas pyocyaneus*, Proteus, Spirochaetes, Borrelia, Bordetella, Chlamydia)

Chapter Outline

- Pseudomonas
- Proteus
- Spirochaetes
- Borrelia
- *Bordetella pertussis*
- Chlamydia

1. PSEUDOMONAS

Pseudomonas are Gram-negative bacilli and are the common cause of hospital infection.

Morphology: This is Gram –ve bacillus. Its size is 1.5–3.0 µm × 0.5 µm. These are non-sporing, non-capsulated bacteria. There is a single polar flagellum of this bacterium which is used for its motility. They produce pigments which are of the following types:

1. Fluorescein which is yellow–green pigment.
2. Pyocyanin which is blue–green pigment
3. Pyorubrin which is reddish–brown pigment.
4. Pyomelanin which is black pigment.

Culture: This is an aerobe. Optimum temperature is 37°C and optimum pH 7.2–7.4. Nutrient agar, MacConkey agar and blood agar are used for these bacteria. On MacConkey agar, these bacteria produce pale, i.e. non-lactose fermenting colonies.

Biochemical reaction: Indole, MR and VP –ve, catalase +ve, oxidase +ve, ferment glucose with the production of acid only.

Structure, classification and antigenic types: ***Pseudomonas*** species are Gram-negative, aerobic bacilli measuring 0.5 to 0.8 µm by 1.5 to 3.0 µm. Motility is by a single polar flagellum. Species are distinguished by biochemical and DNA hybridization tests. Antisera to lipopolysaccharide and outer membrane proteins show cross-reactivity among serovars.

Epidemiology: *Pseudomonas* species normally inhabit soil, water, and vegetation and can be isolated from the skin, throat, and stool of healthy persons. They often colonize hospital food, sinks, taps, mops, and respiratory equipment. Spread is from patient-to-patient via contact with fomites or by ingestion of contaminated food and water.

Pathogenesis: Neutropenia in cancer patients and others receiving immunosuppressive drugs contributes to infection. *Pseudomonas aeruginosa* has several virulence factors, but their roles in pathogenesis are unclear. An alginate is antiphagocytic, and most strains isolated produce toxin A, a diphtheria-toxin-like exotoxin. All strains have endotoxin, which is a major virulence factor in bacteremia and septic shock.

Pseudomonas aeroginosa and *Pseudomonas pyocyaneus* are important members of this genus.

Clinical manifestations: Pseudomonas has established itself as one of the most troublesome agents causing nosocomial infections. *Pseudomonas aeruginosa* and *P. maltophilia* account for 80% of opportunistic infections by Pseudomonas. *Pseudomonas aeruginosa* infection is a serious problem in patients hospitalized with cancer, cystic fibrosis, and burns; the case fatality is 50%. Other infections caused by *Pseudomonas* species include endocarditis, pneumonia, and infections of the urinary tract, central nervous system, wounds, eyes, ears, skin, and musculoskeletal system.

Diagnosis: Pseudomonas can be cultured on most general-purpose media and identified with biochemical tests. Repeated isolation and demonstration of agglutinins in the patient's serum would also help to confirm the diagnosis.

Control: The spread of Pseudomonas is best controlled by cleaning and disinfecting medical equipment. In burn patients, topical therapy of the burn with antimicrobial agents such as silver sulfadiazine, coupled with surgical debridement, has markedly reduced sepsis. Antibiotic susceptibility testing of clinical isolates is mandatory, because of multiple antibiotic resistance; however, the combination of gentamycin and carbenicillin can be very effective in patients with acute *P. aeruginosa* infections.

2. PROTEUS

Morphology: These are Gram-negative rods show great variation in size (pleomorphic) 0.4–0.8 µm × 1–3 µm. It may be in long filaments or in granular form.

Culture characters: It is aerobic and facultative anaerobic. *Proteus vulgaris* and *Proteus mirabilis* show swarming type of growth at 37°C while swarming is absent in other species.

Biochemical reactions: Forms acid and gas from glucose, MR +ve, VP –ve, indole is not produced by *Proteus mirabilis*, citrate is positive in *Proteus rettgeri* and negative in *Proteus morganii*.

Pathogenicity: It may cause urinary tract infection, pyogenic lesions like abscess, infection of wound, ear or respiratory tract.

Laboratory diagnosis: Culture of material (urine, pus, sputum), etc. shows swarming type of growth of bacteria.

Capsular stain: They are not stained with ordinary aniline dyes. In Gram stain, capsules are shown as clear area of halo around bacterium. Methods of capsule staining are:

1. India ink method.
2. Hiss method.

3. SPIROCHAETES

Spirochaetes are elongated, motile, flexible organisms twisted around their long axis: For descriptive purpose, they are classified into Spirochaeta, Cristispira. Spirochaeta possess a central axis around which the body is twisted in a spiral manner. Cristispira possess a band-like membrance (Crista) and body is divided into chambers by septa. Pathogenic spirochaetes belong to family Trepanematecear and include three genera, viz. Treponema, Borrelia, and Leptospira. Treponemes have neither central axis, nor membranes, they have a number of primary spirals, leptospira like treponema do not possess axial fibre or crista, but consist of a large number of closely wound spirals with bend ends.

Treponema

Treponemes are slender spirochaetes with fine spirals and pointed ends. Some of them are pathogenic for man, while others occur as commensals in mouth and genitalia. *Treponema* species pathogenic for man includes the causative agents of venereal syphilis *(T. pallidum)* and non-venereal treponematoses: Yaws *(T. pertenue)*, endemic syphilis *(T. endemicum)* and pinta *(T. carateum)*.

Treponema pallidum

Morphology: It is a thin, delicate, long, motile, flexible organism which is twisted spirally around its long axis. It is 6–14 µm long. Its width is 0.13 µm in dried state, but is about 0.2 µm in the wet living state, which is just great enough for resolution with the light microscope. It has 6–12 coils which are remarkably evenly disposed at 1 µm intervals and the amplitude of spirals is 1–1.5 µm. They have tapering ends. It is actively motile exhibiting flexion and extension, translatory and corkscrew-like motility. As the spirochaete moves across the dark-field of the microscope, it often displays a characteristic tendency to bend at right angle near its midpoint. These secondary curves appear and disappear but its primary spirals remain unchanged.

T. pallidum cannot be seen under the light microscope in wet films. Its morphology and motility can be seen under the dark-ground microscope. It can be stained by silver impregnation methods. Fontana's method is useful for staining films and Levaditi's method for tissue sections. By immunofluorescence method, treponemes can be detected in tissues and body fluids.

Ultrastructurally, *T. pallidum* possesses usually three but occasionally four endoflagella attached subterminally at each end of the cell and extend towards the opposite pole between outer membrane and peptidoglycan layer and cytoplasmic fibrils that run the length of the organism internal to cytoplasmic membrane.

Cultivation: Pathogenic treponemes cannot be cultivated in artificial media and are maintained by subculture in susceptible animals. Nichols strain of *T. pallidum* has been maintained, in rabbit testis, for several decades by serial testicular passages since it was isolated in 1913 from CSF of a patient with neurosyphilis. The mean generation time for growth, *in vivo*, in the rabbit testis appears to be 30 hours. It can be maintained, *in vitro*, for 1–6 days, using maintenance medium (Nelson medium) that contains rabbit serum, reducing agents, vitamins, cofactors, amino acids and salts. Eagle and McCoy cell culture medium supplemented with foetal bovine serum and reducing agents may also be used for the maintenance of the organism. Cultivable treponemes such as *T. phagedenis* (Reiter treponeme) and *T. refringens* are nonpathogenic. They can be grown under strictly anaerobic conditions in Smith-Noguchi medium or in digest broth enriched with serum.

Type of motility is seen in *Treponema pallidum*: *T. pallidum* is actively motile exhibiting flexion and extension, translatory and corkscrew-like motility. As the spirochaete moves across the dark-field of the microscope, it often displays a characteristic tendency to bend at right angle near its midpoint. The secondary curves appear and disappear but its primary spirals remain unchanged.

T. pallidum causes syphilis.

The incubation period of syphilis is about a month (range 10–90 days).

Transmission of syphilis:

- Sexual intercourse
- Blood transfusion.
- Congenital (mother-to-foetus)

Stages of syphilis: There are four stages of syphilis:

- Primary syphilis
- Secondary syphilis
- Latent syphilis
- Tertiary syphilis

Diagnosis of Syphilis

Dark-field examination technique

A. Surface of suspected ulcerated lesion should be cleaned with saline and gauze, then gently abraded further with dry gauze, without bleeding. The lesion is then squeezed to express a serous transudate and a drop of transudate is picked up on the surface of a glass slide. Mix a drop of saline with it. Cover it with coverslip and examine immediately for *Treponema pallidum* with a dark field or contrast microscope. A single examination does not exclude syphilis. Prior use of topical antiseptic may interfere with the examination.

B. In case of secondary syphilis, organism may be demonstrated by saline aspiration of lymph nodes.

Serology

Serology is very important because after primary syphilis it is almost impossible to demonstrate treponemes. At this point, it is necessary to perform serological tests to diagnose the condition.

Serological tests
- Lipoidophil Nonspecific antibody test (STS)
  1. Flocculation (VDRL)
  2. CFT (KarlmanWasserman)
  3. Agglutination
- Specific treponemal antibody tests
  1. FTA-ABS
  2. *Tr. pallidum I* (TPI)
  3. Haemagglutination

Lipoidophil Antibody Tests (STS)

1. **VDRL:** Carried out on 76 × 50 mm slides with ceramic rings or 3 × ½″ tubes

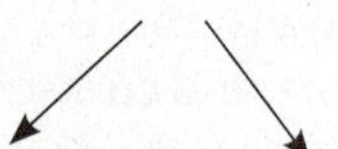

Transfer 0.5 ml of inactivated serum to tube and add 0.5 ml of diluted antigen (cardiolipin). Shake for 5 min in a Kahn shaker Centrifuge at 2000 mp.	Place 0.016 ml serum and 0.01 ml diluted antigen onto the slide with ceramic ring. Rotation is carried out by a mechanical slide rotator.

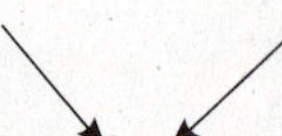

Visible aggregation is taken to be positive.
VDRL titers reach 1.32 during sec. syphilis.

2. **Complement fixation test:** Reagents are added as follows:

Tube 1 (control)— Serum 0.2 ml.
Saline 2 ml
Complement (serum control) 1 ml

Tube 2 (test)— Serum 0.2 ml
Saline 1 ml
Complement (test) 1 ml
Antigen 1 ml

—Place the tubes in waterbath for 1 hr at 37°C

After this, to each tube add 1 vol. of sensitized RBCs and place in waterbath for another 30 minutes.

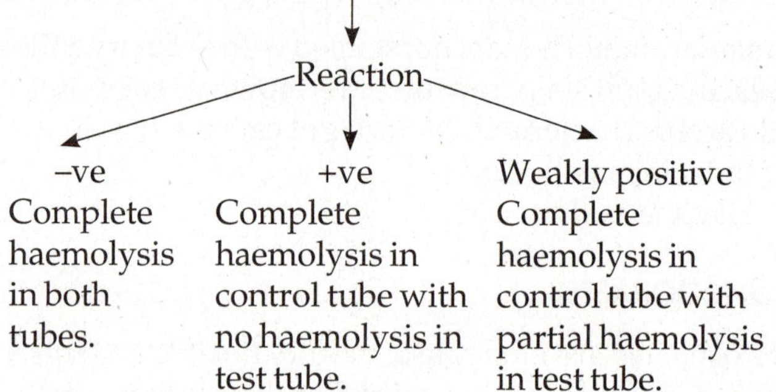

Reaction

–ve	+ve	Weakly positive
Complete haemolysis in both tubes.	Complete haemolysis in control tube with no haemolysis in test tube.	Complete haemolysis in control tube with partial haemolysis in test tube.

This test can be quantitative if doubling dilutions of serum in saline from 1 in 5 to 1 in 160 are used.

Treponemal Antibody Tests

1. **FTA-ABS test (absorbed fluorescent treponemal antibody test):** The patients serum is first absorbed with a non-pathogenic treponemal antigen to remove group specific antibiotics which may be produced against saprophytic treponemes.

   The patients absorbed serum is then placed on a slide containing *T. pallidum* (dried). Any specific Ab, in the serum is fixed to treponemes. It is then detected by addition of fluorescein labelled AHG.

2. **Treponema haemagglutination antibody test:** Formolized tanned sheep RBCs are conjugated with the antigens of a lysate of Nichols strain of *T. pallidum*. Results of the reaction between antibody and coated cells give clear cut and reproducible results.

   Specificity is similar to TPI test and sensitivity comparable to FTA tests.

3. **TPI test:** Points serum is incubated with living virulent treponemes (Nichols strain) in the presence of complement. When specific antibody is present, the spirochaetes are killed and immobilized.

Current routine practice of sera examination

i. VDRL slide test
ii. Treponema haemagglutination antibody test.
iii. Absorbed fluorescent treponemal antibody test.

False +ve serological tests for syphilis

Acute (disappear within 6 months)	*Chronic (persist for 6 months)*
Occur in	Occur in
1. *Mycoplasma pneumoniae*	1. Drug addicts
2. Malaria	2. Autoimmune diseases, e.g. SLE
3. Acute viral infections	3. Ageing
4. Acute bacterial infections	
5. Following smallpox vaccination	

4. BORRELIA

It is large motile, refractive with irregular, wide and open coils. It is 0.3 to 0.7 µm wide and 10 to 30 µm long and is Gram-negative. Borrelia of medical importance are:

1. *Borrelia recurrentis* (relapsing fever)
2. *Borrelia vincentii*

Borrelia recurrentis

Morphology: It is irregular, spiral with one or both ends pointed. It is 8 to 20 µm × 0.2 to 0.4 µm in size. It possesses 5 to 8 loose spiral coils. It is actively motile.

Culture characters: Its culture is difficult. Culture is successfully done in ascitic fluid containing rabbit kidney (Noguchi's medium). Growth occurs on chorioallantoic membrane of chick embryo.

Pathogenicity: It causes relapsing fever. Incubation period is 2 to 10 days. Splenomegaly, jaundice and haemorrhagic lesions in kidney, intestine and meningitis may occur.

Laboratory diagnosis: Blood is collected during rise of fever. Thin and thick blood smears are made. They are stained with Leishman's stain or Giemsa stain. Organism may be demonstrated by dark-field examination of drop of centrifuged blood from buffy coat. However, phase contrast microscope is considered the method of choice.

***Borrelia vincentii*:** It is motile Borrelia about 4 to 20 µm long and 0.2 to 0.6 µm wide having 3 to 8 coils of variable size. It is Gram-negative and is obligatory anaerobic. It is a commensal of oral cavity. Under predisposing condition like malnutrition, etc. It may cause gingiva stomatitis or pharyngitis. Diagnosis may be made by stained smear taken from lesion.

5. *BORDETELLA PERTUSSIS*

It is found in nasopharynx and respiratory tract mucosa.

Morphology: It is small, ovoid coccobacillus, is non-motile, non-sporing and capsulated.

Culture characters: It is aerobic and facultative anaerobic. It grows best at 35°C to 36°C. Bordet-Gengou glycerine potato blood agar medium is used for its isolation.

Biochemical reactions: Oxidase +ve, catalase +ve.

Pathogenicity: These bacteria liberate toxins and other substances that irritate surface cells, causing cough and marked lymphocytosis. It causes whooping cough. In man incubation period is 1 to 2 weeks.

Laboratory diagnosis

i. Microscopic examination is done to demonstrate bacilli from respiratory secretion preferable by fluorescent antibody technique.
ii. Culture:
   a. *The cough plate method*: Culture plate is held 10 to 15 cm away, in front of patient's mouth and patient is asked to cough in front of plate.
   b. *Postnasal swab*: In this method, secretion from post-pharyngeal wall is taken with cotton swab or bent wire passed through mouth.

The swabs are plated on glycerine potato blood agar. After 48 to 72 hours incubation at 35°C to 36°C colonies appear. They are confirmed by microscopy and biochemical reaction.

6. CHLAMYDIA

Chlamydia are obligate intracellular bacteria found worldwide.

Structure, classification and antigenic types: Chlamydiae are obligate intracellular bacteria. They lack several metabolic and biosynthetic pathways and depend on the host cell for intermediates, including ATP. Chlamydiae exist as two stages:

1. Infectious particles called elementary bodies and
2. Intracytoplasmic, reproductive forms called initial bodies.

The elementary body is a spherical particle, 0.25–0.3 µm in diameter with an electron dense nucleoid. An initial body is 0.5–1.0 µm in size and divides by binary fusion to produce a large number of elementary bodies. The chlamydiae consist of three species, *C. trachomatis*, *C. psittaci*, and *C. pneumoniae*. The first two contain many serovars based on differences in cell wall and outer membrane proteins.

Clinical manifestations

Ocular infections: *Chlamydia trachomatis* causes trachoma and inclusion conjunctivitis. Trachoma is characterized by the development of follicles and inflamed conjunctivae. The cornea may become cloudy and vascularized; repeated infections are a common cause of blindness. Inclusion conjunctivitis is a milder inflammatory conjunctival infection with purulent discharge.

Genital infections: Some *C. trachomatis* strains cause genital infections, including non-gonococcal urethritis in men and acute salpingitis and cervicitis in women. Other strains cause lymphogranuloma venereum, a venereal disease with genital lesions and regional lymph node involvement (buboes).

Respiratory infections: *Chlamydia psittaci* causes psittacosis whose manifestations may vary from a mild influenza like illness to fatal pneumonia.

Diagnosis: The clinical presentation is often diagnostic; the diagnosis may be confirmed by serology (complement fixation or microimmunofluorescence tests) on sera and/or tears. The characteristic inclusions are called Halberstaedter-Prowazek (H-P bodies) may be demonstrated in conjunctival scraping as intracytoplasmic inclusions. They can be stained with iodine solution also. The chlamydia may be grown in the yolk sac of 6–8 days eggs. Irradiated McCoy cell cultures can be used for isolation.

Control: Tetracycline and erythromycin are the drugs of choice. Single dose of 1 g of azithromycin in adults has been found useful in a number of studies. Penicillin is not effective. Topical administration of sulfonamides and tetracycline is recommended in ocular disease.

Systemic Bacteriology V

Mycobacterium tuberculosis, Leprosy and Atypical Mycobacteria, Anaerobic Gram-negative Bacteria, Pasteurella and Brucella

Chapter Outline

- Mycobacteria (Acid Fast Bacteria)
- *Mycobacterium tuberculosis*
- Diagnosis of Tuberculosis
- Brucella

MYCOBACTERIA (ACID-FAST BACTERIA)

The acid-fast bacteria are so-called because of their ability when once stained, to resist subsequent decolorization by mineral acids. The degree of acid fastness varies with members of the group. The following are the common types of strains of mycobacteria.

1. *Mycobacterium tuberculosis* of human, bovine.
2. *Mycobacterium leprae* (human leprosy bacilli) and *Mycobacterium Lepramurium* (rats and mice).
3. Saprophytic acid-fast bacilli: *M. tortuitum, M. Chelonae.*
4. **A typical mycobacteria:** These are the newly described mycobacteria. Normally these bacteria are free-living, but a number has an animal host. They are responsible for the prevalence of non-specific sensitivity to tuberculosis, in the inhabitants of certain regions and sometimes they produce lesions just like tuberculosis. Morphologically in comparison to *Mycobacterium tuberculosis* the organisms are either very short, or very long. They are resistant to PAS, INH and streptomycin, non-pathogenic to guinea pigs, can be cultured in ordinary media and produce pigments (chromogenic), e.g. *M. kansasii., M. marinum;* MAC (*M. avium* intracellular complex).

MYCOBACTERIUM TUBERCULOSIS

Morphology and staining characteristics: Organisms are rod-shaped, straight or slightly curved with round ends, they are arranged either singly in small groups or bundles forming characteristic cords. Size varies considerably depending on the medium on which they are grown. Staining is either uniform or granular. In the latter condition, they show beaded form. They are Gram-positive and acid-fast. Acid fastness depends on integrity of the cellular structure.

Cultural characters: The acid-fast bacilli vary in case with which they can be grown under artificial conditions. At one end are saprophytic acid-fast bacilli which grow well in 2–3 days. At the other end are mammalian tubercle bacilli which grow only on special media and may take 3 weeks or even more time to form visible growth. In general use, the most satisfactory solid media are of inspissated serum (Lowenstein-Jensen media).

For mass culture, glycerine broth is used to get a dispersed growth Middle Brook Dubos Tween 80 media is used. Effect of glycerine on growth of tubercle bacilli can differentiate between human and bovine types. Another point of differentiation is that human type often forms yellowish to orange red pigment, whereas bovine type never does.

Metabolism and biochemical reaction: Optimum temperature for growth is 37°C. Human and bovine types not grow below 30°C, saprophytic acid-fast and cold-blooded type grow freely at 20°C, whereas avian type can grow at 40°C. Tubercle bacilli are strict aerobes. Biochemical reactions are of little use in the study of mycobacteria.

Chemical structure

A. **Lipids:** The organisms are mixed in lipids which are intimately bound to protein and polysaccharides. These are thought to be responsible for elicitating characteristic tissue response to tubercle bacilli. Mycolic acid is responsible for acid-fast property. Cord formation by virulent tubercle bacilli is thought to be due to 'Cord factro' a lipid fraction responsible for virulence of organism. The lipids consist of glycerides, phosphatides and wax.

B. **Polysaccharides:** A large number of polysaccharides have been isolated but their role in pathogenicity is uncertain. They can induce anaphylactic type of hypersensitivity.

C. **Proteins:** Soluble protein fractions are responsible for tuberculin type of sensitivity.

Pathogenicity: Human type mainly gives rise to disease under natural conditions in man, monkeys and pigs; bovine type in cattle, pigs, horses and man; murine type in volis; avian type in birds and cold-blooded type of animals, viz. fishes.

Laboratory diagnosis of tuberculosis: Final diagnosis of tuberculosis depends on:

1. **Demonstration of characteristic organism** in exudates and tissues by microscopic examination. Microscopic examination can be done directly after making a smear. In this method, if the number of bacteria is less, then possibility of missing them is always there. So, concentration method is to be preferred.
   Concentration method (Petroff's): One volume of material is mixed with 3 volumes of 4% KOH, which is then incubated at 37°C for half an hour. At the end of this time, the mixture is neutral red with 8% HCl, centrifuged, supernatant discarded, deposit is used for culture, animal inoculation add for preparation of smear.
2. **Culture methods:** Culture is done on LJ medium or Dorset egg medium and examined after 6–8 weeks.
3. **Animal inoculation tests:** Rabbits and guinea pigs are used. Rabbits are resistant to human type where as guinea pigs are highly susceptible to experimental infection with human and bovine types. It has been stated that injection of a single bacillus may succeed in producing disease. Following subcutaneous infection, death occurs from generalised tuberculosis in about 6–16 weeks. At necropsy, there is caseous local lesion, enlarged and caseous lymph nodes. Gross lesions resemble those produced by pasteurella pseudotuberculosis, which should be differentiated by microscopic and cultural examination.

ZN staining: Smear is prepared from morbid material. Fix the smear after drying in air. After ZN staining, smear is examined under oil immersion lens. In case, when direct smear fails to reveal AFB.

Apart from pulmonary tuberculosis, the following varieties are not uncommon:

1. Tubercular meningitis
2. Tubercular lymphadenitis
3. Tubercular peritonitis
4. Renal tuberculosis
5. Tubercular osteomyelitis

Methods of obtaining a sputum specimen are given in Table 33.1.

Diagnosis of Tuberculosis

There are two kinds of tests used to detect TB bacteria in the body: The TB skin test (TST) and TB blood tests.

Tuberculin test: This test is generally positive in persons, either who are suffering from tuberculosis or who had tuberculosis. The test can be performed by two types of antigens.

a. **Old tuberculin (OT):** It is a concentrated filtrate of glycerine broth in which tubercle bacilli have weeks. In addition to tuberculoprotein it contains a variety of constitutes of tubercle bacilli.

Table 33.1: Methods of obtaining a sputum specimen

Method	*Description*	*Advantage*	*Disadvantage*
Spontaneous sputum sample	• Patient coughs up sputum into a sterile container	• Inexpensive • Easy to do	• Patient may not be able to cough up sputum without assistance or may spit up saliva instead of sputum • Health care worker has to coach and supervise the patient when collecting sputum
Sputum induction	• Patient inhales a saline mist which can cause deep cough	• Easy to do • Use to obtain sputum when coughing sputum is not productive	• Specimens may be watery and may be confused with saliva should be labelled induced specimen • Requires special equipment • May cause bronchospasm
Bronchoscopy	• Bronchoscope is passed through the mouth or nose directly into the diseased portion of the lung and sputum or lung tissue is removed	• Use to obtain sputum when coughing or inducing sputum not productive or other diagnoses are being considered	• Most expensive and invasive procedure • Requires special equipment • Must be done by a specialist in a hospital or clinic • Requires anaesthesia
Gastric washing	• Tube is inserted through the patient's mouth or nose and passed into the stomach to get a sample of gastric secretions that contain sputum that has been coughed into the throat and then swallowed	• Use to obtain samples in children, who do not produce sputum when they cough	• Must be done as soon as patient wakes up in the morning patient may be required to stay in hospital • Can be uncomfortable for the patient

b. A purified protein derivtative (PPD) is obtained from OT biochemical fractionations.

The tuberculosis (TB) blood test, also called an interferon gamma release assay or IGRA, is a way to find out if you have TB germs in your body. The TB blood test can be done instead of a TB skin test (Mantoux).

There are two kinds of TB blood tests:

- QuantiFERON®-TB
- T-SPOT® TB

Mantoux test: Erythema or induration in area of 10–15 mm diameter after 48–72 hours indicate a positive test.

A positive TB skin test or TB blood test only tells that a person has been infected with TB bacteria. It does not tell whether the person has latent TB infection (LTBI) or has progressed to TB disease.

QuantiFERON TB Gold (QFT) test is a blood test helpful in detecting *Mycobacterium tuberculosis*. Also, with TB Gold test diagnosis, it is possible to check latent or active tuberculosis infection.

QuantiFERON Gold Plus is the new, improved version of the QuantiFERON Gold TB test. This is the same test with the same fundamental principles, but is more advanced at detecting TB. The Gold Plus test has been optimized in such an innovative way with the TB-specific antigens that elicit CD8 and CD4 T cell responses.

Direct detection of *M. tuberculosis* in clinical specimen using nucleic acid amplification (NAA): NAA tests are used to amplify DNA and RNA segments to rapidly identify the microorganisms in specimen. NAA testing can reliably detect *M. tuberculosis* bacteria in specimens in hours as compared to 1 week or more for culture. Possible benefits of using NAA tests include:

- Earlier laboratory confirmation of TB disease;
- Earlier treatment initiation;
- Improved patient outcomes;
- Interruption of transmission by early diagnosis, respiratory isolation and appropriate treatment;
- Earlier, more efficient use of respiratory isolation;
- Earlier initiation of contact investigation; and
- More effective public health interventions.

BCG: A live vaccine prepared from a bovine strain is used for prophylactic measure. This Bacillius Calmette-Guerin (BCG) vaccine is given by intradermal injection.

The BCG vaccine (TB vaccine) may help protect young children from getting very sick with TB. This protection goes away as people get older. People who have had BCG vaccine still can get latent TB infection and active TB disease.

If you had the BCG vaccine and you have a choice of having a TB blood test or a TB skin test, it is better for you to have the TB blood test. This is because, the TB blood test is not affected by the BCG vaccine. This means that your TB blood test will be "positive" only if you have TB germs in your body.

***Mycobacterium laprae*:** There bacteria produce a chronic granulomatus disease called leprosy. These cannot be stained with Gram-staining so ZN stain is used. These bacteria cannot be grown on artificial medium. Leprosy is caused by these bacteria. Incubation period is 6 months to many years. Leprae bacilli involve the peripheral nerves and damage them, thus producing anaesthetic patches in the body. These bacteria produce various types of injuries in individuals.

Laprae bacilli are demonstrated from specimen collected from nasal secretion and ear lobule. Histopathological examination is conclusive from the lesion of tissue pieces to demonstrate leprae bacilli.

Leprosy

Leprosy (Hansen's disease) is caused by the acid-fast bacillus *Mycobacterium leprae*. Unlike other mycobacteria, it does not grow in artificial media or even in tissue culture. Man is the only natural host of *M. leprae*.

The precise mode of transmission of leprosy is still uncertain but it is likely that nasal secretions play a role. Infection is related to poverty and overcrowding. Once an individual is infected, subsequent progression to clinical disease appears to be dependent on several factors. Males appear to be more susceptible than females.

- Probably the **oldest disease known** to mankind
- Mainly affect **peripheral nerves**, also affects the skin, muscles, eyes, bones, testes and internal organs
- Leprosy is often known as a '**social disease**'
- **Social stigma** is attached to it. Stigma is coupled with physical deformity leads to social isolation and depression.

Types of Leprosy

There are three main types of leprosy, including:

- **Tuberculoid leprosy:** Someone with this type of leprosy usually has mild symptoms, developing only a few sores.
- **Lepromatous leprosy:** People with this type of leprosy have widespread sores and lesions affecting nerves, skin and organs.
- **Borderline leprosy.**

Classification

- **Ridley and Jopling classification:** Based on clinical, bacteriologic, immunologic and histopathologic features
  1. Tuberculoid leprosy
  2. Borderline tuberculoid leprosy
  3. Borderline leprosy
  4. Borderline lepromatous leprosy
  5. Lepromatous leprosy
  6. Histoid leprosy
- **Depending on clinical features, leprosy is classified as:**
  1. Indeterminate leprosy (IL)
  2. Paucibacillary leprosy (PB)
  3. Borderline tuberculoid leprosy (BT)

4. Borderline borderline leprosy (BB)
5. Borderline lepromatous leprosy (BL)
6. Multibacillary leprosy (MB)

Lepromin Test

Antigens

- Mitsuda antigen
- Human source of bacilli lepromin H
- Armadillos source of bacilli lepromin A
- Bacillary lepromin—Dharmendra antigen
- Inject 0.1 ml of lepromin
- Lepromin is boiled emulsified lepromatous tissue—rich in lepra bacilli.
- Lepromins, made from boiled bacilli from lepromatous lesions.
- Leprosins ultrasonic preparation of tissue free bacilli
- Human source, Leprosins-H, Armadillo-Leprosins—A
- Events in the reaction—biphasic reaction

Read for two types of reactions:
1. Early Farnandez reaction
2. Late Mitsuda reaction

1. Fernandez reaction >24–48 hours, remains for 3–5 days, like tuberculin reaction, a little significant.
2. Mitsuda reaction occurs after 1–2 weeks prominent after 4 weeks
   - Infiltration with lymphocytes, epitheloid cells, and giant cells
   - Indicates CMI
   - Differentiates those mount immune response and those cannot
   - Now, antigens are derived from Armadillo-derived lepra bacilli.

Uses of Lepromin Test

- Body will react to the leprosy antigens
- Check injection 3 days and 28 days later
  a. Classification of leprosy:
     - Positive in tuberculoid leprosy
     - Negative in lepromatous leprosy
  b. Assessment of prognosis:
     - Positive lepromin test indicates a good prognosis.
     - Negative lepromin test indicates a bad prognosis.

Vaccine for Leprosy

Leprosy is endemic in several regions of the world. Currently, the only protection has come from vaccination with BCG (Bacillus Calmette-Guérin), a single dose which gives 50% or higher protection against the disease.

Anaerobic Gram-negative Bacilli

Gram-negative bacilli cause foul smelling discharge and are common elements of mucous membrane flora.

Structure, classification, and antigenic types: Some are pleomorphic, whereas others have distinctive morphology. Most are obligate anaerobes. The key characters for classification are motility, arrangement of flagella, organic and volatile fatty acid metabolic, end-products and cellular fatty acid patterns. Antigens are not useful. These include Bacteroides, Fusobacterium, Dialister and Sphaerophorus genus.

Epidemiology: They are part of the normal flora of the mouth, upper respiratory tract, intestine and vagina. Infections arise endogenously from the mucosal flora.

Pathogenesis: They usually invade as opportunistic pathogens through a break in the mucosa. A low redox potential favours infection. Some types produce virulence factors or interfere with host defenses (e.g. by inhibiting phagocytosis).

Host defenses: Antibodies, complement (via both classic and alternative pathways), and cell-mediated immunity (involving both polymorphonuclear leukocytes and T lymphocytes) are important.

Clinical manifestations: Anaerobic Gram-negative bacilli are common elements of the mucous membrane flora throughout the body; they often act as secondary pathogens. They are the most common anaerobes involved in infection and include some of the most antibiotic-resistant species. They are involved in mixed infections, including lung or liver abscess, mastoiditis, intestinal lesions and lesions of mouth and gums.

Diagnosis: Clues suggesting anaerobic infection include foul-smelling discharge, proximity of infection to mucosal surfaces, abscess formation, necrosis and gas in tissues, septic thrombophlebitis, various distinctive clinical pictures (e.g. actinomycosis, gas gangrene), and results of a Gram stain of clinical specimens. Collection of clinical specimens should avoid the mucosal flora, and transport must be anaerobic.

Control: Control involves (1) surgical drainage of abscesses and debridement of necrotic tissue; and (2) use of antimicrobials (particularly metronidazole, imipenem, chloramphenicol, or combinations of amoxicillin, ticarcillin, ampicillin or piperacillin with β-lactamase inhibitors).

Yersinia, Pasteurella

These are Gram-negative, short bacilli showing bipolar staining with methylene blue. They are non-motile except. *Yersinia pseudotuberculosis* and *Y. enterocolitica*. These bacteria are primary pathogens of rodents and men are accidentally infected. They were previously considered together under the genus Pasteurella. Based on their cultural, biochemical and antigenic characters, this group has been divided into three genera—Yersinia, Pasteurella and Francisella (Table 33.2). The genus Yersinia contains three medically important species—*Y. pestis* (the causative agent of plague), *Y. pseudotuberculosis* (a primary pathogen of rodents) and *Y. enterocolitica* (causes human diarrhoeal diseases). The name Yersinia is given after *Alexander Yersin*, who discovered the plague bacillus.

Table 33.2: Diseases caused by species of Yersinia, Pasteurella, Francisella

Genera	Species	Diseases
Yersinia	*Y. pestis*	Plague in man and rodents
	Y. pseudotuberculosis	Pseudotuberculosis of animals
	Y. enterocolitica	Enteritis in man and animals
Pasteurella	*P. multocida*	Haemorrhagic septicaemia in animals
Francisella	*F. tularensis*	Tularaemia

The genus Yersinia now belongs to the tribe Yersinicae and the family Enterobacteriaceae. The genus Pasteurella is now restricted to several related bacteria causing haemorrhagic septicaemia in different species of animals and occasionally producing human infections, grouped under a common species called *P. multocida*. The genus Francisella, consisting of the single species, *F. tularensis* is named after *Francis* for his contribution on tularaemia, caused by this bacterium.

Yersinia pestis

Yersinia pestis, the causative agent of plague, formerly known as *Pasteurella pestis*, was isolated independently and almost simultaneously by *Yersin* (1894) and *Kitasato* (1894).

Morphology: *Y. pestis* is a short, ovoid, Gram-negative bacillus, about 1.5 µm × 0.7 µm in size, with round ends and convex sides, occur singly, in short chains or in small groups. When stained with methylene blue, it shows bipolar staining *(safety pin appearance)* with two ends darkly or densely stained and the central area clear motile, non-sporing and non-acid-fast.

Culture: The organism is aerobic and facultatively anaerobic. The optimum temperature for growth (unlike most pathogens) is 27°C but the envelope develops best at 37°C. It grows on ordinary media.

Biochemical reactions: *Y. pestis* ferments glucose, mannitol and maltose with the production of acid but no gas. Lactose and sucrose are not fermented. It is catalase positive, indole negative, urease negative, methyl red (MR) positive, Voges Proskauer (VP) and citrate negative. Gelatin is not liquefied.

On the basis of fermentation of glycerol and reduction of nitrate, *Devignat* has distinguished three physiological varieties of *Y. pestis*. This typing is of epidemiological significance because of the different geographical distribution of the types.

Antigen structure: Plague bacilli are antigenically homogenous and serotypes do not exist. The antigenic structure is complex and about 20 different antigens have been identified.

Pathogenesis: *Y. pestis* is a natural pathogen of rodents and causes zoonotic disease called *plague*.

Plague is a natural disease of rodents and is transmitted to man via the bite of infected rat flea (*X cheopis*). The incubation period is 2–6 days. In man, plague occurs in three forms: bubonic, pneumonic and septicaemic.

Epidemiology: Plague is a zoonotic disease and may become epidemic in the rat population. The infection may spread to domestic rats and man by flea bites or contact. The commonest vector is *Xenopsiella cheopis* but other fleas like X. *astia*, Ceratophyllus may also transmit the infection.

Plague is the greatest killer known to mankind. In 14th century, plague pandemic known as 'black death' is believed to have killed about a quarter of all mankind.

Antigen detection: F_1 glycoprotein Ag may be detected in aspirated fluid from bubo or sputum by immunofluorescence and ELISA test.

Serological tests: Antibodies to F_1 antigen may be detected by passive haemagglutination or complement fixation tests. Antibodies appear towards the end of first week of the illness. Serological tests are useful for identifying plague foci as the tests remain positive for several years after recovery from plague. It has a limited diagnostic value as the titres reach diagnostic levels (1:16 or four-fold rise) only after 2–3 weeks following onset of disease.

Diagnosis of Plague in Rats

Before examining rats, immerse them in disinfectant to kill any flea. Necropsy reveals enlargement of lymph nodes with periglandular inflammation and oedema. Generally, cervical lymph nodes are involved due to the tendency of the rat flea to bite rat's neck region. Other features include pleural effusion, enlargement of spleen and haemorrhages under the skin and in internal organs.

Specimens (heart blood, lymph nodes and spleen) collected from the animals are utilised for smear examination, culture and animal inoculation test.

Specific measures: Two types of vaccines can be used—killed and live attenuated.

i. **Killed vaccine:** Killed vaccine is widely used for active immunisation. It is a whole bacterial culture antigen of plague bacillus. It is prepared at Haffkine Institute, Mumbai. The plague bacillus (virulent strain) is grown in casein hydrolysate broth for 2–4 weeks at 32°C and killed by 0.05% formaldehyde and preserved with phenyl mercuric nitrate (Sokhey's modification of Haffkine's vaccine).
ii. **Live vaccine:** Live vaccines are prepared from two avirulent strains of *Y. pestis, Otten's Tjiwidej* strain from Jawa and Girard's EV 76 strain from Malagasey. Since live vaccines are difficult to prepares and carry some risk of unacceptable reactions, killed vaccines are recommended for general use. However, mass vaccination is no more recommended.

BRUCELLA

The genus Brucella consists of small, non-motile, aerobic, Gram-negative coccobacilli which are strict parasite of animals (goats, sheep, cattle, pigs, buffaloes). Man acquires infection by contact with infected animals or through their products. The human disease had been recognised from very early times in the Mediterranean countries and had been known under various names such as Mediterranean fever, Malta fever and undulant fever. Bruce (1887) isolated a small microorganism from the spleen of fatal cases in Malta. This has been named *Brucella melitensis (Brucella* after *Bruce; melitensis* after *Melita*, the Roman name for Malta). Bang (1897) described *Br. abortus* in Copenhagen, the cause of contagious abortion in cattle. *Traum* (1914) isolated *Br. suis* from pigs in USA. These three are the major species in the genus. Three additional species *Br. neotomae, Br ovis* and *Br. canis* have been recognised which are animal pathogens and except for *Br. canis*, they do not infect man.

Morphology: Brucellae are Gram-negative, non-motile, coccobacilli or short rods measuring 0.5–0.7 µm × 0.6–1.5 µm. They are arranged singly or in short chains. They are non-sporing and non-capsulated.

Culture: Brucellae are strict aerobes. *Br. abortus* is capnophilic, requiring 5–10% CO_2 for its growth, whereas *Br. suis* growth is unaffected by CO_2. The optimum temperature for growth is 37°C (range 20–40°C) and optimum pH 6.6–7.4.

They may grow on ordinary media, though growth is slow and scanty. Growth is improved by addition of glucose, serum, blood or liver extract. The media employed for culture are serum-dextrose agar, serum-potato-infusion agar, trypticase soy agar or tryptose agar. The addition of bacitracin, cycloheximide, polymyxin B or vancomycin makes these media selective. On solid media, colonies are small, moist and translucent. In liquid media, growth is uniform.

Biochemical reactions (Table 33.3): No carbohydrates are ordinarily fermented but they possess oxidative capacity. They are catalase and oxidase positive (except for *Br. neotomae* and *Br. ovis* which are negative). They are urease positive, nitrate reduction positive, citrate negative, indole is not produced and MR and VP tests are negative. Urease test is very rapidly positive particularly in *Br. suis* which is positive within 30 minutes and *Br. abortus* takes 1–2 hours to become urease positive.

Antigenic structure: Two main somatic antigens of brucellae, A and M are present in different amounts in the three major species. Antigen 'A' is dominant (about 20 times as much as 'M' antigen) in *Br. abortus* and antigen

Table 33.3: Differential features of Brucella species and biotypes

Species	Biotypes	CO_2 requirement	H_2S production	Growth in the presence of		Agglutination by monospecific sera		Anti-rough serum	Lysis by phage		Common host
				Basic fuchsin	Thionin	A	M		RTD	RTD × 10^4	
Br. melitensis	1	–	–	+	+	–	+	–	–	–	Sheep
	2	–	–	+	+	+	–	–	–	–	Goats
	3	–	–	+	+	+	+	–	–	–	
Br. abortus	1	±	+	+	–	+	–	–	+	+	
	2	±	+	–	–	+	–	–	+	+	
	3	±	+	+	+	+	–	–	+	+	
	4	±	+	+	–	–	+	–	+	+	Cattle
	5	–	–	+	–	–	+	–	+	+	
	6	–	±	+	–	+	–	–	+	+	
	9	±	+	+	–	–	+	–	+	+	Pigs
Br. suis	1	–	+	–	+	+	–	–	–	+	Pigs, hare
	2	–	–	±	+	+	–	–	–	±	Pigs
	3	–	–	+	+	+	–	–	–	+	Reindeer
	4	–	–	+	+	+	+	–	–	+	Rodents
	5	–	–	–	+	–	+	–	–	+	
Br. canis		–	–	–	+	–	–	+	–	–	Dogs
Br. ovis		+	–	+	+	–	–	+	–	–	Sheep
Br. neotomae		–	+	–	–	+	–	–	–	+	Wood rat

Dannish strains of *Br. suis* differ from American strains in not producing H_2S.

'M' is dominant in *Br. melitensis* (about 20 times of antigen). *Br suis* has an intermediate antigenic pattern. Absorption of the minor antigenic components of antiserum will leave most of the major antibody components.

Biotypes

i. *Br. abortus*—7 biotypes (1 to 9, number 7 and 8 are deleted)
ii. *Br. melitensis*—3 biotypes
iii. *Br. suis* strains which produce H_2S are called *American strains* and those not producing H_2S are called *Danish strains*.

Types of infection: Human infection may be of three types:

i. *Subclinical or latent infection:* There is no clinical evidence of disease but is detectable only by serological tests.
ii. *Acute brucellosis:* It is also known as *undulant fever* or *Malta fever*. It is associated with prolonged bacteraemia.
iii. *Chronic brucellosis*: It is usually non-bacteraemic. The symptoms are generally related to a state of hypersensitivity.

Pathogenesis: All the three major species of brucellae are pathogenic to human beings. *Br. melitensis* is the most pathogenic species followed by *Br. suis* of intermediate pathogenicity and *Br. abortus* is the least pathogenic. Brucellosis is a zoonotic disease.

Laboratory diagnosis: Brucellosis is a febrile disease with varied clinical manifestations and clinical diagnosis is often difficult and laboratory aid is, therefore, essential. Laboratory methods include culture of brucellae, serology and hypersensitivity test.

i. **Serology:** Serological methods are more useful as cultures are negative in high percentage of cases. Antibodies (IgG and IgM) appear in 7–10 days after clinical infection. As the disease progresses, IgM antibodies decline, while the IgG antibodies persist or increase. In chronic brucellosis, only IgG can be demonstrated and IgM may often be absent. The agglutination test identifies mainly the IgM antibody, while both IgM and IgG can fix complement.
ii. **Standard tube agglutination test:** This is a tube agglutination test in which equal volumes of serial two-fold dilutions (1:20 to 1: 640) of patient's serum and the standardised antigen (heat-killed Brucella suspension) are mixed and incubated at 37°C for 24 hours. A single titre of more than 1:160 is presumptive evidence of Brucella infection.
   A positive agglutination test may also be produced by cholera, tularaemia or Yersinia infection or vaccination. Cholera-induced antibodies may be removed by absorption with 2-mercaptoethanol.
iii. **Complement fixation test (CFT):** It is more useful in chronic cases as it detects both IgG and IgM.
iv. **ELISA and RIA:** These tests are very sensitive and helpful to distinguish acute and chronic brucellosis.
v. **Indirect immunofluorescent test:** It is specific and sensitive method for detecting antibodies and may be positive even when the agglutination test is negative.

Hypersensitivity test (brucellin test): It is delayed (type IV) hypersensitivity to Brucella antigen. It is an intradermal test using protein extract of the organisms, called *brucellin*. Positive reaction is indicated by an erythema and induration of 6 mm diameter within 24 hours. This test is not useful for diagnosis of acute infections because test may remain positive for years after acquiring infection. It may be helpful in chronic brucellosis where a positive skin test may sometimes be the only indicator of infection. Persistent negative skin test helps to exclude brucellosis.

Detection of animal infection: The methods used for the laboratory diagnosis of human infections may also be employed for the diagnosis of animal infections. Culture of milk and urine may give positive results. In addition, rapid methods such as 'rapid plate agglutination test' and the 'Rose Bengal card test' have been employed for the diagnosis of brucellosis in herd of cattle. For detection of infected animals in dairies, besides culture, pooled milk samples may be tested for antibodies by *milk ring test*.

- **Milk ring test:** It detects brucella agglutinins in the milk of infected dairy cattle.

  Method

  1. A sample of whole milk is mixed well with a drop of the stained brucella antigen (a concentrated suspension of *Br. abortus* or *Br. melitensis* stained with haematoxylin) in a narrow test tube.
  2. This mixture of milk and bacterial suspension is incubated in a water bath at 70°C for 40–50 minutes.

  Result: In a positive test, the bacilli are agglutinated and rise with the cream to form a blue ring at the top, leaving the milk unstained. When antibodies are absent (negative test), no coloured ring is formed and the milk remains uniformly blue.

  Whey agglutination test is another useful test for detecting antibodies in milk.

Prophylaxis

1. Persons handling the animals should use protective clothing and gloves.
2. Pasteurisation or boiling of milk should be done.
3. Vaccination: Cattle should be vaccinated with live attenuated *Br. abortus strains* 19 vaccine. Goats and sheep with *Br. melitensis* revived vaccine 19–BA attenuated vaccine.

Section

3B

Virology

34. Virology (General Virology, RNA, DNA Virus)
35. AIDS and HIV (Retrovirus)
36. Hepatitis Viruses
37. Rabies Virus (Rhabdovirus)
38. Arboviruses and Rubella (Dengue, Chikungunya, Rubella)
39. Rotavirus
40. Coronavirus (COVID-19)

Chapter 34

Virology
(General Virology, RNA, DNA Virus)

INTRODUCTION

Viruses occupy the transitional zone that separates the 'living' from 'nonliving'.

Viruses do not fall into the category of unicellular micro-organisms, as they do not possess a cellular organization.

As the smallest 'living units, viruses offer the best prospects for understanding the chemistry of life. The medical importance of viruses lies in their ability to cause a very large number of human diseases. They can cause diseases ranging from common cold to yellow fever, measles, influenza, corona infection, etc. Viruses can also cause—cancers in animals, birds as well as human beings.

Viruses have different sizes and shapes and are classified accordingly. Their multiplication is typical, having six phases.

Viruses are particles that are in between animate and inanimate sphere. They are inert in extracellular environment but become vegetative when come in contact with animal cells. Viruses are ultramicroscopic entities. They reproduce inside living cells, pass through filters and are covered by protein coat. They do not possess cellular organisation. They contain either RNA or DNA. They lack enzymes necessary for protein and nucleic acid synthesis. They depend on synthetic machinery of host cells. They multiply by complex process. They are sensitive to interferon.

NOMENCLATURE

Aside from physical data, genome structure and mode of replication are criteria applied in—the classification and nomenclature of viruses, including the chemical composition and configuration of the nucleic acid, whether the genome is monopartite or multipartite. The genomic RNA strand of single-stranded RNA viruses is called sense (positive sense, plus sense) in orientation. If it can serve as mRNA, and antisense (negative sense, minus sense) if a complementary strand synthesized by a viral RNA transcriptase serves as mRNA. Also considered in viral classification is the site of capsid assembly and, in enveloped viruses, the site of envelopment.

Viruses were earlier known as 'filterable viruses' due to their small size and filterability and 'ultramicroscopic' as they could not be seen under the light microscope. Their size varies from 300 nm (smallpox) to over 20 nm (foot and mouth disease virus). Viruses are inert outside the host cell. Small viruses, e.g. polio and tobacco mosaic virus, can even be crystallized. Viruses are unable to generate energy. As obligate intracellular parasites, during replication, they fully depend on the complicated biochemical machinery of eukaryotic or prokaryotic cells. The main purpose of a virus is to deliver its genome into the host cell to allow its expression (transcription and translation) by the host cell.

Some virus families have an additional covering, called the envelope, which is usually derived in part from modified host cell membranes. The outer capsid and the envelope proteins of viruses are glycosylated and important in determining the host range and antigenic composition of the virion.

Structure

Viruses are small obligate intracellular parasites, which by definition contain either a RNA or DNA genome surrounded by a protective, virus-coded protein coat. Viruses may be viewed as mobile genetic elements, most probably of, cellular origin and characterized by a long co-evolution of virus and host. For propagation; viruses depend on specialized host cells supplying the complex metabolic and biosynthetic machinery of eukaryotic or prokaryotic cells. A complete virus particle is called a virion. The main function of the virion is to deliver its DNA or RNA genome into the host cell so that the genome can be expressed (transcribed and translated) by the host cell. The viral genome often with associated basic proteins, is packaged inside a symmetric protein capsid. The nucleic acid-associated protein, called nucleoprotein, together with the genome, forms the nucleocapsid. In enveloped viruses, the nucleocapsid is surrounded by a lipid bilayer derived from the modified host cell membrane and studded with an outer layer of virus envelope glycoproteins.

Morphological Features of Viruses

a. **Size:** (i) Largest virus measuring 300 nm, (ii) smallest virus measuring 20 nm.
b. **Shape:** (i) Rabies virus are bullet-shaped, (ii) poxviruses are brick-shaped, (iii) polioviruses are spherical in shape.
c. **Structure:** (i) Central core consists of nucleic acid (RNA or DNA), (ii) protein coat around central core is called capsid, (iii) subunits of capsid are known as capsomers, (iv) envelope, (v) protein subunits on surface of envelope known as peplomers.

Cultivation of Virus

Viruses are obligate intracellular parasite, so they do not grow on artificial culture media.

i. **Animal inoculation:** It is one of the oldest methods. Growth of virus in animals may be known by the disease.
ii. **Chick embryo:** It is better than animal inoculation.
iii. **Tissue culture:** Tissue culture of human or animal cells are used for cultivation of viruses.
(i) Organ culture, (ii) explant culture, (iii) cell culture

Viruses are classified on the basis of morphology, chemical composition, and mode of replication. The viruses, that infect humans are currently grouped into 21 families, reflecting only a small part of the spectrum of the multitude of different viruses whose host ranges extend from vertebrates to protozoa and from plants and fungi to bacteria.

Morphology: Viruses are grouped on the basis of size and shape, chemical composition and structure of the genome, and mode of replication. Helical morphology is seen in nucleocapsids of many filamentous and pleomorphic viruses. Helical nucleocapsids consist of a helical array of capsid proteins (protomers) wrapped around a helical filament of nucleic acid. Icosahedral morphology is characteristic of the nucleocapsids of many "spherical" viruses. The number and arrangement of the capsomeres (morphologic subunits of the icosahedron) are useful in identification and classification. Many viruses also have an outer envelope (Fig. 34.1).

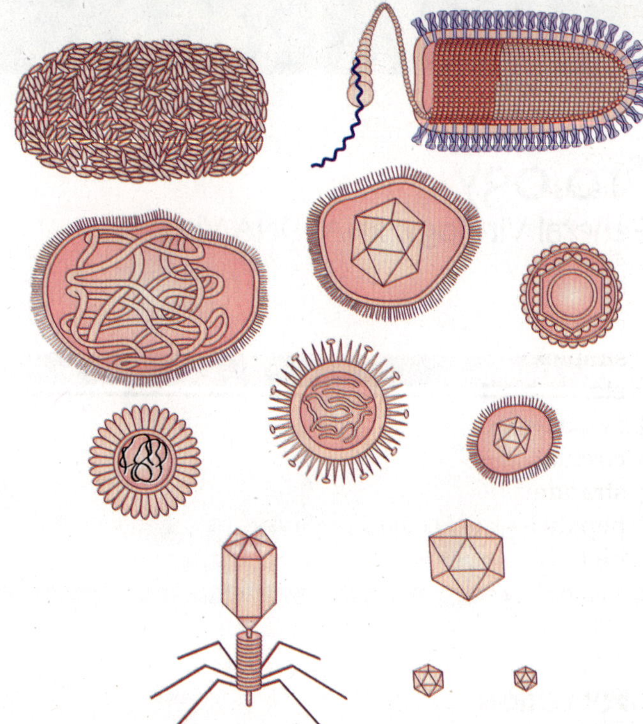

Fig. 34.1: Size and shape of various sub-types of viruses: (A) Poxvirus, (B) Rhabdovirus, (C) Herpesvirus, (D) Retrovirus, (E) Togavirus, (F) Adenovirus, (G) Parvovirus, (H) Picornavirus, (I) Bacteriophage, (J) Coronavirus, (K) Orthomyxovirus, (L) Paramyxovirus

Virus core structure (Fig. 34.2): Except in helical nucleocapsids, a little is known about the packaging or organization of the viral genome within the core. Small virions are simple nucleocapsids containing 1 to 2 protein species. The larger viruses contain in a core the nucleic acid genome complexed with basic protein(s) and protected by a single- or double-layered capsid (consisting of more than one species of protein) or by an envelope.

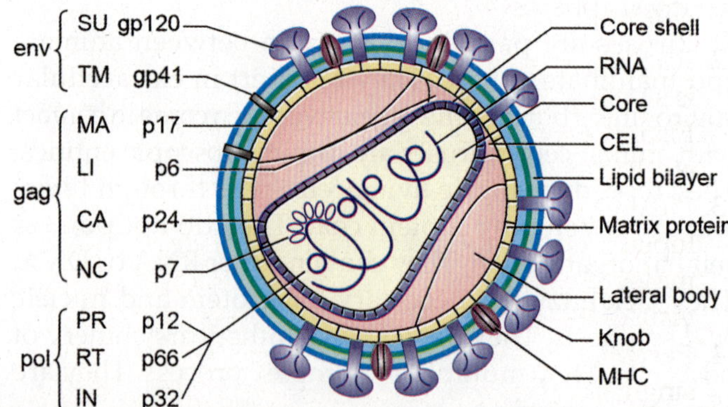

Fig. 34.2: Two-dimensional diagram of HIV-1 correlating (immuno-) electron microscopic findings with the recent nomenclature for the structural components in a 2-letter code and with the molecular weights of the virus structural (glyco-) proteins

Classification of Virus

Viruses are majorly divided into two groups, i.e. DNA viruses and RNA viruses.

Major Groups of DNA Virus

1. **Adenovirus:** Its size is 70–90 nm (1 nm = 10^9 meters). The core consists of double-stranded DNA and envelope is absent. This virus multiply in nucleus. This is ether resistant. Adenovirus causes acute respiratory disease, pharyngitis and conjunctivitis.
2. **Herpesvirus:** Its size is 100–200 nm. There is double-stranded DNA. It is surrounded by a ether sensitive envelope. Herpesvirus causes vesicular skin lesions, encephalitis, chickenpox, etc. Examples are herpes simplex virus, varicella zoster virus, cytomegalovirus, etc.
3. **Hepadnavirus:** Small virus (42 to 48 nm) containing circular DNA molecules that are partially double-stranded. Hepadnavirus causes acute and chronic hepatitis. Persistent infections are associated with a high risk of developing liver cancer.
4. **Poxvirus:** Large, brick-shaped or ovoid virus (230–300 × 200–250 nm) containing double-stranded DNA, with a lipid containing envelope. All poxviruses tend to produce skin lesions. Examples of poxvirus are variola, vaccinia, molluscum contagiosum, avian pox, etc.
5. **Papovaviruses:** Small (40–50 nm) ether stable. They may cause human warts, papillomata of rabbits and polyoma of mice they produce chronic infections in natural hosts.
6. **Parvoviruses:** Very small virus (20 nm) contain single-stranded DNA. They do not have envelopes. Some members of the family cause gastroenteritis while others are associated with haemolytic disease.

Major Groups of RNA Virus

1. **Retrovirus:** Enveloped virus 90–120 nm containing single-stranded RNA. The family has many tumour producing viruses such as the sarcoma virus. Human immunodeficiency virus (HIV) which is the causative agent of acquired immunodeficiency syndrome (AIDS) belongs to the family.
2. **Rhabdovirus:** Its size is 50–95 × 130–390 nm. There is single-stranded RNA and envelope is present in it. Examples are rabies virus, vesicular stomatitis virus, etc. Rabies virus causes infection of nervous system.
3. **Orthomyxovirus:** Medium sized, 80–120 nm, enveloped virus containing single-stranded RNA. They may cause influenze, etc. Examples are influenza viruses type A, B, C, etc.
4. **Paramyxoviruses:** Its size is 150–300 nm. There is single-stranded RNA and envelope is present in this virus. They may cause respiratory infections, bad cold, measles, mumps, etc. Examples are parainfluenza virus 1 to 4, measles virus, distemper virus, rinderpest virus, mumps virus, Newcastle virus, etc.
5. **Togavirus:** Its size is 40–70 nm. Envelope is present and there is single-stranded RNA present in this virus. This virus causes meningoencephalitis, lymphadenopathy, bleeding and purpuric rashes, yellow fever, etc. Examples are yellow fever, Sindbis and dengue viruses.
6. **Arenavirus:** Its size is 85–120 nm. Envelope is present and there is single-stranded RNA in this virus. These are ether sensitive causing benign meningitis and encephalitis, e.g. lymphocytic choriomeningitis virus, etc.
7. **Reovirus:** Its size is 60–80 nm. Envelope is present and there is double-stranded RNA in this virus. This is ether resistant. This causes gastroenteritis.
8. **Picornavirus:** Its size is 20–30 nm. This is ether resistant virus containing single-stranded RNA. The groups infecting humans are rhinoviruses (causing common cold) and enterovirus (causing polio).
9. **Coronavirus:** Its size is 80–130 nm. This is ether resistant virus containing envelope and single-stranded RNA. It causes cold, acute respiratory infection, mouse hepatitis, etc. Examples are human, murine and avian virus.

Multiplication of Viruses

The genetic information necessary for viral replication is contained in the viral nucleic acid, but due to lack of biosynthetic enzymes, they depend on the host's synthetic machinery for replication. The multiplication cycle can be divided into six sequential phases:

- **Adsorption or attachment:** This depends on the presence of specific receptor sites for the virions on the host cell surface.
- **Penetration:** The intact virion can enter the animal cells as they lack cell walls, but, only the viral genome is introduced in case of bacteria due to the presence of cell wall.
- **Uncoating:** This is the process of stripping the virus of its outer layers and capsid, so that the nucleic acid is released into the cell.
- **Biosynthesis:** This includes synthesis of viral nucleic acid and capsid protein and enzymes necessary in various stages of viral synthesis, assembly and release. Maturation: This step involves the assembly of daughter virions, from the products of the last step.
- **Release:** The release of progeny can occur with or without the lysis of host cells.

Viral Genetics and Pathogenesis

In order to understand virology, it is essential to study viral genetics and pathogenesis.

Genetic Change in Viruses

Viruses are continuously changing as a result of genetic selection. They undergo subtle genetic changes through mutation and major genetic changes through recombination. Mutation occurs when an error is incorporated in the viral genome. Recombination occurs when co-infecting viruses exchange genetic information, creating a novel virus.

Mutations

Mutation Rates and Outcomes

The mutation rates of DNA viruses approximate those of eukaryotic cells, yielding in theory one mutant virus in several hundred to many thousand genome copies. RNA viruses have much higher mutation rates, perhaps one mutation per virus F (detected in 1990 linked to viral hepatitis) genome copy mutations can be deleterious or occasionally favourable.

Only mutations that do not interfere with essential virus functions can persist in a virus population.

Phenotypic variation by mutations: Mutations can produce viruses with new antigenic determinants. The appearance of an antigenically novel virus through mutation is called antigenic drift. Antigenically altered viruses may be able to cause disease in previously resistant or immune hosts.

Vaccine strains from mutations: Mutations can produce viruses with a reduced pathogenicity, altered host range, or altered target cell specificity but with intact antigenicity. Such viruses can sometimes be used as vaccine strains.

Recombination

Recombination involves the exchange of genetic material between two related viruses during co-infection of a host cell.

Recombination by independent assortment: Recombination by independent assortment can occur among viruses with segmented genomes. Genes that reside on different places of nucleic acid are randomly assorted. This can result in the generation of viruses with new antigenic determinants and new host ranges. Development of viruses with new antigenic determinants through independent assortment is called antigenic shift.

Recombination of incompletely linked genes: Genes that reside on the same piece of nucleic acid may undergo recombination. The closer the two genes are, the rarer the recombination between them (partial linkage).

Phenotypic variation from recombination: Development of viruses with new antigenic determinants by either type of recombination may allow viruses to infect and cause disease in previously immune hosts.

Vaccines through recombination: Vaccine strains of viruses can be used to create recombinant viruses that carry extra genes coding for a specific immunogen. During viral vaccination, the replicating virus will express the specific immunogen. Specific antibody production will be stimulated, and the host will be protected from the immunogen as well as from the vaccine virus.

Pathogenesis of Viral Infection

Pathogenesis is the process by which an infection leads to disease. Pathogenic mechanisms of viral disease include (1) implantation of virus at the portal of entry, (2) local replication, (3) spread to target organs (disease sites), and (4) spread to sites of shedding of virus into the environment.

Factors that affect pathogenic mechanisms are (1) accessibility of virus to tissue, (2) cell susceptibility to virus multiplication, and (3) virus susceptibility to host defences. Natural selection favours the dominance of low-virulence virus strains.

Diseases Produced by Some Important Viruses

1. **Measles virus:** This is responsible for bronchopneumonia, stomatitis, diarrhoea, conjunctivitis, encephalitis, etc. diseases.
2. **Influenza virus:** This produces epidemic influenza disease.
3. **Rotavirus:** This produces gastroenteritis disease.
4. **Poliovirus:** This is responsible for poliomyelitis.
5. **Herpesvirus:** This is responsible for ulceration in the gums, inflammation of conjunctiva, inflammation of cornea. An other species of this virus is also responsible for chickenpox.
6. **Rabies virus:** This virus is responsible for encephalomyelitis.
7. **Hepatitis virus:** This produces acute hepatitis.
   a. *Immune defences*
   b. *Control of viral infections and diseases*
   c. *Chemotherapy*

Most viral infections are limited by defences that are antigen nonspecific and/or specific. Nonspecific defences act sooner than specific defences. Some are always in place (anatomic barriers, nonspecific inhibitors, and phagocytic cells), others are evoked by the infection (fever, inflammation and interferon).

1. Immune Defences

There are various immune defence mechanisms which protect our body from viral attack. Some of these are given below:

- **Anatomic barriers:** Anatomic barriers are located at body surfaces (skin and mucosa) or within the body (endothelial cells and basement membranes). They are partly emotive in preventing virus spread but may be breached by large numbers of virus, by trauma, by increased permeability, by replication of virus in endothelial cells, or by transportation of virus in leukocytes.
- **Non-specific inhibitors:** Body fluids, and tissues normally contain soluble viral inhibitors. Most prevent viral attachment, some directly inactivate viruses, and others act intracellularly. These inhibitors may be overwhelmed by sufficient virus load.
- **Phagocytosis:** Viruses may be phagocytosed to different degrees by polymorphonuclear leukocytes and macrophages. The effect of phagocytosis may

be virus inactivation, persistence, or multiplication; consequently, the result may be clearance of virus, transportation to distant sites, or enhanced infection.

- **Fever:** Replication of most viruses is reduced by even a modest rise in temperature. During viral infection, fever can be initiated by several endogenous pyrogens, such as interleukins-1 and -6, interferon, prostaglandin E_2, and tumour necrosis factor.
- **Inflammation:** Inflammation inhibits viral replication through (1) elevated local temperature, (2) reduced oxygen tension, (3) metabolic alterations, and (4) acid production. The effects of these mechanisms are often additive.
- **Viral interference and interferon:** Viral interference occurs when infection by one virus renders cells resistant to the same or other superinfecting viruses. Interference is usually mediated by newly induced host cell proteins designated as the interferon systems. Secreted interferon binds to cells and induces them to block various stages of viral replication. Interferon also (1) inhibits growth of some normal and tumour cells and of many intracellular parasites, such as rickettsiae and protozoa; (2) modulates the immune response; and (3) affects cell differentiation. There are three main types of interferons, alpha, beta, and gamma. Alpha interferon is produced mainly by certain leukocytes (dendritic cells, macrophages and B cells), beta interferon by epithelial cells and fibroblasts, and gamma interferon by T and natural killer cells. Two other interferon types are related to alpha interferon. Omega interferons share about 70% identity with alpha interferons. Tau interferons also are related structurally to alpha interferons but are unusual by (a) being produced for only a few days by normal placental trophoblasts and (b) not being inducible by viruses.
- **Viral activation of immunity:** Immunity to viral infection is caused by a variety of specific and nonspecific mechanisms. The activation of different immune functions and the duration and magnitude of the immune response depend on how the virus interacts with host cells (on whether it is a cytolytic, steady-state, latent, and/or integrated infection) and on how the virus spreads (by local, primary haematogenous, secondary haematogenous and/or nervous system spread). Therefore, viral antigens may be present in different parts of the body depending on the route of spread and phase of infection. Local infections at surfaces such as the mucosa can elicit local cell-mediated and humoral (IgA) immune responses, but not necessarily systemic immunity.
- **Humoral immunity:** Virus and/or virus-infected cells can stimulate B lymphocytes to produce antibody (specific for viral antigens). Antibody neutralization is most effective when virus is present in large fluid spaces (e.g. serum) or on moist surfaces (e.g. the gastrointestinal and respiratory tracts). IgG, IgM, and IgA have all been shown to exert antiviral activity. Antibody can neutralize virus by: (1) blocking virus–host cell interactions or (2) recognizing viral antigens on virus-infected cells which can lead to antibody-dependent cytotoxic cells (ADCC) or complement-mediated lysis. IgG antibodies are responsible for most antiviral activity in serum, while IgA is the most important antibody when viruses infect mucosal surfaces.
- **Cell-mediated immunity:** The term cell-mediated immunity refers to (1) the recognition and/or killing of virus and virus-infected cells by leukocytes and (2) the production of different soluble factors (cytokines) by these cells when stimulated by virus or virus-infected cells. Cytotoxic T lymphocytes, natural killer (NK) cells and antiviral macrophages can recognize and kill virus-infected cells. Helper T cells can recognize virus-infected cells and produce a number of important cytokines. Cytokines produced by monocytes (monokines). T cells and NK cells (lymphokines) play important roles in regulating immune functions and developing antiviral immune functions.
- **Virus-induced immunopathology:** Immune-mediated disease may develop in certain virus infections in which viral antigens and uncontrolled immune hypersensitivity to them persist for a long period. Immune-mediated disease can be mediated by both humoral and cell-mediated immune functions. Immune-complex syndrome can be mediated by virus/virus antigen–antibody complexes. T cells (cytotoxic and helper) can also mediate, immunopathologic injuries via a number of mechanisms. Immunopathology can result from tissue/organ damage via cytotoxic T cells, inflammation induced via cytokines, antibody plus complement, antigen–antibody complexes and/or ADCC.

2. Control of Viral Infections and Diseases

Viral infections and diseases are controlled by following:

- **Immunoprophylaxis:** Immunoprophylaxis against viral illnesses includes the use of vaccines or antibody containing preparations to provide immune protection against a specific disease.
- **Active prophylaxis (vaccines):** Active immunization involves administering a virus preparation that stimulates the body's immune system to produce its own specific immunity. Viral vaccines now available for use include the following types: (1) Attenuated live viruses; (2) killed viruses; (3) recombinant produced antigens. A vaccinee is a person who has been vaccinated.
- **Immune response to vaccines:** Vaccination evokes an antibody response and stimulates T lymphocytes. Vaccine effectiveness is assessed in terms of percentage of recipients protected and the duration

and degree of protection. Most effective viral vaccines protect more than 90% of recipients and produce fairly durable immunity.

- **Passive prophylaxis:** Passive immunity is conferred by administering antibodies formed in another host. Human immunoglobulins remain a mainstay of passive prophylaxis (and occasionally therapy) for viral illnesses; they are usually used to protect individuals who have been exposed to a disease and cannot be protected by vaccination.
- **Sanitation and vector control:** Many viral diseases are controlled (1) eliminating non-human reservoirs, (2) eliminating the vector, and (3) improving sanitation.
- **Antiviral chemotherapy:** There are three types of antiviral agents: (1) virucidal agents, which directly inactivate viruses, (2) antiviral agents, which inhibit viral replication, and (3) immunomodulators, which boost the host immune response.
- **Interferons:** Virus-infected cells and cells induced with other agents, e.g. double-stranded polynucleotides, can secrete proteins called interferons, which protect normal cells from viral infection. Therapeutic administration of interferon-alpha has proven effective for several human viral illnesses.
- **Cytokines:** Cytokines are molecules produced by cells which modify the biological responses of the same or other cells.

3. Chemotherapy

Details of chemotherapy will be discussed in the block dealing with pharmacology. Basic mechanisms and main targets are described below.

- **Basic mechanisms:** Antiviral drugs specifically inhibit one or more steps of virus replication without causing unacceptable side effects.
- **Main targets for antiviral drugs:** Specific events in virus replication identified as targets for antiviral agents are viral adsorption: Penetration, uncoating, and viral nucleic acid synthesis as well as viral protein synthesis. Specificity for infected cells may occur when virus-specific enzymes (e.g. thymidine kinase-induced by herpes simplex virus or varicella-zoster virus) activate drugs (e.g. acyclovir).
- **Limitations of antiviral drugs:** Limitations include a narrow antiviral spectrum, ineffectiveness against the latent virus, development of drug-resistant mutants and toxic side effects.

Chapter 35

AIDS and HIV (Retrovirus)

ACQUIRED IMMUNODEFICIENCY SYNDROME (AIDS)

Definition

AIDS is a disabling or life-threatening disease caused by human immunodeficiency virus (HIV) characterized by HIV encephalopathy, HIV wasting syndrome, or certain diseases resulting from immunodeficiency in a person with laboratory evidence for HIV infection or without other causes of immunodeficiency.

CDC defined AIDS according to type of infections grouped accordingly as shown in Table 35.1.

WHO defined AIDS according to major and minor signs shown in Table 35.2.

Aetiology

This syndrome is caused by infection with HIV, a retrovirus of the lentivirus subgroup. The usual cause is the HIV-1 virus (Fig. 35.1). A second retrovirus, HIV-2 has also been associated with AIDS in Africa and Europe. These viruses are closely associated with a family of animal lentiviruses which cause immunodeficiency in lower primates (simian immune deficiency), neurological degenerative diseases in sheep, anaemia in horses and rheumatic disorders in goats. The geographical origin of the HIV virus is still unclear, but some evidence suggests it was present in Africa a decade before its appearance in the USA and Europe.

Following the initial recognition of cases in the USA in 1979, the epidemic has expanded rapidly. The World Health Organization has estimated that by the year 2023 there may be 39.9 million people infected with HIV.

Table 35.1: CDC cases definition of AIDS
Protozoal infections × *Pneumocystis carinii* pneumonia × Toxoplasmosis of brain × Cryptosporidiosis with diarrhoea of over 1 month's duration
Viral Cytomegalovirus (CMV)—retinitis, pneumonitis and colitis are encephalitis
Fungal Candidiasis—esophageal, tracheal, bronchial or pulmonary cryptococcal meningitis (or other extrapulmonary site)
Bacterial × *Mycobacterium avium-intracellulare* or × *M. kansasii*-disseminated + *Mycobacterium tuberculosis* (if extrapulmonary, and not confined only to lymph glands, in a patient who is HIV antibody positive) + Recurrent non-typhoid Salmonella septicaemia (if patient HIV antibody positive)
Tumours × Kaposi's sarcoma: Any age if HIV antibody +ve (<60); if HIV status unknown × Primary CNA lymphoma × Non-Hodgkin's lymphoma of B cell type (only if patient is HIV antibody +ve)
Others × HIV encephalopathy (HIV brain and spinal cord disease/AIDS dementia complex)—if patient is HIV antibody +ve × HIV wasting syndrome (slim disease)—if patient is HIV antibody +ve × Lymphoid interstitial pneumonia (LIP) in a child <13 years.

Table 35.2: WHO case definition of AIDS
Major signs
1. Weight loss >10% of body weight
2. Chronic diarrhoea >1 month
3. Fever >1 month (intermittent or constant)
Minor signs
1. Persistent cough >1 month
2. General pruritic dermatitis
3. Recurrent herpes zoster
4. Oropharyngeal candidiasis
5. Chronic progressive and disseminated herpes simplex infections
6. Generalised lymphadenopathy

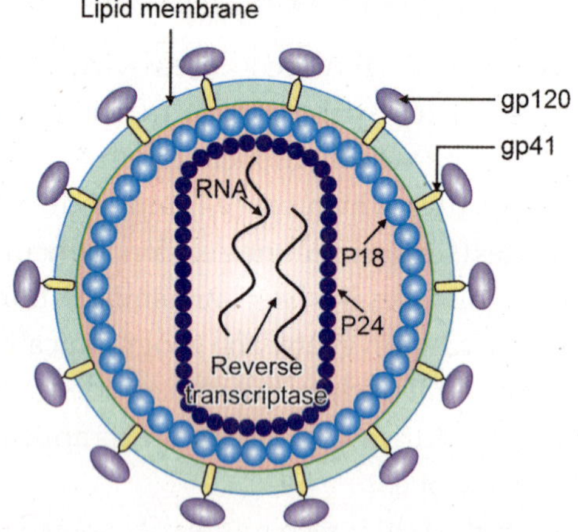

Fig. 35.1: Virocid structure of HIV, 1. gp120; 2. gp41; 3. p18; 4. Lipid envelope; 5. p24; 6. RNA; 7. Reverse transcriptase

Virus Structure

The virus contains RNA encoding three groups of structural genes encoding virion proteins and other genes which code for proteins which regulated viral replication. The three groups of structural genes are:

1. gag (group-specific antigen) coding for proteins within the viral particle, e.g. p24 which can be detected in serum of some patients with HIV infection.
2. pol coding for reverse transcriptase which converts the RNA to DNA in the host cell and for other enzymes.
3. env which codes for envelope proteins.

The virus also contains LTK (long terminal repeat) segments at either end involved in viral expression and open reading frames for other regulatory genes, e.g. tat and rev.

The structure of the HIV genome and virus (gp—glycoprotein; p—protein; numbers are molecular weight kDa).

Epidemiology

The virus is transmitted in semen, blood and other body fluids. Most infection occurs during intimate sexual contact or from blood or blood products. Homosexual activity and unprotected anal intercourse are dominant risk factors. AIDS is also seen frequently in intravenous drug abusers, haemophiliacs, thalassaemics and other patients who have been transfused with HIV-infected blood or blood products and in the heterosexual partners of those infected with HIV.

Initially, the CDC defined AIDS as a "disease at least moderately predictive of a defect in cell-mediated immunity, occurring in a person with no known cause for diminished resistance to that disease." Although this definition is still of some value for epidemiologic and surveillance studies, it does not take into account the established role of human immunodeficiency virus (HIV) in the pathogenesis of AIDS, nor that HIV infection may present with a variety of other manifestations not included in the original definition. In recognition of these new developments and in an effort to provide uniformity to the diagnosis of AIDS and other HIV-related syndromes, the CDC has proposed a revised classification effective (January 1, 1988) that divides the spectrum of HIV infections into three categories:

- **Group I:** HIV infection with specified secondary infections of malignant neoplasms.
- **Group II:** HIV infection with other specified manifestations in the absence of the secondary infections and neoplasms included in the first category (this includes patients previously referred to as having pre-AIDS and AIDS-related complex, or ARC).
- **Group III:** HIV infections not classifiable in the above two categories (this includes certain manifestations of acute HIV infection such as acute lymphadenitis, aseptic meningitis, and a syndrome resembling infectious mononucleosis).

Pathology

The pathological features of this acquired immune deficiency may be reflected in various tissues of the body such as lymph nodes, thymus, spleen, bone marrow, lymphoid elements of the gastrointestinal tract, testes and kidneys. The morphologic manifestation of infections and neoplasms occurring in AIDS of course, will also show their own characteristic pathology displayed in the target organs.

The opportunistic infections, for example, may affect the central nervous system, gastrointestinal system or the respiratory system, and thus, will cause their specific pathological alterations in these tissues, with demonstration of the causative microbes from within the tissues. In the same way, the bizarre malignancies, such as B cell lymphomas and Kaposi's sarcomas will demonstrate their own histopathologic characteristics. An unmost precaution is, however, required for handling these tissues of the AIDS patients, as these can infect the dealing personnel.

Lymphadenopathy and fever may be seen by the end of the second stage. The AIDS-related symptoms (ARS) are wide. Since the immunity is deficient, non-pathogenic microorganisms enter into the body and produce lesions in skin, gastrointestinal tract, lungs, urinary tract and brain. Gastroenteritis and tuberculosis are the predominant pattern in India. In all the cases, there will be weight reduction.

Selected secondary infections and neoplasms found in patients with HIV infection are summarized in Table 35.3.

Natural Course of the Disease

1. **Window period:** When the virus enters the body, it is multiplied in the body cells, but it cannot be detected easily. This is called the window period. The viral capsid antigen p24 can be detected in the blood during this time.
2. **Seropositive stage:** After a few months, antibodies are seen in circulation. This is called seropositivity. During this period, the person is completely normal. However, this person is a carrier of the disease, and can transmit the disease to others. About 10% seropositive individuals will go for the 3rd stage of AIDS disease within 5 years, about 50% will get AIDS within 10 years and about 90% enter into the disease state within 15 years. For each AIDS patient, there are 100 seropositive persons in the general population.
3. **AIDS disease:** The third stage is when the clinical manifestations start. By this time, the immune status of the individual is depressed. Therefore, commensal microbes will start multiplication inside the body. Patient usually succumbs to death within about 2 years after entering this stage.

Salient features of HIV are shown in Table 35.4. CDC classification of HIV is given in Table 35.5.

Transmission

1. 80% of the total patients got the infection as a sexually transmitted disease.
2. In about 15% of patients, the disease was transmitted through blood. The drug abusers usually use the same needle without any sterilization for intravenous injection. The risk of getting HIV is high in patients who receive blood transfusion many times, e.g. haemophilia patients.
3. In the rest 5% cases, virus may be transmitted from mother to foetus through placenta. About 30% of infants born to HIV positive mothers may get the infection.
4. Clinical presentations

Immunology of AIDS

1. The CD4 (T-helper) lymphocytes are decreased in number, leading to immunodeficiency. The gp120 surface unit could specifically attach with CD4 molecule present on the surface of T-helper cells. Therefore, HIV preferentially enters into the T-helper cells and they are lysed.
2. Macrophages and monocytes act as the reservoir of HIV infection, which disseminate the virus to various organs, including CNS. In turn, macrophage activity is also reduced.

Table 35.3: Selected secondary infections and neoplasms found in patients with HIV infection
Protozoal and helminthic infections
▪ Cryptosporidiosis or isosporidiosis (enteritis) ▪ Pneumocystosis (pneumonia or disseminated infection) ▪ Toxoplasmosis (pneumonia or CNS infection) ▪ Strongyloidosis (pneumonia, CNS infection, or disseminated infection)
Fungal infections
▪ Candidiasis (mouth, lung, skin or nails, disseminated) ▪ Cryptococcosis (CNS infection) ▪ Coccidioidomycosis (disseminated) ▪ Histoplasmosis (disseminated) ▪ Other opportunistic mycoses ▪ Bacterial infections ▪ Mycobacteriosis ("atypical," e.g. *M. avium-intracellulare* and *M. tuberculosis* infections, disseminated) ▪ Nocardiosis (pneumonia, meningitis, disseminated) ▪ Salmonella infections
Viral infections
▪ Cytomegalovirus (pulmonary, intestinal, or CNS infections) ▪ Herpes simplex virus (localized or disseminated) ▪ Varicella zoster virus (localized or disseminated) ▪ Progressive multifocal leukoencephalopathy
Malignant neoplasms
▪ Burkitt's lymphoma ▪ Kaposi's sarcoma ▪ Immunoblastic lymphoma (B cells) ▪ Primary CNS lymphomas

Table 35.4: Salient features of HIV
A member of the lentivirus subfamily of Retroviridae
Genetic information is encoded in 2 RNA strands The RNA is surrounded by p18 and p24, the two protein coats
It possesses a spiked envelope, whose outer portion is gp120, while the stalk that penetrates gp41
The 3 genes common to all retroviruses are *gag*, *pol* and *enn gag* codes for p24 and p18, *pol* codes for the enzyme reverse transcriptase and *env* codes for the synthesis of gp120 and gp41 It also contains non-structural genes *tat*, *art*, *3′ off*. *tat* is essential for viral replication (transactivation factor) acting both on transcription and post-transcriptional modification of all viral proteins. *art* acts to enhance the synthesis of viral structural proteins by promoting active translation of viral mRNA
HIV chiefly infects cell bearing CD4 receptors: gp120 virus projections bind to CD4 receptors on T-helper lymphocytes. The virus then enters the target cell by fusing directly with host cell membrane
A double-stranded DNA (provirus) is formed from viral provirus; integrates into host cell's DNA and remains sequestered from host immune defences
Mitogens, antigens, and cytokines such as tumour necrosis factor alpha, IL-6, and granulocyte-macrophage colony stimulating factor (GM-CSF) may induce the active replication of the latent virus, when new viruses but out from the host cell membrane.
The newly formed gp120 spikes bind to surrounding CD4 molecules on adjacent cells, and die their membrane. The punctured cells swell and die. Syncytium may form when the gp120 of infected cell binds to CD4 receptor on healthy cells. Thus, many cells fuse to form the giant cell "Syncytium". Syncytia die soon after formation

Table 35.5: CDC classification of HIV infection	
Group I	Initial infection Symptomatic (e.g. mononucleosis-like syndrome, mild meningoencephalitis)
Group II	Asymptomatic seroconversion
Group III	Persistent generalized lymphadenopathy Laboratory test abnormalities as in group II may or may not be present
Group IV	Other diseases a. Constitutional disease—fever, weight loss, diarrhoea b. Neurological disease—either central (e.g. dementia or myelopathy) or peripheral neuropathies c. Secondary infectious disease, e.g. *Pneumocystis carinii*, toxoplasmosis, Cryptococcus, cryptosporidiosis, atypical mycobacteria, herpes simplex or zoster, oral hairy leucoplakia, histoplasmosis, candidiasis, cytomegalovirus, Salmonella d. Secondary cancers, e.g. Kaposi sarcoma, non-Hodgkin's lymphoma, squamous cell carcinoma of the mouth or rectum e. Other conditions—clinical problems related to HIV and decreased cellular immunity not included above

3. Since T-helper cells play a pivotal role in the immunological system, their deficiency will lead to suppression of almost all the immunological effectors.
4. T-helper (CD4) count is less than 400/cu mm of blood. T-killer cytotoxic activity is reduced.
5. Antibody response against a foreign antigen is poor. Lymphokines such as interferon, interleukin-2, etc. are lowered.
6. When all the effector mechanisms of immunity are thus paralysed, opportunistic pathogens get entry into the body.

Immunological aberrations of AIDS and pre-AIDS are given in Table 35.6.

The sera of AIDS patients also show certain alterations, which are recounted in Table 35.7.

Table 35.6: Aberrations of cell-mediated immunity
Lymphocytopenia
T-lymphocyte dysfunction
T_4-depletion (CD_4, helper/inducer lymphocytes)
T_4: T_4 ratio alteration (CD_4: CD_4, ratio inversion)
Defective response to mitogens and antigens
Thymic involution and epithelial destruction
Aberrations of humoral immunity
Spontaneous B-cell proliferation and differentiation
Decreased B-cell response to mitogens
Lack of *de novo* antigen response
Circulating acid-labile alpha interferon and immune complexes (CIC)
Non-specific anti-lymphocyte antibodies
Elevated alpha-1 microglobulin levels
Defects in monocyte functions
Elevated beta-2 microglobulin levels
Decreased serum-thymulin levels
Increased soluble interleukin-2 receptor level
Presence of circulating and inducible suppressor factors.

Laboratory Diagnosis

Principles of Laboratory Diagnosis of HIV Infection and Related Disorders

Ever since the discovery of the aetiologic agent of AIDS, array of technologically advanced diagnostic tests have been developed to detect HIV infection. Subsequent years

Table 35.7: Serological alterations in AIDS
1. Elevation of alpha-1 thymosin
2. Elevation of beta-2 microglobulin
3. Presence of acid-liable alpha interferon
4. Demonstration of suppressive factors
5. Demonstration of anti-lymphocyte antibodies
6. Decreased serum thymulin levels

witnessed immense improvements and innovations in such techniques, which now help in providing accurate diagnosis of the disease. Most of the antigen–antibody based tests, due to their potential value, have been commercialised and are being marketed world-over.

While most laboratories essentially use a widely known enzyme immunoassay technique for initial testing. Followed by confirmation by Western blot or IF test research and clinical laboratories also consider a number of other parameters for confirming the diagnosis. A cascade of various laboratory tests in practice are categorised below.

Specific tests

- Serology by ELISA and Western blot/immuno-fluorescence test
- Antigen detection test
- Virus isolation/culture in neoplastic T cell line or by co-cultivation
- Polymerase chain reaction (PCR) or gene amplification method/dot-blot hybridisation/molecular hybridisation.
- Assays in which conjugated anti-HIV competes with anti-HIV in the specimen for HIV antigen bound to the solid phase.
- Assays in which anti-human immunoglobulin on the solid phase is used to capture antibody from the specimen, the specificity of which is then determined for HIV. Visual HIV screening assays are shown in Table 35.8.

The salient laboratory abnormalities thus include: Anaemia, leukopenia, lymphopenia and thrombocytopenia, but an apparently normal bone marrow. Liver enzymes may be slightly raised, but kidney functions are usually normal. A rapid deterioration of kidney functions may be a feature of focal/segmental glomerulosclerosis. Further, raised immunoglobulin levels are present, where IgG is usually over 2000 mg/dl and IgA over 350 mg/dl. IgM ordinarily remains unaltered.

Table 35.8: Visual HIV screening assays

Types	*Advantages*	*Disadvantages*
• Particle agglutination (RBC, latex gelatin)	• Rapid, simple, reader not needed	• Reading subjective, lot of material for safe disposal
• Colloidal gold	• Small number of samples can be tested	• Time consuming if a large number of samples tested
• Immuno dot Immuno strip	• Cost effective in small centres, sensitive and specific, less skilled person needed, longer shelf life	• Reading subjective, not suited for a large number of samples

Currently available EIAs have one of the following formats:

- Assays in which an anti-human immunoglobulin is used in the final step to detect binding of antibody to HIV antigen.
- Assays in which conjugated anti-HIV competes with anti-HIV in the specimen for HIV antigen bound to the solid phase.
- Assays in which anti-human immunoglobulin on the solid phase is used to capture antibody from the specimen, the specificity of which is then determined for HIV.

SUMMARY OF AIDS (HIV INFECTION)

Diagnosis

1. The blood count reveals a progressive lymphopenia. The depletion of helper T cells results in a fall of the CD4 : CD8 (helper : suppressor) ratio from the normal value of 1.5–2.5: 1 to less than 1:1. An absolute CD4 count of less than 0.2×10^9/L is usually associated with clinical disease and a bad prognosis.
2. A polyclonal rise in serum immunoglobulin is often found.
3. HIV infection is confirmed by serological detection of antibodies to one of the HIV antigens by enzyme-linked immunosorbent assay (ELISA) or by immunoblotting (Western blot assay). Confirmation may also be provided by detection of HIV antigen in the blood or positive culture of the virus. The lag period between infection and a positive antibody test is usually several months.
4. AIDS patients show depressed delayed-type skin reactivity to common antigens.
5. Examination of the lymph nodes reveal a spectrum of changes. In the type I pattern there is follicular and paracortical hyperplasia with attenuation of mantle zones. In the type I pattern there is follicular and paracortical hyperplasia with attenuation of mantle zones. In type II there is a loss of germinal centres but diffuse lymphoid hyperplasia and in type III, and end stage, lymphocyte depletion predominates.

HIV, the virus causing AIDS, can be inactivated (Table 35.9) by the following:

Prevention: Since there is no cure for AIDS, and vaccines are still decades away, public education and awareness are the only means to limit the spread of HIV infection. Since the major method of transmission is through sexual contact avoidance of extramarital relationships will stop the spread. All the blood samples should be tested

Table 35.9: Measures for inactivation of HIV	
Boiling	Inactivated in a second
Ethanol	70% (700 gm/L)
Glutaraldehyde	2% (available commercially CIDEX (registered) as 2% solution).
Household	1% solution (it is available in the market as a 3.5% readymade solution (Polar®. Dilute it with 2.5 volume of tap water to give 1.0% solution
Formaldehyde	5% (50 gm/L)
Chlorine-sodium hypochlorite	10% solution
Hydrogen peroxide	3% solution
Isopropyl alcohol	35% solution
Lysol	0.5% solution
Tween-20	2.5% solution

for the presence of HIV antibodies before transfusion. Syringes and needles should be properly sterilized. Disposable syringes and needles are to be used and destroyed immediately after use. Boiling for 10 minutes will inactivate the virus. Ordinary autoclaving at 120°C for 20 minutes is effective to sterilize instruments and gloves. Blood spills can be decontaminated by washing with 1% sodium hypochlorite solution, containing 10,000 ppm chlorine. Heat sensitive instruments may be decontaminated by immersing in 2% glutaraldehyde (CIDEX) for 3 hours.

Transmission of HIV infection and AIDS can be prevented if workers adopt the blood and body fluid precautions which one practice to avoid hepatitis B virus (HBV) such as

- All blood, body fluids and objects contaminated with them must be regarded as infected.
- Precautions must be taken to avoid their accidental inoculation or accidental exposure to areas with broken or unhealthy skin, wounds or cut.
- Precautions must be taken to avoid their accidental splashes on mucous membrane (viz. the eye, mouth, nose, etc.)
- All such accidental exposures must be immediately reported to the authorities.
- All contaminated objects must be properly disposed and/or appropriately decontaminated.
- Hands must always be washed immediately before and after the procedure.

Therefore, avoid direct contact with blood and/or body fluids of the patients. Use gloves, masks, protective eye shields (goggles or simple clear plastic sheets on the top of the mask), when contact with blood or body fluids of any patients is anticipated.

ANTIRETROVIRAL THERAPY (ART)

Specific treatment with antiretroviral drugs is the mainstay in the management of HIV infection. *Highly active antiretroviral therapy (HAART)* is effective in inhibition of HIV replication in most of the HIV-infected individuals but major drawback with this therapy is the selection of resistant mutants. Antiretroviral drugs include both nucleoside and non-nucleoside inhibitors of enzyme reverse transcriptase, nucleotide inhibitor, viral protease inhibitors and fusion inhibitor (Table 35.10). These drugs have been used as monotherapy or in various combinations. Adverse reactions and high cost restrict their wide use in developing countries.

Apart from specific antiretroviral therapy, other measures in the treatment of AIDS include: (i) Treatment and prophylaxis of opportunistic infections and tumours, (ii) general management and (iii) immunorestorative measures.

Postexposure Prophylaxis (PEP)

Exposure to blood, body fluid, other potentially infected material or an instrument contaminated with one of these materials may lead to risk of acquiring HIV infection. The risk of infection varies with the type of exposure and other factors. Most exposures do not result in infection. Health workers are normally at very low risk of acquiring infection during management of infected patients. Following exposure, postexposure prophylaxis (PEP) may be required depending upon the exposure code (EC) and HIV status code (HIV SC) of exposure source. Zidovudine 300 mg BD and Lamivudine 150 mg BD are used in combination for a period of four weeks. In selected cases, indinavir 800 mg TDS is added to this combination of drugs according to PEP guidelines. To be effective these drugs must be started within an hour or two. Both risk of infection and possible side-effects of antiretroviral drugs should be carefully considered when deciding to start

Table 35.10: Antiretroviral drugs

Nucleoside reverse transcriptase inhibitors (NRTIs)	*Non-nucleoside reverse transcriptase inhibitors (NNRTIs)*	*Nucleotide inhibitor*	*Protease inhibitors (PIs)*	*Fusion inhibitor*
Zidovudine (AZT, azidothymidine)	*Nevirapine (viramune)*	*Tenofovir*	*Saquinavir*	*Enfuvirtide*
Didanosine (ddl)	Delaviridine (rescriptor)		*Ritonavir*	
Zalcitabine (ddc)	Efavirenz (sustiva)		Indinavir	
Stavudine (d4T)	Loviride		Nelfinavir	
Lamivudine (3TC)			Amprenavir	
Abacavir (1592)			Tipranavir	

PEP. Besides PEP, injured site on the wound should be thoroughly washed with soap and water. Antiseptics may also be used.

Universal Precautions

Concerns about transmission of the hepatitis B virus (HBV) and human immunodeficiency virus (HIV) led to the introduction of 'universal precautions', to minimise the infections in medical laboratory workers and health care personnel. These universal precautions include:

1. Assume that all specimens/patients are potentially infectious for HIV and other bloodborne pathogens.
2. All blood specimens or body fluids should be placed in a leak-proof impervious bags for transporation to the laboratory.
3. Use gloves while handling blood and body fluid specimens and other objects exposed to them. If there is a likelihood of spattering, use face masks with glasses or goggles.
4. Wear laboratory coats or gowns while working in the laboratory. Wrap-around gowns should be preferred. These should not be taken outside.
5. Never pipette by mouth. Mechanical pipetting devices should be used.
6. Decontaminate the laboratory work surfaces with an appropriate disinfectant after the spillage of blood or other body fluids and when the procedures are completed.
7. Limit use of needles and syringes to situations for which there are no other alternatives.
8. Biological safety hoods should be used for laboratory work.
9. All the potentially contaminated materials of the laboratory should be decontaminated before disposal or reprocessing.
10. Always wash hands after completing laboratory work and remove all protective clothings before leaving the laboratory.

Chapter 36

Hepatitis Viruses

Chapter Outline

HEPATITIS VIRUSES

Hepatitis A (Fig. 36.1A to C)

The disease formerly called infectious hepatitis, or short incubation hepatitis, almost always results from oral ingestion of the HA virus. Infected patients shed virus in faeces for several weeks before clinical illness appears and for 1 to 2 weeks thereafter. During the prodromal and early jaundiced period, there may be viraemia at low and unpredictable levels, but chronic viraemia does not occur. Epidemic spread often occurs in outbreaks related to contaminated water supplies or uncooked shellfish harvested from contaminated beds. Interpersonal spread, especially between children in institutions or in close family settings, allows widespread exposure and is undoubtedly responsible for much subclinical illness.

Structure of Hepatitis A Virus (Fig. 36.1A to C)

Hepatitis A virus differs from other picornaviruses in that it is non-cytopathogenic and particles are released within membranous structures containing 1–4 virions. The virus infects the epithelial cells of the small intestine and hepatocytes of primates. Viral replication predominantly occurs in the liver, is excreted via the bile into the colon, and transmitted faecal–oral. Clinical manifestations include jaundice, fever, abdominal pain, light stools, and diarrhoea. The infection is generally of a limited nature, and does not persist chronically. The virus is very stable, resistant to acid pH, and stable at elevated temperatures (60°C) for short durations.

Epidemiology

Hepatitis A is usually a fairly mild, self-limited illness that rarely causes prolonged debility or persisting liver damage. Many persons who have never knowingly had hepatitis have anti-HA. Worldwide, the incidence of anti-HA positivity increases with declining socioeconomic levels and standards of sanitation.

Laboratory Tests

Diagnosis of hepatitis A depends on clinical and laboratory observations:

1. The patient experiences malaise, anorexia, fever, and nausea.
2. Elevated aminotransferases and bilirubinuria are almost universal; alkaline phosphatase and serum direct bilirubin are often high.
3. Definitive diagnosis rests on serologic demonstration of viral exposure.

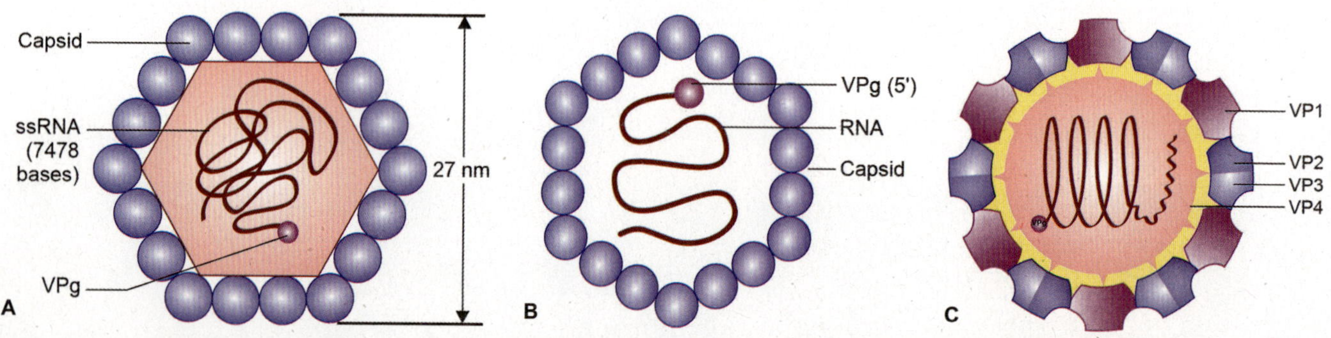

Fig. 36.1: (A) Capsid, ssRNA, a 27 nm structure, (B) RNA, VPg (5'), (C) Polypeptides VP_1, VP_2, VP_3 and VP_4

4. Tests for viremia are not clinically feasible, and immunoelectron microscopy is the only way to demonstrate virus in the faeces.
5. Anti-HA antibodies, however, are easily demonstrated by radioimmunoassay. An acute illness is considered to be hepatitis A if anti-HA antibody titers rise between acute and convalescent serum samples; or if post-illness serum contains antibody in a person whose pre-illness serum was known to lack antibody; or if there is a high level of IgM anti-HA relative to the level of IgG antibody (Fig. 36.2).

Hepatitis B

The disease formerly called serum hepatitis, or long incubation hepatitis, is now called hepatitis B. Infective HB virions circulate in the blood for prolonged periods, and can at times be found in faeces, urine, semen, saliva, and virtually any body fluid. Spread can occur by blood transfusion or parenteral exposure to materials containing blood, or instruments contaminated with body fluids; by faecal–oral transmission; and by person-to-person contact, including sexual activity. Vertical transmission from mother to child is common, producing a persistent state of viral infection in the infant. Although mild and subclinical hepatitis B infections do occur, the disease is usually more severe than hepatitis A and may be fatal, especially in the very old or persons with other illnesses. Chronic active hepatitis may follow the acute illness. In some patients with minimal or no evidence of continuing liver damage, viral material may remain in the circulation for months or years, or for life.

Laboratory Testing

Intense laboratory scrutiny of the HB virus has uncovered numerous aspects susceptible to clinical or research testing. Highly sensitive tests for hepatitis B antigen (HBsAg) are widely available. Testing for HBsAg allows specific diagnosis of hepatitis B even in mild, subclinical, or persistent cases. All blood destined for transfusion must be tested and found negative for HBsAg because HBs antigenemia carries a strong, though not absolute association with infectivity. Tests for anti-HBs are also widely available and are useful for retrospective diagnosis and for epidemiologic studies. Some workers believe that anti-HBc, testing might provide still further safeguard against hepatitis transmission in blood transfusion. Tests for HBeAg and anti-HBe are used mostly in research settings, to attempt prediction or prognosis in acute and chronic infection (Figs 36.3 to 36.5).

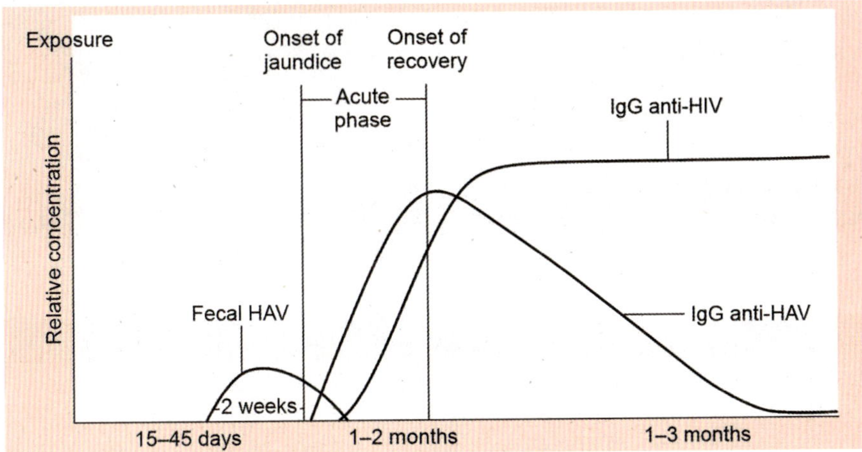

Fig. 36.2: Sequence of serologic changes in acute hepatitis A

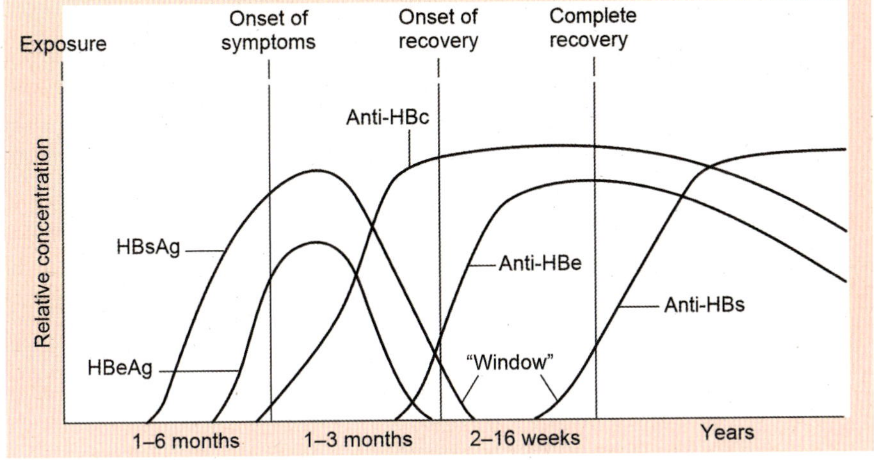

Fig. 36.3: Sequence of serologic changes in acute hepatitis B

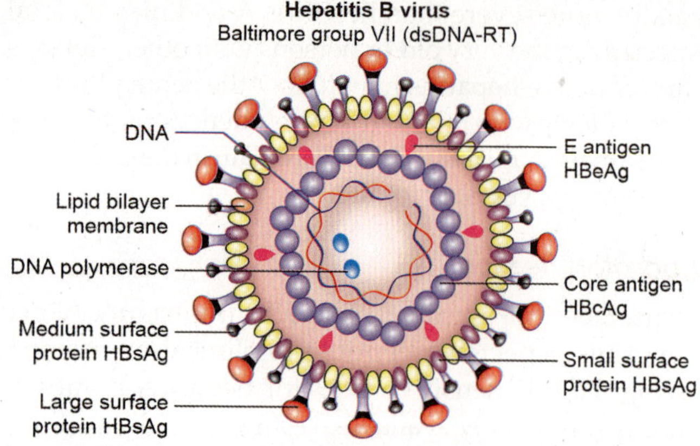

Fig. 36.4: Structure of hepatitis B showing HBcAg, HBsAg, HBeAg

Fig. 36.5: Structure of hepatitis B illustrating HBsAg, HBeAg and DNA polymerase in the centre

Hepatitis C (Non-A, Non-B Hepatitis Virus (NANBV))

Hepatitis C virus is a small, enveloped, icosahedral, positive ssRNA virus that belongs to the Flaviviridae family. The Flaviviridae are vector-borne RNA viruses that cause a wide spectrum of diseases including hepatitis; encephalitis, vascular shock, acute flaccid paralysis, congenital abnormalities, and foetal death. The family is subdivided into three genera. Flavivirus, Pestivirus, and Hepacivirus. The Flavivirus genus are zoonotic and insect-borne viruses, and responsible for Yellow fever, Dengue fever, Japanese encephalitis, West Nile encephalitis, and tick-borne encephalitis. The Pestivirus genus includes animal viruses causing bovine viral diarrhea and classical swine fever. The Hepacivirus genus (hepatitis C) causes viral hepatitis and hepatocellular carcinoma in humans (Fig. 36.6).

Contrasting features of various types of hepatitis are shown in Table 36.1.

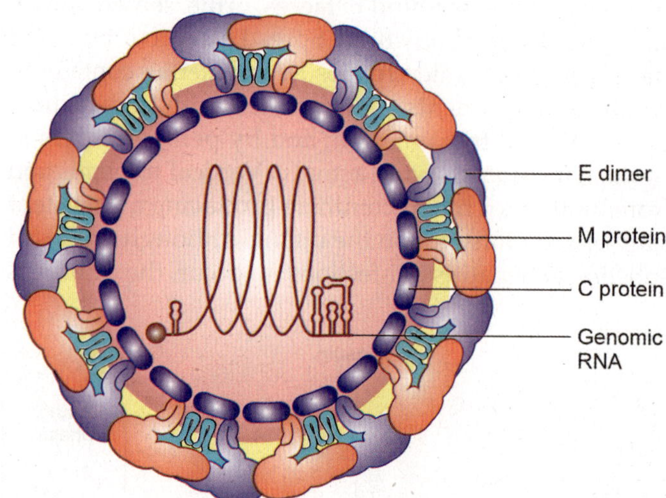

Fig. 36.6: Structure of hepatitis C showing E dimer, M protein, C protein

Table 36.1: Contrasting features of various types of hepatitis

Feature	*Hepatitis A*	*Hepatitis B*	*Hepatitis D*	*Hepatitis C (non-A, non-B hepatitis)*
1. *Etiologic agent*	HAV, 27 nm RNA	HBV, 42 nm DNA	HDV, 36 nm HBsAg-coated RNA Parenteral	HCV (NANBV), 50–60 nm RNA Mainly parenteral, some by enteric route
2. *Spread*	Faecal–oral	Parenteral		
3. *Incubation period*	15–45 days	30–180 days	30–50 days (in superinfection)	42–56 days
4. *Major antigens*	HAAg	HBsAg, HBcAg, HBeAg	HDAg	Unknown
5. *Antibodies*	Anti-HAV, Anti-HBe	Anti-HB, Anti-HBc	Anti-HD	Anti-HCV
6. *Virologic marker*	None	HBV-DNA	HDV particle	HCV-RNA
7. *Severity and complications*	Mild	Marked	Marked	Mild to marked
8. *Carrier state*	None	Yes	Yes	Yes
9. *Chronic hepatitis*	No	Yes (10%)	Yes (10–40% in superinfection)	Yes (40–60%)
10. *Liver cancer*	No	Yes	Rare	Yes

Hepatitis delta virus (HDV) which is sometimes associated as superinfection with hepatitis B infection

Hepatitis B terminology illustrations are given in Table 36.2.

Serologic and virologic markers for HCV infection available presently are as under:

1. **Anti-HCV antibody** appears after a delay of about 4–12 months in post-transfusion hepatitis C (windows period). Because of this reason, anti-HCV detection is worthless for diagnosis of acute hepatitis C as blood remains infectious during window period while the test is negative.
2. **HCV-RNA test** which is at present a research test only. These tests are commercially not available yet. Thus, much knowledge is yet to be acquired about hepatitis C.

Hepatitis D

Hepatitis delta virus (HDV) is a defective RNA virus that depends upon the expression of the hepatitis B virus surface antigen (HBsAg) in the same cell in order to complete its life cycle. HDV can infect hepatocytes that do not contain HBsAg, and can replicate its genome and express the hepatitis delta antigen, however, is unable to secreted infectious viral particles. When co-infection occurs with HBV, chronic hepatitis D is the most aggressive form of viral hepatitis, and is associated with cirrhosis, liver failure, and hepatocellular carcinoma. Co-infection can occur simultaneously with HBV, or can occur as a superinfection of a chronic carrier of HBV. Co-infection causes acute hepatitis, but most cases resolve both infections, although the chance of liver failure is higher than with HBV infection alone. In the case of superinfection, most progress to chronic dual infection with both viruses. There are no significant therapies that are successful in treating HDV infection, and nucleoside analogues that are useful for treating HBV have no effect on HDV replication (Fig. 36.7).

The virions are 35–37 nm, and comprised of an envelope and ribonucleoprotein. Similar in structure to HBV, both viruses use HBV surface proteins S, M (Fig. 36.7) and HBsAg for assembly. The capsid is formed from

Table 36.2: Hepatitis B terminology illustrations	
Dane particle	The 42 nm particle consisting of DNA core and protein coat; thought to be the infective HB virion
HBcAg (Fig. 36.4)	The core antigen of the HB virus, found only in the core of the intact virion and naturally demonstrable only in the nucleus of infected hepatocytes. Artificially stripping the protein coat from the Dane particle reveals HBcAg in laboratory material
HBeAg (Fig. 36.5)	An antigen that does circulate in blood, associated more with the core than the surface of the virus. Persistence of HBeAg in a patient's serum suggests continuing infectivity, because antigen is usually promptly cleared from serum as antibodies develop
HBsAg	The protein-containing surface material manufactured in the cytoplasm of infected hepatocytes. Circulates in blood before and during acute infection and, in chronic carriers, after acute illness. HBsAg is not, by itself, infective but does elicit antibodies that protect against subsequent infection. Used as a marker for infectivity, because Dane particles often accompany HBsAg in body fluids. Formerly called hepatitis-associated antigen (HAA) or Australian antigen
Anti-HBc	Antibody to core antigen; develops earlier than anti-HBs and persists for months or years
Anti-HBs	Antibody to HBsAg that develops during or shortly after clinically apparent illness and persists lifelong. Has some but not total protective immunity. Presence of anti-HBs in a person not deliberately immunized is evidence of prior infection

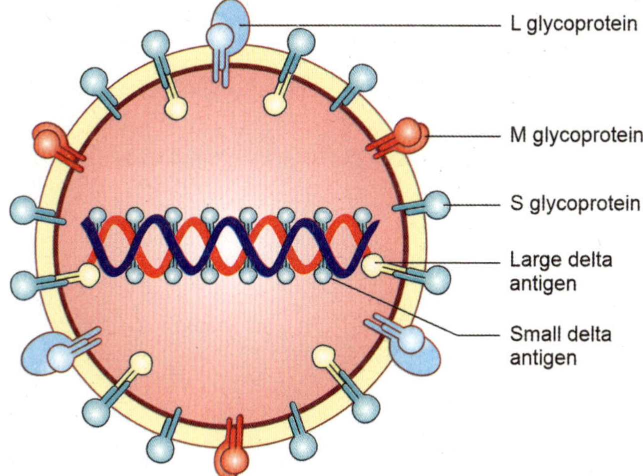

Fig. 36.7: Structure of hepatitis D virus (HDV) showing L, M, S glycoproteins with large delta antigen and small delta antigen

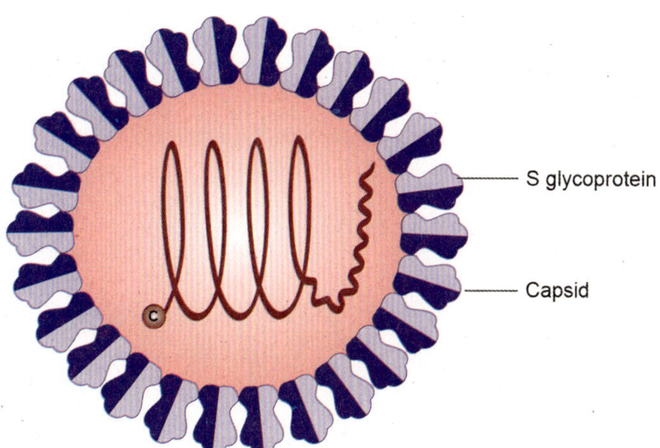

Fig. 36.8: Structure virus hepatitis E virus (HEV) showing icosahedral capsid, and single-stranded RNA

multimerisation of core protein HBcAg, and contains one copy of the viral circular, ssRNA genome, enclosed by large and small delta antigens which form the viral ribonucleoprotein. The HDV genome is a circular, closed ssRNA which folds into a partially double-stranded rod.

Hepatitis E

Hepatitis E virus (HEV) is the most common cause of hepatitis globally. A member of the Orthohepevirus family with four species (A to D), human disease is caused by strains of species A. HEV is a non-enveloped virus with an icosahedral capsid (Fig. 36.8), a size of 27–34 nm, and contain a positive-sense, single-stranded, 7.2 kb RNA genome which is 5′ capped and 3′ polyadenylated.

Clinical Manifestations

HEV infection causes an acute, self-limited hepatitis in 5% of patients who contract the virus, but can have high mortality in pregnant women, the elderly, or those with pre-existing liver disease. Chronic infection can occur in the immunosuppressed or organ transplant patients. The virus can also cause extrahepatic manifestations including glomerulonephritis, pancreatitis, thrombocytopenia, autoimmune condition, and neurological conditions such as neuritis, neuropathy, Guillain-Barré syndrome, and encephalitis/myelitis.

Chapter 37

Rabies Virus (Rhabdovirus)

Chapter Outline

RHABDOVIRUSES

Rhabdoviruses are bullet- or rod-shaped (*rhabdos*, meaning rod) enveloped viruses with single-stranded RNA genome. They are included in the family Rhabdoviridae.

The family Rhabdoviridae consists of more than 100 single-stranded, negative-sense, nonsegmented viruses that infect a wide variety of hosts, including vertebrates, invertebrates, and plants. Common to all members of the family is a distinctive rod- or bullet-shaped morphology.

Human pathogens of medical importance are found in the genera Lyssavirus and Vesiculovirus. Only rabies virus, medically the most significant member of the genus Lyssavirus.

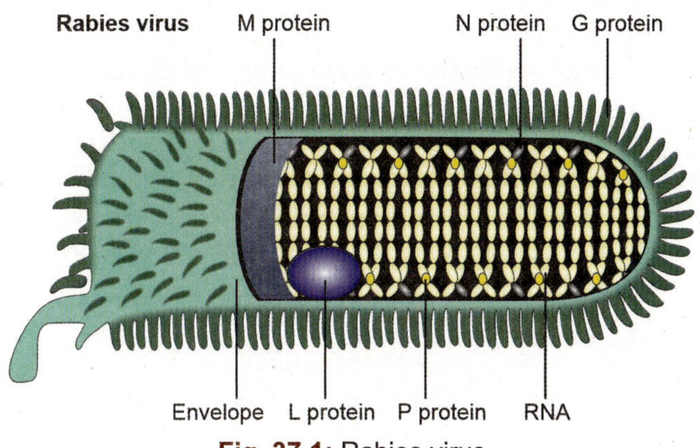

Fig. 37.1: Rabies virus

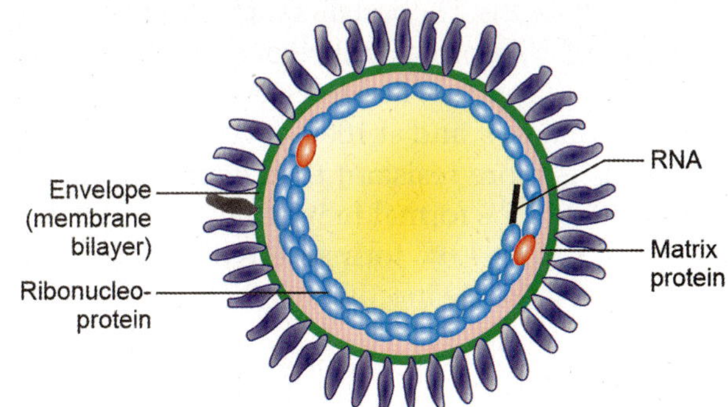

Fig. 37.2: Cross section rabies virus

RABIES VIRUS

Structure

Morphology

1. Bullet-shaped, 75 × 180 nm, with one end round and the other end planar or concave.
2. The outer lipoprotein envelope contains haemagglutinating peplomer spikes.
3. Beneath the lipoprotein envelope is the matrix (M) protein layer.
4. Nucleocapsid shows helical symmetry containing a single-stranded, RNA genome and a RNA-dependent RNA polymerase. The genome is unsegmented (Fig. 37.1).

The cross-sectional diagram demonstrates the concentric layers: Envelope membrane bilayer, M protein, and tightly coiled encased genomic RNA.

The virus genome encodes five proteins associated with either the ribonucleoprotein (RNP) complex or the viral envelope (Fig. 37.2).

The L (transcriptase), N (nucleoprotein), and NS (transcriptase-associated) proteins comprise the RNP complex, together with the viral RNA. These aggregate in the cytoplasm of virus-infected neurons and compose Negri bodies, the characteristic histopathologic finding of rabies virus infection. The M (matrix) and G (glycoprotein) proteins are associated with the lipid envelope. The G protein forms the protrusions that cover the outer surface of the virion envelope and is the only rabies virus protein known to induce virus-neutralizing antibody.

Host Range and Cultivation

There is a wide range of susceptible animals, including man and almost all mammals; the outcome of infection is nearly always fatal, with the exception that vampire bats are known to be able to transmit the virus for several months without showing any signs of the disease themselves. The virus invades blood and the central nervous system of the host and is excreted in the saliva, milk and urine. These materials can be used to transmit the infection to laboratory animals, including rabbits, mice and guinea pig. Freshly isolated strains of the virus are known as "street virus" and will fill laboratory animals with a severe encephalitis after an incubation period which varies from one to twelve weeks according to the species inoculated. Multiple eosinophilic inclusions known as Negri bodies are found in the nerve cells especially in the hippocampus, and measure 0.5 micron to 20 micron diameter. Negri bodies are specific in rabies infection and their detection in nerve tissue enables a diagnosis of rabies to be made.

Serial brain-to-brain passage of the virus in rabbits yields an attenuated or "fixed" strain of the virus which is no longer able to multiply in extraneural situations. Negri bodies are scanty in the brains of animals inoculated with the fixed virus. The virus grows in the tissues of 7-day-old chick embryos inoculated by any of the usual routes; the maximum yield of virus is obtained nine days after inoculation. The virus has been grown in monolayer cultures of the following cells, chick or mouse embryo, suckling hamster kidney and embryo rabbit brain. Most strains appear to grow poorly and do not produce any cytopathic effect.

Viability

The infectivity of the virus in tissues kept at room temperatures is gradually lost in 7–14 days at 4°C, the virus survives several weeks and in 50% glycerol saline at 4°C for many months. The best diluent for the preservation of the virus is 2.5% normal guinea pig serum in saline.

At 37°C, the virus survives five days, at 50°C one hour, at 60°C five minutes, and at 100°C two to three minutes. Rabies virus is more resistant than vegetative bacteria to disinfectant; 0.5% formaldehyde fails to kill it in two months at 4°C, but 1.0% formaldehyde, 3% cresol and 0.1% mercuric chloride inactivate in 15 minutes.

Pathogenesis

Rabies virus is most commonly transmitted through the bite of an infected mammal, all of which may be susceptible, but to greatly varying degrees. The virus may enter the peripheral nervous system directly, or may replicate in muscle tissue after entering the host, remaining at or near the site of introduction for most of the incubation period. However, the precise sites of viral sequestration remain unknown, since neither antigen nor virus can usually be found in any organ during this phase.

Rabies is a natural infection of dogs, foxes, cats, wolves and bats. Man is infected by the bite of rabid dog or other animals. Saliva containing viruses are deposited in the wound. The rabies virus multiplies in muscle or connective tissue at or near the site of introduction before it attaches to nerves.

After inoculation, rabies virus may enter the peripheral nervous system directly and migrates to the brain or may replicate in muscle tissue, remaining sequestered at or near the entry site during incubation, prior to central nervous system invasion and replication. It then spreads centrifugally to numerous other organs. The case: fatality ratio approaches unity, but exact pathogenic mechanisms are not fully understood.

Virus may enter the peripheral nervous system via the neuromuscular junctions, and moves rapidly centripetally to the central nervous system for replication; symptoms may develop shortly thereafter. The virus then begins to pass centrifugally to many tissues and organs, such as the salivary glands.

In general, gross examination of the brain shows mild congestion of the meningeal vessels; microscopic examination usually demonstrates slight perivascular cuffing, limited tissue necrosis, acidophilic intracytoplasmic neuronal inclusions, and rarely, neuronophagia.

Host Defenses

The host animal species, viral variant, inoculum concentration, body location and severity of exposure, and host immune status have been associated with overt susceptibility to infection and with different incubation periods. The association of virus-neutralizing antibody. principally IgG, and protective immunity is well-known.

Susceptibility to lethal infection is related to the animal species, viral variant, inoculum concentration, location and severity of exposure, and host immune status.

Multiplication

The viral RNA uncoats in the cytoplasm of infected cells. The genome is transcribed by a virion-associated RNA-dependent RNA polymerase. Viral RNA is then translated into individual viral proteins. Replication occurs with synthesis of positive-stranded RNA templates for the production of progeny negative-stranded RNA.

Transmission

Rabies is most common in countries where stray dogs are present in large numbers, with Asia and Africa accounting for 95% of cases.

As saliva carries the virus, rabies can develop if an infected animal bites someone. It can also occur if saliva from an infected animal gets into an open wound or through a mucous membrane, such as the eyes or mouth. However, the virus cannot pass through unbroken skin.

The portal of entry is the bite and the rabies virus in the infected saliva is introduced into the depths of the wound. Occasionally, the virus may gain access through a preexisting scratch or abrasion if this has been contaminated by saliva. The virus multiplies locally in the tissues, invades damaged nerve fibres, and spreads centrally to reach the brain and spinal cord. It is not yet decided whether the virus travels along the axons of nerves or along perineural lymphatics. There is no evidence that the virus is spread through the blood stream or lymphatic channels, and it has only rarely been isolated from the cerebrospinal fluid (CSF).

There have been no confirmed instances of human-to-human transmission of rabies virus aside from those attributable to organ/tissue transplantation.

People usually get rabies from the bite of a rabid animal.

Incubation Period

The incubation period varies from ten days to two years after the bite of a rabid animal; its duration may depend on the distance the virus has to move from the point of entry to reach the brain. Average figures are: For bites on the leg 60 days, on the arm 40 days and on the heel 30 days. The incubation period is shorter in children than in adults.

Clinical Manifestations

There are three clinical phases of the disease:

1. **Prodromal phase:** The onset of clinical rabies in man includes 2–4 days of prodromal.
2. **Excitation phase:** The excitation phase begins gradually and may persist to death.
3. **Paralytic phase:** Hydrophobia, if present, disappears and swallowing becomes possible.

Rabies virus causes acute infection of the central nervous system. Five general stages are recognized in humans: Incubation, prodrome, acute neurologic period, coma, and death. The incubation period is exceptionally variable, ranging from fewer than 10 days to longer than 2 years, but is usually 1–3 months.

These symptoms are often non-specific (general malaise, fever, and fatigue) or suggest involvement of the respiratory system (sore throat, cough, and dyspnoea), gastrointestinal system (anorexia, dysphagia, nausea, vomiting, abdominal pain, and diarrhoea), or central nervous systems (headache, vertigo, anxiety, apprehension, irritability, and nervousness).

More remarkable abnormalities (agitation, photophobia, priapism, increased libido, insomnia, nightmares, and depression) may also occur, suggesting encephalitis, psychiatric disturbances, or brain conditions. Pain or paresthesia at the site of virus inoculation, combined with a history of recent animal bite, should suggest a consideration of rabies.

Lastly, however, high fever, difficulty in swallowing and a fear of water (hydrophobia) become the dominant symptoms, and the patient passes into delirium with generalised convulsions. The outcome is invariably fatal.

Diagnosis

Early diagnosis is difficult. Rabies should be suspected in human cases of unexplained viral encephalitis with a history of animal bite. Unvaccinated persons are often negative for virus-neutralizing antibodies until late in the course of disease. Virus isolation from saliva, positive immunofluorescent skin biopsies or virus-neutralizing antibody (from cerebrospinal fluid, or serum of a non-vaccinated patient), establish a diagnosis.

Laboratory Diagnosis

Diagnosis in Humans

i. **Immunofluorescence test:** Viral antigens can be detected in corneal impression smears and facial skin biopsies or saliva by direct immunofluorescence using antirabies serum tagged with fluorescein isothiocyanate. Diagnosis may be made postmortem using brain as a specimen.
ii. **Demonstration of Negri bodies:** This is demonstrated in brain. Negri bodies appear as intracytoplasmic, oval or round, purplish pink (3–27 mm) bodies with characteristic basophilic inner granules. *Seller's technique* is used to demonstrate these bodies.
iii. **Isolation of the virus:** The virus can be isolated from specimens like CSF, saliva and urine, by intracerebral inoculation in mice. However, during postmortem, brain tissue is also used. The inoculated mice are examined for signs of illness, and their brains are examined at death or at 28 days after inoculation for Negri bodies. Brains can also be examined by immunofluorescence technique.
   A more rapid and sensitive method is isolation of the virus by tissue culture. Diagnosis is made by detection of rabies virus in inoculated tissue culture cells by immunofluorescence.
iv. **Antibody detection:** High titre antibodies in the CSF can be used for diagnosis.
v. **PCR:** PCR can be used for detection of rabies virus RNA. It is a sensitive method.

Vaccination

Vaccines are of two main categories—neural and non-neural. Non-neural (Table 37.1) vaccines are being used increasingly because neural vaccines are associated with serious risk of neurological complications.

(i) Neural Vaccines

The following are some of the infected brain vaccines being used.

a. **Semple vaccine:** It was developed by Semple (1911) at the Central Research Institute (CRI), Kasauli, India. It is a 5% suspension of infected sheep brain and inactivated by 5% phenol at 37°C, leaving no residual live virus.
b. **Beta-propiolactone (BPL) vaccine:** It is modified Semple vaccine with BPL as inactivating agent instead of phenol.
c. **Infant brain vaccine:** Brain tissue vaccines are associated with neurological complications due to the presence of myelin. It is scanty or absent in non-

Table 37.1: Antirabies vaccines

Vaccine	Type	Use
Neural		
1. Semple vaccine	Inactivated by 5% phenol at 37°C	Widely used
2. Beta-propiolactone (BPL) vaccine	Inactivated by BPL instead of phenol	Most of the Indian laboratories manufacture this vaccine
3. Infant brain vaccine	Inactivated by UV radiation, BPL or phenol	Used widely in South America
Non-neural		
1. Duck egg vaccine	–	Discontinued
2. Tissue culture vaccine	Inactivated by BPL	Highly antigenic, free from side effects, but costly

myelinated neural tissue of infant brain and thus may reduce neurological complications.

(ii) Non-neural Vaccines

a. **Duck egg vaccine:** It is beta-propiolactone inactivated vaccine. It has a poor immunogenicity and is therefore discontinued.
b. **Cell culture vaccines:** The human diploid cell strain (HDCS) vaccine is prepared by growing rabies virus on human diploid cells and is inactivated with beta-propiolactone. This vaccine is highly antigenic and free of side effects. The only disadvantage is its high cost.
   Other equally effective but more economical cell culture vaccines have been developed. The purified chick embryo cell (PCEC) culture vaccine is now widely used in the trade name of Rabipur. Purified vero cell (PVC) vaccine is the another economical cell culture vaccine.

Commonly used vaccines against rabies are shown in Table 37.2.

Table 37.2: Commonly used antirabies vaccines

S. No.	Vaccine	Substrate to grow virus	Type
1.	Semple vaccine	Sheep brain	Inactivated by phenol
2.	BPL vaccine	Sheep brain	Inactivated by BPL
3.	HDCS vaccine	Human diploid cell	Inactivated by BPL
4.	PCEC vaccine	Chick embryo cells	Inactivated by BPL
5.	PVC vaccine	Vero cells	Inactivated by BPL

VACCINATION SCHEDULES

When the biting animal can be observed for ten days and the animal remains healthy, rabies may be excluded and vaccine, if already started, may be discontinued.

a. **Neural vaccines:** The vaccine schedule varies according to the degree of risk to which patient has been exposed.
   The vaccine is given subcutaneously on the anterior abdominal wall. It requires seven to fourteen injections depending on the degree of risk.
b. **Cell culture vaccines:** All three cell culture vaccines available in India (HDCS, PCEC and PVC vaccines) have the same dose schedule. It is also same for both adults and children.
   Postexposure vaccination: 1.0 ml is given by intramuscular route in the deltoid region, on days 0, 3, 7, 14 and 30, with a booster dose (optional) on day 90.

Chapter 38

Arboviruses and Rubella

(Dengue, Chikungunya, Rubella)

Chapter Outline

- Arboviruses
- Dengue
- Chikungunya
- Rubella
- Pathophysiology
- Congenital Rubella Syndrome (CRS)

ARBOVIRUSES

Arbovirus, any of a large group of viruses, that develop in arthropods (chiefly mosquitoes and ticks). The name derives from *arthropod-borne virus*. The spheroidal virus particle is encased in a fatty membrane (Fig. 38.1) and contains RNA; it causes no apparent harm to the arthropod host. Arboviruses are transmitted by bites to vertebrate hosts, in which they establish infections and complete their growth cycle.

Taxonomically, arboviruses belong to five families: Togaviridae, Flaviviridae, Bunyaviridae, Reoviridae and Rhabdoviridae.

Structure of Arbovirus Shape

The majority of the arboviruses are **spherical in shape although a few are rod-shaped**. They are 17–150 nm in diameter and most have an RNA genome (Figs 38.2 and 38.3) (the single exception is African swine fever virus, which has a DNA genome).

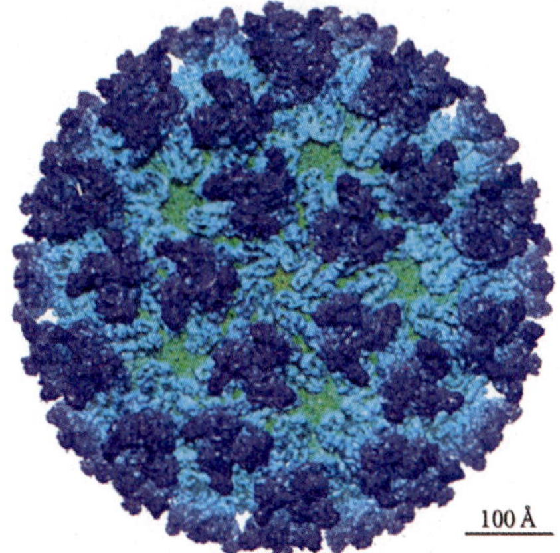

Fig. 38.1: Structure of arbovirus in general

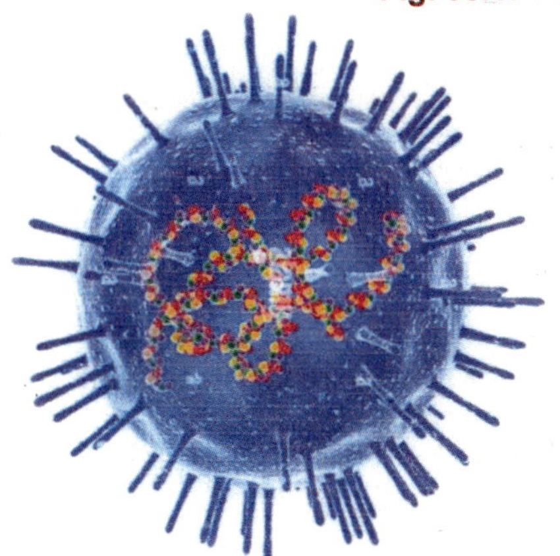

Fig. 38.2: Arbovirus spherical shape

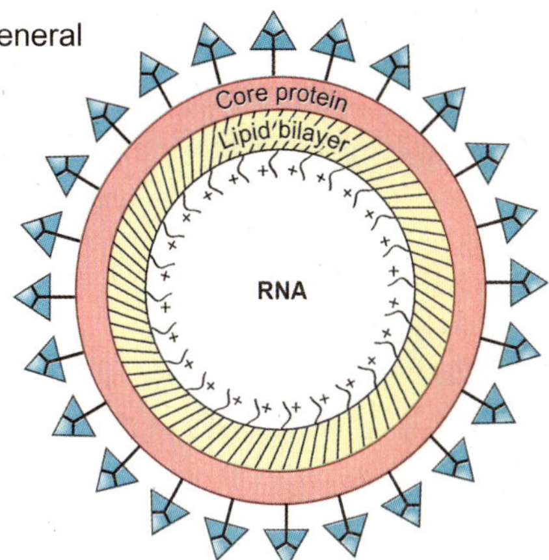

Fig. 38.3: Arbovirus showing spikes lipid bilayer core proteins and RNA

Diseases caused by Arboviruses are shown in Table 38.1.

Laboratory Diagnosis of Arboviruses

Diagnosis may be established by virus isolation or serology.

A. **Specimens:** Blood, CSF and brain may be used for isolation of virus. As all arboviruses are viraemic, blood is collected during the acute phase of the disease. CSF is useful in encephalitis cases but the best specimen is the brain.

B. **Virus Isolation**
   1. *Suckling mice:* Specimens are inoculated intracerebrally into suckling mice. The animal develops fatal encephalitis.
   2. *Tissue culture:* Some viruses may also be isolated in tissue cultures. Growth of virus in cell cultures is identified by immunofluorescence, haemagglutination inhibition, complement fixation, ELISA or neutralisation tests.

C. **Serology:** Using ELISA, serotype specific IgM antibody may be detected in patient serum. The detection of a fourfold rise or more in antibody titre provides a good evidence of infection.

DENGUE

Dengue is characterised by fever of sudden onset, headache, retrobulbar pain, conjunctival infection, pain in the back and joints (also called break-bone fever), lymphadenopathy and maculopapular rash.

Dengue virus has four serotypes: Dengue 1 (DEN1), dengue 2 (DEN 2), dengue 3 (DEN 3) and dengue 4 (DEN4). It is transmitted by *Aedes aegypti* (Fig. 38.4).

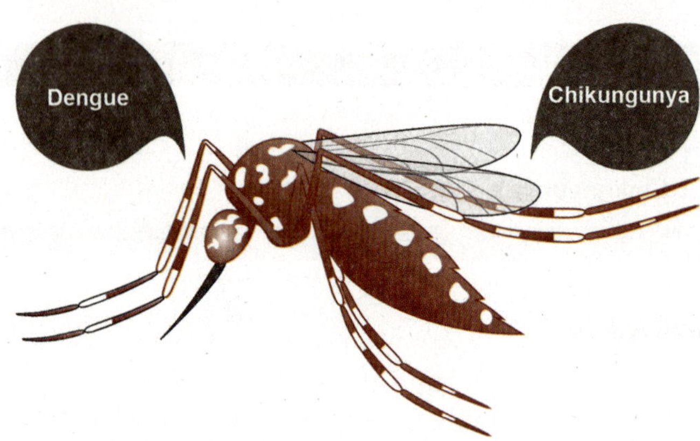

Fig. 38.4: *Aedes aegypti* showing alternate white and barred appearances over body, legs and arms

Table 38.1: Diseases caused by arboviruses

Family and genus	*Encephalitis*	*Viruses causing febrile illness*	*Haemorrhagic fever*
I. Togaviridae *Alphavirus* (mosquito-borne)	• Western equine encephalitis • Eastern equine encephalitis • Venezuelan equine encephalitis	• Chikungunya • O'nyong-nyong • Semliki forest • Sindbis • Ross river virus	Chikungunya
II. Flaviviridaet *Flavivirus*			
i. Mosquito-borne	• St. Louis encephalitis • Ilheus • West Nile • Murray valley encephalitis • Japanese B encephalitis	Dengue, type 1–4	• Dengue • Yellow fever
ii. Tick-borne	• Russian spring summer encephalitis • Powassan		• Kyasanur forest disease • Omsk haemorrhagic fever
III. Bunyaviridae			
a. *Bunya virus* (mosquito-borne)	• California encephalitis • La Crosse	Chittor virus	
b. *Phlebovirus* (phlebotomus or mosquito-borne)		• Sandfly fever • Rift-valley fever	
c. Nairovirus (tick-borne)		• Nairobi sheep disease • Ganjam virus	
IV. Reoviridae Orbivirus (tick-borne)		• Colorado tick-borne virus	
V. Rhabdoviridae *Vesiculovirus* (mosquito- borne, sandfly-borne)		• Vesicular stomatitis virus • Chandipura virus	

Structure: Dengue virus (Figs 38.5 and 38.6).

Dengue fever is a mosquito-borne disease. It is spread by numerous species of the Aedes mosquito. Dengue has become a global cause of concern ever since the commencement of the Second World War.

Dengue and chikungunya are both viral diseases spread by the bite of the Aedes mosquito. Historically, chikungunya was identified as dengue but after an outbreak of chikungunya in Makonde Plateau near Tanzania, it was recognised as a separate disease.

Both chikungunya and dengue are mosquito-borne diseases spread by the Aedes mosquito. The *Aedes aegypti* is more likely to spread dengue while the *Aedes albopictus* is more likely to pass on the chikungunya virus. However, both the types can spread both the diseases.

Clinical features: The disease may occur in two forms: Classical dengue fever and dengue in more serious forms with haemorrhagic manifestations.

i. *Classical dengue fever:* This usually affects older children and adults. It has relatively benign course with fever, headache and pain in muscles and bones. The fever is typically biphasic (saddle back). Incubation period is 5–8 days. The febrile illness lasts for about 10 days after which recovery is generally complete. It is rarely fatal.

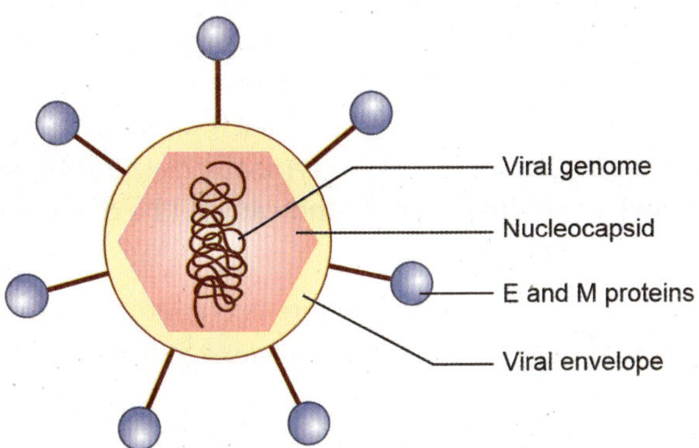

Fig. 38.5: Dengue virus showing viral genome E and M proteins

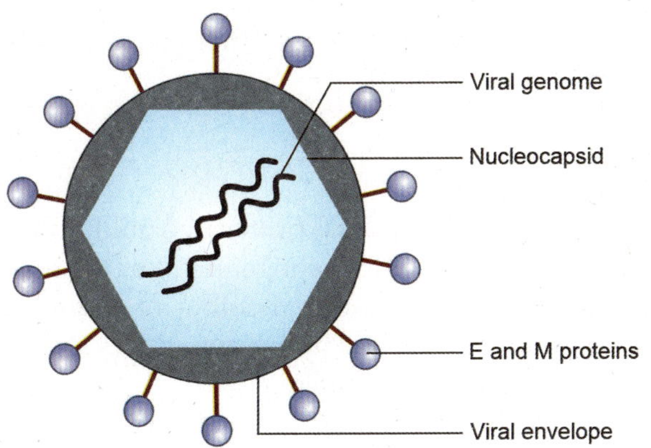

Fig. 38.6: Dengue virus showing viral envelope, E and M proteins, nucleocapsid, and viral genome

ii. *Other manifestations:* Dengue may also occur in more serious forms, with haemorrhagic manifestations or with shock. These are known as dengue haemorrhagic fever (DHF) and dengue shock syndrome (DSS). DHF/DSS remains mostly confined among children of 5–10 years age group in area where multiple dengue viruses cause disease. It is seen in patients previously infected with dengue virus. On reinfection with a different serotype of dengue virus, antibody formed against the first virus reacts with the second serotype virus forming immune complexes (virus–antibody complex).

Initial symptoms are like those of dengue fever but associated with haemorrhagic rash, thrombocytopenia and shock. The mortality rate is 5–10%.

Dengue symptoms in severe cases are as follows:

1. Bleeding from the nose, gum, mouth or bruises on the skin
2. Excessive thirst
3. Pale and cold skin
4. Black stool
5. Restlessness

Dengue epidemics: In 1963, extensive outbreaks affected Calcutta and Madras. In the 1990s, Surat and Delhi had major epidemics with deaths due to DHF and DSS. All four types of dengue virus are present in India.

Laboratory diagnosis: Isolation of the virus is difficult but serology plays a major role in diagnosis. Demonstration of IgM antibody in serum provides early diagnosis. IgM antibody appears within 2–5 days of the onset of illness and persists for one to three months. ELISA is used for detection of IgM antibody. A strip immunochromatographic test for IgM is also available for rapid diagnosis.

Prophylaxis: Control measures include elimination of mosquitoes. No effective vaccine is available.

CHIKUNGUNYA

The name chikungunya derives from a word in the Kimakonde language, meaning "to become contorted".

Chikungunya is a disease transmitted to humans by mosquitoes in Africa, Asia, and the Americas; sporadic outbreaks have been reported in other regions.

Chikungunya is a mosquito-borne viral disease caused by the chikungunya virus (CHIKV), an RNA virus in the Alphavirus genus of the family Togaviridae.

The morphology and structure of chikungunya virus (CHIKV) is shown in Figs 38.7 and 38.8.

Morphology and Structure of Chikungunya Virus (CHIKV) (Togaviridae)

Dengue and Zika have similar symptoms to chikungunya, making chikungunya easy to misdiagnose.

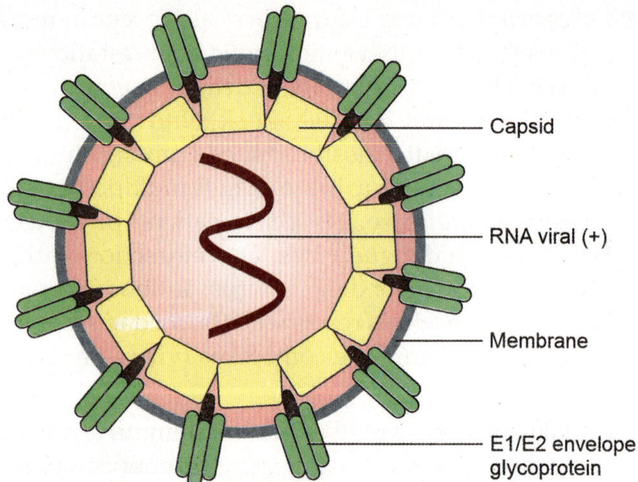

Fig. 38.7: CHIKV spherical virion with spikes on surface and E1/E2 envelope glycoprotein

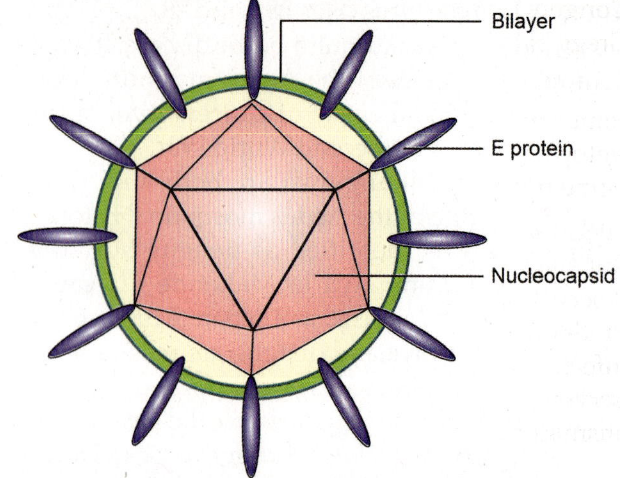

Fig. 38.8: CHIKV virion showing nucleocapsid (NC) core of ~35 nm in diameter, E protein and bilayer membrane

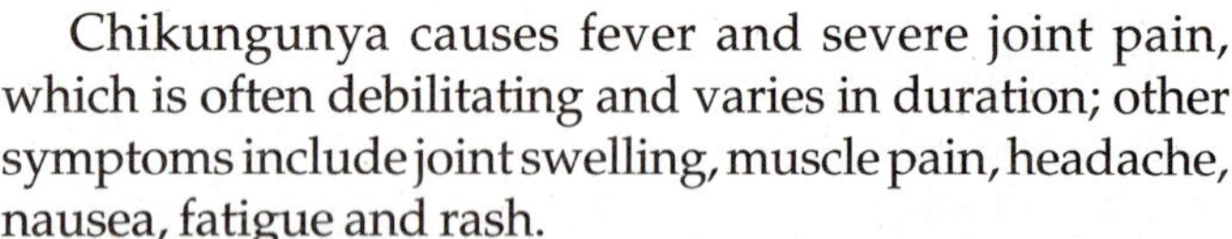

Chikungunya causes fever and severe joint pain, which is often debilitating and varies in duration; other symptoms include joint swelling, muscle pain, headache, nausea, fatigue and rash.

Dengue and chikungunya diseases are more common in the tropical and sub-tropical climates. India is one such country where it rains and rains continuously for many months. This is the reason people in India face the threat of these vector-borne diseases.

Despite being quite similar, both the diseases are very much different. Due to sharing quite similar signs, it becomes difficult in identifying the exact problem. Some of the differences in both the viral infections are:

1. Dengue and chikungunya, though carried by the same mosquito type, but are caused by different viruses. While chikungunya is caused by a Togaviridae alphavirus. Dengue is caused by Flaviridae flavivirus.
2. The incubation period of chikungunya is of 1–12 days and the duration varies from 1 to 2 weeks. However, signs such as joint pain may stay for a long time. The incubation period for dengue is of 3–7 weeks while it stays from about 4 to 7 weeks.
3. Swelling and pain is high in chikungunya as compared to that in dengue.
4. Chikungunya can cause tremendous joint pain, whereas dengue can cause bleeding in some cases, breathing problems, etc.
5. In chikungunya, rashes all across the face, palms, feet, limbs can be found, whereas in dengue, rashes are limited to limbs and face.
6. Complications such as chronic arthritis and rare neurological problems are possible in chikungunya. In severe cases of dengue, respiratory problems, organ failure or shock can be caused. Arthritis is absent in dengue.

Transmission: Chikungunya virus is transmitted by mosquitoes, most commonly *Aedes* (Stegomyia) *aegypti* and *Aedes* (Stegomyia) *albopictus*, which can also transmit dengue and Zika viruses. These mosquitoes bite primarily during daylight hours. They lay eggs in containers with standing water. Both species feed outdoors, and *Aedes aegypti* also feeds indoors.

Diagnostics: Chikungunya virus may be detected directly in blood samples collected during the first week of illness using tests such as reverse transcriptase–polymerase chain reaction (RT–PCR).

Other tests can detect a person's immune response to chikungunya virus infection. These are typically used after the first week of infection to test for antibodies to the virus. The antibody levels are typically detectable by the first week after illness onset and can still be detected for about 2 months.

Prophylaxis and vaccines: There is currently no approved and vaccine or specific treatment for chikungunya virus infections.

Due to the challenges in reporting and diagnosis, the number of people affected by chikungunya is underestimated.

Severe symptoms and deaths from chikungunya are rare and usually related to other coexisting health problems.

RUBELLA

Rubella or German measles is primarily a mild childhood disease. It may be acquired congenitally or postnatally. Although rubella virus is a member of Togaviridae family, it is not transmitted by arthropods.

- From Latin meaning "little red".
- Discovered in 18th century—thought to be variant of measles.
- First described as distinct clinical entity in German literature.

- Congenital rubella syndrome (CRS) described by Gregg in 1941.

Morphology (Figs 38.9 to 38.11): Rubella virus is a pleomorphic, roughly spherical, 50–70 nm in diameter, enveloped RNA virus. It has single-stranded RNA genome and envelope carries haemagglutinin peplomers.

Epidemiology

- Rubella is worldwide in distribution
- It occurs round the year
- Epidemics occur every 20–25 years
- Infection is transmitted by respiratory route

Reservoir	Human
Transmission	Respiratory Subclinical cases may transmit
Temporal pattern	Peak in late winter and spring
Communicability	7 days before to 5–7 days after rash onset Infants with CRS may shed virus for a year or more

Pathogenesis and Pathology (Fig. 38.12)

- Respiratory transmission of virus
- Replication in nasopharynx and regional lymph nodes
- Viraemia 5–7 days after exposure with spread to tissues
- Placenta and foetus infected during viraemia
- *Transmission:* Respiratory droplets.
- Primary implantation and replication in the nasopharynx are followed by spread to the lymph nodes. Subsequent viraemia occurs, which in pregnant women often results in infection of the placenta. Placental virus replication may lead to infection of foetal organs.
- Individuals with acquired rubella may shed virus from 7 days before rash onset to 5–7 days.
- Infants with CRS may shed large quantities of virus from bodily secretions, particularly from the throat and in the urine, up to 1 year of age. Outbreaks of rubella, including some in nosocomial settings, have originated with index cases of CRS. Thus, only individuals immune to rubella should have contact with infants who have CRS.

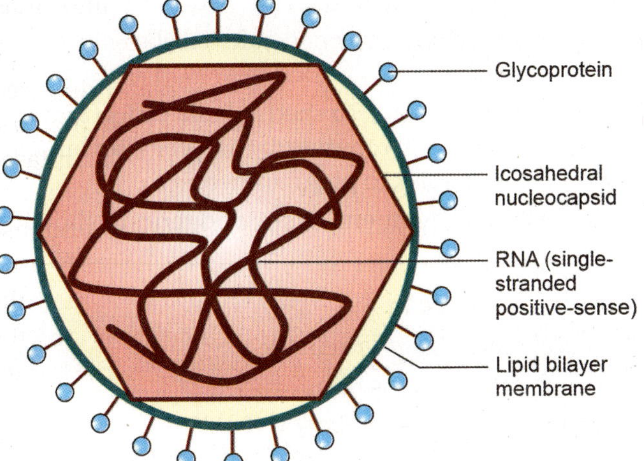

Fig. 38.9: Rubella virus showing icosahedral nucleocapsid

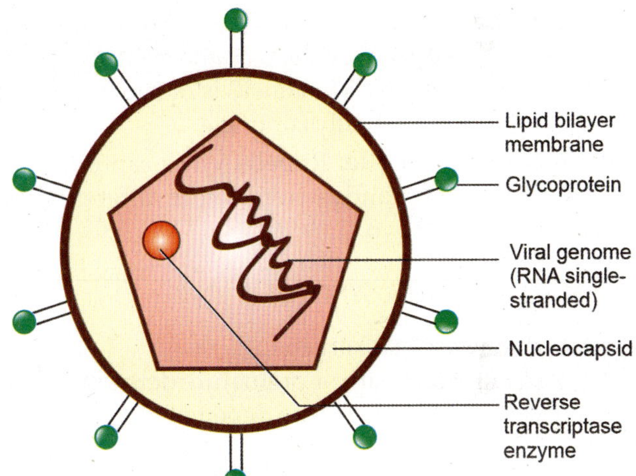

Fig. 38.11: Rubella virus showing lipid bilayer membrane, reverse transcriptase enzyme and RNA single-stranded

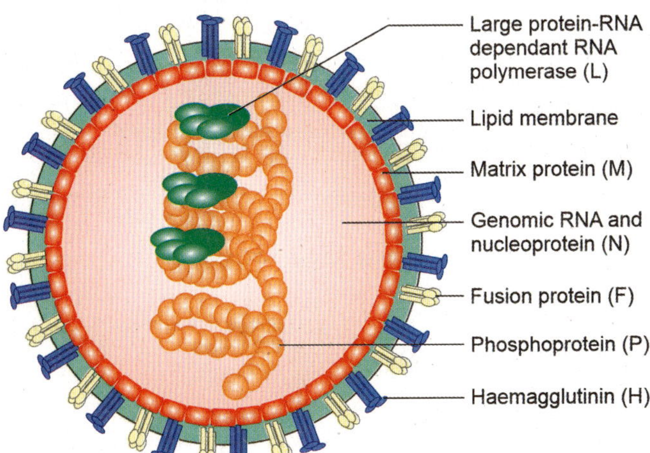

Fig. 38.10: Rubella virus showing large protein RNA, phosphoprotein, fusion protein and heamagglutinin

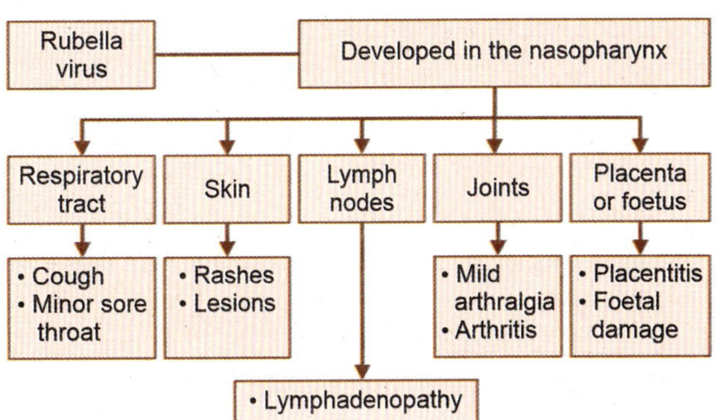

Fig. 38.12: Pathogenesis

B. Pathophysiology

Measles enters by **droplets or by fomites** through the upper respiratory tract, with initial replication taking place locally and in regional lymph nodes. Then, primary viraemia sets in and infects the reticuloendothelial system.

After 5–7 days, secondary viraemia follows:

- An incubation period of **9–12 days** culminates in fever, upper respiratory symptoms, and pathognomonic **Koplik's spots** (red spots with bluish to white centers on the buccal mucosa).
- Followed 1–2 days later by a **rash** that begins on the head and descends to the trunk and limbs.
- Invasion of the respiratory, urinary, and gastrointestinal tracts, as well as the CNS, leads to a variety of symptoms. Sequelae can be acute or chronic.
  i. **Postnatal rubella:** Infection is acquired by inhalation. Virus multiplies locally and in the cervical lymph nodes. After an incubation period of 2–3 weeks, viraemia occurs. The virus is disseminated throughout the body by blood stream. Patient develops fever, and fine, pink, macular rash, which first appears on the face and then spreads to the trunk and legs. The illness is of short duration and recovery is usually complete.
  ii. **Congenital rubella:** Rubella virus can cross the placental barrier and can replicate in differentiating cells of the embryo.

CONGENITAL RUBELLA SYNDROME (CRS)

- Infection may affect all organs
- May lead to foetal death or premature delivery
- Severity of damage to foetus depends on gestational age
- Up to 85% of infants affected if infected during first trimester
- Since the virus can cross the placenta, it can cause congenital rubella syndrome in the newly born.
- Congenital infection may be mild and asymptomatic or severe, causing cataracts, glaucoma, deafness, heart abnormalities, mental retardation or death.

Congenital Rubella (Fig. 38.13)

Pathogenesis of Congenital Rubella

a. Infection of foetus during first trimester of pregnancy
b. At least 20% of infants have severe birth defects
   i. Neurosensory deafness
   ii. Blindness (total or partial; cataracts are especially common)
   iii. Congenital heart disease
   iv. Microcephaly with mental retardation
c. Other symptoms associated with CRS
   i. Bone translucency and retarded growth

Congenital rubella

Rubella virus infection in the early weeks of pregnancy
↓
Enzymatic slowing of the metabolism and catabolism of vitamin A, leading to its accumulation in the liver
↓
Acute liver damage and cholestasis
↓
Spillage of retinoic acids in bile and leakage of retinyl esters into the circulation from damaged hepatocytes
↓
Mitochondrial damage, apoptosis and alteration in DNA
↓
Congenital rubella syndrome

Fig. 38.13: Congenital rubella syndrome

   ii. Hepatosplenomegaly
   iii. Intrauterine growth retardation
d. 10–20% of babies with CRS die within 1 year
e. 20% will develop insulin dependent diabetes mellitus as young adults
f. CRS babies continue to shed rubella virus from their throats for several months up to a year after birth and pose a serious risk to pregnant women.

General derangement of organogenesis shown in Fig. 38.14.

Diagnosis of Rubella

- Clinical diagnosis is unreliable
- Many viral infections mimic rubella
- Specific diagnosis of infection with
  1. Isolation of virus
  2. Evidence of seroconversion

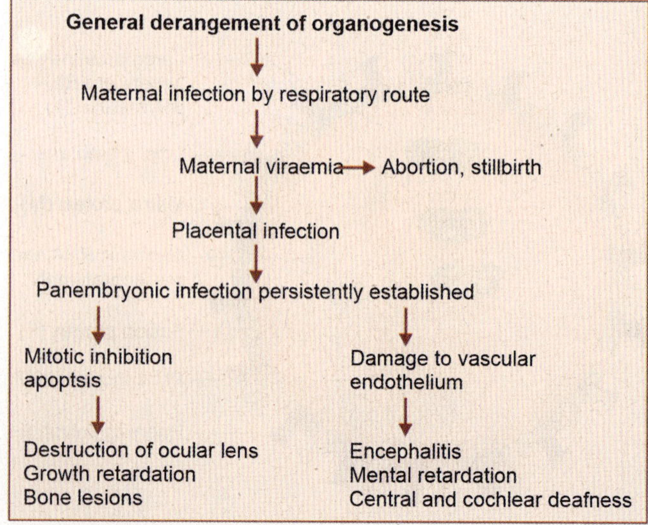

Fig. 38.14: General derangement of organogenesis

Laboratory Diagnosis

Routine diagnosis of rubella is not called for but the laboratory diagnosis becomes important in pregnant women suspected to have rubella. Diagnosis can be established by virus isolation or serology.

i. **Virus isolation:** Rubella virus can be isolated from adult throat swab. In infants with congenital rubella, the throat swab, urine or CSF can be used for isolation. The virus isolation is not commonly employed for rubella diagnosis because of the difficulties and the delay involved.

ii. **Serology:** Serological diagnosis is the method of choice in rubella. Antibodies in blood are detected by ELISA. Demonstration of rubella IgM antibody in a single specimen of blood has a diagnostic value. In case of rubella IgG antibody, fourfold rise in titre must be demonstrated between two serum samples collected at 10 days interval. In a newborn baby, rubella specific IgM antibody is diagnostic of congenital rubella as IgM antibodies do not cross the placenta.

Chapter 39

Rotavirus

Chapter Outline

ROTAVIRUSES

Introduction

Rotaviruses are the commonest cause of gastroenteritis in children. Rotavirus (*rota*, meaning wheel) is a double-shelled icosahedral capsid resembling a wheel with short spokes radiating from a wide hub to a clearly defined outer rim. The genome consists of double-stranded segmented RNA. There are seven serogroups (A to G). Most human rotaviruses fall into serogroup A.

Acute diarrhoeal diseases are still a major health problem throughout the world, causing 25–30% of all deaths among children younger than 5 years of age in developing countries.

Diarrhoeal diseases are also of public health importance in developed countries and are associated with considerable morbidity and a substantial number of hospitalizations among children and the elderly. Acute diarrhoea can be caused by many different agents including parasites, bacteria and viruses.

Rotaviruses are recognized as the single most important cause of severe infantile gastroenteritis worldwide and have been estimated to be responsible for > 600, 000 deaths annually.

Transmission of rotaviruses occurs primarily by the fecal–oral route, providing a highly efficient mechanism for universal exposure that circumvents differences in national cultural practices and public health standards.

Nearly all children less than 5 years of age have experienced at least one rotavirus infection.

Structure

Rotaviruses are double-stranded RNA viruses, with a diameter of 75 nm, which is relatively large among the enteric viruses. Unlike the other enteric viruses, which are generally icosahedral in shape, rotaviruses have a more complex morphology. The capsid consists of three concentric layers of protein, inside of which is the dsRNA genome, which range from approximately 670 to 3300 base pairs in length.

Rotaviruses are icosahedral (Fig. 39.1), nonenveloped viruses with a genome consisting of 11 segments of double-stranded RNA. They are the leading causes of severe diarrhoea in young children worldwide and important pathogens of many animal species. Approximately 1600 children die daily due to rotavirus (RV) diarrhoea, primarily in developing countries.

Schematic representation of a rotavirus virion. The virus is composed of **three protein shells, an outer capsid, an inner capsid, and an internal core**, that surround the 11 segments of double-stranded RNA. The outer capsid proteins VP4 and VP7 are neutralization antigens and define the P and G serotypes, respectively (Figs 39.2 and 39.3).

The following diagram shows complex and interlacing RNA segment (VP1/VP3), outer capsid (VP4-VP7) and inter-mediate capsid (VP5) (Fig. 39.4).

The genome of rotaviruses is located inside the inner core and consists of 11 segments of double-stranded RNA. All segments, except one, code for only one virus-specific protein (VP).

Classification: Rotaviruses have been classified into at least seven antigenic groups (A to G) based on antigenic epitopes on the internal structural protein VP6. These can be detected by immunofluorescence, ELISA, and immune electron microscopy (IEM). Multiple serotypes have been identified among human and animal rotaviruses.

- **Group A strains** cause the majority of human infections and have been classified into subgroups (I and II) by ELISA, CFT or immune adherence agglutination, and into many serotypes (1, 2, 3, etc.) by neutralization tests.
- **Group B strain:** The Chinese adult diarrhoea rotavirus (ADRV) is of group B.
- **Group C rotaviruses** cause occasional outbreaks in humans.

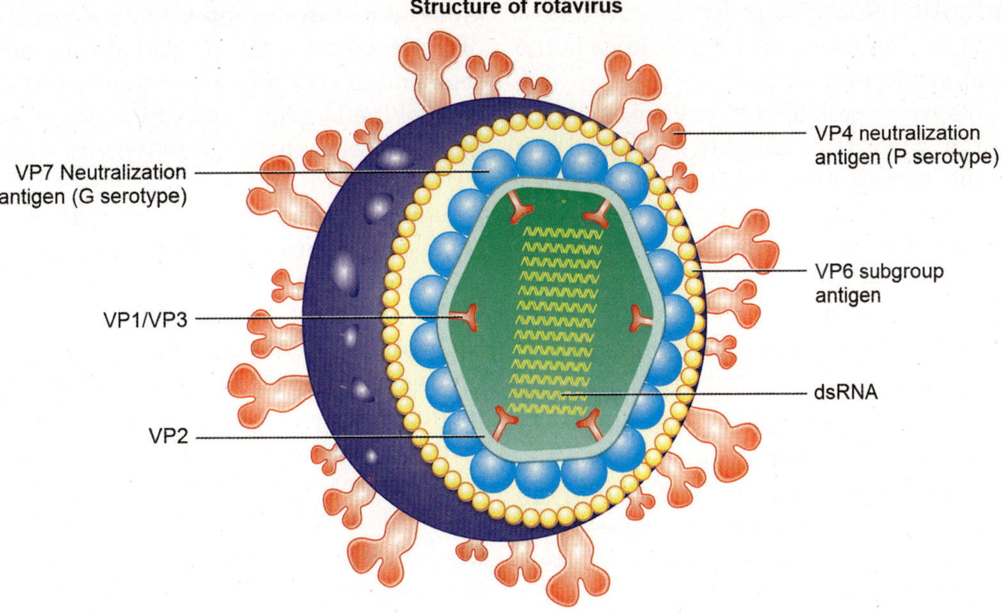

Fig. 39.1: Structure of rotavirus showing icosahedral shape and various antigens

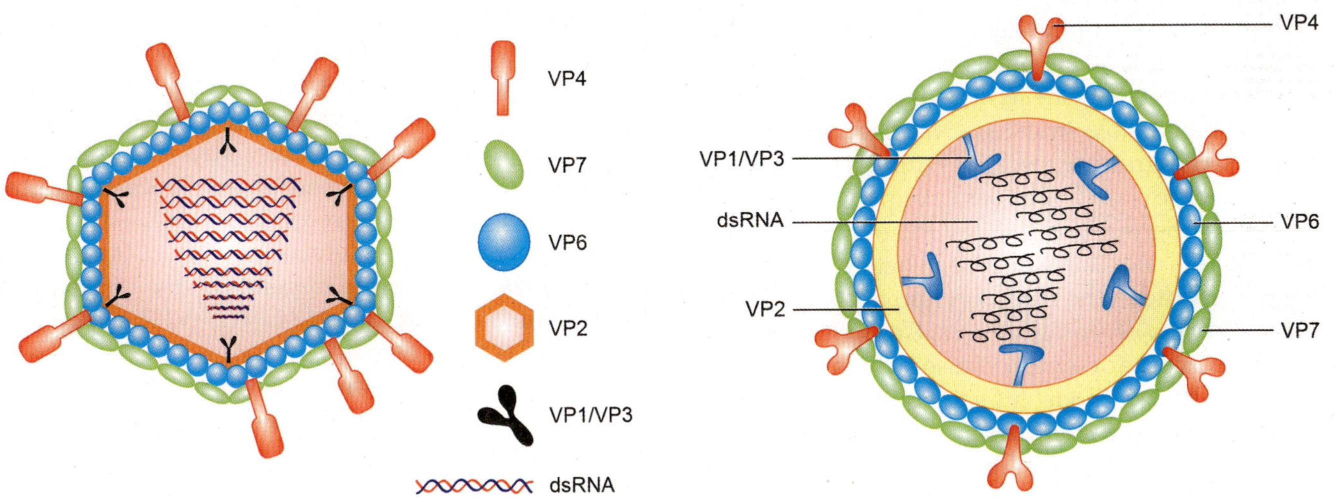

Fig. 39.2: Protein shells and capsids

Fig. 39.3: VP4 and VP7 neutralization antigens

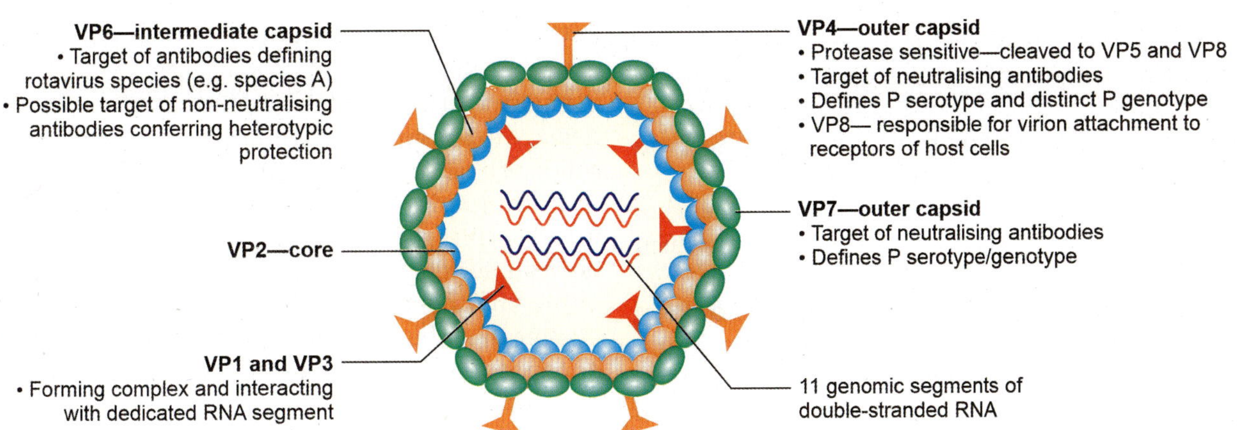

Fig. 39.4: Rotavirus showing illustrations of VP1–VP7 along with 11 genomic segments of double-stranded RNA

Animal susceptibility: Rotaviruses have a wide host range and are a class of viruses causing diarrhoea in the young of many animals and some birds.

The human rotavirus is related to the viruses of epidemic diarrhoea of infant mice (EDIM), Nebraska calf diarrhoea and the simian virus SAI1. Cross-species infections can occur in experimental inoculations. Human rotavirus infection has been transferred to piglets, calves and monkeys. It is not known whether human infection can be caused by animal rotaviruses. Swine rotavirus infects both newborn and weaning piglets.

Propagation in cell culture: Rotaviruses are fastidious agents to culture. Most group A human rotaviruses can be cultivated if pretreated with the proteolytic enzyme trypsin and if low levels of trypsin are included in the tissue culture medium. As calf and simian viruses grow readily in cell cultures, they have been used as antigens for serological studies.

Etiology: Rotaviruses, astroviruses, caliciviruses such as the Norwalk agent, and enteric adenoviruses are the medically important pathogens of human viral gastroenteritis.

Rotaviruses are in the Reoviridae family and cause disease in virtually all mammals and birds. These viruses are wheel-like, triple-shelled icosahedrons containing 11 segments of double-stranded RNA. The diameter of the particles on electron microscopy is approximately 80 nm. Rotaviruses are classified by serogroup, (A, B, C, D, E, F, and G) and subgroup (I or II). Rotavirus strains are species specific and do not cause disease in heterologous hosts. Group A includes the common human pathogens as well as a variety of animal viruses. Group B rotavirus is reported as a cause of severe disease in infants and adults in China only. Occasional human outbreaks of group C rotavirus are reported. The other serogroups infect only nonhumans.

Subgrouping of rotaviruses is determined by the antigenic structure of the inner capsid protein, VP6. Serotyping of rotaviruses, described for group A only, is determined by classic cross-neutralisation testing and depends on the outer capsid glycoproteins, VP7 and VP4. The VP7 serotype is referred to as the G type (for glycoprotein). There are ten G designated groups A–G. The most important species causing infection in humans is group A rotavirus, although people have also been infected with rotavirus groups B and C.

Group A rotaviruses are serotyped on the basis of antibody reactivity to either VP6 or VP7, both of which are proteins on the outer shell of the virion.

The 11-segmented rotavirus genome, in addition to coding for the structural proteins, encodes six non-structural proteins. It is believed that non-structural proteins 1 and 3 are involved in the virulence of rotaviruses. In addition, non-structural protein 4 acts as an endotoxin.

General features of rotavirus: Rotaviruses are members of the Reoviridae family and are characterised by their segmented (11 segments) double-stranded RNA genome. Each of the 11 genes codes for a single gene product. Six of the proteins are found in the virus particle (VP1, VP2, VP3, VP4, VP6 and VP7), whereas the remaining five proteins are non-structural (NDP1-NSP5). Rotavirus is classified into serogroups A–E based on antigenic properties. Only groups A–C have been shown to infect humans and most human rotavirus disease is caused by group A rotavirus. The group A rotaviruses are further classified into G (serotypes) and P types based on identification of antigens on the outer capsid proteins. Of the 14 serotypes (G types) that have been identified in various species, nine have been recognized in humans, and of these, four serotypes (1–4) are dominant globally.

Classification: Rotaviruses most commonly are classified according to group and serotype. Six groups of rotavirus have been described (A–F), and are based on differences in the VP6 protein. Only those viruses in groups A, B, and C are known to cause disease in humans. Group A rotaviruses are the principal cause of human disease and the subject of most of this chapter. Group B rotaviruses have been associated with epidemic gastroenteritis in Asia, and group C rotaviruses with sporadic mild gastroenteritis. Limited evidence that group C rotaviruses might be associated with biliary atresia has not been confirmed. Groups B and C are of less clinical and public health significance compared with group A viruses.

Group A only, is determined by classic cross-neutralisation testing and depends on the outer capsid glycoproteins, VP7 and VP4. The VP7 serotype is referred to as the G type (for glycoprotein). There are ten G serotypes, of which four cause most illness and vary in occurrence from year to year and region to region. The VP4 serotype is referred to as the P type. There are eleven P serotypes. Although both VP4 and VP7 elicit neutralising immunoglobulin G antibodies, the relative role of these systemic antibodies compared with that of mucosal immunoglobulin A antibodies and cellular responses in protective immunity remains unclear.

Pathophysiology: The pathophysiology of rotavirus diarrhoea is clearly multifactoral. There is a malabsorptive component of the diarrhoea that seems related to primary damage to intestinal epithelium by virus infection and the action of a secreted viral enterotoxin (NSP4) (Fig. 39.5).

Pathogenic mechanisms include an osmotic malabsorptive diarrhoea, stimulation of the enteric nervous system by the virus, and the enterotoxic effect of the viral nonstructural protein NSP4. Two new RV vaccines have been recently approved for use in a variety of countries and may help reduce the disease burden due to this pathogen.

Mechanisms involved in rotavirus-associated diarrhoea (Fig. 39.6): Rotavirus is predominantly transmitted by the

Ingestion of rotavirus

Infects intestinal apical cells

NSP4 and enterotoxin

Decreased water and electrolyte absorption

Impaired disaccharide activity

Water and electrolyte secretion

Water and electrolyte loss

Carbohydrate malabsorption

Osmotic diarrhoea

Metabolic acidosis

Fig. 39.5: Rotavirus gastrointestinal pathophysiology

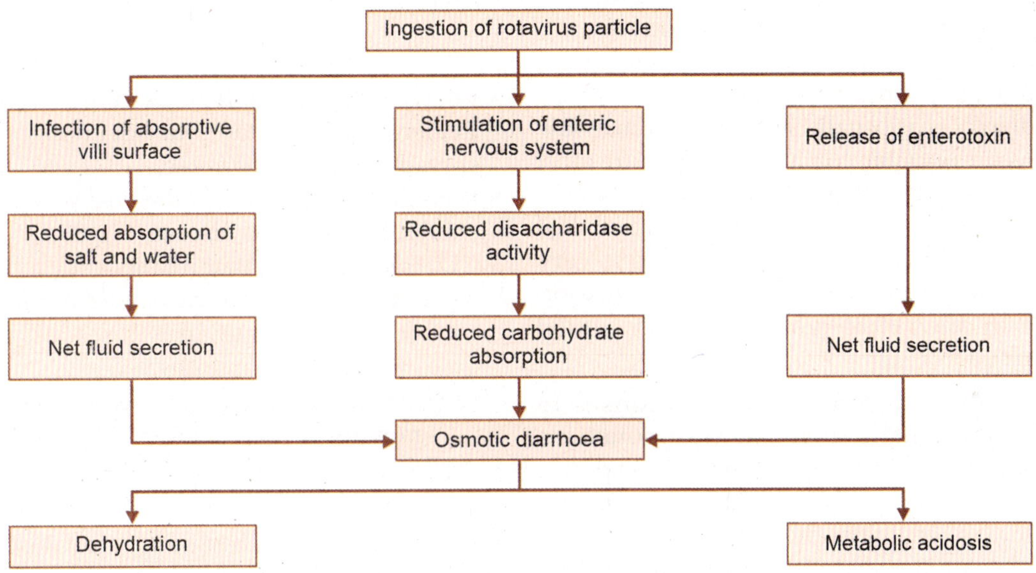

Fig. 39.6: Mechanism of rotavirus diarrhoea

faecal–oral route, although airborne transmission has been suggested in some situations. After ingestion, the virus primarily infects mature villi tip (apical) cells in the upper two-thirds of the small intestine. Viral replication kills these cells causing atrophy and blunting of the villi. Subsequently there is repopulation of the villous tips with immature secretory cells (crypt hyperplasia) that cannot efficiently absorb carbohydrates and other nutrients. Thus, rotavirus infection causes an osmotic diarrhoea. In addition, the non-structural rotavirus protein, NSP4, appears to act as an enterotoxin, stimulating water and electrolyte secretion from the epithelial cells.

Rotaviruses cause enteric disease with symptoms characterised by **diarrhoea, vomiting, abdominal discomfort, and fever, or any combination**. The virus affects mainly infants and young children. Diarrhoea ranges from mild to severe and can cause fatal dehydration.

Clinical features (manifestations): Infection is by the faecal–oral route. The incubation period is 2–3 days. Vomiting and diarrhoea occur with a little or no fever. Stools are usually greenish yellow or pale, with no blood or mucus. The disease is self-limited and recovery occurs within 5–10 days. Mortality is low. Group B rotaviruses have been implicated in large outbreaks of severe gastroenteritis in adults in China.

The manifestations of rotavirus infection range from subclinical infection through mild diarrhoea to severe, occasionally fatal dehydrating illness. The incubation period is relatively short, 1 to 3 days. More than 80% of affected children develop vomiting followed by diarrhoea. Generally, the vomiting lessens by the second or third day as the diarrhoea increases. Perhaps the greatest dehydration risk occurs when both vomiting and diarrhoea are present, as the child cannot ingest hydrating fluids. Other common symptoms include abdominal pain and irritability, and about a third of hospitalised children have a fever higher than 39°C.

The diarrhoea is usually watery. Mucus is commonly found in the stool but white and red blood cells are only occasionally present. Diarrhoea usually last 3–7 days but may be longer in malnourished and immunocompromised children. Also, persisting lactose intolerance may prolong symptoms.

The severity of diarrhoea depends on previous exposure to rotavirus, intestine sensitivity, the amount of virus ingested (as little as 10,000 viral particles are sufficient) immune system integrity, and other factors that are still unknown. The first rotavirus infection is usually the most severe with subsequent infections having progressively milder symptoms.

Epidemiology: Rotaviruses are the commonest cause of diarrhoea in infants and children the world over and typically account for about half the cases of children hospitalised for diarrhoea. Rotavirus infections usually predominate during the winter season. In tropical areas, infections occur evenly throughout the year.

Rotavirus diarrhoea is usually seen in children below the age of five years but symptomatic infections are most common in children between ages 6 months and 2 years. By the age of five years, most children have had clinical or subclinical infection, so rotavirus diarrhoea is very uncommon in older children and adults. Transmission appears to be by the faecal–oral route. Nosocomial infections are frequent.

Humoral and cell-mediated immune responses to rotavirus: A symptomatic infection with rotavirus stimulates a strong humoral IgG immune response which lasts for the lifetime. While the IgG responses are easily recorded, it is generally thought that protection from rotavirus disease is mediated by local IgA antibodies. Several studies have shown that local IgA is important or at least a good predictor of protection.

Two proteins on rotavirus, VP4 and VP7, are thought to play a critical role in mounting a protective immune response. Both proteins are constituents of the outer capsid and have been found, independently of each other, to stimulate production of neutralizing antibodies. Children infected with a particular serotype of rotavirus are more likely to be protected against challenge with the same serotype than against reinfection with a different serotype.

Laboratory diagnosis: Laboratory diagnosis rests on demonstration of virus in stool collected early in the illness and on a rise in antibody titer.

Demonstration of virus: At the peak of the disease, as many as 10 virus particles per milliliter of faeces are present. Therefore, the diagnosis is not difficult. Virus in stool is demonstrated by immune electron microscopy (IEM), latex agglutination tests, or ELISA.

Rotavirus can be detected by numerous techniques, including a variety of commercial antigenic assays, RT-PCR, electron microscopy, immune electron microscopy, polyacrylamide gel electrophoresis (PAGE) for viral genomic RNA, and viral culture. Detection of viral antigen in stool or rectal swabs, most commonly using enzyme-linked immunosorbent assay or latex agglutination formats, forms the basis for practical, commercially available, and widely used diagnostic kits. Latex agglutination is particularly suitable for use in areas with limited resources, although a confirmatory technique is desirable to evaluate indeterminate results because of the limited sensitivity of the test.

Multiplexed RT-PCR has become a major diagnostic technique used in epidemiologic studies. RT-PCR allows determination of P and G types and permits finer definition of strain differences. Real-time RT-PCR provides greater sensitivity and speed than conventional or nested PCR diagnosis.

Prevention Tips

- Rotavirus is very contagious. Hand washing and good hygiene are important but not enough to control the spread of rotavirus disease.
- Rotavirus vaccination is the best way to protect your child from rotavirus disease (Fig. 39.7).
- CDC recommends that infants get vaccinated against rotavirus disease. Two vaccines are available:
  - i. RotaTeq® is given in 3 doses at ages 2 months, 4 months, and 6 months.
  - ii. Rotarix® is given in 2 doses at ages 2 months and 4 months.

The first dose of the rotavirus vaccine can be given as early as 6 weeks of age and should be given before 15 weeks of age. Infants should get all doses by 8 months of age.

Rotavirus vaccines will not prevent diarrhoea or throwing up caused by other viruses, but they are very effective against rotavirus infection.

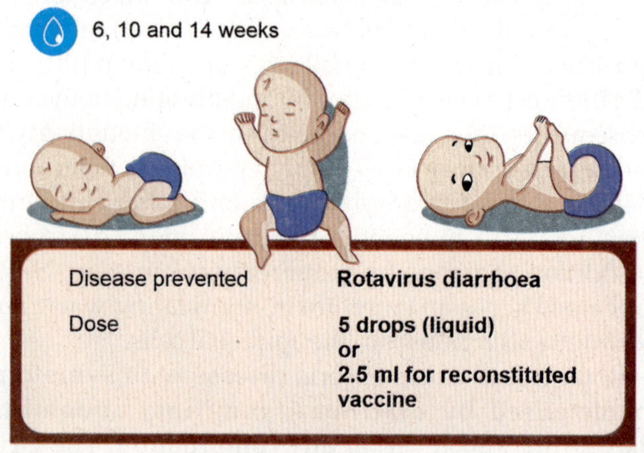

Fig. 39.7: Rotavirus vaccine

Chapter 40

Coronavirus
(COVID-19)

Chapter Outline

- Introduction
- Morphology: Structure CoV-2
- Pathogenicity and Pathophysiology of COVID-19 Infection
- Spread of COVID-19
- COVID-19 Infection in India and Pandemic Wave
- COVID-19 Pandemic
- Tracking SARS-CoV-2 Variants
- Immunity and Host Defence CoV-2
- COVID-19 Variants
- Classes of Variants being Monitored
- Consequence (VOHC)
- Mu Variant
- Side-effects
- Laboratory Diagnosis

Introduction

SARS-CoV-2 (severe acute respiratory syndrome coronavirus 2) is a beta-coronavirus responsible for the COVID-19 disease. It is the seventh coronavirus causing infection in humans, and the third, after SARS-CoV-1 and MERS, that triggered the epidemic and have pandemic potential. The infection spreads mainly through the droplet route and can be asymptomatic, mild or acute, with fever, cough and runny nose, and respiratory illness, which in some cases have a fatal outcome. It is estimated that mortality affects 3–9% of all cases.

The first appearance of the pathogen was recorded in 2019 in Wuhan, China, most likely as a result of an adaptation of the virus transmitted from bats to humans.

The official date is 17 November 2019. Over time, it spreads to all continents, resulting in WHO (World Health Organization) announcing the pandemic state on 11 March 2020.

COVID-19, which started as an outbreak in Wuhan, China, in December 2019 was initially reported as "pneumonia of unknown origin." The subsequent studies revealed that SARS-CoV-2 is the causative agent. As a huge amount of study has been conducted, it has been clarified that COVID-19 patients present with various pathological conditions in various organs throughout the body including thrombosis, renal dysfunction.

Pathological analyses have played a major role in elucidating the pathogenesis of COVID-19, and autopsies have provided many valuable insights. Furthermore, immunological analyses have not only started to clarify the host's protective mechanism against SARS-CoV-2, but it also helped to understand the pathogenic mechanism of COVID-19. We hope that the insight into the mechanism of COVID-19 pathogenesis from the viewpoints of pathology and immunology will lead to the development of effective therapeutics.

Since the first case of COVID-19 was reported in Wuhan, China, in December 2019, the SARS-CoV-2 epidemic has spread all over the world and has become a significant public health issue. The development of treatments for COVID-19 is currently in progress; however, their effects remain limited, and the development of more effective therapeutics is desired. Thus, sufficient understanding of the pathophysiology of COVID-19 is essential to develop effective therapeutics for this disease.

Morphology: Structure of CoV-2

CoVs are RNA viruses and have the largest genomes (26–32 kb) among all RNA virus families. Each viral transcript has a 5′-cap structure and a 3′-poly(A) tail. The diameter of a single virion is 50–200 nm. Most often, the virion of SARS-CoV-2 has a spherical form, but also pleomorphic and oval shapes occur. The viral envelope is built of three proteins: the S-spike protein that forms the peplomers and gives the virus a characteristic crown shape, M-membrane protein, and E-envelope protein (Fig. 40.1), which provide the ring structure fourth protein, N-nucleocapsid protein, a phosphoprotein, which is a structural component of the nucleocapsid.

SARS-COV-2 contains 4 main structural proteins: spike (S) glycoprotein, small envelope (E) glycoprotein, membrane (M) glycoprotein and nucleocapsid (N) protein. Most COVID-19 vaccines target the spike protein, which contains 2 subunits: S1 and S2 (Fig. 40.2A and B).

Since the emergence of SARS-CoV in 2002 and its spread throughout 32 countries and areas, the world has

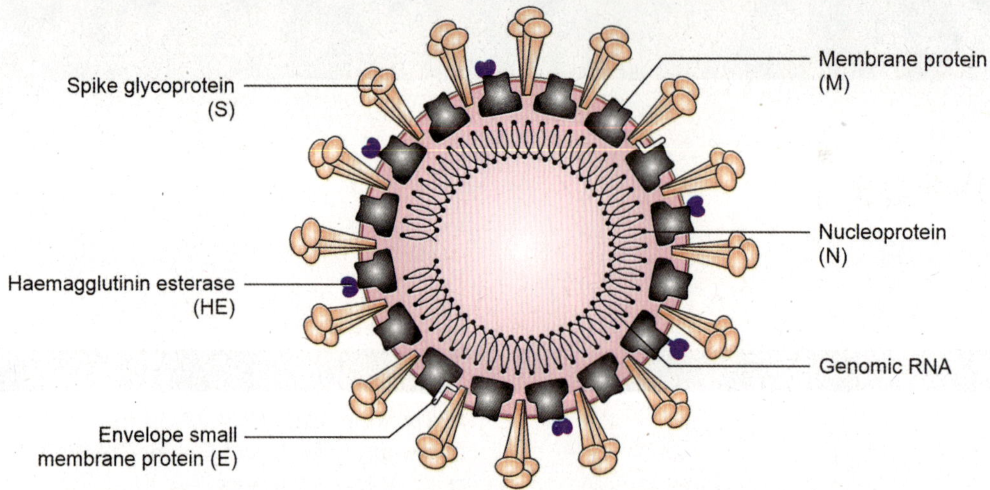

Fig. 40.1: CoV-2 crown shape, membrane protein (M) and haemagglutinin esterase (HE)

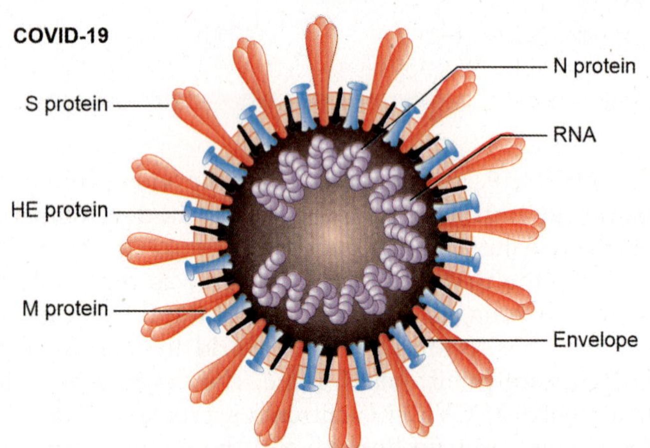

Fig. 40.2A: Structural proteins

Fig. 40.2B: Neucleocapsid (N) protein and other proteins S, M, and E with RNA viral genome

experienced the outbreak of MERS-CoV and now, the 2019-nCoV. All these viruses belong to the subfamily Coronavirinae in the family Coronaviridae. Since CoVs emerge periodically and unpredictably, spread rapidly, and induce serious infectious diseases, they become a continuous threat to human health. This is especially true when there are no approved vaccines or drugs for the treatment of CoV infections and there exists a range of animal reservoirs for CoVs and recombinant CoVs. In recent years, profound understandings of the innate immune response to viruses have been made.

The seven stages of virus replication are categorized as follows:

1. Attachment
2. Penetration
3. Uncoating
4. Replication
5. Assembly
6. Maturation
7. Release

Viruses like SARS-CoV-2 continuously evolve as changes in the genetic code (caused by genetic mutations or viral recombination) occur during replication of the genome. A lineage is a genetically closely related group of virus variants derived from a common ancestor. A variant has one or more mutations that differentiate it from other variants of the SARS-CoV-2 viruses. A recombinant is a variant created by the combination of genetic material from two different variants. As expected, multiple variants of SARS-COV-2 have been documented organs in most COVID-19 cases.

Pathogenicity and Pathophysiology of COVID-19 Infection

Respiratory organs are identified as the major affected organs in most COVID-19 cases; also, various lesions were noted in other organs (Fig. 40.3).

Pathology of COVID-19 from a histopathological and immunological perspective focusing on the mechanisms of COVID-19 pathogenesis.

Various lesions were noted in other organs. Further, there have been increasing reports that show that the immune responses of the host contribute to the deterioration of the pathological condition of body

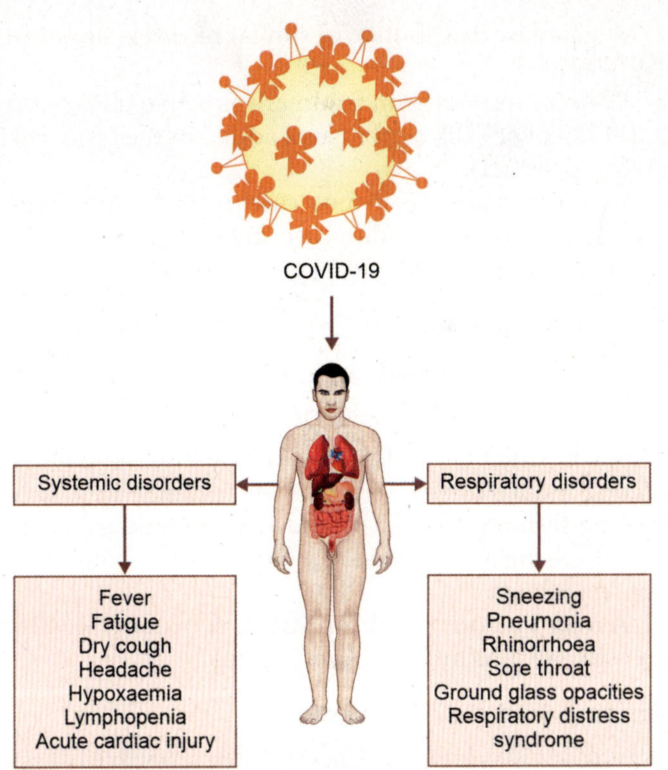

Fig. 40.3: Systemic and respiratory disorders in COVID-19 infection

including thrombosis, renal dysfunction, cardiovascular complications, and neurological dysfunction in addition to pneumonia, and that the host immune response causes damage to various organs. However, there are still many unclear points about the mechanism of development of these pathological conditions. There is controversy over whether or not the SARS-CoV-2 is directly involved, especially regarding pathological conditions other than pneumonia.

Pathophysiology of COVID-19 is essential to develop effective therapeutics for this disease. Pathological analyses in particular play an important role to demonstrate the causal link between an infectious disease and the pathogen and elucidate the mechanism of pathogenesis. As per pathological analyses to date.

Spread of COVID-19

Humans are primarily infected by consuming suspected reservoirs (bats or snakes). The possibility of COVID-19 is increased because of close contacts, such as handshaking from human to human (Fig. 40.4).

COVID-19 Infection in India and Pandemic Wave

First wave of infection came in September 2020 after the first appearance of pathogen recorded in 2019 in

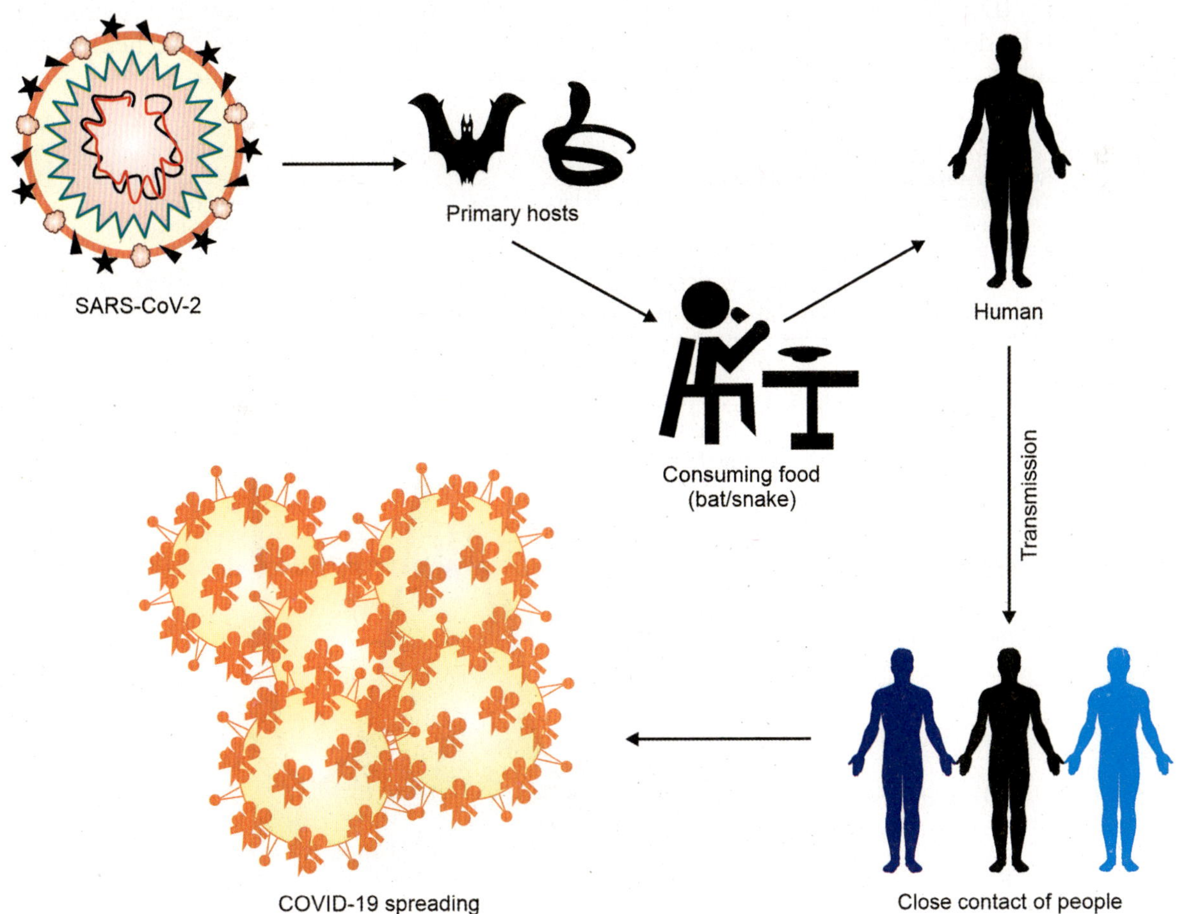

Fig. 40.4: Spread of COVID-19 (SARS-CoV-2)

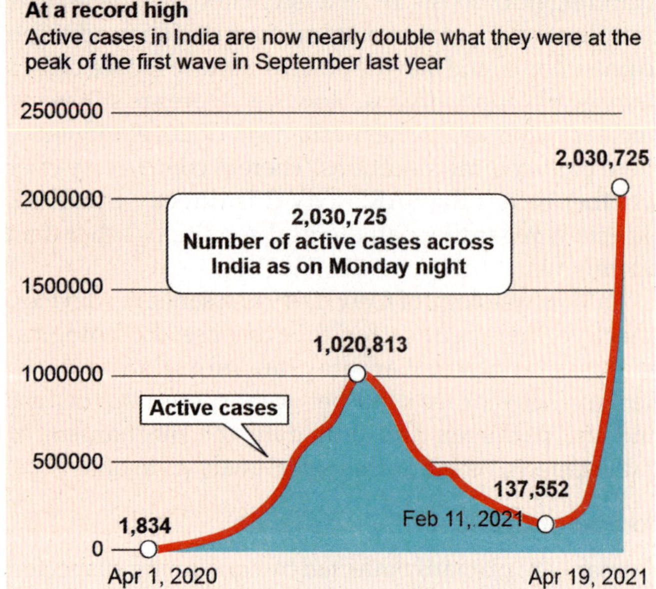

Fig. 40.5: Country record of cases

Wuhan, China. A record high active cases reported as on 19th April 2021 (Fig. 40.5) as 2,030,725, numbers of cases across India. Second wave soars to record high, 315, 904 daily cases in India with new deaths in India as 2,102 daily (Fig. 40.6).

A COVID Tracker Published on 29th May 2021 for record of total COVID cases, total doses of vaccine administered and total doses administered on 28th May (Friday) 2021 (Fig. 40.7).

A statewise distribution of similar record is shown in Fig. 40.7 also.

Country records grim landmark as active cases reach 2,030,725 over 770k active cases added in the last week (10th April 2021).

India overtakes U.S. in most cases recorded in a single day and the highest 7-day case trajectory seen in any country during the COVID-19 pandemic.

COVID-19 Pandemic

COVID Tracker (Fig. 40.7)

COVID impact: India during pandemic

Mumbai, Chennai, Delhi, Hyderabad and Bengaluru, among India's largest and most important cities, have been badly hit by COVID-19 and all five would appear to be witnessing a prolonged run if the disease, with some ebbs and flows.

A recent report of 16th Jan 2023 is shown in Fig. 40.8, showing all time total cases and deaths.

Tracking SARS-CoV-2 Variants

All viruses, including SARS-CoV-2, the virus that causes COVID-19, change over time. Most changes have a little to no impact on the propertie of virus. However, some changes may affect the properties of virus, such as how easily it spreads, the associated disease severity, or the performance of vaccines, therapeutic medicines, diagnostic tools, or other public health and social measures.

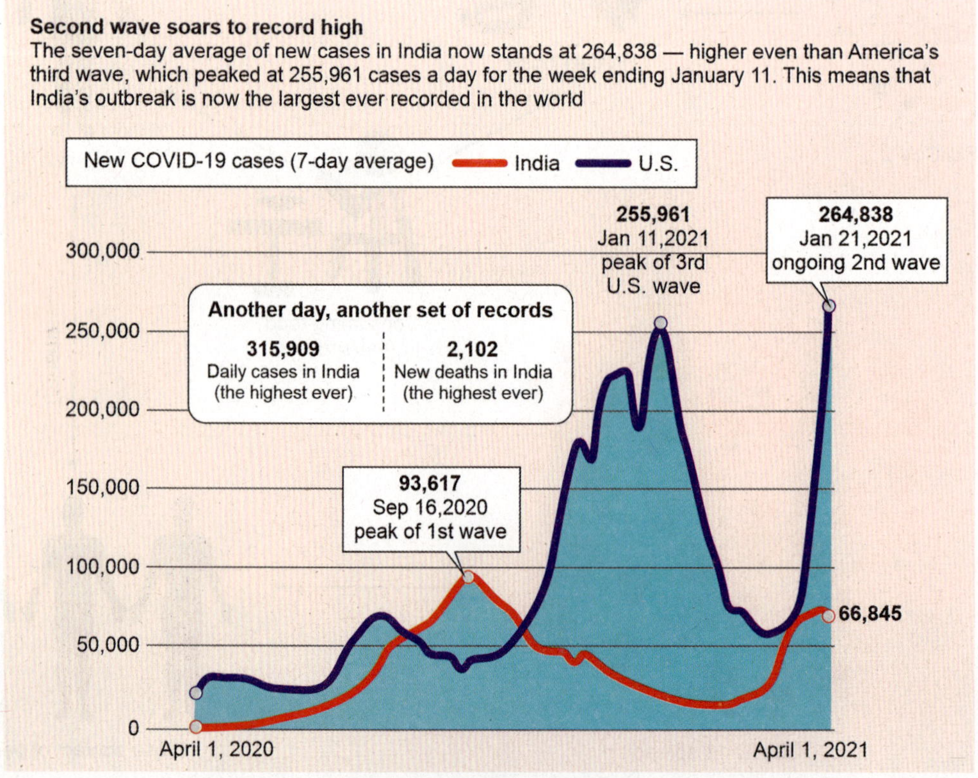

Fig. 40.6: Second wave record

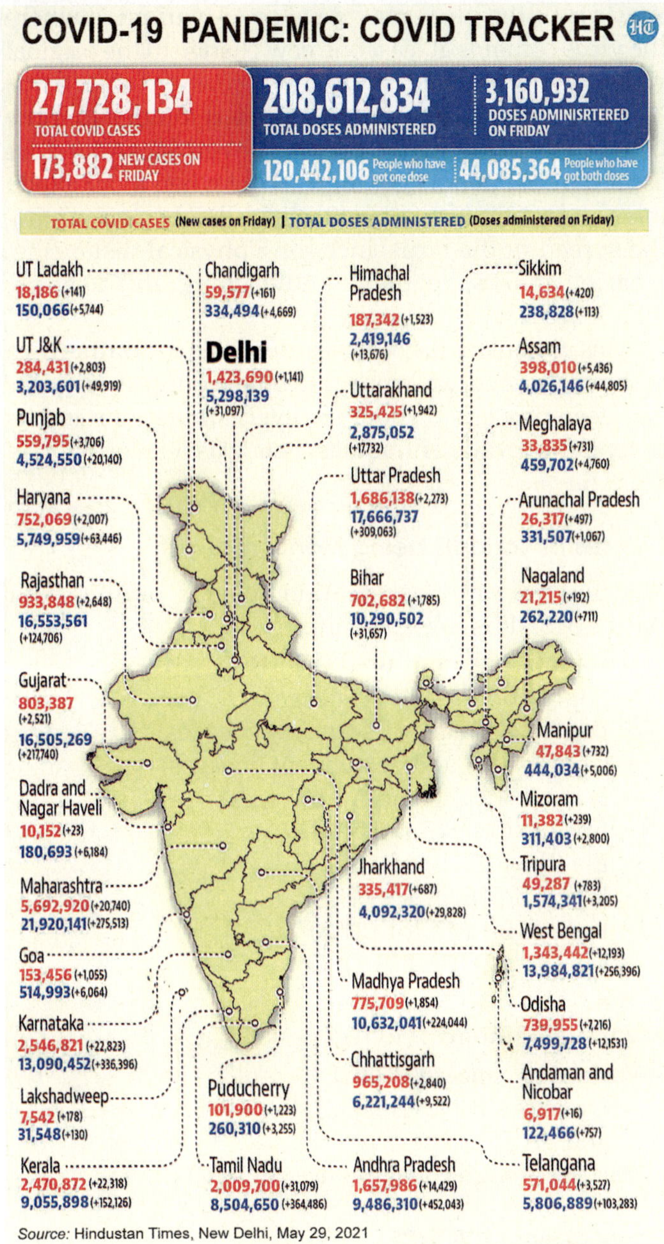

Fig. 40.7: COVID tracker report dated 29th May 2021

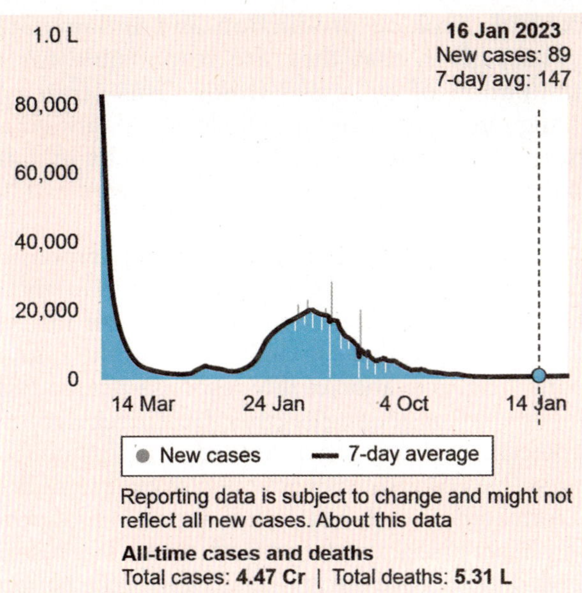

Fig. 40.8: All time cases after 2nd wave and overall coverage of vaccines administration

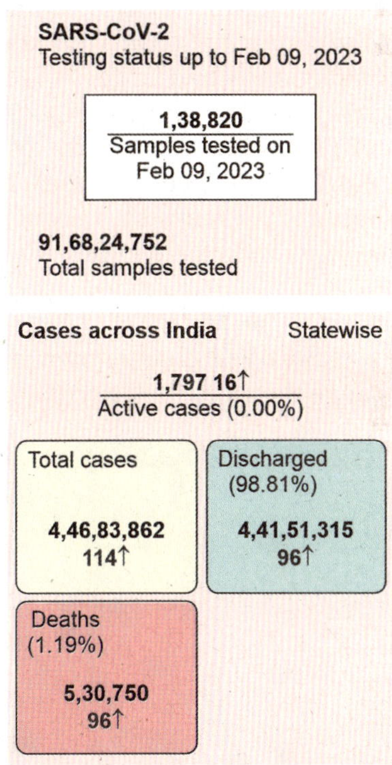

Fig. 40.9: The cases across India statewise total and active cases with a minimum deaths as 1.19%

A Tracking Report of 9th Feb 2023 (Fig. 40.9) showing cases across India, total samples tested and fall in death rate as 1.19 %.

Immunity and Host Defence CoV-2

This type of immune response inhibits virus replication, promotes virus clearance, induces tissue repair, and triggers a prolonged adaptive immune response against the viruses. In most cases, pulmonary and systemic inflammatory responses associated with CoVs are triggered by the innate immune system when it recognizes the viruses. Although a broadly protective, universal vaccine is considered the ultimate protection against the virus spread, vaccine development can be time-consuming. To fulfil the pressing need, we should propose effective therapeutic measures using the accumulated knowledge of the innate immune response system.

Targeted immunotherapy is a good alternative to some antivirals that have narrow treatment windows and meet with drug resistance easily. In 2003, glucocorticoid was widely used in SARS treatment to control pulmonary infection by regulating inflammatory responses. Except for viral pathogenicity, the inflammatory response of the body also plays a crucial role in SARS-induced lung injury cases. Therefore, in CoV pneumonia cases, it is important to control cytokine production and inflammatory response, given that they are responsible for the accumulation of cells and fluids. This strategy is challenging as we have not yet clearly identified any features in an immune response that can be inhibited specifically without compromising the beneficial host defense.

However, accomplishing this is not impossible. Notable achievements have been made in analyzing detrimental and protective mechanisms. For instance, completely blocking a proximal event in the immune response (e.g. activation of IFN response-related PRRs) seems unwise considering its general role in regulating the host defense. In contrast, more limited and specific effector arms, such as controlled production of oxygen radicals, NET formation, IL-1, IL-4, IL-6, IL-8, and IL-21 production, are probably practicable targets. At last, further research is needed to improve the understanding of the temporal features of CoV-induced inflammatory response in relation to the timing of therapeutic interventions.

Further, there have been increasing reports that show that the development of herd immunity in large population of the country. A return gift after successful vaccination completion by and large.

That it would and it is another reason why India should carry out widespread antibody tests at regular intervals to assess the spread of the disease. The proportion of the population that must be vaccinated against COVID-19 to begin inducing herd immunity is not known.

COVID-19 Variants (Fig. 40.10A and B)

Viruses, like SARS-CoV-2, change over time and will continue to change the more they circulate. Sometimes, variants of the virus may develop. A variant is where the virus contains at least one new change to the original virus.

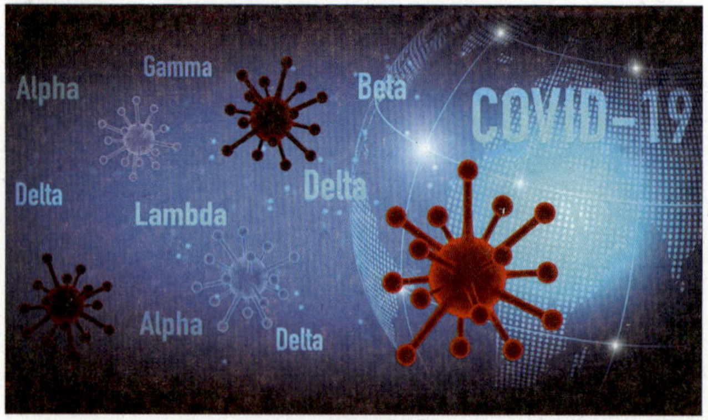

Fig. 40.10A: COVID-19 variants pandemic

Variants of SARS-CoV-2

α	β	γ	δ	o
Alpha	**Beta**	**Gamma**	**Delta**	**Omicron**
B.1.1.7	B.1.351	P.1	B.1.617.2	B.1.1.529

Fig. 40.10B: Variants of SARS-CoV-2 alpha, beta, gamma, delta, omicron

New variants like omicron are a reminder that the COVID-19 pandemic is far from over. It is therefore essential that people get the vaccine when available to them and continue to follow existing advice on preventing the spread of the virus, including physical distancing, wearing masks, regular handwashing and keeping indoor areas well ventilated.

This variant, or B.1.351, was identified in South Africa at the end of 2020 and spread to other countries. Experts had been concerned about its several mutations and its potential to evade antibodies. Beta was not common in the U.S.

Classes of Variants being Monitored

The SIG variant classification scheme defines four classes of SARS-CoV-2 variants:

- **Variant being monitored (VBM)**
  - Alpha (B.1.1.7 and Q lineages)
  - Beta (B.1.351 and descendent lineages)
  - Gamma (P.1 and descendent lineages)
  - Delta (B.1.617.2 and AY lineages)
  - Epsilon (8.1.427 and B.1.429)
  - Eta (B.1.525)
  - Iota (B.1.526)
  - Kappa (B.1.617.1, 1.617.3)
  - Mu (B.1.621, B.1.621.1)
  - Zeta (P.2)
- **Variant of interest (VOI)**
- **Variant of concern (VOC)**
  - Omicron (B.1.1.529, BA.1, BA.1.1, BA.2, BA.3, BA.4 and BA.5 lineages)
- **Variant of high consequence (VOHC)**

Consequence (VOHC)

To date, no variants of high consequence.

Alpha (B.1.1.7) was the first of the highly publicized variants. Alpha first appeared in Great Britain in November 2020 and infections surged in December of that year. It soon surfaced around the world and became the dominant variant in the U.S., where the CDC classified it as a variant of concern. Then, alpha faded away with the rise of the more aggressive delta variant.

Delta (B.1.617.2) was first identified in India in late 2020; it soon spreads throughout the world, becoming what was the predominant version of the coronavirus—until omicron took its place in mid-December.

Omicron's subvariants are considered to be especially efficient spreaders of the disease, and while scientists are still learning about XBB. 1.5, they say it is the most transmissible strain of the virus so far. The original strain of omicron was more transmissible than delta was.

Currently circulating variants of concern (VOC): The omicron variant, B.1.1.529 of SARS-CoV-2, was designated by the United States as a variant of concern (VOC) on November 30, 2021. Since the first confirmed case of omicron in the United States was identified on December 1, 2021, this variant and its subvariants.

Although it still spreads from person-to-person through air (within 6 feet through respiratory droplets), research shows that the omicron variant likely spreads easier and faster than the original COVID-19 virus.

Omicron spreads more easily than earlier variants, including the delta variant. Anyone with omicron infection, regardless of vaccination status or whether or not they have symptoms, can spread the virus to others. Data suggest that omicron can cause reinfection, even in people who have recovered from COVID-19.

Symptoms of the omicron subvariants include:
- Sore throat
- Hoarse voice
- Cough
- Fatigue
- Nasal congestion
- Runny nose
- Headache
- Muscle aches

MU VARIANT

"The Mu variant has a constellation of mutations that indicate potential properties of immune escape," the bulletin said.

There is widespread concern over the emergence of new virus mutations as infection rates are ticking up globally again, with the highly transmissible. Delta variant taking hold—especially among the unvaccinated—and in regions where anti-virus measures have been relaxed. Mu, known scientifically as B.1.621, has been classified as a "variant of interest".

Government of India is taking all necessary steps to ensure that we are prepared well to face the challenge and threat posed by the growing pandemic of COVID-19 the Coronavirus. The most important factor in preventing the spread of the virus locally is to empower the citizens with the right information and taking precautions as per the advisories being issued by Ministry of Health and Family Welfare (Fig. 40.11).

WHO, in collaboration with partners, expert networks, national authorities, institutions and researchers have been monitoring and assessing the evolution of SARS-CoV-2 since January 2020. During late 2020, the emergence of variants that posed an increased risk to

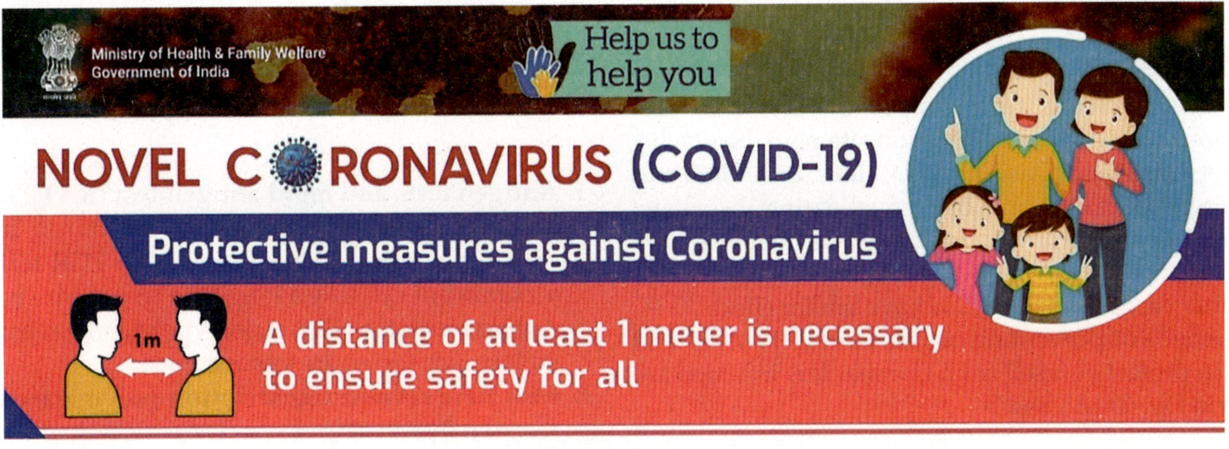

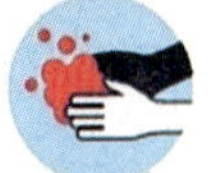
Wash your hands with soap and water regularly

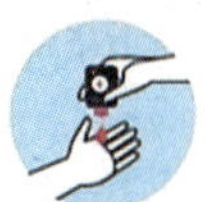
If soap and water is not available, use hand sanitizer with at least 60% alcohol

Wash hands before touching eyes, nose and mouth

Throw used tissues into closed bins immediately after use

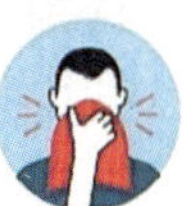
Cover your nose and mouth with handkerchief/tissue while sneezing and coughing

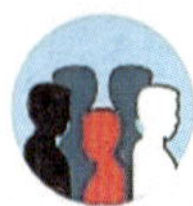
Avoid mass gathering and crowded places

davp 17102/13/0028/1920

If you are experiencing symptoms like fever, cough or difficulty in breathing, please call the state helpline number or 24x7 helpline numbers of Ministry of Health and Family Welfare, Government of India and follow the instructions.

1075 (Toll Free) | 011-23978046

Email to: ncov2019@gov.in , ncov2019@gmail.com

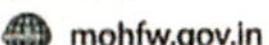

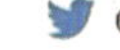
@MoHFW_INDIA mohfwindia

Fig. 40.11: Protective measures against Coronavirus (COVID-19), issued by Govt of India; MOH and FW, New Delhi

global public health prompted the characterisation of specific variants of interest (VOI) and variants of concern (VOC), in order to prioritise global monitoring and research, and ultimately to inform the ongoing response to the COVID-19 pandemic.

COVID-19 vaccines are used in the country at present for COVID-19 vaccination

1. Covishield® vaccine, manufactured by the Serum Institute of India, is a viral vector-based technology which is also used to manufacture Ebola vaccine.
2. Covaxin® vaccine, manufactured by the Bharat Biotech, is a whole-virion inactivated Coronavirus vaccine which is also used to manufacture vaccines like influenza, rabies and hepatitis A.
3. Sputnik V is manufactured by Gamaleya Research Institute in Russia and is imported by Dr Reddy's Laboratories for Gam-COVID-Vac combined vector vaccine (component I and II).
4. Corbevax is developed by Biological E Ltd. is a protein subunit vaccine which has receptor binding domain of SARS-CoV-2 gene.
5. Cavovax vaccine, manufactured by Serum Institute of India, is a SARS-CoV-2 rS protein COVID-19 recombinant spike protein nanoparticle vaccine.
6. ZyCoV-D vaccine, manufactured by Zydus Cadila, is recombinant DNA novel Coronavirus, 2019—nCoV vaccine.

Side-effects

Covishield®: Some mild symptoms may occur like injection site tenderness, infection site pain, headache, fatigue myalgia, malaise, pyrexia, chills, arthralgia and nausea. Very rare events of demyelinating disorders, thrombosis with thrombocytopenia syndrome (TTS) have been reported.

Other vaccines in India also have similar effects.

Methods of prevention of spread of COVID-19 and steps to protect yourself from Coronavirus infection are given in Fig. 40.12A and B.

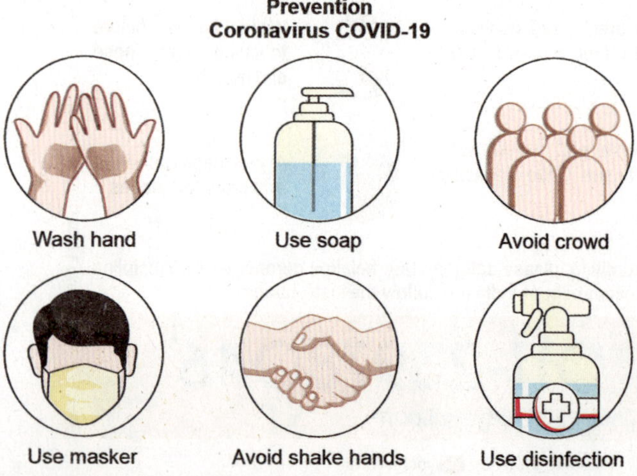

Fig. 40.12A: Methods of prevention of spread of COVID-19

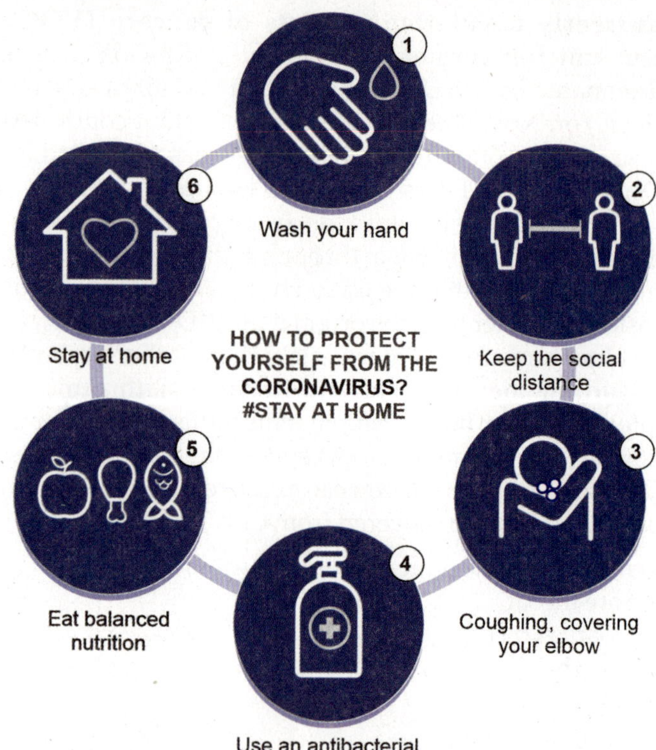

Fig. 40.12B: Steps 1–6. How to protect yourself from Coronavirus infection?

Laboratory Diagnosis

A. Direct tests
B. Indirect tests

A. Direct Tests

i. **Antigen tests and rapid antigen test (RAT)**: Rapid, accurate tests are essential to contain a highly contagious virus like SARS-CoV-2. PCR tests are accurate but can take a long time to produce results. Antigen tests, the other major type of coronavirus test, while much faster, are less accurate.
ii. **Real time reverse transcription polymerase chain reaction (RT-PCR).**

B. Indirect Tests

- For antibody tests.
- Indicates presence of antibody after infection.

The RT-PCR test detects the presence of the RNA of virus in a sample, while the rapid antigen test looks for the presence of surface antigen.

Antigen tests do have some drawbacks. Depending on the situation, they can be less accurate than PCR tests. When a person is symptomatic or has a lot of virus in their system, antigen tests are very accurate. However, unlike molecular PCR tests, antigen tests do not amplify the thing they are looking for. This means there need to be enough viral antigen in the sample for the antibodies on the test strip to generate a signal. When a person is in the early stages of infection, not a lot of virus is in the nose and throat, from which the samples are taken. So, antigen tests can miss early cases of COVID-19. It is also during this stage that a person has no symptoms, so they are more likely to be unaware they are infected.

Due to **low sensitivity**, majority of times **RAT** produces **false negative** results.

Rapid antigen test for COVID-19 variant (omicron) available (Fig. 40.13).

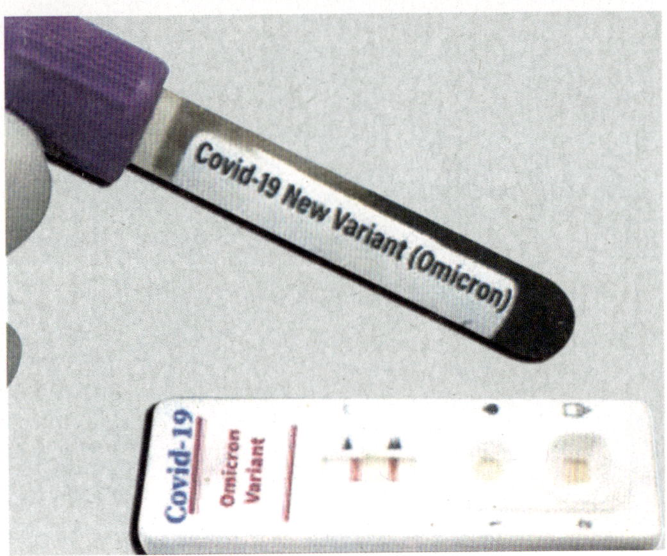

Fig. 40.13: RAT (omicron) showing 2 lines (control + positive antigen)

Section 3C

Mycology

41. Mycology (General)
42. Candida (Candidiasis and *Cryptococcus neoformans*—Cryptococcosis)
43. *Aspergillus* Species (Aspergillosis and Mucormycosis)
44. Dermatophytes (Dermatophytosis)

Mycology
(General)

Chapter Outline

INTRODUCTION AND GENERAL CONCEPTS OF MYCOLOGY

Definition

The branch of biology that deals with the study of fungi is known as mycology, which is derived from mykes, a Greek word for mushroom. The medical mycology is the study of fungi, their ecology and epidemiology in relation to diseases produced in man and other mammals. Although Augustino Bassi in 1835, observed that muscardine, a silk work disease was caused by a fungus (*Beauveria bassiana*) but the discipline of medical mycology gained recognition in world sciences when the monumental work on dermatophytes was published in 1910 by Raymond Sabouraud (1984–1938). He has been rightly called the Father of Medical Mycology. The fungi were initially classified with the plants and hence much of botanical influence is still seen on the subject. That is why mycology has been a subject of interest to the botanists. However, these organisms have now been transferred to a separate, *fifth kingdom*, based on the cell morphology and nutritional behaviour. After the recent rise in the fungal infections, particularly in the immunocompromised patients, it has now become the subject of much interest to the medical community.

Classification of Fungus (Table 41.1)

Fungi are eukaryotic organisms that do not contain chlorophyll, but have cell walls, filamentous structures, and produce spores. These organisms grow as saprophytes and decompose dead organic matter. There are between 100,000 and 200,000 species depending on how they are classified. About 300 species are presently known to be pathogenic for man.

Table 41.1: There are five kingdoms of living things. The fungi are in the Kingdom Fungi

Kingdom	*Characteristic*	*Example*
Monera	Prokaryocyte	Bacteria Actinomycetes
Protista	Eukaryocyte	Protozoa
Fungi	Eukaryocyte*	Fungi
Plantae	Eukaryocyte	Plants, Moss
Animalia	Eukaryocyte*	Arthropods
		Mammals
		Man

*This common characteristic is responsible for the therapeutic dilemma in anti-mycotic therapy

The taxonomy of the Kingdom Fungi is evolving and is controversial. Formerly based on gross and light microscopic; morphology, studies of ultrastructure, biochemistry and molecular biology provide new evidence on which to base taxonomic positions. Medically important fungi are in four phyla:

1. **Ascomycota:** Sexual reproduction in a sac (ascus). With the production of ascospores.
2. **Basidiomycota:** Sexual reproduction on a base (basidium), with the production of basidiospores.
3. **Phycomycetes:** Lower fungi which have non-septate hyphae and form endogenous asexual spores called 'sporangiophores' within sac-like structures called 'sporangia'.

4. **Deuteromycetes or hyphomycetes (fungi imperfecti):** No recognizable form of sexual reproduction. Includes most pathogenic fungi.

Fungi: Fungi are eukaryotes microorganisms. They may be unicellular or multicellular. Disease produced by fungi is known as mycosis.

Classification

1. **Yeast:** This is unicellular fungi. They multiply by budding. Bud is called blastospore. *Cryptococcus neoformans* is only pathogenic and important yeast.
2. **Yeast like:** This is unicellular organism. They multiply by budding but daughter cell is attached with parent cell and give appearance of long thread-like. This thread is called pseudohyphae.
3. **Molds:** This is multicellular fungi and multiply by branching. One single multicellular is called hyphae. Group of hyphae is called mycelium.
4. **Dimorphic:** Dimorphic fungi occur as yeast and molds at different temperature. These fungi can grow at 37°C like yeast. At room temperature these fungi grow like mycelium forms.

Clinical classification of the mycoses

Fungal diseases may be discussed in a variety of ways. The most practical method for medical students is the clinical taxonomy, which divides the fungi into:

- Superficial mycoses
  - Surface
  - Cutaneous
- Deep mycoses
  - Subcutaneous
  - Systemic
- Opportunistic mycoses
- **Superficial mycoses:** The superficial mycoses can be of two types—surface and cutaneous mycoses. In surface mycoses, fungi live exclusively on the dead layers of the skin and its appendages. They elicit no inflammatory response as there is no contact with the living tissues. The only changes are cosmetic effects, e.g. tinea versicolor. The cutaneous mycoses are fungal diseases that are confined to the outer layers of the skin, nail, or hair (keratinized layers), rarely invading the deeper tissue or viscera. The fungi involved are called dermatophytes.
- **Deep mycoses:** The deep mycoses can be of two types—the subcutaneous and the systemic mycoses. The subcutaneous mycoses are confined to the subcutaneous tissue and only rarely spread systemically. They usually form deep, ulcerated skin lesions or fungating masses, most commonly involving the lower extremities. The causative organisms are soil saprophytes which are introduced through trauma to the feet or legs. The systemic mycoses may involve deep viscera and become widely disseminated.
- **Opportunistic mycoses:** The opportunistic mycoses are infections due to fungi with low inherent virulence. The etiologic agents are organisms which are common in all environments. These are seen in hosts with lowered immunity states due to debilitating diseases or use of drugs.

Diagnosis of Fungal Infections and Processing of Clinical Specimens

Laboratory diagnosis: The laboratory procedures may confirm a clinical suspicion to establish a fungal cause in a disease of unknown etiology or exclude fungal involvement where there are many differential diagnosis. When a diagnosis of fungal infection has been established, the laboratory may help with the choice of therapeutic agents, monitoring the course of the disease and successful mycological cure.

Processing of specimens: Pretreatment of specimens is sometimes necessary before examination by microscopy and culture. The samples of CSF and urine are best centrifuged and the deposit resuspended in a small volume of saline to detect the scanty numbers of sites and types of specimens.

1. Superficial Mycoses

The diagnosis of superficial mycoses may be strongly suspected on clinical grounds and it is usually prudent and sometimes essential to seek laboratory aid. Both, direct microscopic examination and the culture on selective media should be made whenever possible.

a. **Respiratory specimens:** The specimens from the respiratory system for fungal culture are sputum, tracheal secretions and the bronchial washings. A sufficient amount of specimen should be inoculated on each medium. The interpretation of the results with opportunistic pathogens such as Candida, is more difficult because it is commonly present in sputum specimens, as an oropharyngeal contaminant.

b. **Cerebrospinal fluid:** Cerebrospinal fluid collected for culture should be centrifuged and one drop of the sediment should be placed onto several areas on the agar surface. The media used for the recovery of fungi from CSF should contain no antimicrobial agents because it is a sterile fluid.

c. **Blood:** The disseminated fungal infections are more prevalent than previously recognised. The blood cultures provide an accurate method for establishing the diagnosis.

d. **Skin, nail and hair:** These specimens are usually taken for dermatophyte infection and may be obtained by scraping the skin. The nail clippings should be taken from discoloured, dystrophic or brittle parts of the nails. Fungus in the distal part of the nail is often non-viable and although it may be visible on microscopy, it fails to grow in culture. The hairs are removed by plucking them with forceps. The specimen should be placed in a sterile Petri dish or paper envelope and it should not be refrigerated. The Sabouraud's dextrose agar with chloramphenicol and cycloheximide, is satisfactory for culturing dermatophytes. The cultures should be incubated at 25°C, 30°C and 37°C for a minimum of four weeks before being reported as negative.

e. **Urine:** Urine specimens collected for fungal culture should be processed as early as possible after collection.
f. **Tissue, bone marrow and sterile body fluids:** All tissues should be processed before culture by mincing or grinding. After processing, at least 1 ml of specimen should be spread on the surface of appropriate culture media and incubation should be for four weeks at 37°C.
g. **Vaginal secretions:** The diagnosis of vaginal candidiasis is better established with the help of clinical features.
h. **Hair and nail:** The material is best collected into folded squares of paper, thereby permitting drying of the specimen, reducing bacterial contamination and providing conditions under which specimens can be stored for long periods without appreciable loss in viability of the fungal agents.

The dermatophytic lesion usually spreads outward in a concentric fashion with healing in the central region. Therefore, the material should be collected by scraping outward from the edges of the lesions with a scalpel blade held at 90′ to the skin surface. When there is least scaling, as with the lesions of the glabrous skin, it is preferable and sometimes necessary to use cellophane tape to take adequate material for laboratory examination.

The specimens from the scalp are best obtained by scraping with a blunt scalpel so that they include hair stubs, contents of plugged follicles and scales. Hairs that have been cut rather than plucked are seldom satisfactory. In kerion, the hairs which resist pull of the epilation forceps can be left which come away easily are preferably selected. The ringworm of the scalp, especially if caused by anthropophilic species, may cause small lesions that are difficult to detect clinically. This type of infection may produce fluorescence of infected hair and may be detected by Wood's light. The Wood's lamp examination is helpful to detect scalp ringworm or to select material for culture when the infection is caused by species which produce fluorescence of the infected hair. The hairbrush sampling technique may be utilised to obtain cultures. This involves thoroughly brushing the scalp and using the hairbrush to inoculate on the culture media.

Nail specimens should be clipped from the free edge, taken as far back in the nail as possible and should include its full thickness. The fungus in the distal portion of nail is often non-viable and if culture does fail, success can sometimes be obtained by culturing "borings" taken from the base of the nail.

2. Subcutaneous Mycoses

The scrapings or crusts from the superficial parts of subcutaneous lesions may be satisfactory for microscopy and culture.

3. Systemic Mycoses

The patients with suspected deep-seated mycoses should have specimens taken from as many sites as possible. The sources include tissue removed for biopsy, pus, faeces, urine, sputum, spinal fluid, blood and scrapings or swabs from the edges of lesions. It is important to ensure that specimens such as sputum and urine are freshly collected.

Incubation of Culture

i. The media inoculated with specimen for fungal cultures are incubated at 25–30°C. The cultures are examined every 2–3 days for evidence of growth. If no growth is observed in four weeks, the specimen is reported as negative for fungi.
ii. When an infection with a dimorphic fungi is suspected, an enriched medium such as BHIBA should be incubated at 37°C and examined every 2–3 days for at least up to six weeks. If there is growth, examine microscopically for a yeast or tissue form.

Staining Methods

1. **Potassium hydroxide (KOH) preparation:** The KOH preparation is ideal for determining fungal morphology because even though it readily dissolves the clinical material, fungal elements remain intact for a longer period due to the chitin in their cell walls.
   Reagent: Prepare a 10% solution of KOH. A few drops of permanent blue-black ink may be added to the solution to highlight fungal walls.
2. **Negative staining using India ink or 10% nigrosin:** For specimens such as cerebrospinal fluid, the negative staining procedure using India ink or 10% nigrosin is very useful. In this technique, i.e. ink is used as a dark background to highlight the hyaline yeast cells and capsular material around them.
   Reagent: 10% nigrosin or India ink.
3. **Giemsa stain:** Giemsa stain is excellent for demonstrating the presence of intracellular yeast cells of *Histoplasma capsulatum* in specimens such as bone marrow or peripheral blood. The intracellular yeast forms of *H. capsulatum* stain light to dark blue with Giemsa stain.
4. **Periodic acid–Schiff (PAS) stain:** In some specimens such as nail or skin, fungi are not readily visible in the clinical specimens by KOH preparation. PAS staining is a very useful technique for the detection of fungi.
5. **Other staining methods**
   a. Gram stain is useful for demonstrating the presence of Gram-positive filaments of Actinomyces and yeasts such as *Candida* species.
   b. Acid-fast stain using 1% sulphuric acid for decolourization, can detect *Nocardia* species.
   c. Calcofluor white fluorescent stain can detect fungi very easily as they fluoresce under UV light.

Serology

Serology may be helpful when it is applied to a specific fungal disease; there are no screening antigens for fungi in general. Because fungi are poor antigens, their efficacy of serology varies with different fungal infections. The most common serological tests for fungi are based on latex agglutination, double immunodiffusion, complement fixation and enzyme immunoassays. While latex agglutination may favour the detection of IgM antibodies, double immunodiffusion and complement fixation usually detect IgG antibodies. Some EIA tests are being developed to detect both IgG and IgM antibodies. There are some tests which can detect specific fungal antigens, but they are just coming into general use.

Direct Fluorescent Microscopy

Direct fluorescent microscopy may be used for identification, even on non-viable cultures or on fixed tissue sections. The reagents for this test are difficult to obtain.

Biopsy and Histopathology

A biopsy may be very useful for the identification and as a source of the tissue evading fungi. Usually the Gomori methenamine silver (GMS) stain, is used to reveal the organisms which stain black against a green background. The H&E stain not always tint the organism, but it will also stain the inflammatory cells.

Culture

A definitive diagnosis requires a culture and identification. Pathogenic fungi are usually grown on Sabouraud dextrose agar. It has a slightly acidic pH (~5.6). Cyclohexamide, penicillin, streptomycin or other inhibitory antibiotics are often added to prevent bacterial contamination and overgrowth. Two cultures are inoculated and incubated separately at 25°C and 37° C to reveal dimorphism. The cultures are examined macroscopically and microscopically. They are not considered negative for growth until after 4 weeks of incubation.

Mechanism of Fungal Pathogenicity

The basic mechanism of fungal pathogenicity is its ability to adapt to the tissue environment, physiological barriers and temperature (37°C) and withstand the lytic activity of hosts' cellular defense. Based on their wide spectrum of adaptability, various fungi causing human mycoses can be categorised into the following groups:

a. **Pathogenic:** The ability to adapt to tissue environment is quite marked and is expressed as thermal dimorphism.
b. **Opportunist pathogenic:** (i) A defect in the normal defences of the host is required for the establishment of the fungal agent. Such fungi do not exhibit thermal dimorphism. (ii) Causal agents of subcutaneous mycosis require mechanical introduction of the organism into the tissue through traumatic implantation.
c. **Toxic:** Species which cause illness or death of patients or animals after ingestion of the contaminated food with toxin is produced by fungi.
d. **Allergenic:** Species which act as allergens and cause allergic manifestations in the human beings.

Immunology and Serology

The immunological tests are also used in the diagnosis of fungal diseases and to identify patients whose fungal cultures have been non-productive. Serology is helpful in interpreting the clinical significance of positive cultures of Aspergillus because this organism may be a laboratory contaminant.

The specific immune response that results from exposure to cell/wall, cytoplasmic or extracellular fungal antigen during infection, can be used for diagnosis.

Significance of Fungi

The fungi have recently gained more importance due to the increased incidence of various fungal diseases. Normally, most of these organisms are found as soil saprobes but whenever there is some underlying cause, the same very organisms become substantially pathogenic.

The fungus is a diverse group of heterotrophic organisms that exist as saprobes, commensals or parasites. Most of them are found on decaying vegetative material and in the soil. At an ambient temperature the fungus grows as spore-bearing mold, which is the infectious form to man and animals.

Salient differentiating features between fungi and bacteria are given in Table 41.2.

Yeast

The yeasts are unicellular and reproduced by asexual process known as budding, i.e. blastospore formation or fission transverse septum formation. The cell develops a protuberance which enlarges and eventually separates from the parent cell. The yeasts may produce chains of elongated cells known as pseudohyphae which resemble the mycelia of the molds. Some species produce true mycelia also. The yeasts are ubiquitous in the environment being found on fruits, vegetables and other plant materials (exogenous). Some live as normal inhabitants in the human body (endogenous). Therefore, they may be found in specimens without any clinical significance.

Pathogenic fungi can exist as yeasts or as hyphae. A mass of hyphae is called mycelia. Mycelia are multicellular filamentous structures, constituted by tubular cells with cell walls. Thus on the basis of morphology, fungi can be four types: Yeasts, yeast-like fungi, moulds and dimorphic fungi. Some fungi occur in both the yeast and mycelial forms. Yeasts are unicellular organisms which occur as spherical or ellipsoidal cells and reproduce by budding. The only pathogenic yeast is *Cryptococcus neoformans*. Yeast like fungi grow partly as yeast and partly as elongated cells resembling hyphae (pseudomycelium), *Candida albicans* is a pathologic yeast like fungus.

Table 41.2: Salient differentiating features between fungi and bacteria

Properties	*Fungi*	*Bacteria*
1. Cell structure	Eukaryotic	Prokaryotic
2. Cell wall composition	Multilayered; chitin, mannan, other polysaccharides and peptides; capsules in some members	Muramic and teichoic acids; lipopolysaccharides, capsule present in some members
3. Cytoplasmic membrane	Sterols present	Lack sterols (except Mycoplasma)
4. Cytoplasmic contents	Include mitochondria, endoplasmic reticulum	Lack mitochondria, endoplasmic reticulum
5. Nucleus	True nucleus with nuclear membrane, paired chromosomes	Nuclear body equivalent to a single chromosome without nuclear membrane
6. Diameter	5–10 µm may be > 100 µm in length	<2 µm
7. Morphology	Yeast: Ovoid, round Mold: Filamentous branching, septate, nonseptate	Coccal, bacillary; some branching (Actinomyces, Nocardia), spirochaetal
8. Spores	Asexual and sexual reproductive spores	Endospores (non-reproductive)
9. Staining attributes	Gram-positive, mostly non-acid fast stain with methenamine silver and periodic acid-Schiff	Gram-positive, Gram-negative; acid-fast (*Mycobacterium*, *Nocardia*)
10. Mode of reproduction	Either sexual or asexual, both stages result in spore formation	Binary fission

Vegetative Structures

Several structures are formed by the vegetative mycelium which have no reproductive significance but are of considerable value in the differentiation of most of the clinically important fungi. These arise following modifications of single vegetative cells or hyphae, for instance, chlamydospores develop from cells which become enriched with nutritive materials and form a thick resistant wall to tide over adverse conditions. They are usually larger than other cells and may be formed singly or in groups and in an intercalary, terminal or sessile position.

Another unicellular vegetative spore is the arthrospore. Here many septa in the hypha are formed to give chains of small cuboidal spores with slightly thickened wall which disarticulate when mature. Arthrospore production is a characteristic of parasitic phase of the dermatophyte.

Spiral hyphae are corkscrew-like turns of mycelium which are similar to the coiled filaments of actinomycetes, e.g. *Streptomyces* species. These are observed in several pathogenic fungi.

The mycelial forms branch and the pattern of branching is an aid to the morphological identification. If the mycelia do not have septa, they are called coenocytic (nonseptate).

The terms "hypha" and "mycelium" are frequently used interchangeably.

Dimorphic fungi can occur as yeasts or filament, depending on the growth conditions. In host tissue or cultures at 37°C, they occur as yeasts, while in soil and in cultures at 22°C, they appear as moulds. Most fungi causing systemic diseases, are dimorphic. Conversion to the yeast form appears to be essential for pathogenicity. Fungi are identified by several morphological or biochemical characteristics, including the appearance of their fruiting bodies. The asexual spores may be large (macroconidia, chlamydospores) or small (microconidia, blastospores, arthroconidia).

Molds

The molds are composed of branching filaments known as hyphae. They grow by apical extension, forming an interwoven masses, i.e. mycelia. The hypha is a structural unit of the mycelium. In most of the fungi the hyphae have regular cross-wall, i.e. septate but in lower fungi these are aseptate. Usually the hyphae that grow horizontally along the surface of the culture medium or submerged in the liquid medium are called vegetative hyphae and they are largely responsible for absorbing nutrients. The hyphae which project above the surface of the medium are called aerial hyphae and produce specialised structures called conidia or sporangiospores. Homothallic fungi are self-fertile in which sexual reproduction can take place within the thallus, whereas heterothallic fungi require two compatible thalli for the sexual reproduction. The diagrammatic representation of the fungal thallus is given in Fig. 41.1. In higher fungi the hyphae are variously compacted together to form a variety of fungal tissues which give rise to macroscopic structures known as sporophorus or fruiting bodies.

Representation of fungal thallus is shown in Fig. 41.1.

Diagrammatic representation of vegetative forms of fungi (A–E) is shown in Fig. 41.2.

Vegetative structures of dermatophytes are shown in Fig. 41.3 (A–E).

Types of sexual spores produced by molds are shown in Fig. 41.4 (A–F).

Mold
Mycelia
Germ
(True)
hyphae
Yeast
Solitary
Budding
Pseudohyphae

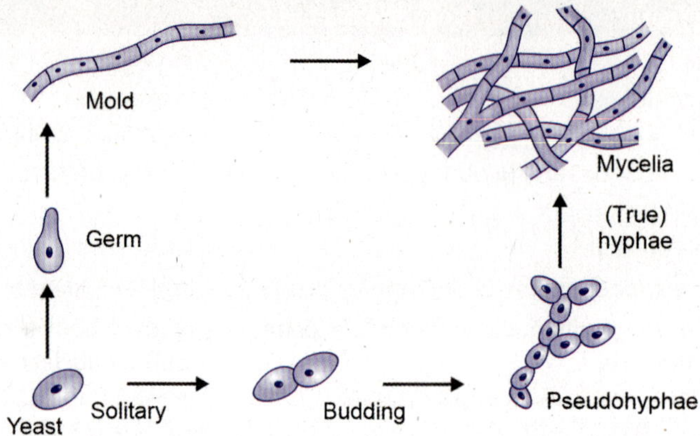

Fig. 41.1: Diagrammatic representation of the fungal thallus

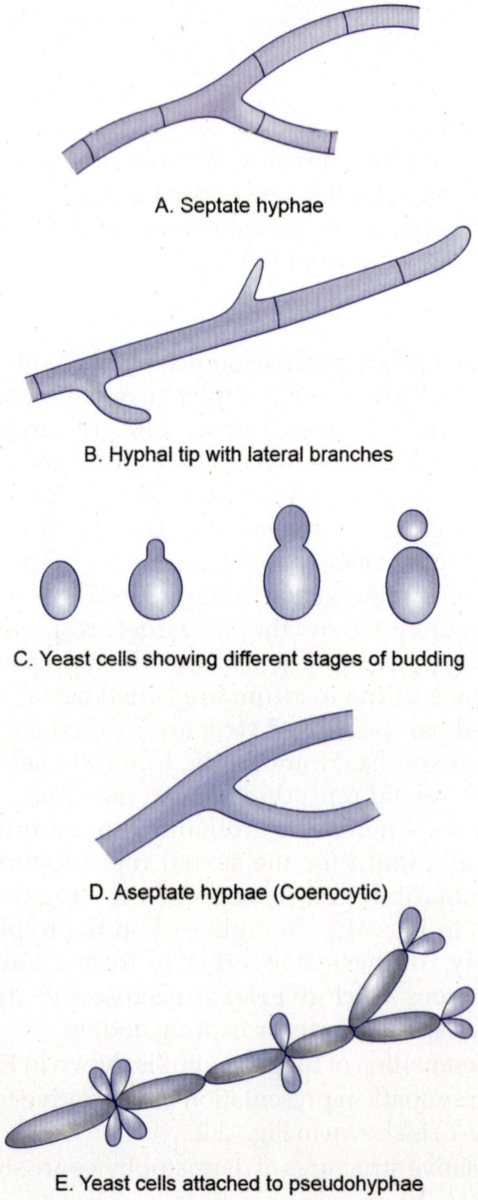

A. Septate hyphae
B. Hyphal tip with lateral branches
C. Yeast cells showing different stages of budding
D. Aseptate hyphae (Coenocytic)
E. Yeast cells attached to pseudohyphae

Fig. 41.2: (A–E)

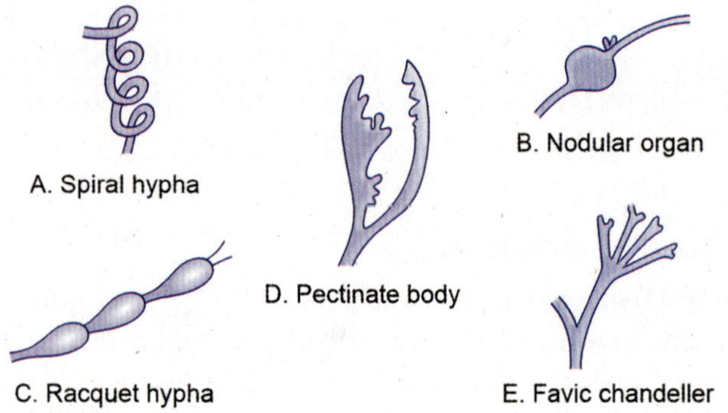

A. Spiral hypha
B. Nodular organ
C. Racquet hypha
D. Pectinate body
E. Favic chandeller

Fig. 41.3: Vegetative structures of dermatophytes (A–E)

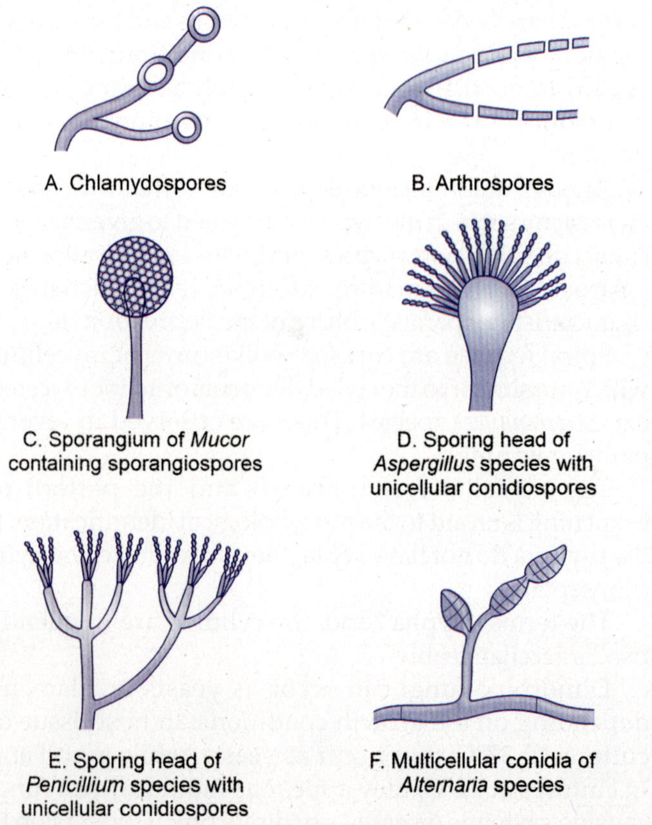

A. Chlamydospores
B. Arthrospores
C. Sporangium of *Mucor* containing sporangiospores
D. Sporing head of *Aspergillus* species with unicellular conidiospores
E. Sporing head of *Penicillium* species with unicellular conidiospores
F. Multicellular conidia of *Alternaria* species

Fig. 41.4: Types of asexual spores produced by molds (A–F)

Chapter 42

Candida

(Candidiasis and *Cryptococcus neoformans*—Cryptococcosis)

Chapter Outline

- *Candida albicans*: Yeast and Hyphae
- *Cryptococcus neoformans*
- Cryptococcosis
- Diagnosis of Cryptococcosis

CANDIDA ALBICANS: YEAST AND HYPHAE

- Family: Saccharomycetaceae
- Phylum: Ascomycota
- Approx 200 species
- About 20 associated with pathology in humans and animals.

Introduction

Candida albicans is an oval or spherical budding yeast cell 3–5 g in diameter. It produces pseudohyphae when the buds continue to grow but fails to detach, producing chains of elongated cells that are pinched or constricted at the septation between cells. It can also produce true hyphae. The yeast is a common commensal of the gastrointestinal tract, mucous membranes and skin. Since Candida is normally present on skin and mucosa, therefore, it is significant only when it is present in large numbers. In addition, presence of pseudohyphae indicates colonization. Gram-stained smears from lesions, exudates and skin and nail scrapings show budding Gram-positive yeast cells and pseudohyphae (Fig. 42.1).

Out of more than 200 species, the most commonly encountered in medical practices are *C. albicans*, *C. guilliermondii*, *C. krusei*, *C. tropicalis*, *C. parapsilosis*, *C. pseudotropicalis*, *C. lusitaniae*, *C. dubliniensis* and *C. glabrata*.

Pathogens

Candida spp are asexual yeast of genus Ascomycetes and genetically diploid with presence of 8 chromosomes.

They are small (4 to 6 µm), thin walled, ovoid cells (blastospores) that reproduce by budding (Fig. 42.2).

They grow well invented routine blood culture bottles and on agar plate and do not require special fungal media for cultivation.

About 8–15% of nosocomial blood stream infections are reported to be caused by Candida species.

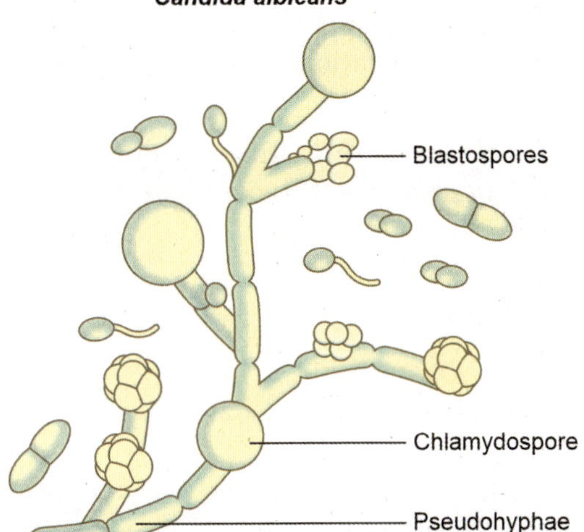

Fig. 42.1: *Candida albicans*, spore and hyphae

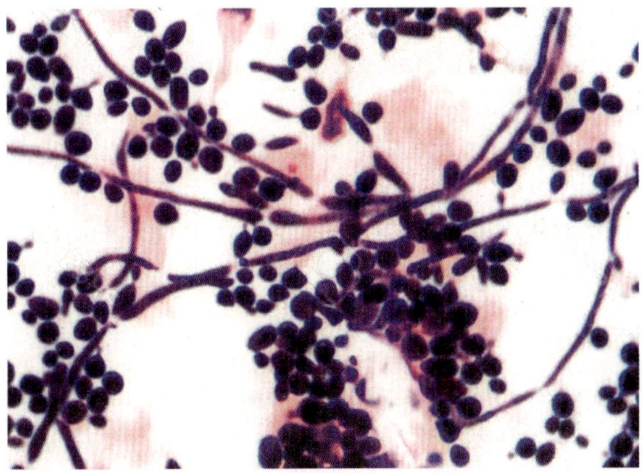

Fig. 42.2: Thin wall ovoid cells blastospores with budding and hyphae

Cultural Characteristics

Sabouraud's dextrose agar (SDA): *C. albicans* grows well on SDA. Cream-coloured, smooth, pasty colonies appear in 1–2 days at 25–37°C. Lactophenol cotton blue (LCB) preparation and Gram-stained smears show budding yeast cells and pseudohyphae.

Corn meal agar: *C. albicans* produces large spherical chlamydospores which may be intercalary, terminal or sessile.

Test for Presumptive Identification of *C. albicans*

Germ tube test: A germ tube is a filamentous outgrowth from a yeast cell. The filament lacks a constriction at the point of origin which differentiates it from the pseudohyphae.

Method

- Take 0.5 ml of pooled human serum into a small test tube.
- Using a sterile wire, inoculate the serum with a yeast colony from the culture plate. Place the tube in a water-bath or incubator at 35–37°C for 2–3 hours.
- Using a sterile wire loop or Pasteur pipette, transfer a drop of the serum yeast culture to a glass slide and cover it with a coverslip.
- Examine the preparation under low and high power objectives for germ tube.

C. albicans can also be differentiated from other species by sugar fermentation and sugar assimilation reactions.

Epidemiology

Habitat

- Human commensal
- Major reservoir: GI tract
- Can invade into bloodstream from GI tract after damaging GI mucosa.

Source of infection

- Endogenous:
  - Primarily
  - Can spread hematogenously into various organs
- Exogenous:
  - Introduction into the body through medical device catheters
  - Important in the development of deep-seated and systemic infections

Candidiasis

Candidiasis is the commonest fungal disease in human being. The causative agent of the disease is *Candida albicans* and non-albicans *Candida*.

Typically, *C. albicans* live as harmless commensals in the gastrointestinal and genitourinary tract and are found in over 70% of the population. Overgrowth of these organisms, however, will lead to disease.

It usually occurs in the mouth and pharynx but may also occur in the esophagus.

Candidiasis can become a source of systemic dissemination, particularly in high-risk persons.

Several different clinical forms:

- Acute pseudomembranous candidiasis (oral thrush)
- Acute atrophic candidiasis
- Chronic atrophic candidiasis
- Chronic hyperplastic candidiasis
- Angular cheilitis

Types of Candidiasis (Fig. 42.3)

Deep-seated Candidiasis

Candidiasis of GI tract

- Gastrointestinal candidiasis
- Though being normal flora of GI tract, clinical involvement of mucosal surfaces of the stomach and/or intestine with mucosal white plaques and ulcerations are found.
- Plays an important role in the pathogenesis of disseminated candidiasis.

Pathogenesis: Candidiasis is caused by the abnormal growth in *C. albicans*, which is usually due to an imbalance in the environment.

Usually, this imbalance occurs in a woman's vagina this infection less likely to occur for men.

Several events can spark an imbalance. For example, antibiotic use can decrease the amount of lactobacillus bacteria, which decreases the amount of acidic products and the pH of the vagina. Other events are pregnancy, uncontrolled diabetes, impaired immune system, and irritation of the vagina.

C. albicans are able to take advantage of the conditions and outcompete the normal microflora, resulting in candidiasis or a yeast infection.

Surface molecules that permit adherence of the organism to other structures (e.g. human cells, extracellular matrix, prosthetic devices).

Acid proteases and phospholipases that involve penetration and damage of cell envelopes.

Ability to convert to a hyphal form (phenotypic switching).

Stages of disseminated infection (Fig. 42.4)

Laboratory diagnosis of Candida: Depends on the nature of infection, whether mucocutaneous or deep-seated forms

Mucocutaneous Candidiasis

- Sample: Skin, nail or mucosal surface swabs
- Includes 2 steps:
  - Direct examination of the specimen to demonstrate fungal presence
  - Isolation of the fungus and its identification

Microbiology methods

- Recovery of Candida species from sterile sites (e.g. blood. peritoneal fluid) is diagnostic of IC and recovery from multiple non-sterile sites is highly suggestive of IC in the at-risk patient.

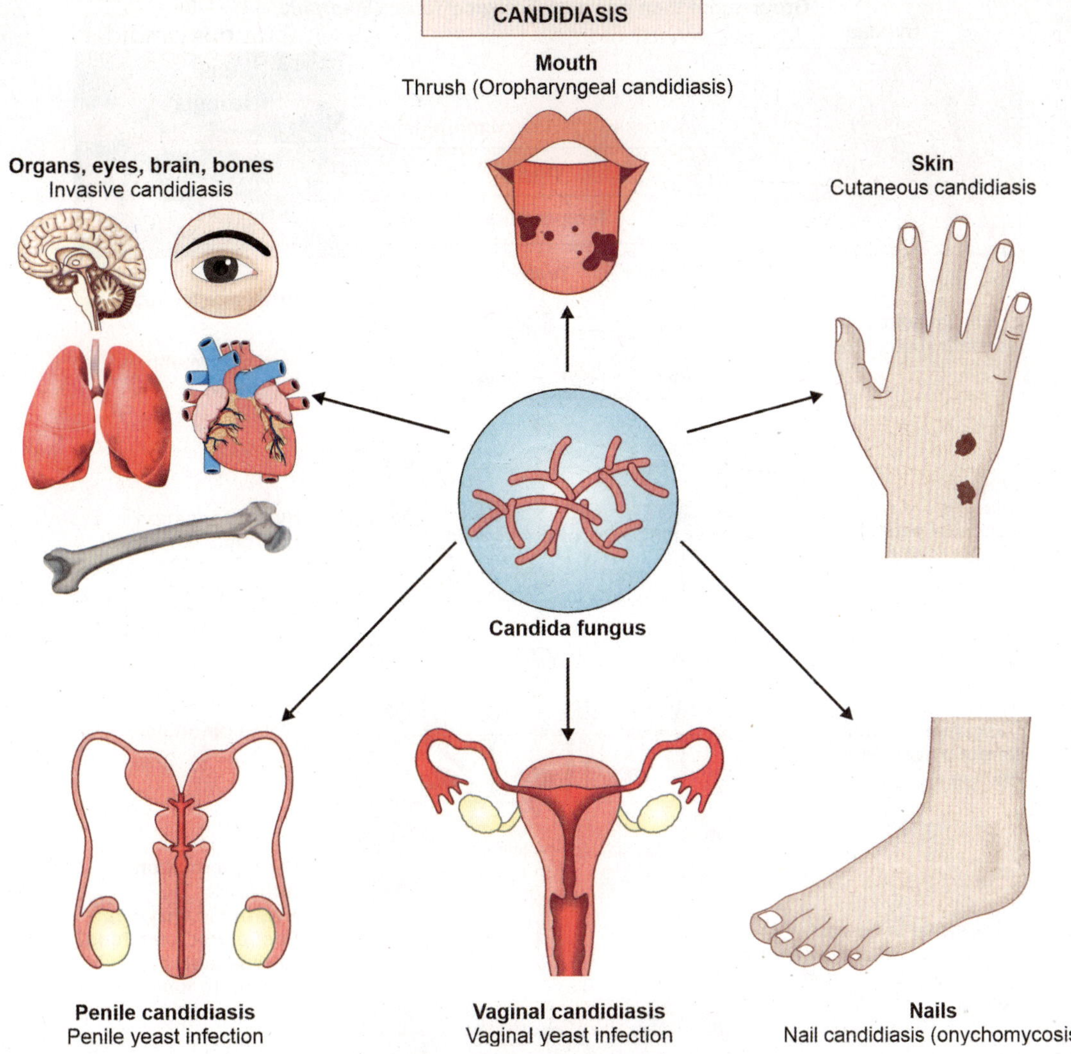

Fig. 42.3: Various types of candidiasis

- Blood culture is positive in less than 50% of patients with autopsy proven IC.

Molecular methods: Early identification ex PNA FISH.

Serological methods: Early diagnosis ex 1, 3 beta D glucan assay.

Histopathologic methods.

1. **Direct examination (wet mount method)**
   - Treat specimen with keratinolytic substance (10–30% KOH) to facilitate the microscopic examination of the specimen
   - Demonstration of fungi enhanced by
     - the addition of cotton blue or acid Parker's ink
     - the use of calcofluor white, a fluorochrome with an affinity for chitin and glucan which makes a demonstration of fungal elements with a fluorescent microscope relatively simple.
   - Gram's staining for nail and skin specimens—not generally done.

Pathogenetic mechanism: Overgrowth of *C. albicans* results in mucosal colonisation resulting to micro-invasion and finally candidemia and disseminated diseases (Fig. 42.5).

Candida albicans is the commonest cause of candidiasis (moniliasis). Candidiasis is an opportunistic endogenous infection. Predisposing factors for candidiasis are AIDS, diabetes mellitus, neutropaenia and prolonged administration of antimicrobial agents.

Microscopic examination of specimens from vulvovaginitis or oral candidiasis will reveal the presence of budding yeast cells, pseudohyphae and hyphae.

Presence of hyphal elements in direct microscopic examination is important (vagina and mouth normally colonised by *Candida* spp).

Presence of hyphal elements indicates infection (Fig. 42.6).

Immunodiagnosis

- For deep-seated infection, microscopy and culture methods not sufficient as in case of mucocutaneous infection.
- Based on
  - Detection of antibody production

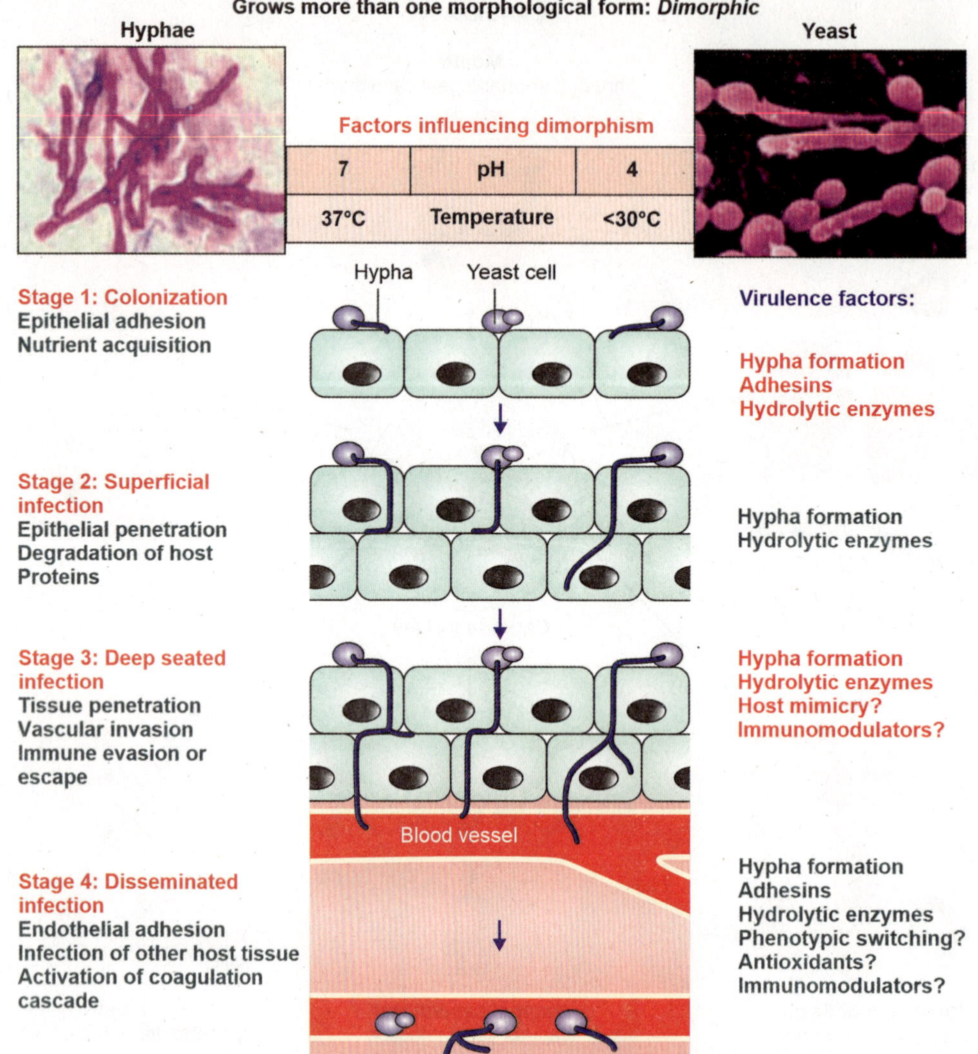

Fig. 42.4: Stages of disseminated infection

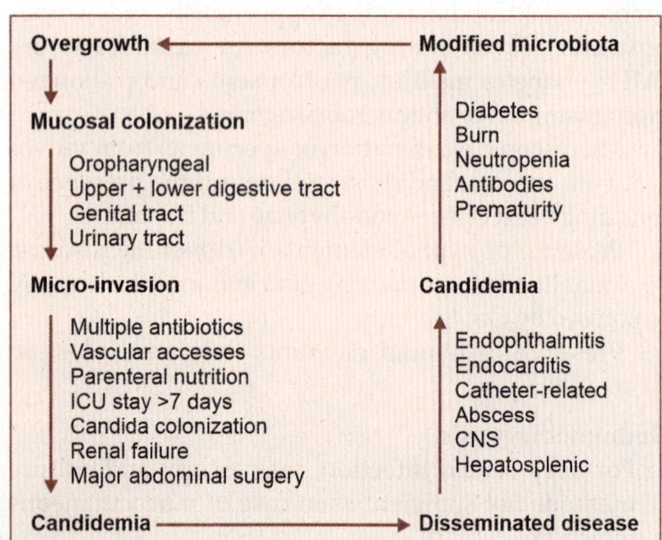

Fig. 42.5: Pathogenetic mechanism candidemia and dissemination

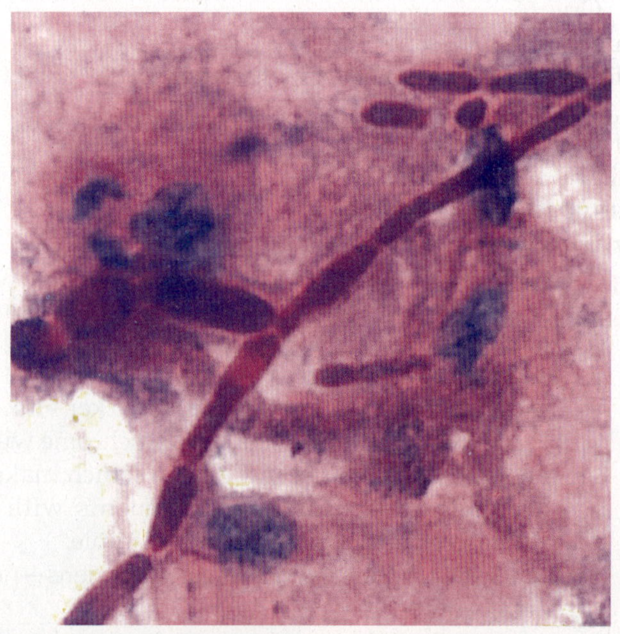

Fig. 42.6: Presence of yeast cells and hyphal elements in vulvo-vaginal lesion

- Detection of fungal antigens in body fluids and in serum.

Antibody Detection

- Agglutination technique representing anti-mannan antibodies, can also be found in healthy individuals and with superficial infections not useful for diagnosis of deep-seated infection.
- Antibody detection for the presence of antibodies to candidal internal antigens released into patient's body during invasion.
  - Techniques gel immunodiffusion CCIE ELISA latex.

CRYPTOCOCCUS NEOFORMANS

Introduction

Cryptococcus neoformans is dimorphic, existing in the asexual yeast form characterized by oval to spherical cells with a polysaccharide capsule, and in the sexual or perfect state characterized by the presence of basidiospores.

C. neoformans is readily cultured in the laboratory, producing mucoid colonies within 36–72 hours, although growth is inhibited at 37 °C.

Colonies are white to cream in colour, but characteristic dark brown colonies are formed when grown on birdseed agar.

C. neoformans is present worldwide; it is acquired by inhaling dust from soil contaminated with bird droppings, particularly those of pigeons.

In immunocompetent patients, infection is typically asymptomatic anti self-limited.

In immunocompromised patients, *Cryptococcus* may disseminate to many sites, commonly to the brain and meninges, and to the skin.

Diagnose using culture staining, and/or serum and cerebrospinal fluid testing for cryptococcal antigen.

Cryptococcosis is a pulmonary or disseminated infection acquired by inhalation of soil contaminated with the encapsulated yeasts *Cryptococcus neoformans* or *C. gattii*. Symptoms are those of pneumonia, meningitis, or involvement of skin, bones, or viscera. Diagnosis is clinical and microscopic, confirmed by culture or fixed-tissue staining. Treatment, when necessary, is with azoles or amphotericin B, with or without flucytosine.

Morphology

- Spherical budding cell (5–15 µm diameter) having a prominent polysaccharide capsule.
- It is a true yeast and is Gram-positive.
- Capsule may be demonstrated by India ink or nigrosin staining (Fig. 42.7).
- The disease is usually seen in immunocompromised host.
- Most infections are asymptomatic.
- Pulmonary cryptococcosis may lead to a mild pneumonitis.
- Cryptococcal meningitis occurs by haematogenous spread. It is often seen in AIDS patients.

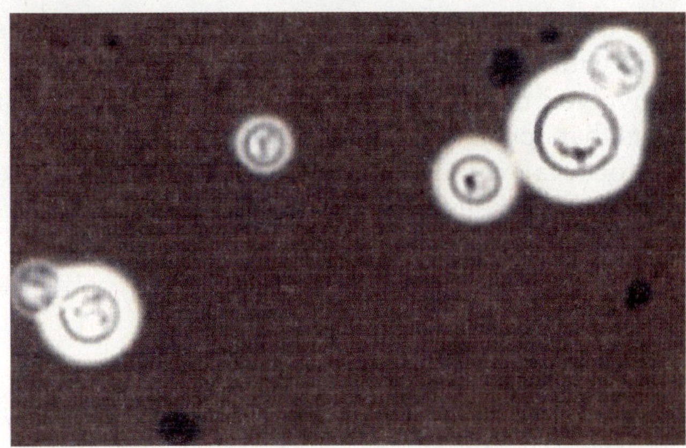

Fig. 42.7: *Cryptococcous neoformans* India ink positive capsule demonstration

- Skin, lymph nodes, bones and other organs may be involved when dissemination of infection occurs. Cutaneous cryptococcosis varies from small ulcers to large granulomas.
- Visceral forms of cryptococcal infection simulate tuberculosis and cancer clinically.

Antigenicity: On the basis of cryptococcal polysaccharide antigen, *C. neoformans* has four serotypes (A, B, C and D).

Source of infection: Infection is usually acquired by inhalation of dust containing yeast cells.

Pathogenesis

- *C. neoformans* is pathogenic in humans and animals.
- Gram staining shows Gram-positive yeast cells.
- The histopathological examination of tissue can be done by staining with H and E, PAS and mucicarmine stains.

C. neoformans has ability to

- grow at 37°C.
- hydrolyse urea.

CRYPTOCOCCOSIS

Cryptococcus is the most common fungus that causes serious infection worldwide. Both types of fungi are found in soil. If you breathe the fungus in, it infects your lungs. The infection may go away on its own, remain in the lungs only, or spread throughout the body (disseminate).

Causative fungus: *Cryptococcus neoformans*, a capsulated yeast.

It is a soil saprophyte and is particularly abundant in the faeces of pigeons.

C. neoformans does not appear to infect birds, probably because of their high body temperature. Cryptococcal infection occurs throughout the world. Several cases of cryptococcosis have been identified in India. This is the only deep mycosis common in India.

Pathophysiology of cryptococcosis: Focal sites of dissemination may also occur in skin, the ends of long bones, joints, liver, spleen, kidneys, prostate, and other tissues. Except for those in the skin, these lesions usually cause a few or no symptoms. Rarely, pyelonephritis occurs with renal papillary necrosis.

Involved tissues typically contain cystic masses of yeasts that appear gelatinous because of accumulated cryptococcal capsular polysaccharide, but acute inflammatory changes are minimal or absent.

Risk factors for cryptococcosis include:

- AIDS
- Hodgkin lymphoma
- Other lymphomas
- Sarcoidosis
- Long-term corticosteroid therapy
- Solid organ transplantation

Cryptococcosis is a defining opportunistic infection for AIDS (typically associated with CD4 cell counts <100/µl).

C. gattii is primarily associated with trees, especially the Eucalyptus and, unlike *C. neoformans*, is not associated with birds and is more likely to cause disease in immunocompetent hosts.

Symptoms and signs of cryptococcosi: Manifestations of cryptococcosis depend on the affected area.

Lungs: Many patients with cryptococcal pulmonary infection are asymptomatic. Those with pneumonia usually have cough and other nonspecific respiratory symptoms. However, AIDS-associated cryptococcal pulmonary infection may manifest as severe, progressive pneumonia with acute dyspnea and an X-ray pattern suggesting Pneumocystis infection.

Skin: Dermatologic spread can manifest as pustular, papular, nodular, or ulcerated lesions, which sometimes resemble acne, molluscum contagiosum, or basal cell carcinoma.

Central nervous system: Because inflammation is not extensive, fever is usually low grade or absent, and meningismus is uncommon.

In patients with AIDS, cryptococcal meningitis may cause minimal or no symptoms, but headache frequently occurs and sometimes slowly progressively altered mental status.

Because most symptoms of cryptococcal meningitis result from cerebral edema, they are usually nonspecific (e.g. headache, blurred vision, confusion, depression, agitation, other behavioral changes). Except for ocular or facial palsies, focal signs are rare until relatively late in the course. Blindness may develop because of cerebral oedema or direct involvement of the optic tracts.

Diagnosis of Cryptococcosis

Laboratory diagnosis

- **Specimens**
  - CSF
  - Sputum pus
  - Brain tissue

Direct microscopy: Specimen mixed with a drop of India ink or nigrosin shows round budding yeast cells. In India ink, capsule appears as a clear halo around the yeast cells.

Culture

- Sediment from a centrifuged CSF is inoculated on SDA and incubated at 37°C. Other specimens may also be inoculated on SDA.
- *C. neoformans* grows to form smooth, mucoid, cream coloured colonies.
- Lactophenol cotton blue mount shows budding yeast cells.
- Niger seed (bird seed) agar is a differential medium for presumptive identification of *C. neoformans*. It produces brown colonies on this medium within one week when incubated at 30°C. *C. neoformans* produces phenoloxidase, which oxidises the caffeic acid in the niger seed into melanin.

Immuno-biochemical and serology: Elevated CSF protein and a mononuclear cell pleocytosis are usual in cryptococcal meningitis. Glucose is frequently low, and encapsulated yeasts forming narrow-based buds can be seen on India ink smears in most patients, especially in those who have AIDS (who typically have a higher fungal burden than those without HIV infection). In some patients with AIDS, CSF parameters are normal, except for the presence of numerous yeasts on India ink preparation.

The latex test for cryptococcal capsular antigen is positive in CSF or blood specimens or both in >90% of patients with meningitis and is generally specific although false-positive results may occur, usually with titers ≤1:8, especially if rheumatoid factor is also present.

Animal inoculation test: Intracerebral or intraperitoneal inoculation into mice leads to a fatal infection in case of *C. neoformans*. Capsulated budding yeast cells can be demonstrated in the brain of the infected mice.

Other tests: *C. neoformans* hydrolyses urea.

Chapter 43

Aspergillus Species
(Aspergillosis and Mucormycosis)

Chapter Outline

- Aspergillus
- Airway Colonization
- Symptoms and Signs of Aspergillosis
- Zygomycois (Mucormycosis)

ASPERGILLUS

Introduction

Aspergillus species are globally ubiquitous saprophytes found in a variety of ecological niches. Almost 200 species of aspergilli have been identified, less than 20 of which are known to cause human disease. Among them, *Aspergillus fumigatus* is the most prevalent and is largely responsible for the increased incidence of invasive aspergillosis (IA) in the immunocompromised patient population. IA is a devastating illness with mortality rates in some patient groups reaching as high as 90%. Studies identifying and assessing the roles of specific factors of *A. fumigatus* that contribute to the pathogenesis of IA have traditionally focused on single-gene deletion and mutant characterization.

Some Aspergillus species cause serious disease in humans and animals. The most common pathogenic species are *A. fumigatus* and *A. flavus*, which produces aflatoxin which is both a toxin and a carcinogen, and which can contaminate foods such as nuts.

Aspergillosis

Aspergillosis is an opportunistic infection that usually affects the lower respiratory tract and is caused by inhaling spores of the filamentous fungus *Aspergillus*, commonly present in the environment. The spores germinate and develop into hyphae, which enter blood vessels and, with invasive disease, cause haemorrhagic necrosis and infarction. Symptoms may be those of asthma, pneumonia, sinusitis, or rapidly progressing systemic illness. Diagnosis is primarily clinical but may be aided by imaging, histopathology, and specimen staining and culture.

Major risk factors for aspergillosis include:

- Neutropenia when prolonged (typically > 7 days)
- Long-term high-dose corticosteroid therapy
- Organ transplantation (especially bone marrow transplantation with graft-vs-host disease [GVHD])
- Hereditary disorders of neutrophil function (e.g. chronic granulomatous disease).

1. Aspergilli are ubiquitous in nature.
2. *Aspergillus fumigatus* is the main opportunistic pathogen.
3. Other important species are *A. niger*, *A. flavus*, *A. terreus* and *A. nidulans*.

Aspergillus fumigatus (Figs 43.1, 43.2A and B)

The colonies of *A. fumigatus* are granular to cottony and usually have some shades of green, green-grey or green-brown pigmentation. Microscopically, the conidiophores are relatively long (300–500 pm), the vesicles are 30–50 pm in diameter, club-shaped and covered on top half with only a single row of sterigmata (uniseriate), giving rise to long chains of spherical to slightly ovoid conidia that tend to sweep towards the central axis.

Structure, Morphology of Aspergillus (Fig. 43.1).

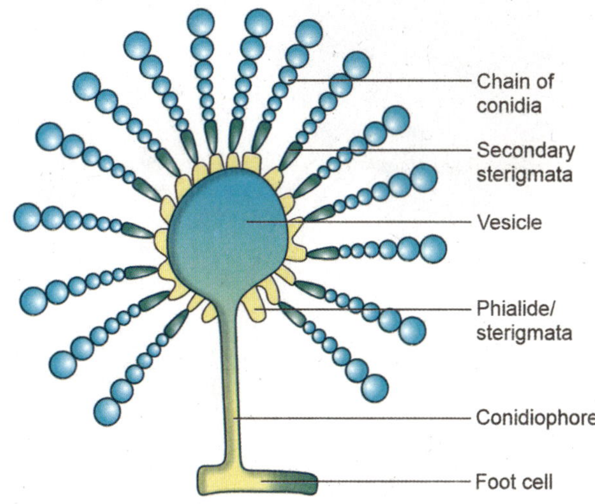

Fig. 43.1: Diagrammatic representation of morphology of Aspergillus

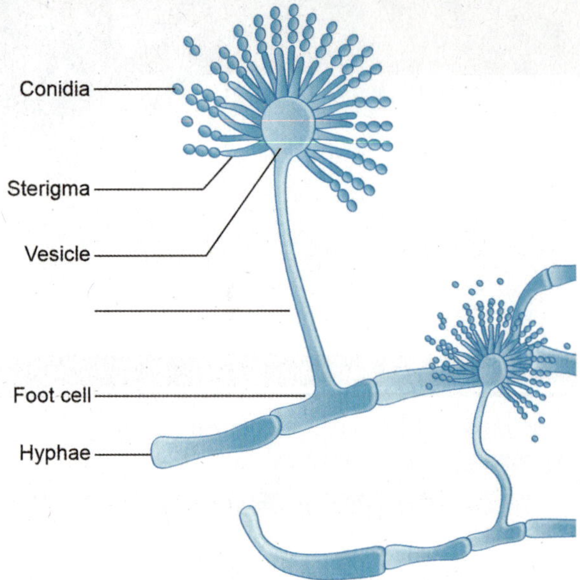

Fig. 43.2A: *Aspergillus fumigatus* labelled photographs

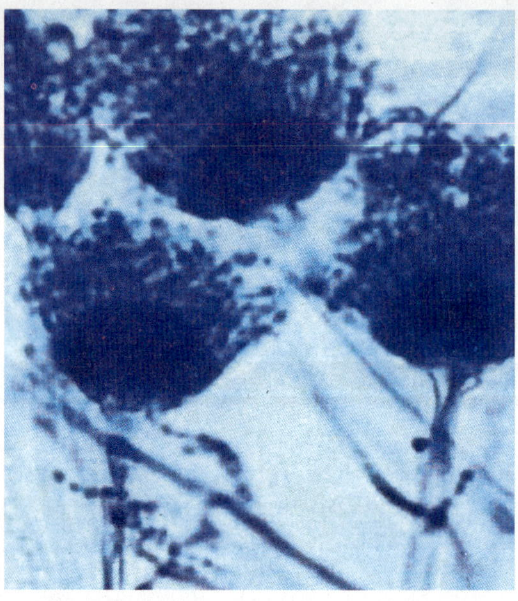

Fig. 43.2B: Photomicrograph of *Aspergillus fumigatus* from culture

Aspergillus niger

The surface of the colonies of *A. niger* is covered by a dense aggregate of jet black conidia. The underside of the colony is buff or yellow-grey, distinguishing *A. niger* from the dematiaceous fungi. Microscopically, the vesicles are globose and measure up to 75 pm in diameter. They bear a double row of sterigmata covering the entire surface. Conidiation is extremely profuse, to the extent that the vesicles are obscured by dense aggregates of 3–5 pm diameter, spherical, black conidia that become roughened with maturity (Fig. 43.3).

The fungus *Aspergillus niger* is a type of mould, which can sometimes be attributed to the cause of some cases of pneumonia. It is also the causative agent of 'black mould' on the outsides of certain foods, such as apricots, onions, grapes, etc. therefore making *Aspergillus niger* a food 'spoilage' organism.

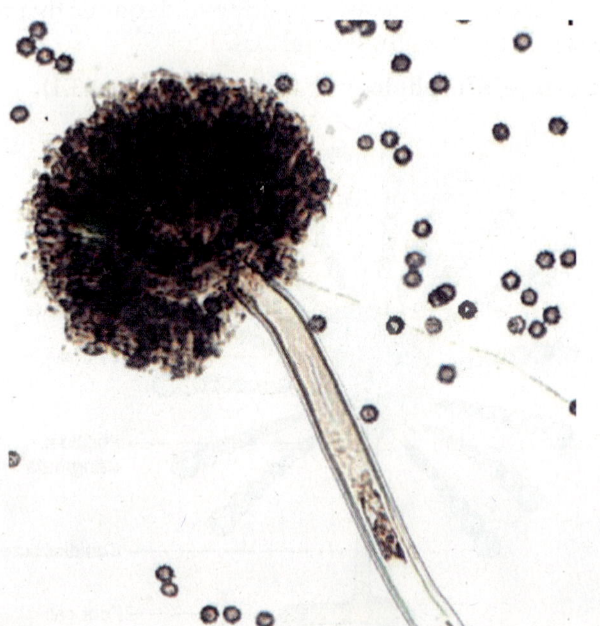

Fig. 43.3: Photomicrograph of *Aspergillus niger* showing jet black conidia

Some strains of *Aspergillus niger* are known to secrete ochratoxins—mycotoxins which can give rise to nephrotoxicity and renal tumours in a variety of animal species and are potentially hazardous to human health through their consumption. They are released by *Aspergillus* and Penicillium fungi species. Ochratoxin A, for example, is a problem organism during the bulk storage of grains if the conditions are in any way wet or damp.

A. niger could be removed more easily by mucociliary clearance of the upper respiratory tract. Furthermore, *A. fumigatus* is more thermotolerant than other disease-causing species, growing well at 37°C and withstanding temperatures above 50°C, such as those encountered in decaying vegetation, a frequently inhabited niche.

Aspergillus flavus

The colonies of *A. flavus* are granular to woolly and have some shade of yellow or yellow-brown. Microscopically, the conidiophores are long (400–800 pm) and the vesicles are 25–45 pm in diameter. The sterigmata arise from three-fourths or the entire circumference of the vesicle and may have one row (umseriate), or more characteristically two rows (biseriate) of sterigmata. Conidia are spherical, smooth, are slightly roughened with maturity and form long chains (Fig. 43.4).

A. fumigatus is the most common cause of invasive pulmonary disease; *A. flavus* most often causes invasive extrapulmonary disease, probably because it tends to occur in patients who are more severely immunosuppressed than patients infected with *A. fumigatus*.

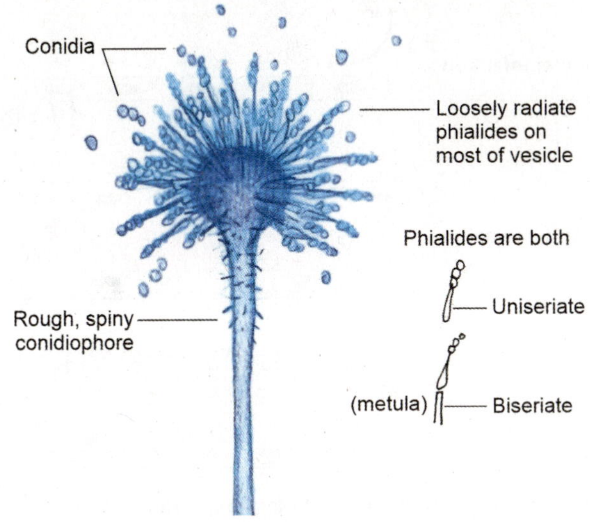

Fig. 43.4: *Aspergillus flavus*

Focal infections, typically in the lung, sometimes form a fungus ball (aspergilloma), a characteristic growth of tangled masses of hyphae, with fibrin exudate and a few inflammatory cells, typically encapsulated by fibrous tissue. Occasionally, there is some local invasion of tissue at the periphery of the cavity, but usually the fungus just resides within the cavity with no appreciable local invasion.

Aspergillus nidulans

A. nidulans may rarely be recovered from the cases of human infections. The vesicles bear two rows of sterigmata on their upper half surface. *A. nidulans* may form sexually derived ascospores contained within sac-like structures called cleistothecia.

Aspergillus terreus

The colonies of *A. terreus* are cinnamon buff, brown or orange-brown. Radial folds emanating from the centre of the colony are often observed. Microscopically, the vesicles are relatively small (10–16 pm in diameter) flask-shaped or hemispherical. They produce biseriate sterigmata on the upper half only. The proximal, primary sterigmata are shorter (5–8 pm) than the secondary sterigmata (8–12 pm). Conidia are smooth, elliptical, measure 2–2.5 pm in diameter.

Pathology and pathogenesis aspergillosis: *Aspergillus* species tend to infect open spaces, such as pulmonary cavities caused by previous lung disorders (e.g. bronchiectasis, tumour, tuberculosis), the sinuses, or external auditory canals (otomycosis). Such infections tend to be locally invasive and destructive, although systemic spread sometimes occurs, particularly in immunocompromised patients with neutropenia or immunosuppression due to corticosteroid use. However, aspergillosis is unusual in those with HIV infection.

A. fumigatus is the most common cause of invasive pulmonary disease; *A. flavus* most often causes invasive extrapulmonary disease, probably because it tends to occur in patients who are more severely debilitated.

AIRWAY COLONIZATION

Inhalation of *Aspergillus* conidia is a common occurrence due to their ubiquitous presence in the environment; estimates suggest that the average person may inhale up to 200 conidia per day. In IA-susceptible patient populations, the mucosal defenses of the lung are compromised, leading to fungal colonization and growth (Fig. 43.5).

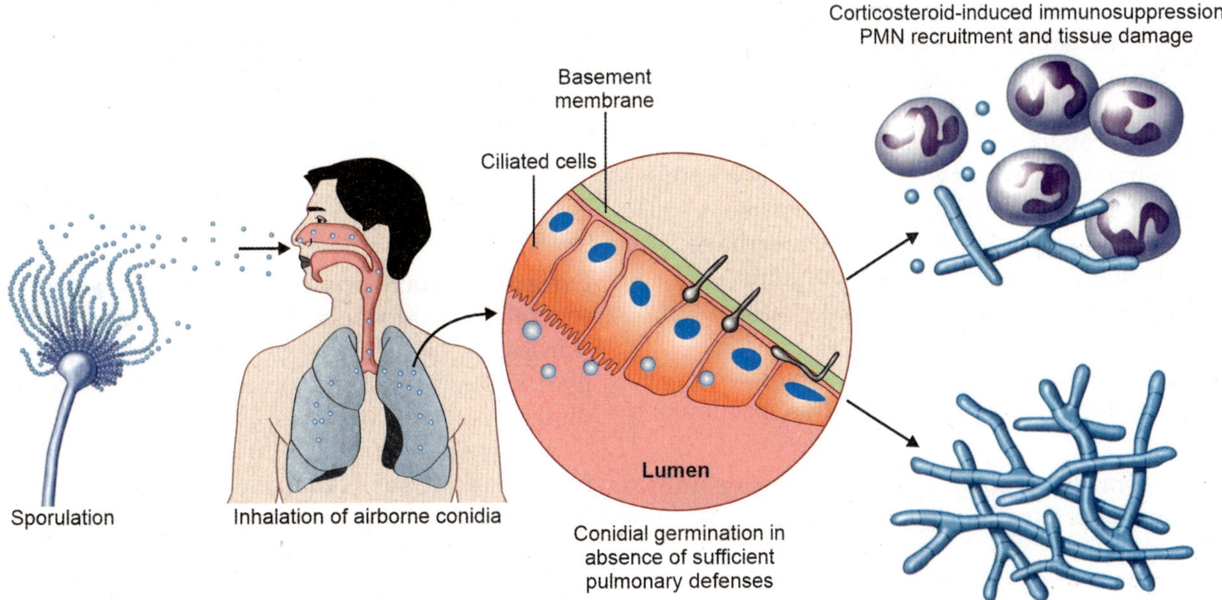

Fig. 43.5: Pathogenesis of aspergillosis sporulation to dissemination

The primary route of infection with Aspergillus is via the inhalation of airborne conidia and deposition in the bronchioles or alveolar spaces. The average size of *A. fumigatus* conidia (2 to 3 μm) is ideal for infiltrating deep into the alveoli, whereas larger conidia of other human pathogens including *A. flavus* and *A. nidulans*.

Transmission occurs through inhalation of airborne conidia. Hospital-acquired infections may be sporadic or may be associated with dust exposure during building renovation or construction. Occasional outbreaks of cutaneous infection have been traced to contaminated biomedical devices.

Following inhalation. *A. fumigatus* conidia immediately encounter the airway mucosa comprised of the fluid lining the respiratory tract and airway epithelia. This pulmonary fluid is comprised of mucus, proteins, lipids, ions, water, and other cellular secretions that contribute to the mucociliary clearance of inhaled particles or pathogens. Also within this complex fluid are opsonic PRRS that coat inhaled pathogens and contribute to host defense.

There are three clinical forms of systemic aspergillosis.

a. **Respiratory disease**
   - *Aspergillus asthma:* Hypersensitivity to aspergilli may occur in atopic individuals following inhalation of spores of aspergilli.
   - *Bronchopulmonary aspergillosis:* The fungus grows within the lumen of the bronchioles, which may be occluded by fungus plugs. Some patients may expectorate mucus plugs containing fungus.
   - *Aspergilloma:* The fungus colonises in the pre-existing pulmonary cavities such as in tuberculosis or cystic disease. It is often called *fungus ball*.

b. **Invasive aspergillosis:** Invasive or disseminated aspergillosis occurs in severely immunocompromised individuals. The fungus first establishes in lung tissue and then disseminate to involve other organs particularly brain, kidney and heart.
   Pathology is mainly due to angioinvasion resulting in wedge-shaped infarcts or well-circumscribed nodules around a vessel. The inflammation is sparse because of severe neutropenia. Necrosis, hemorrhage, and invasion of tissue/vessels with Aspergillus.

c. **Superficial infections**
   - Sinusitis: *A. flavus* and *A. fumigatus*
   - Mycotic keratitis: *A. flavus* and *A. fumigatus*
   - Otomycosis: Species of Aspergillus, particularly *A. niger*.

Mechanism of alveolar infection causing angioinvasion and dissemination (Fig. 43.6).

Symptoms and Signs of Aspergillosis

Symptoms: May include unilateral (one-sided) facial swelling, headaches, nasal or sinus congestion or pain, serosanguinous (bloody) nasal discharge, and fever.

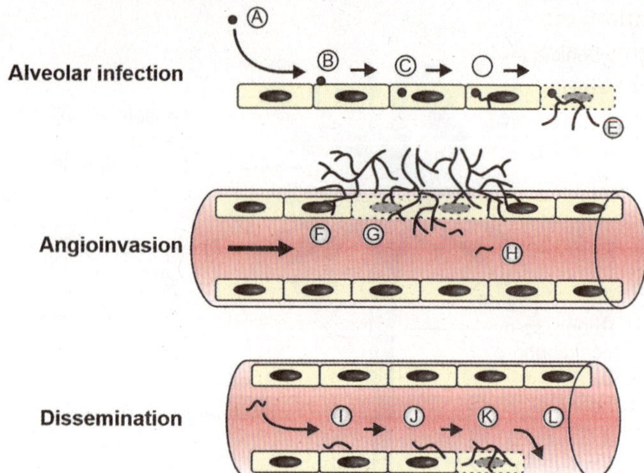

Fig. 43.6: Angioinvasion and dissemination in aspergillosis

As the infection spreads, ptosis ("drooping eyelid"), proptosis (eye dislocation), loss of extraocular muscle function, and vision disturbance may occur.

Acute invasive pulmonary aspergillosis usually causes cough, often with hemoptysis, pleuritic chest pain, and shortness of breath. If untreated, invasive pulmonary aspergillosis may lead to rapidly progressive, ultimately fatal respiratory failure.

Spores are small enough to be carried to the terminal parts of the bronchial tree. Mycelial growth may extend into blood vessels, leading to vasculitis. thrombus formation and dissemination to other parts of the body.

Chronic pulmonary aspergillosis may manifest with mild, indolent symptoms despite significant disease.

A chronic form of invasive aspergillosis occasionally occurs, particularly in patients taking corticosteroids long-term and those with chronic granulomatous disease, which is characterized by a hereditary phagocytic cell defect.

Granulomas can develop in many body organs and are visible as yellowish-grey nodules.

If *A. fumigatus* breaks out into an air space in the body, such as the air sacs in chickens, distorted fruiting heads can be formed.

Extrapulmonary invasive aspergillosis occurs in severely immunocompromised patients. It begins with skin lesions, sinusitis, or pneumonia and may involve the liver, kidneys, brain, and other tissues via hematogenous dissemination; it is often rapidly fatal.

Aspergillus species tend to infect open spaces, such as pulmonary cavities caused by previous lung disorders (e.g. bronchiectasis, tumour, tuberculosis), the sinuses, or external auditory canals (otomycosis).

Aspergillosis in the sinuses can form an aspergilloma or cause allergic fungal sinusitis or a chronic, slowly invasive granulomatous inflammation with fever, rhinitis, and headache. Patients may have necrosing cutaneous lesions overlying the nose or sinuses, palatal or gingival ulcerations, signs of cavernous sinus thrombosis, or pulmonary or disseminated lesions.

Aspergillus species can also cause endophthalmitis after trauma or surgery to the eye or by haematogenous seeding and can infect intravascular and intracardiac prostheses.

Primary superficial aspergillosis is uncommon but may occur in burns; beneath occlusive dressings; after corneal trauma (keratitis); or in the sinuses.

Laboratory Diagnosis

i. **Specimens**
   - Sputum
   - Bronchoalveolar lavage
   - Biopsy
ii. **Direct microscopy:** KOH preparation of the specimen reveals non-pigmented septate hyphae.

Specimens

- Pneumonic lung
- Granulomatous nodules
- Centrifuged mastitic milk
- Foetal lesions
- Foetal stomach contents, cotyledons
- Ear swabs, skin scrapings and biopsies from nasal granulomas
- Fungal plaques in the guttural pouch.

Isolation

- Sabouraud dextrose agar, with and without 0.05 g/L chloramphenicol, is used.
- The surface of the agar should be crosshatched to a depth of about 2 mm in four to five well-separated areas on the plate.
- Small pieces of tissue (about one-quarter the size of a finger nail) are placed on the cross-hatched areas and gently pushed into the agar.
- Incubated aerobically at 37°C for up to five days.

Identification: On the basis of colony pigmentation; the size and length of the conidiophores; the shape and size of the vesicles; presence or absence of metulae; position of phialides; size, shape and appearance of the conidia; the length of the chains of spores and other criteria.

Culture and histopathology of a tissue sample are usually necessary for confirmation; histopathology helps distinguish invasive infection from colonization. The sample is typically taken from the lungs via bronchoscopy or percutaneous needle biopsy and from the sinuses via anterior rhinoscopy. Because cultures take time and histopathology results may be false-negative, most decisions to treat are based on strong presumptive clinical evidence. Blood cultures are almost always negative, even in rare cases of endocarditis. In aspergillus endocarditis, large vegetations often release sizable emboli that may occlude blood vessels and provide specimens for diagnosis.

ZYGOMYCOSIS (MUCORMYCOSIS)

Introduction

Zygomycosis or mucormycosis is an opportunistic infection caused by saprophytic fungi, notably species of *Mucor, Rhizopus* and *Absidia* of the family Mucoraceae. These fungi are common saprophytes of soil, manure and decaying vegetables, and fruits. These are essentially opportunistic fungi. The major predisposing factors to zygomycosis are diabetes mellitus, leukaemia or lymphoma and immunosuppression. The characteristic pathological changes in zygomycosis are suppuration and necrosis. Invasion of thrombosed blood vessels by the fungus is a conspicuous feature.

Zygomycosis

1. Zygomycosis includes mucormycosis and entomophthoramycosis. The latter is an infection of the subcutaneous tissue or paranasal sinuses.
2. Three genera of class *Zygomycetes, Mucor, Rhizopus* and *Absidia* are associated with zygomycosis.
3. These fungi are saprophytes of soil, manure and decaying vegetables.
4. These are normally avirulent and are able to cause disease only when general resistance is extremely low.
5. The primary infection is usually in upper respiratory tract or nose.
6. Rhinocerebral form of disease is characterised by spreading lesion from nasal mucosa to turbinate bone, paranasal sinuses, orbit and brain.
7. *Mucor* and *Absidia* are most commonly isolated from mucormycosis.
8. Rhizopus causes zygomycosis and otomycosis.
9. Absidia may also cause keratitis.
10. Pulmonary mucormycosis is a progressive severe pneumonia. The fungi may spread haematogenously to other areas of the lung and to other organs such as brain.
11. Gastrointestinal mucormycosis may occur in malnutrition, uraemia and diarrhoeal diseases.

Laboratory diagnosis

1. **Specimens**
   - Scrapings from the lesions
   - Pus
   - Sputum
   - Nasal discharge

Direct Microscopy

KOH preparation: KOH preparation of scrapings from the lesions, pus, sputum and nasal discharge shows irregularly branched, non-septate, thin-walled very broad hyphae (7–15 µm in diameter). True septa are rarely seen in the hyphae but under low magnification, cross folds in the walls of the hyphae may resemble septa.

Histological sections: The fungi are deeply stained with routine H and E stain. On the other hand, colouration by special fungal stain such as Gridley, PAS and in some cases GMS may be very poor.

Histological sections stained with H and E stain reveal the presence of hyphae.

Cultural characteristics: Fungi can be readily grown on SDA without cycloheximide at 37°C.

Fungi can be readily isolated on SDA at 37°C. *Rhizopus* has rhizoids and sporangiophores that arise in groups directly above the rhizoids. *Aspergillus mucor* does not possess rhizoids and shows branched sporangiophores arising randomly along aerial mycelium. *Absidia* has rhizoids and sporangiophores that arise from the aerial mycelium in between the rhizoids (Fig. 43.7).

Lactophenol cotton blue preparation of colonies shows branched sporangiophores arising randomly along aerial mycelium. In the case of mucor rhizoids are absent, Rhizopus has rhizoids, and sporangiospore arise in groups directly above the rhizoids.

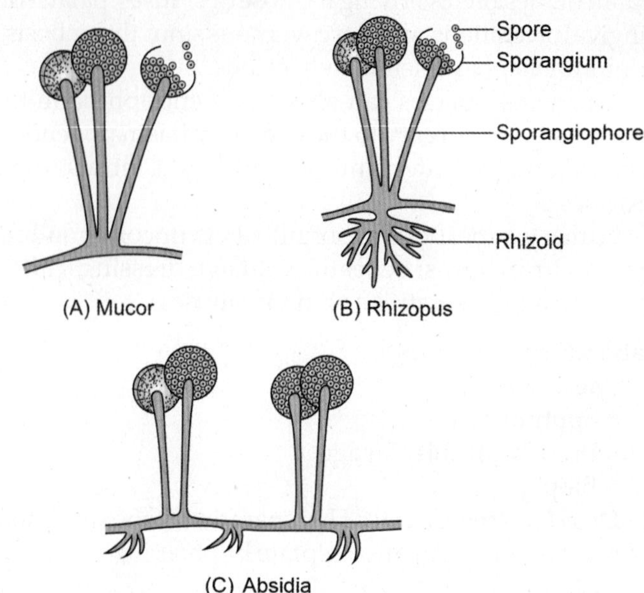

Fig. 43.7: Zygomycetes. (A) Mucor (B) Rhizopus (C) Absidia

Chapter 44

Dermatophytes
(Dermatophytosis)

Chapter Outline

- Symptoms of Dermatophytoses
- *Trichophyton rubrum*
- *Trichophyton mentagrophytes*
- *T. tonsurans*
- *Microsporum audouinii*
- *M. canis*
- *M. gypseum*
- *Epidermophyton floccosum*
- Dermatophyte infections

Introduction

Dermatophytes are a closely related homogeneous clade of keratinophilic filamentous fungi that are associated with the stratum corneum of the skin, as well as hair and nails on the living host. They possess similar appearance, physiology, antigenicity, growth requirements, infectivity, and pathology. These fungi are classified in the anamorphic genera *Epidermophyton, Keratinomyces, Microsporum,* and *Trichophyton*. Some dermatophytes may reproduce sexually when the opposite mating types are crossed with each other.

Definition

Dermatophytes are a unique group of fungi that infect keratinous tissue and are able to invade the hair, skin, and nails of a living host.

Dermatophytes are the most common agents of superficial fungal infections in humans and animals, but they also cause serious infections in patients with solid organ transplant or congenital immune disorders. The reduced size of their genome with the expansion of particular gene families indicate that these fungi are highly specialized and have the ability to degrade hard keratin and escape the immune system during infection. The ability of dermatophyte to switch from a saprophytic to a parasitic lifestyle is achieved through significant reprogramming of gene expression. Research on dermatophytes has generated renewed interest with the emergence of cases of dermatophytosis resistant to standard treatments.

Dermatophytoses are fungal infections of the skin and nails caused by several different fungi and classified by the location on the body. Dermatophyte infections are also called ringworm or tinea.

Tinea pedis, onychomycosis, tinea cruris, and tinea capitis are among the most common dermatophyte infections and are seen in all socioeconomic groups.

The common anthropophilic dermatophytes include lower body dermatophytes associated with sites other than the scalp, and dermatophytes strongly adapted for tinea capitis, less commonly causing other tineas. *Trichophyton rubrum, T. mentagrophytes* complex and *Epidermophyton floccosum* are the common lower body species. Tinea capitis dermatophytes consist of two major groups distinguished by their colonization of hair.

Tinea capitis agents primarily cause new infections in children, and may cause dramatic outbreaks. *Microsporum audouinii* infections spontaneously resolve at 15–19 years of age, but most endothrix agents cause lifelong asymptomatic infections in some adult carriers.

Lastly dermatophytes are

i. Dermatophytes are a group of fungi that infect only superficial keratinised tissue (skin, hair and nails) without involving the living tissue.
ii. They break down and utilise keratin.
iii. They are incapable of penetrating subcutaneous tissue.
iv. They cause dermatophytoses, also known as tinea (Latin for worm or ringworm) or ringworm.
v. Hypersensitivity to fungus antigens is probably responsible for the sterile vesicular lesions sometimes seen in sites distant from the ringworm. These lesions are named dermatophytids (or the 'id' reaction).

Classification: Dermatophytes are classified into three genera as follows:

Genus		*Infection of*
1. Trichophyton	—	Hair, skin, nail
2. Microsporum	—	Hair, skin
3. Epidermophyton	—	Skin, nail

On the basis of their natural habitat and host preferences, these can be classified into three groups:

Anthropophilic — Man
Zoophilic — Animals
Geophilic — Soil

T. rubrum, *E. floccosum* and *M. audouinii* are examples of anthropophilic dermatophytes. Example of zoophilic dermatophytes is *M. canis* in dogs and cats. *M. gypseum* is a geophilic species, which occurs naturally in soil.

Important species

Trichophyton:
- *T. rubrum*
- *T. mentagrophytes*
- *T. tonsurans*
- *T. schoenleinii*
- *T. violaceum*
- *T. verrucosum*

Microsporum:
- *M. gypseum*
- *M. canis*
- *M. audouinii*

Epidermophyton:
- *E. floccosum*

Dermatophytoses are fungal infections of the skin and nails caused by several different fungi and classified by the location on the body. Dermatophyte infections are also called ringworm or tinea. Symptoms of dermatophytoses include rashes, scaling, and itching.

The dermatophytes have the ability to invade keratinized tissue (skin, hair, and nails) but are usually restricted to the nonliving cornified layer of the epidermis because of their inability to penetrate viable tissue of an immunocompetent host.

Clinical types: Clinically, ringworm can be classified depending on the site involved. These include tinea capitis (scalp), tinea corporis (non-hairy skin of the body), tinea cruris (groin), tinea pedis (foot) or athlete's foot and tinea barbae or barber's itch (bearded areas of the face and neck). Favus is a chronic type of ringworm involving the hair follicles. It leads to alopecia and scarring.

Some of the clinical types of dermatophytosis and their common causative agents are listed in Table 44.1.

Table 44.1: Clinical types of dermatophytosis and causative agents

Clinical type	*Causative agents*
Tinea capitis	Microsporum any spp. Trichophyton most spp.
Favus	*T. schoenleinii* *T. violaceum* *M. gypseum*
Tinea corporis	*T. rubrum* and other dermatophytes
Ectothrix	Microsporum spp. *T. rubrum* *T. mentagrophytes*
Endothrix	*T. schoenleinii* *T. tonsurans* *T. violaceum*

Symptoms of Dermatophytoses

Symptoms of a dermatophyte infection vary depending on the location of the infection. Most often, there is a little or no inflammation and the infected areas are mildly itchy with a scaling, slightly raised border. These patches can come and go intermittently. Occasionally, inflammation is more severe and suddenly causes large and small fluid-filled spots to appear (usually on the foot) or an inflamed, swollen patch on the scalp that sometimes oozes pus (kerion).

The fungus can cause mild scaling with or without redness and itching. The scaling may involve a small area (particularly between the toes) or the entire sole of the foot. Sometimes scaling is severe, with breakdown and painful cracking (fissuring) of the skin. Fluid-filled blisters can also form. Over time, the skin on the soles may thicken. Because the fungus may cause the skin to crack, tinea pedis can lead to bacterial infections, especially in older people and in people with inadequate blood flow to the feet.

Pathogenicity: Dermatophytes differ in their host interactions. Anthropophilic dermatophytes, specific to human disease, are distinguished from zoophilic dermatophytes, which have specific animal associations but may be transmitted to humans, and from geophilic dermatophytes, which are occasionally pathogenic to humans.

Dermatophytes normally infect only the keratinized stratum corneum of the epithelial skin layers. They are restricted to the stratum corneum by cellular immune components. An indication of the relative importance of lymphocytes in host defense is seen in HIV infection, in which helper T-cell counts below 100 cells/ml correlate with a marked increase in onychomycosis, including the unusual 'proximal white' form.

Pathogenesis: Dermatophytes prefer to invade keratinized surfaces. In animals, dermatophytosis manifests as a contagious pruritic dermatologic disease resulting in round focal areas of alopecia, 'ringworm.' In humans, dermatophytosis is referred to as tinea and can result in several clinical syndromes such as tinea pedis ('athlete's foot'), tinea capitis (ringworm of the scalp), tinea corporis (ringworm of the body), or onychomycosis (nail-associated disease). A thorough description of variation in clinical presentation has been reviewed elsewhere. The infective stage of dermatophytosis is an arthrospore formed by segmentation of fungal hyphae.

Laboratory diagnosis

- Specimens
  - Skin
  - Hair
  - Nail

The laboratory diagnosis of ringworm is based on direct demonstration of fungal hyphae and arthrospores in the keratinized tissue by microscopy and on colonial appearances and hyphal and conidial morphology in culture. Genera are distinguished according to the morphology of the macroconidia and species by a combination of microscopic and colonial features. Metabolic activities are rarely relevant and skin tests, serology and animal inoculation are not used.

It is particularly important to collect appropriate material with as little contamination as possible. Cleansing of the area should be followed with 70% ethanol, especially for nails. From skin lesions, scales, preferably 2 to 3 mm in diameter, should be scraped outwards with a blunt scalpel from the active periphery of the lesion and the domes of any vesicles snipped off.

Good material from nails is not easy to obtain. It is best to take scrapings from the nail with a scalpel but discard the most superficial samples. Some of the friable material from under the nail may be taken but ordinary nail clippings are not satisfactory; they often fail to yield any fungus.

For good results from hairs careful selection is important. The dusty stumps of ectothrix infections and the black dots of some endothrix infections can be recognized by the naked eye and if suspicious hairs are scanty, a Wood lamp may show the fluorescence of hair infected by Microsporum spp. and *T. schoer leinii*. The hairs when located should be plucked from the follicles with fine forceps. Specimens should be folded up in black paper, which makes it easier not to lose any material.

Direct microscopy: Direct 10% KOH mount may show fungal hyphae (Fig. 44.1).

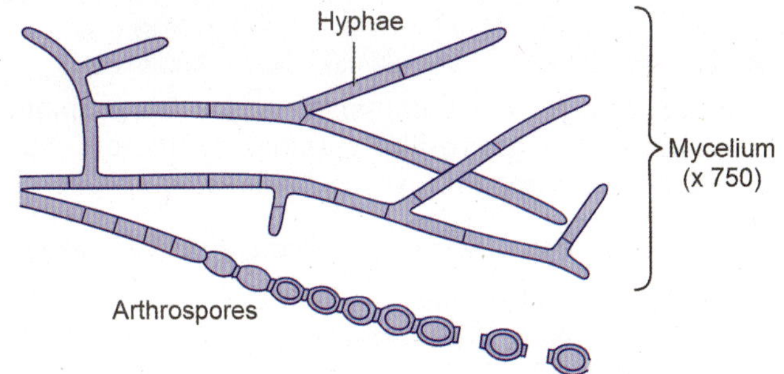

Fig. 44.1: Fungal hyphae and arthrospores diagrammatic representation

In favus, there is sparse hyphal growth and formation of air spaces within the hair shaft.

Two types of hair infection may be present, ectothrix and endothrix. In ectothrix, a sheath of arthospores is present on the surface of hair shaft, while the arthospore formation occurs entirely within the hair shaft in endothrix (Fig. 44.2).

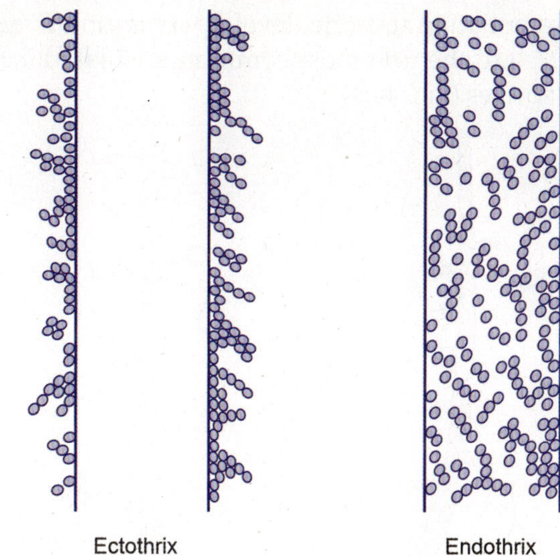

Fig. 44.2: Fungi seen *in vivo* in skin, nail or hair, ectothrix and endothrix arthrospores

Culture

- SDA and SDA with antibiotics are used.
- Culture media are incubated at 25–30°C for three weeks.
- Identification of dermatophytes is based on
  - colony morphology
  - pigment production
  - microconidia and macroconidia
- Colony characters
  - White to creamy, cottony growth
  - Reverse of media is red in *T. rubrum*.

Microscopy

- Lactophenol cotton blue preparation from colony reveals microconidia, macroconidia or both. The following are the characteristics of three genera:
  - Genus *Trichophyton*: More microconidia, very few macroconidia
  - Genus *Microsporum*: Predominant macroconidia (Fig. 44.3).
  - Genus *Epidermophyton*: Macroconidia

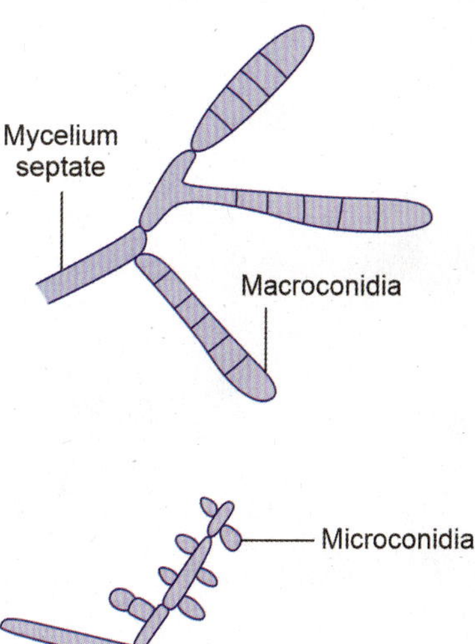

Fig. 44.3: Diagrammatic representation of macroconidia and microconidia

Differentiation at species level *T. rubrum* and *T. mentagrophytes* are the two most commonly isolated *Trichophyton* species (Fig. 44.4).

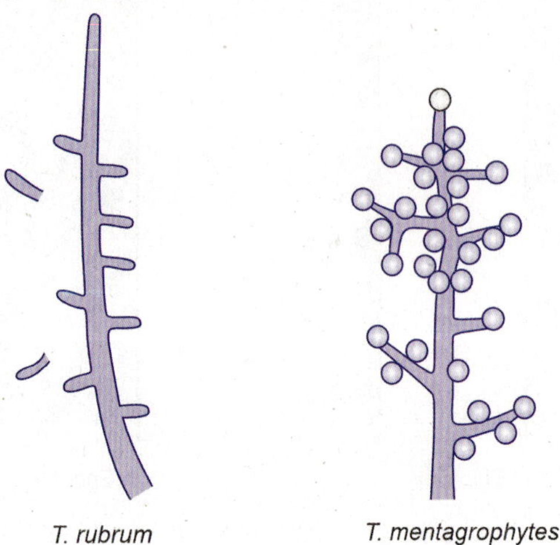

Fig. 44.4: *T. rubrum* and *T. mentagrophytes*

Trichophyton rubrum

- Tear-shaped microconidia along the hyphae (Fig. 44.5).
- 3–8 celled cylindrical which is somewhat same size with *T. mentagrophytes*.
- Appear as thin-walled, smooth-walled, multicelled, cigar-shaped conidia with 3–8 septa.

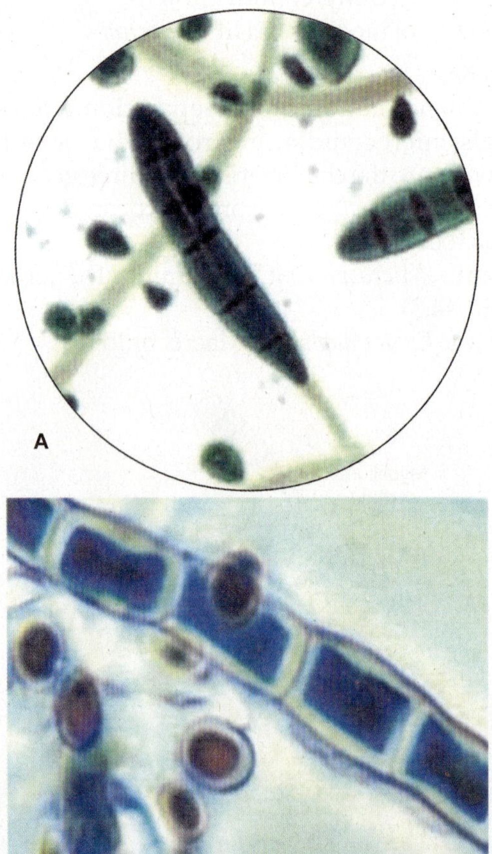

Fig. 44.5A and B: *T. rubrum.* (A) Showing tear shape microconidia and club-shaped thin-walled macroconidia; (B) Showing septate hyphae with reverse red hue conidia

- Red pigment on the reverse side of the medium
- Urease negative
- Club-shaped, thin-walled macroconidia—scanty

Trichophyton mentagrophytes

- Grape-like clusters of microconidia (Fig. 44.6).
- No red pigment
- Urease test is positive and hair perforation test is positive.
- Cigar-shaped macroconidia

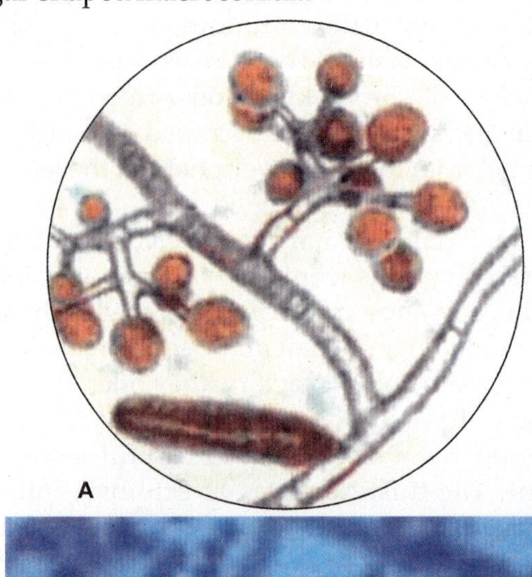

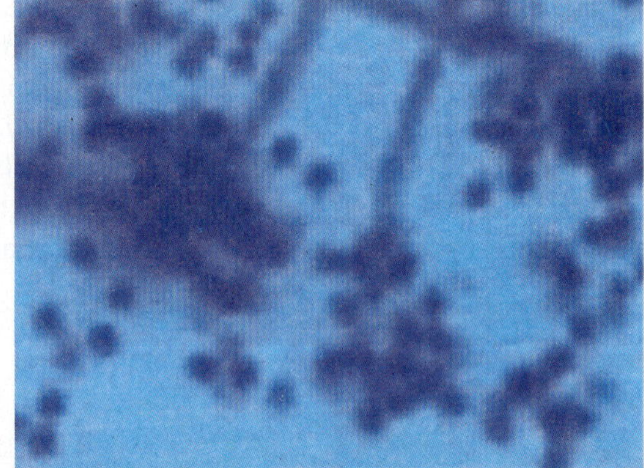

Fig. 44.6A and B: *T. mentagrophytes*. (A) Diagrammatic representation of grape-like clusters of microconidia; (B) Culture photograph microscopy *T. mentagrophytes*

T. violaceum, T. schoenleinii and T. verrucosum (Fig. 44.7)

- These are slow growing.
- Conidia are usually not present.
- Only hyphae are seen.

Apart from the above mentioned common features, these three species have also some specific characteristics. *T. violaceum* has violet coloured colonies.

Antler hyphae (favic chandelier) are present in *T. schoenleinii*. Colony of *T. verrucosum* is partially submerged in media and it contains chain of chlamydospore.

T. tonsurans

Microconidia

Balloon-shaped (Fig. 44.8) (cornmeal agar) numerous clavate varying in size (balloon forms and matchstick forms) if old.

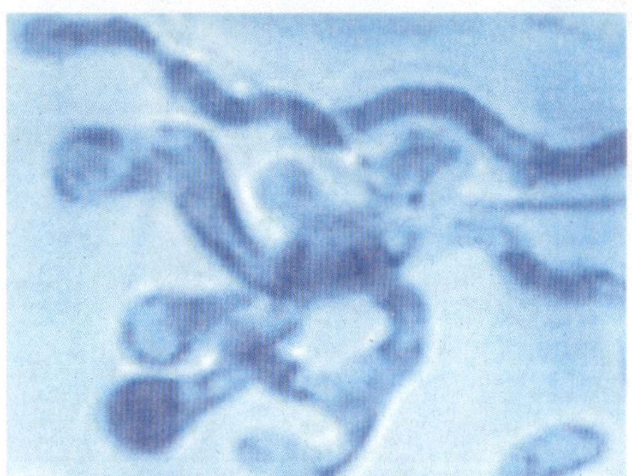

Fig. 44.7: *T. violaceum*, *T. schoenleinii*, *T. verrucosum* showing hyphae conidia is sparsely seen in these fungi

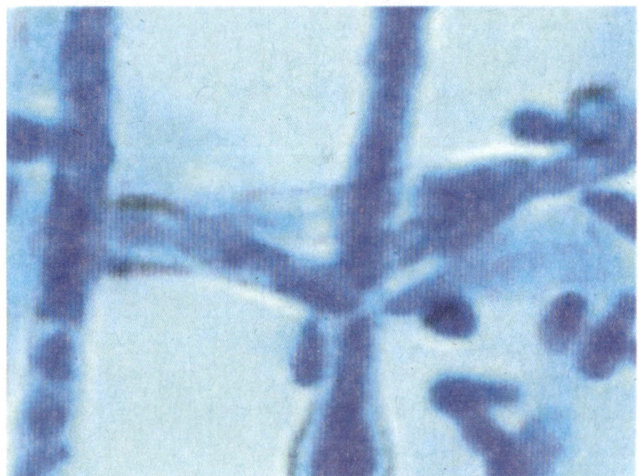

Fig. 44.8: *T. tonsurans* showing *microconidia balloon* shape numerous clavate of varying size, matchstick form

Chlamydoconidia (intercallary) are abundant in old cultures swollen and fragmented hyphal cells resembling arthroconidia may be seen.

Microsporum audouinii

- Anthropophilic
- Hair fluoresce yellow-green when examined under Wood's lamp.
- Velvety, brown coloured colony
- Macroconidia—distorted shape or absent
- Terminal chlamydospore present

M. canis (Fig. 44.9)

- Zoophilic (dogs and cats)
- Hair fluoresce yellow-green.
- Spindle-shaped, rough-walled, multisegmented, curved end, warty projections macroconidia (Fig. 44.9) are abundant.
- Microconidia are very few.

M. gypseum

- Geophilic
- Hair do not fluoresce.

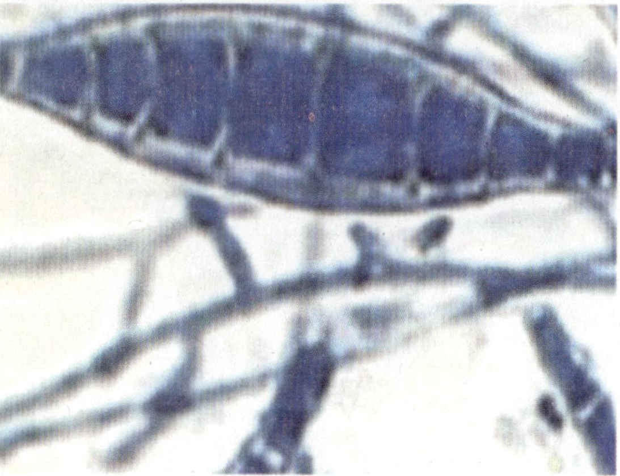

Fig. 44.9: *M. canis*, showing spindle shape, rough-walled, multisegmented macroconidia with curve end

- Spindle-shaped, round end macroconidia (Fig. 44.10) are abundant. There is no curve at the end of macroconidia.

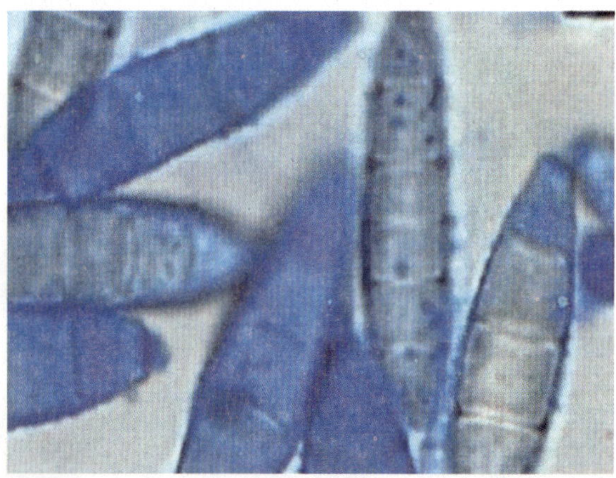

Fig. 44.10: *M. gypseum* showing spindle shape, round macroconidia, no curve at the end

Epidermophyton floccosum

- Macroconidia are numerous. These are smooth, thin-walled, club-shaped, multiseptate and round at tip.
- Microconidia are absent.
- Chlamydospores are numerous.

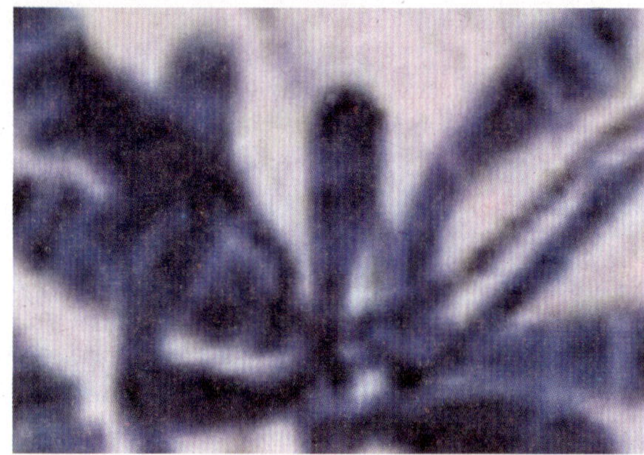

Fig. 44.11: *E. floccosum* showing macroconidia club-shaped round at tip

Comparison of macroconidia of *M. canis, M. gypseum* and *E. floccosum* (Fig. 44.12).

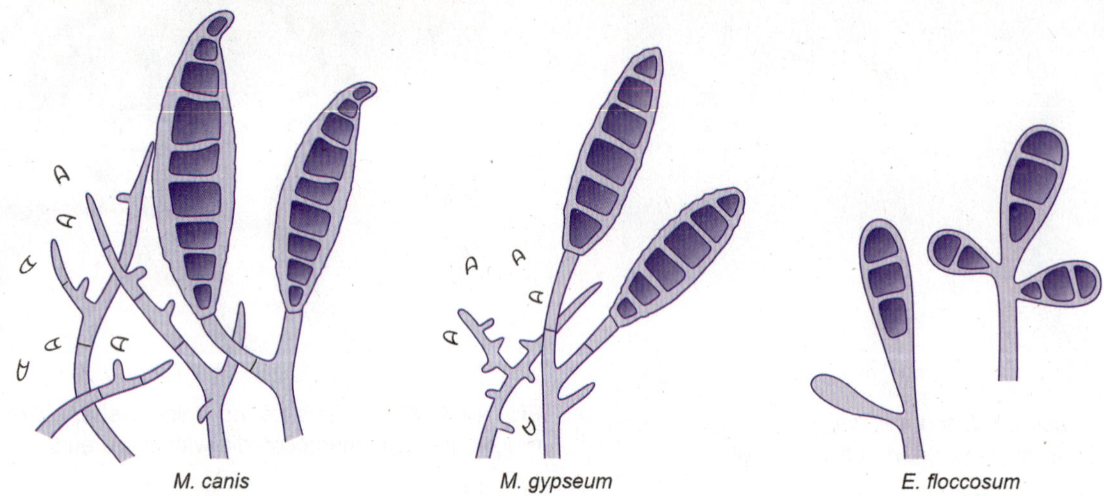

Fig. 44.12: Macroconidia of *M. canis, M. gypseum* and *E. floccosum*

Comparison and macroconidia of Microsporum, Trichophyton and Epidermophyton (Fig. 44.13).

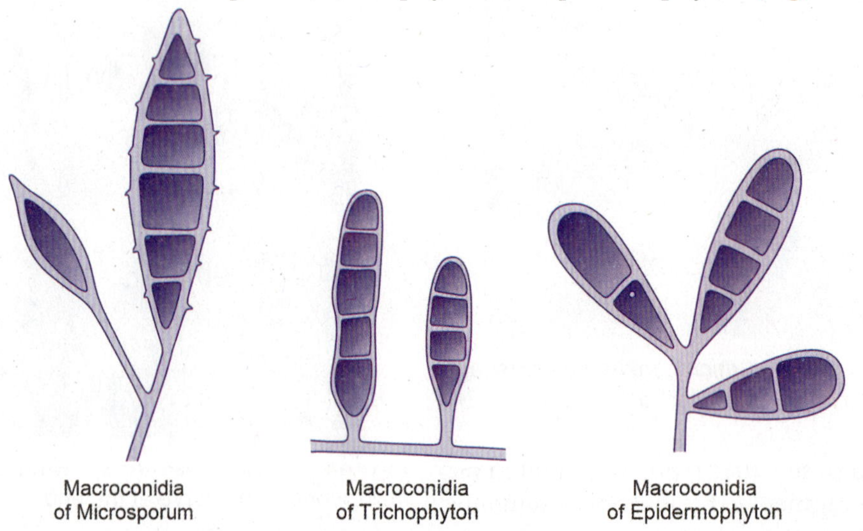

Fig. 44.13: Diagrammatic representation of macroconidia comparison, Microsporum, Trichophyton and Epidermophyton

Table 44.2 shows general distribution of macroconidia and microconidia.

Table 44.2: General distribution of macroconidia and microconidia of dermatophytes

General	*Macroconidia*	*Microconidia*
1. *Trichophyton*	Rare, thin-walled, smooth	Abundant
2. *Microsporum*	Numerous, thick-walled, rough	Rare
3. *Epidermophyton*	Numerous, smooth-walled	Absent

Dermatophyte Infections

Ringworm or tinea: These very common infections of skin, hair and nails are caused by members of a group of some 30 to 40 related filamentous fungi that can digest keratin.

Infection may occur almost anywhere on the skin, including the

- Feet (athlete's foot [tinea pedis])
- Beard area (beard ringworm [tinea barbae])
- Body (body ringworm [tinea corporis])
- Groin (jock itch [tinea cruris])
- Scalp (scalp ringworm [tinea capitis])

Complications that can develop as a result of dermatophytosis are:

- Alopecia
- Superimposed bacterial infections leading to cellulitis.
- Lymphangitis.
- Kerion.
- Bullae formation.
- Erythema nodosum.

Section 3D

Parasitology

45. Protozoa (Protozoa—Plasmodium)
46. Leishmania (Leishmaniasis)
47. *Entamoeba histolytica* (*Giardia lamblia*, Trichomonas)
48. Helminthology I (Nematodes)
49. *Ancylostoma duodenale* (Hookworms), *Strongyloides stercoralis*, Filariodeae (Filaria Worms)
50. *Dracunculus medinensis* (Guinea Worm) and *Trichinella spiralis*
51. Helminthology II (Cestodes)
52. *Echinococcus granulosus* (Hydatid Cyst)
53. *Hymenolepis nana*
54. Trematodes (Schistosomes)

Chapter 45

Protozoa

(Protozoa—Plasmodium)

Chapter Outline

- Classification
- Malarial Parasite
- Typical Attack of Malaria
- Complicated Malaria
- Demonstration of Malarial Parasite in Blood
- Diagnosis of Malaria
- Images of *Plasmodium vivax* and *falciparum*

CLASSIFICATION

Without going into details of zoological classification, a simplified classification of protozoa of medical importance has been designed mentioning the diseases caused by them.

Organism	Disease
I. **Flagellates**	
1. Leishmania	Leishmaniasis or Kala azar
2. Trypanosoma	Sleeping sickness
3. Giardia	Giardiasis
4. Trichomonas	Vaginitis
5. Naegleria	
6. Choilomaslix	
7. Enteromonas	
II. **Amoebae**	
1. Entoamoeba	Amoebic dysentery Amoebic abscess
2. Dientamoeba	
3. Iodamoeba	
4. Hartmanella	
III. **Sporozoa**	
1. Plasmodium	Malaria
2. Toxoplasma	Toxoplasmosis
3. Babesia	Babesosis
4. Pneumocystis	Pneumonitis
5. Sarcocystis	
IV. **Ciliates**	
1. Balantidium	

MALARIAL PARASITE

Introduction

Malaria is a very important disease for two prime reasons:

1. Nearly 15–20 million people all over the world are affected by malaria every year, especially in Africa, Asia and South America where it is an important cause of morbidity and mortality.
2. It is potentially eradicable, but is still rampant for a number of reasons. We say it is eradicable because there is (i) a single reservoir of injection—humans, (ii) a single vector responsible—female anopheline mosquito.

   It has not been eradicated due to numerous medical and administrative problems and also the extent of disease. Malaria is caused by genus Plasmodium, which is transmitted to man by female of the anopheles species of mosquito. (Details will be discussed under life cycle.) Four species of Plasmodium are of importance to man. Differentiation are shown in Table 45.1.

1. *Plasmodium falciparum* (by far the most dangerous)
2. *Plasmodium vivax* (by far the commonest)
3. *Plasmodium malariae* (rare in India).
4. *Plasmodium ovale* (not found on the Indian sub-continent).

Life Cycle (Fig. 45.1)

Life cycle, merozoites are released in the blood in cycles repeated every 48–72 hours, depending upon the infecting species. On the basis of periodicity of these cycles, malaria has been classified into:

I. Tertian—cycle is repeated after 36–48 hours
   A. Benign—caused by *Plasmodium vivax*
   B. Malignant—caused by *Plasmodium falciparum*.
II. Quartan—cycle is repeated after 72 hours caused by *Plasmodium malariae*.

Occasionally, Quotidian (cycles of 24 hours) malaria may be seen with a double infection—some parasites maturing on days 1, 3, 5 and some on days 2, 4 and 6.

Also nowadays most of the cases of malaria do not follow any of the above, fixed courses. In fact, it may present as irregular or even continuous features.

Life Cycle of Plasmodium (Fig. 45.1)

Typical Attack of Malaria

After an incubation period of 1–2 weeks depending on the infecting species, a typical attacks of malaria follows 4 labelled phases.

1. **Prodromal phase:** Characterised by nonspecific malaise and prostration accompanied by bodyaches and headache. There may be a chilly sensation. Lasts for 2–3 days.
2. **Stage of heat:** Most prominent feature of an acute malarial attack characterised by shaking chills and rigors: Following which the temperature mounts steadily to reach up to as much as 40°C (104°F) or more, lasts for a few hours.
3. **Stage of lysis:** Characterised by profound sweating and decline of temperature to normal or even subnormal. May be accompanied by vomiting.
4. **Stage of recovery:** Patient is afebrile but is markedly prostrated. He feels extremely weak.

Clinical signs: May consist inconsistently of the following:

1. Mild to moderate pallor
2. Mild icterus

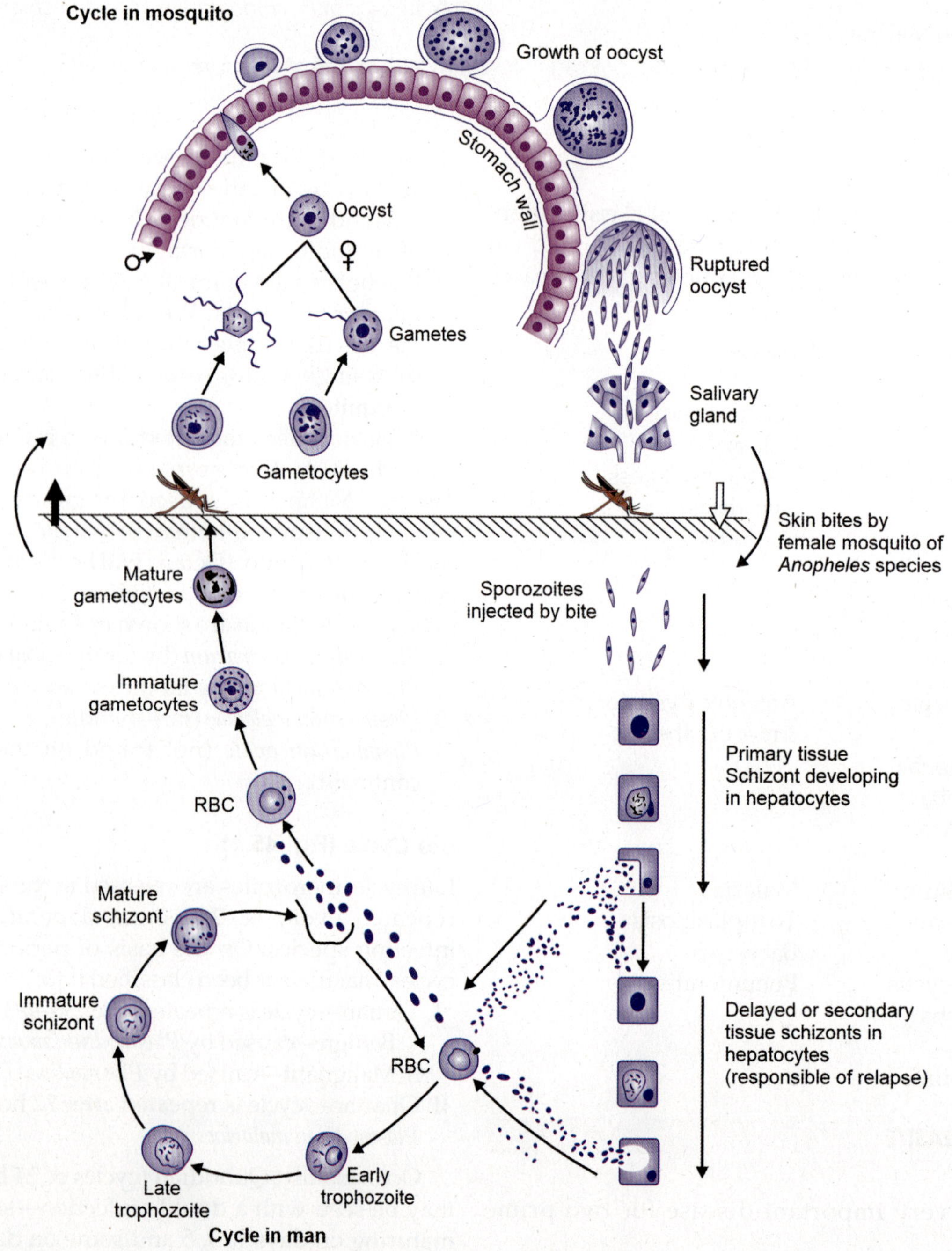

Fig. 45.1: Life cycle of Plasmodium

3. Fever
4. Hepato- and/or splenomegaly
5. Lymphadenopathy.

Complicated Malaria

This generally occurs with *Plasmodium falciparum* and is the fatal form of malaria, which can kill a non-immune person within no time. Here we will be discussing primarily 4 conditions.

1. **Pernicious malaria:** Pernicious malaria carries high number of parasites in the peripheral blood (1,00,000 parasites/mm^3). It may result in death rates of 20% or more.
2. **Cerebral malaria:** It is a severe form of pernicious malaria characterised by:
   1. Hyperpyrexia (41.6°C or 107°F)
   2. Infection of ≥5% erythrocytes
   3. Delirium and coma which may come on very early in disease
   4. Behavioural changes
   5. Conclusions (epileptiform)

   CSF is under pressure, with increased lymphocytes and proteins.
3. **Algid malaria:** It results from an overwhelming infection, with collapse and peripheral vascular failure, possibly resulting from acute adrenal failure. Patient is hypothermic and hypotensive and coma supervenes very fast.
4. **Blackwater fever (malarial haemoglobinuria):** Characterised by sudden, extensive intravascular haemolysis, which results in:
   1. Haemoglobinuria
   2. Icterus
   3. Hepatosplenomegaly
   4. Epigastric pain
   5. Vomiting and diarrhoea

All the 4 conditions listed above are potentially life-threatening and early diagnosis and immediate treatment is absolutely indispensable.

Demonstration of Malarial Parasite in Blood

This consists in staining peripheral smears and identifying malarial parasite in erythrocytes. Two types of methods are used for making blood films.

1. **Thin films:** These are made any other blood smear and stained with Romanowsky stains.
2. **Thick films:** This has the advantage of having increased volume of blood on the slide, the probability of positive diagnosis increases. However, it is difficult to identify the infecting species in thick smears.

Thick smears are prepared as follows:

- Place a good sized drop of blood on a clean slide and spread it with a glass rod until it covers an area of approximately 2 cm diameter.
- Ideal thick smears are ones through which newspaper print can be just read.
- For staining the smears various stains are used. Some of these are:
  1. Giemsa stain
  2. Leishman's stain
  3. Field's stain
  4. JSB stain

i. **Giemsa stain:** Fix smear by dipping it in acetone free methyl alcohol for a few seconds. Air dry and cover it for 10–20 minutes with 5% Giemsa stain. Wash with distilled water and air dry. Used both for thin and thick films.

ii. **Leishman's stain:** Fix smear as above. With slide on a level bench, add 7–8 drops of Leishman's stain. Leave for 20 seconds. Add 12–15 drops (double the amount of stain) of distilled water (pH 7.2). Leave for 20 minutes. Wash with distilled water and air dry. Used for both thin and thick films.

iii. **Field's stain:** Field's stain consists of 2 solutions, solution 1 and 2. Used only for thick films. Immerse dried, unfixed film for 1–3 seconds in solution 1. Remove and rinse immediately for about 5 seconds in clean tap water. Immerse in solution 2 for 2 seconds. Rinse for 2–3 seconds in clean tap water. Allow to air dry.

iv. **JSB (Jasbir Singh Bhattacharya) staining:** It can be used for both thin and thick films. JSB stain also consists of 2 solutions. JSB I and II (it is a modified Romanowsky's stain). Take the smear, dip in JSB I, leave for 2–3 minutes. Then dip in methanol. Take out immediately. Dip in JSB II and take out immediately. Wash it with running water and dry in air.

Basic difference between thin and thick films staining is that thin films have to be fixed before staining while there is no need to fix thick films.

Diagnosis of Malaria

Diagnosis depends primarily on demonstration of malarial parasite in peripheral blood. Ideally blood should be taken in the stage of heat (i.e. when patient is febrile) (Fig. 45.2).

Images of *Plasmodium vivax* and *falciparum*

A. Blood smears showing *Plasmodium vivax* (Fig. 45.3A to D)—ring stage—merozoite formation.

B. Blood smears showing stages of *Plasmodium falciparum*. Ring stage to gametocyte (Figs 45.4 to 45.6).

Table 45.1: Identification of various *Plasmodium* species (both clinical and laboratory features)

No.	*P. vivax*	*P. malariae*	*P. falciparum*
1. Incubation period	12–17 days	½ to 1 month	9–14 days
2. Exo-erythrocytic phase	+	+	–
3. Merozoites in tissue schizont	>10,000	2000	≥40,000
4. Erythrocytic cycle	48 hours	72 hours	36–48 hours
5. Parasitemia (no. of parasites/cu mm)	20–30,000	6000–20,000	20,000–50,000
6. Primary attack severity	Mild to severe	Mild	Severe
7. Relapses	+ + +	+	–
8. Febrile paroxysm (duration—hours)	8–12	8–10	16–36 or even more
9. Infected erythrocyte	Larger than normal and slightly distorted Schuffner's dots present. Infection usually single	Normal in size or smaller Ziemman's granules seen Infection always single	Normal in size or multiple infection common. Maurer's dots seen
10. Trophozoite (ring stage)	Irregular cytoplasm which scatters away chromatin bead	Regular compact with deep blue cytoplasm around single bead	Not common in peripheral blood, regular rings, broken rings and comma shapes seen
11. Mature schizont	12–24 merozoites, relatively large, pigment, granular and clumped	6–12 merozoites, pigment, compact with clump of granules	12–24 or more merozoites, pigment, a single dark mass
12. Gametocyte	Round or oval, relatively large with uniform cytoplasm frayed at edges	Rounded, compact with abundant peripheral pigment in round granules	Distinct crescentic shape with central pigment and chromatin

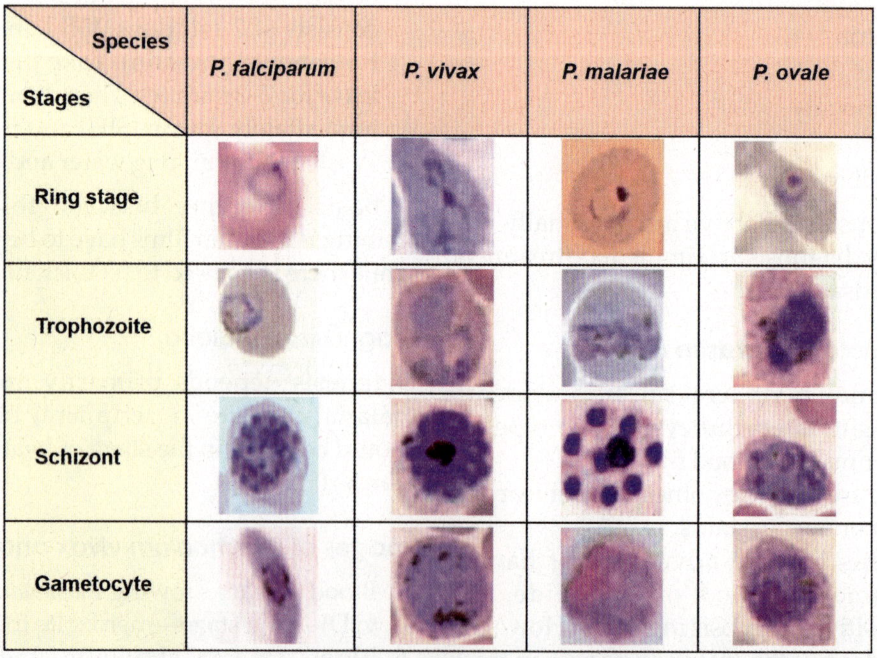

Stages \ Species	*P. falciparum*	*P. vivax*	*P. malariae*	*P. ovale*
Ring stage				
Trophozoite				
Schizont				
Gametocyte				

Fig. 45.2: Development stages of *Plasmodium* species

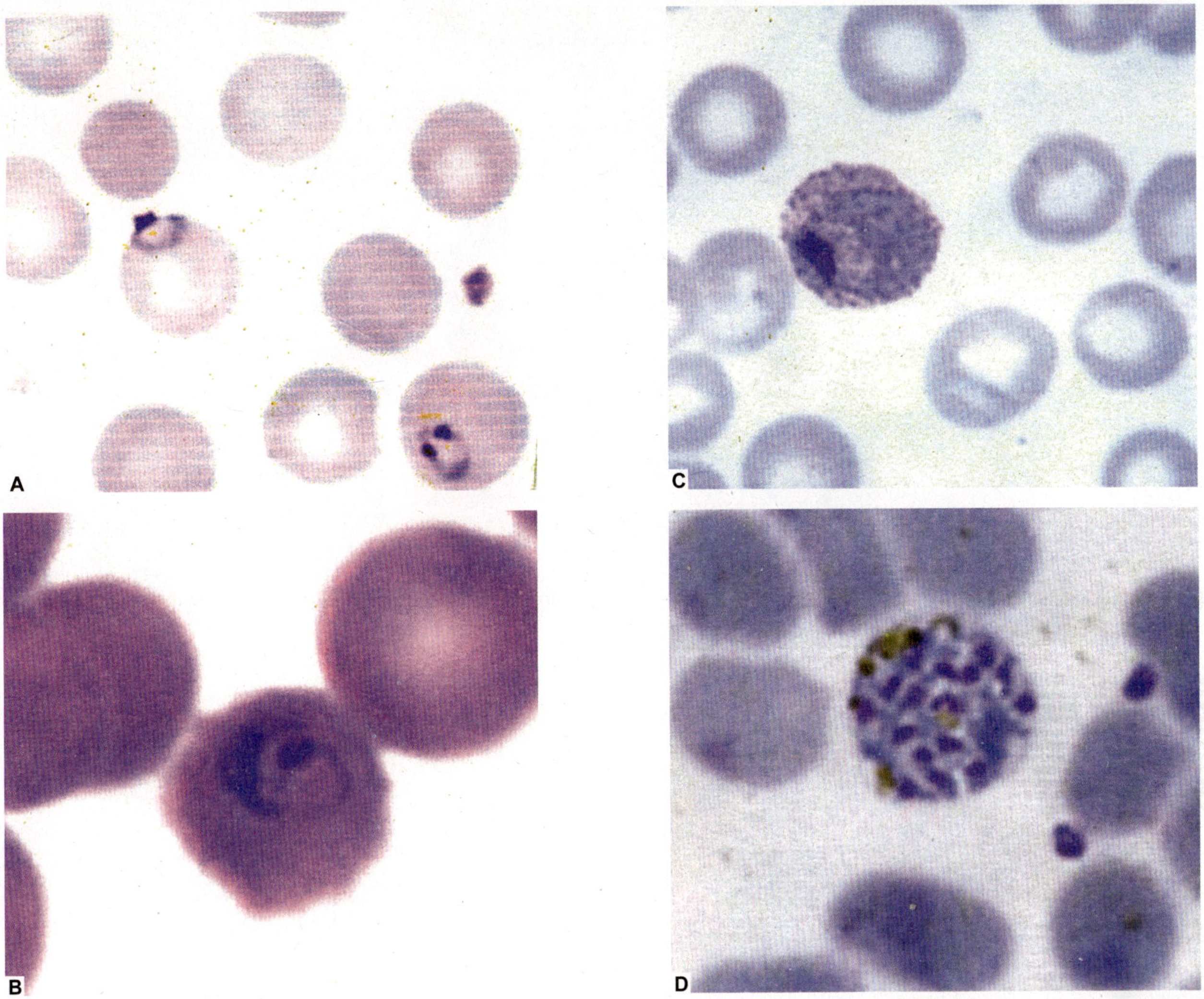

Fig. 45.3: (A) *Plasmodium vivax* ring stages, (B) amoeboid stage vivax, (C) schizont stage vivax, (D) schizont to merozoite vivax

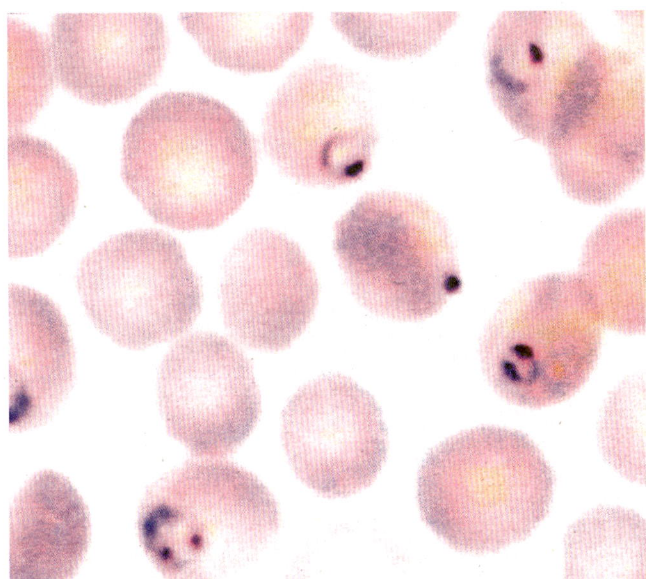

Fig. 45.4: Ring stage: Multiple parasitization falciparum

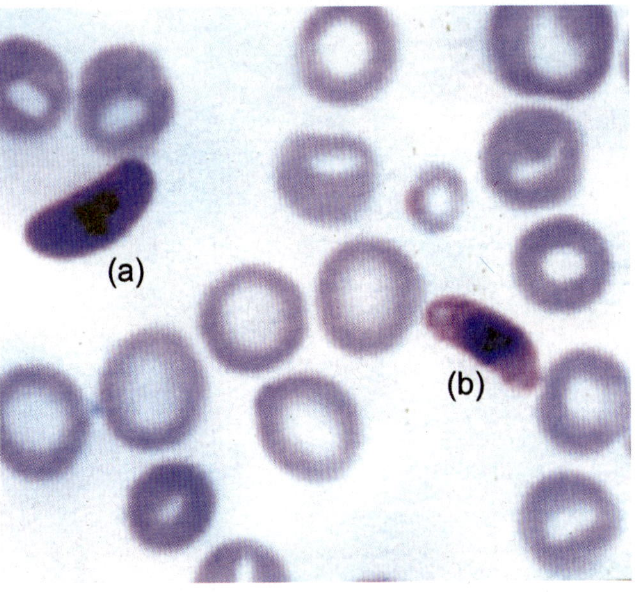

Fig. 45.5: Gametocytes: Falciparum—(a) male with thick round short plumpy, (b) spindle shape with tapering ends

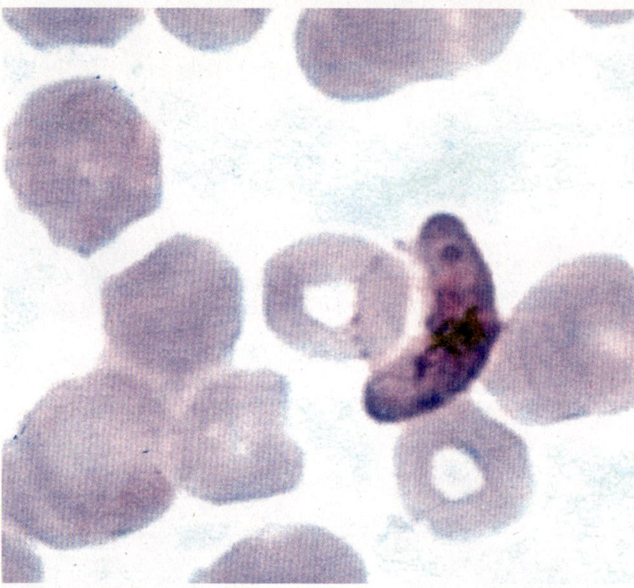

Fig. 45.6: Blood smear showing female gametocyte—spindle shape, showing plenty of haemozoin brown pigments

Chapter 46

Leishmania (Leishmaniasis)

Chapter Outline

- Leishmaniasis
- Etiology of Leishmaniasis
- Symptoms and Signs of Leishmaniasis
- Manifestations
- Culture of *L. donovani*
- Serological Test
- Stages of Leishmaniasis
- Life Cycle: *Leishmania* Species
- Pathophysiology
- Parasitic Pathogenesis
- Prevention of Leishmaniasis

LEISHMANIASIS

Introduction

Leishmaniasis is present in scattered areas worldwide. Human infection is caused by 20 *Leishmania* species that are morphologically indistinguishable but can be differentiated by laboratory analysis.

Table 46.1 shows genus or spices of Leishmania of the Kingdom Protista.

Table 46.1: *Leishmania* species

Kingdom	*Protista*
Subkingdom	Protozoa
Phylum	Sarcomastigophora
Subphylum	Mastigophora
Class	Zoomastigophora
Order	Kinetoplastida
Family	Trypanosomatidae
Section	Salivaria
Genus	Leishmania
Species	donovani, tropica, braziliensis, infantum

There are 3 main forms of leishmaniases: Visceral (the most serious form because it is almost always fatal without treatment), cutaneous (the most common, usually causing skin ulcers), and mucocutaneous (affecting mouth, nose and throat).

- *Leishmania tropica* causes oriental sore
- *Leishmania braziliensis* causes Espundia

Genus Leishmania was created by Ross in 1903. In 1900, Sir William Leishman discovered the parasite in spleen smears of a soldier who died in Calcutta. In same year Charles Donovan found the same parasite in a spleen biopsy in Madras. The parasite has 2 forms:

1. Aflagellate or amastigote
2. Flagellate or promastigote

Leishmania are protozoan parasites of macrophages and are thus in a position to both influence and be influenced by host cytokines. One such cytokine, IL-10, is of particular interest because of its antagonistic effects on IFN-γ, a potent activator of macrophages for intracellular killing of Leishmania. The production of IL-10 could influence the outcome of infection by partially blocking production of IFN-γ. Perhaps more importantly, IL-10 also has powerful effects on macrophages. These include downregulation of antigen presentation, cytokine production, and of metabolic events associated with macrophage activation.

Human visceral leishmaniasis, caused by *L. donovani or L. infantum* in Africa, India, and Europe, or by *L. chagasi* in Latin America, is most often recognized as an acute infection with severe morbidity and high mortality in untreated cases. These patients are characterised immunologically as having high levels of anti-Leishmania antibody and low or absent Leishmania-elicited T cell proliferation and cytokine (IL-2 and IFN- γ) production, responses which become positive upon recovery from acute disease. Delayed hypersensitivity responses to Leishmania antigens parallel the *in vitro* lymphocyte response patterns.

Cutaneous leishmaniasis is a major public health problem and causes a range of diseases from self-healing infections to chronic disfiguring disease. Currently, there is no vaccine for leishmaniasis, and drug therapy is often ineffective.

Etiology of Leishmaniasis

Leishmania promastigotes are transmitted by sand flies *(Phlebotomus, Lutzomyia)* to vertebrate hosts. Vector sand flies are infected by biting infected humans or animals. Animal reservoirs vary with the *Leishmania* species and geographic location and include dogs, other canines, rodents, and other animals. In the Indian subcontinent, humans are the reservoir for *L. donovani*.

Rarely, infection is spread by blood transfusion, shared needles, congenitally, or sexually.

Symptoms and Signs of Leishmaniasis

Leishmaniasis is caused by species of *Leishmania*. Manifestations include cutaneous, mucosal, and visceral syndromes.

Manifestations

The type of leishmaniasis infections depends on the species of *Leishmania* involved HIV-related leishmaniasis has also been reported caused by *L. donovani* in Africa and South Asia.

Cutaneous leishmaniasis, which is caused by several protozoal parasites of the genus *Leishmania,* is endemic to South and Central America, Northern Africa, the Middle East and parts of Asia, and an estimated 1 million new cases arise each year. Of particular interest to immunologists is the wide range of clinical manifestations associated with this disease, which, similar to tuberculosis and leprosy, is dictated largely by the type and magnitude of the immune response of the host.

Cutaneous leishmaniasis causes painless chronic skin lesions ranging from nodules to large ulcers that can persist for months to years but eventually heal. Mucosal leishmaniasis affects nasopharyngeal tissues and can cause gross mutilation of the nose and palate.

In *cutaneous leishmaniasis,* a well-demarcated skin lesion develops at the site of a sandfly bite, usually within several weeks to months. Multiple lesions may occur after multiple infective bites or with metastatic spread. Their appearance varies. The initial lesion is often a papule that slowly enlarges, ulcerates centrally, and develops a raised, erythematous border where intracellular parasites are concentrated. Ulcers are typically painless and cause no systemic symptoms unless secondarily infected. Lesions heal spontaneously after several months but may persist for years. They leave a depressed, burn-like scar. The course depends on the infecting *Leishmania* species and the host's immune status:

- The initial sign of cutaneous leishmaniasis is commonly caused by *L. tropica*, a **red papule** (tiny red bump on the site of the fly's bite) that appears in **2 weeks to 2 months** after exposure.
- The lesion becomes enlarged and ulcerated and it is intensely pruritic (itching).
- The outer crust of the **ulcer** becomes hard and releases a serous substance which is **thin** watery exudates, this acts as a substrate for **secondary infections** which complicate the case, the lesion self recover without any treatment in a few months but leaves rigid scars.
- Mucocutaneous leishmaniasis is initial symptoms and appearance of cutaneous ulcers is similar to the cutaneous leishmania, the only difference is **destruction in mucous membranes and tissues are involved,** 80% of untreated cases turns into mucocutaneous form because primary lesions are accompanied by the nasal and oral mucous spread of leishmania even after the lesion is healed.
- Mucosal lesions do not easily heal, and secondary infections are prevalent cause **severe disfiguring facial form** and occasionally fatal.

Mucosal leishmaniasis due to *L. braziliensis* and related organisms typically starts with one or more primary cutaneous ulcers. Spread to the mucosa via lymphatics and the bloodstream probably occurs early in infection. The skin lesions heal spontaneously, but progressive mucosal lesions may not become apparent for months to years. Typically, patients have nasal stuffiness, discharge, and pain. Over time, the infection may progress, resulting in gross mutilation of the nose, palate, oral pharynx, or face.

Diffuse cutaneous leishmaniasis, a rare syndrome, results in widespread nodular skin lesions resembling those of lepromatous leprosy. It results from cell-mediated energy to the organism.

Oriental sore: Also called dermal leishmaniasis caused by *Leishmania tropica*. Initially a small, red papule develops at the site of bite. It develops a thin crust that hides a spreading ulcer underneath. 20 or more ulcers may coalesce to form a large sore. Secondary infection may occur as:

Yaws—by spirochaetes

Myiasis—by maggots

If no infection occurs; the sore heals in 2 months time, leaving a depressed unpigmented scar.

Espundia: It is a disease, essentially of South America and resembles oriental sore in many ways. Only difference being that espundia is characterised by secondary mucocutaneous lesions which involve larynx, buccal cavity and lips.

In **visceral leishmaniasis**, the clinical manifestations usually develop gradually over weeks to months after inoculation of the parasite but can be acute. Irregular fever, hepatosplenomegaly, pancytopenia, and polyclonal hypergammaglobulinemia with a reversed albumin:globulin ratio occur. In some patients, there are twice-daily temperature spikes. Cutaneous skin lesions rarely occur. Emaciation and death occur within months to years in patients with progressive infections. Those with asymptomatic, self-resolving infections and survivors (after successful treatment) are resistant to further attacks unless cell-mediated immunity is impaired (e.g. by AIDS). Relapse may occur years after initial infection.

Visceral leishmaniasis occurs sudden and severe, and it is fatal as it progresses slowly or can be asymptomatic, self recovering infections. The onset of symptoms such as **fever, diarrhea, and anaemia is gradual,** and chill and sweating are common at the initial stage of infection, the incubation period may range from **several weeks to a year.**

The invasion and proliferation of the organisms in the reticuloendothelial system lead to the **enlargement of visceral organs,** i.e. liver and spleen, weight loss, and loss of flash occur, if glomeruli are infected, it may cause **kidney damage.**

The post-kala-azar dermal leishmaniasis occurs after the persistence of the disease, it appears as **dark pigmented, regions of the skin consist of granuloma.**

Kala-azar (Black Fever)

Dry and scaly skin of hands, abdomen, feet and face gives the Indian name kala-azar which means **'Black Fever'.**

It is transmitted through the bite of the sandfly *(Phlebotomus argentipes)* infected with the parasite *Leishmania donovani*. It causes emaciation, enlargement of the spleen and liver, anaemia and fever, and in chronic cases leads to darkening of the skin, hence the name.

Post-kala-azar dermal leishmaniasis (PKDL) may develop after treatment for visceral leishmaniasis in patients in the Sudan and India. It is characterised by flat or nodular cutaneous lesions that contain many parasites. In patients in the Sudan, these lesions develop at the end of or within 6 months of therapy and spontaneously resolve a few months to a year later. In patients in India and adjacent countries, skin lesions typically develop 1 to 2 years after therapy ends and can last for many years. PKDL lesions are thought to be a reservoir for the spread of infection in these areas.

In India, the only reservoir is man. In India, the disease is primarily active in Eastern belt including Eastern UP, Bihar, Assam, West Bengal, etc.

Incubation period: 2–4 months usually. Kala-azar is characterised by:

1. Malaise
2. Low grade fever (occasionally fever is high grade with chills and rigors).
3. Wasting and marked emaciation
4. Anaemia
5. Protrusion of abdomen
6. Oedema of face and feet

Clinical signs

1. Patient is febrile
2. There is marked pallor, and patient may be icteric
3. Marked splenomegaly
4. Mild to moderate hepatomegaly
5. Lymphadenopathy may occur since immunity in kala-azar is markedly diminished, there is marked susceptibility to secondary infection of:
   A. Respiratory tract
   B. Gastrointestinal tract.

Diagnosis

Investigations

Diagnosis of kala-azar

- Direct evidence
  - Peripheral blood
  - Blood culture
  - Biopsy
    i. Lymph node aspirate
    ii. Bone marrow
    iii. Liver biopsy
    iv. Splenic puncture (surest method of diagnosis)
- Indirect evidence
  - Hemogram (reveals anaemia with leucopenia)
  - Serological tests
    1. Aldehyde test
    2. Complement fixation test
    3. Immunoglobulin assay
    4. Counter immunoelectrophoresis (CIEP)
    5. ELISA (enzyme-linked immunosorbent assay).

Identification in blood and biopsies: Amastigote form appears as an ovoid or rounded body measuring 2–3 mm in length and living intracellularly in monocytes, polymorphs or endothelial cells. Cyloplasm of these stains light blue and nucleus and kinetoplast red (Fig. 46.1).

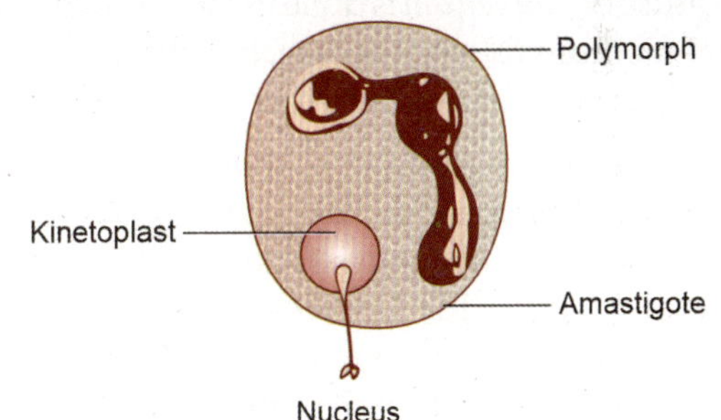

Fig. 46.1: Amastigote form in polymorph appears as ovoid, rounded body

Demonstration in biopsy specimens: Biopsy specimen smears are fixed and stained.

Detection of amastigotes by smear stained of the sample obtained from the lesions or biopsy specimen. It is used for **cutaneous and mucocutaneous leishmaniasis.**

Demonstration of amastigote forms (Donovan bodies) in peripheral blood: This may practically be very difficult. Owing to small number of Leishmania parasites in peripheral blood, casual examination of thin smear may often be negative. Chances of finding *L. donovani* are greatly increased by adopting any one of the following procedures:

1. By making a thick film.
2. By producing a straight leucocytic edge. When a thin blood film is being drawn and before the blood is almost exhausted, spreading slide is abruptly lifted off to prevent tailing.
3. By centrifuging citrated blood. Sediment at the bottom is collected.

As amastigote, it exists in the reticuloendothelial system, especially spleen, liver and marrow. It may also be rarely found in peripheral blood.

Bone marrow showing LD bodies (Fig. 46.2).

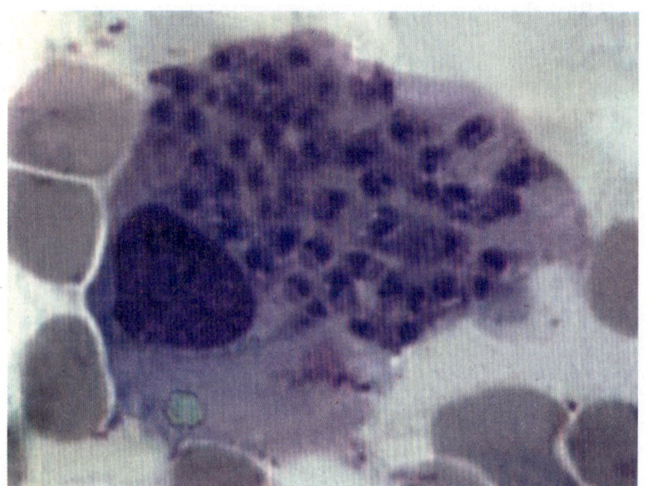

Fig. 46.2: Bone marrow showing plenty of amastigote form of LD bodies in marrow cell

Culture of *L. donovani*

Blood culture of *L. donovani* is done in the following media:

1. NMN medium (Novy, McNeil, Nicolle)
2. Grace's insect tissue culture medium

1–2 ml of venous blood is mixed with 10 ml of citrated saline. Incubate at 22°C overnight, centrifuge. Inoculate into water of condensation of NMN medium. Incubate at 22–26°C for 1–4 weeks. Positive cultures may appear in 3 days or may take as long as 4–6 weeks. Promastigote forms are found in this culture.

Serologic tests can help diagnose visceral leishmaniasis, high titers of antibodies to a recombinant leishmanial antigen (rk39) are present in most immunocompetent patients with visceral leishmaniasis. But antibodies may be absent in patients with AIDS or other immunocompromising conditions. Serologic tests for antileishmanial antibodies are not helpful in the diagnosis of cutaneous leishmaniasis.

Serological Test

1. **Aldehyde test (formal test):** I drop commercial formalin solution is added to 1 ml clear serum—look for solidification and opacity.
   i. Opacity in 20 minutes + 3
   ii. Opacity in 2 hours + 2
   iii. Opacity in 24 hours + 1
   iv. No solidification –ve test
2. **Complement fixation test:** Antigen is prepared from Kedrowsky's acid fast bacillus. Antibodies appear during first 3 months of infection and disappear within 6 months of cure. Titres of 1/10 or more are significant. Cross reaction's occur with Chagas disease, leprosy and TB.
3. **Immunoglobulin assay:** Immunoglobulin, mainly IgG, is markedly raised up to 4400 mg/dl. This leads to a reversal of A : G ratio.
4. **CIEP:** It is 100% negative in non-kala-azar fevers, 80% positive in early and 100% of later kala-azar cases.
5. **ELISA (enzyme-linked immunosorbent assay):** It is highly sensitive and more specific.

Polymerase chain reaction (PCR)-based assays of aspirates from bone marrow, the spleen, or lymph nodes in patients with visceral leishmaniasis or of biopsy, aspirates, or touch preparations from a skin lesion help diagnose leishmaniasis.

Diagnosis is by demonstrating parasites in smears or cultures and increasingly by polymerase chain reaction (PCR)-based assays at reference centers. Serologic testing can be helpful in diagnosing visceral but not cutaneous leishmaniasis.

- **For visceral leishmaniasis**, the specimen is obtained by splenic puncture, liver biopsy, lymph nodes aspirates. The specimen is examined under microscopy, and cultured.
- **Molecular detection** is also used for the diagnosis, to detect nucleic acid (DNA or RNA) of Leishmania.
- **Detection of the antigens** present in the urine sample is also helpful for the **diagnosis of visceral leishmaniasis**.

Stages of Leishmaniasis

The two life stages of Leishmania: Amastigote (A) and Promastigotes (B) (Fig. 46.3). Leishmaniasis is a parasitic disease caused by hemoflagellate, *Leishmania* spp.

The parasite is transmitted through the bites of an infected female phlebotomine sandfly.

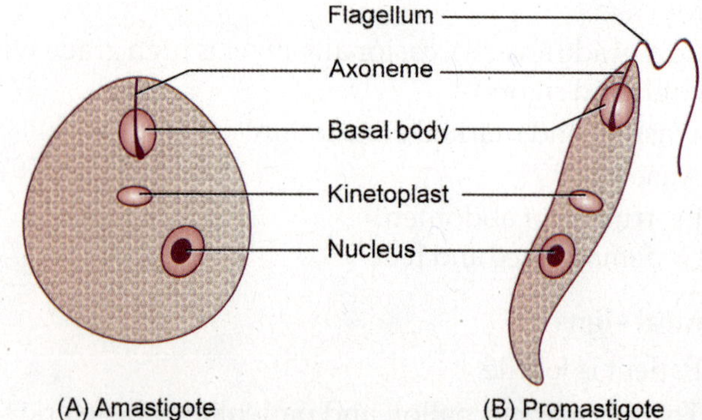

Fig. 46.3: (A) Amastigote, (B) promastigote

Life Cycle: *Leishmania* Species (Fig. 46.4)

As shown in Fig. 46.4 the amastigote stage is both diagnostic in humans and infectious stage in the sandflies.

The amastigote is ingested by sandflies and transforms into a promastigote, it multiplies in the fly midgut by **binary fission**.

During the life cycle, the parasite undergoes two stages: **promastigote stage** and **amastigote stage**:

- In the promastigote stage, it appears as the long, slender form having a free flagellum, which exists in the sale of the infected sandflies.
- The amastigote stage takes place when the infected sandfly bites the human, injecting promastigotes that lose the flagella while entering the skin which helps them to escape the host immune response.
- The amastigote multiplies in reticuloendothelial cells, which cause ruptures in the cells, specific tissues (cutaneous tissues or visceral organs, e.g. liver and spleen) destruction takes place.
- As shown in Fig. 46.4 the amastigote stage is both diagnostic in humans.
- The promastigote migrates to fly proboscis (mouthpart used for piercing to feed) after development, which can be introduced in humans while feeding.
- The only exception in all life cycles of leishmaniasis is, in visceral leishmaniasis, throughout the body, infected **reticuloendothelial cells can be found**.

Pathophysiology

- Transmitted by the bite of infected female phlebotomine sandflies (infective stage: promastigotes).
- Promastigotes phagocytized by macrophages and other types of mononuclear phagocytic cells.
- Promastigotes transform in these cells into the tissue stage of the parasite (i.e. amastigotes).
- Parasite, host and other factors affect whether the infection becomes symptomatic and whether it results in cutaneous or visceral leishmaniasis.
- Sandflies become infected by ingesting infected cells during blood meals.
  - In sandflies, amastigotes transform into promastigotes, develop in the gut, then migrate to the proboscis.

The parasites may remain localized in the skin or spread to the mucosa of the nasopharynx or disseminate to bone marrow, the spleen, the liver, and occasionally other organs, resulting in 3 major clinical forms of leishmaniasis:

i. Cutaneous
ii. Mucosal
iii. Visceral

i. **Cutaneous leishmaniasis** is also known as oriental or tropical sore, Delhi or Aleppo boil, Uta or Chiclero ulcer, or forest yaws. The major causative species are:

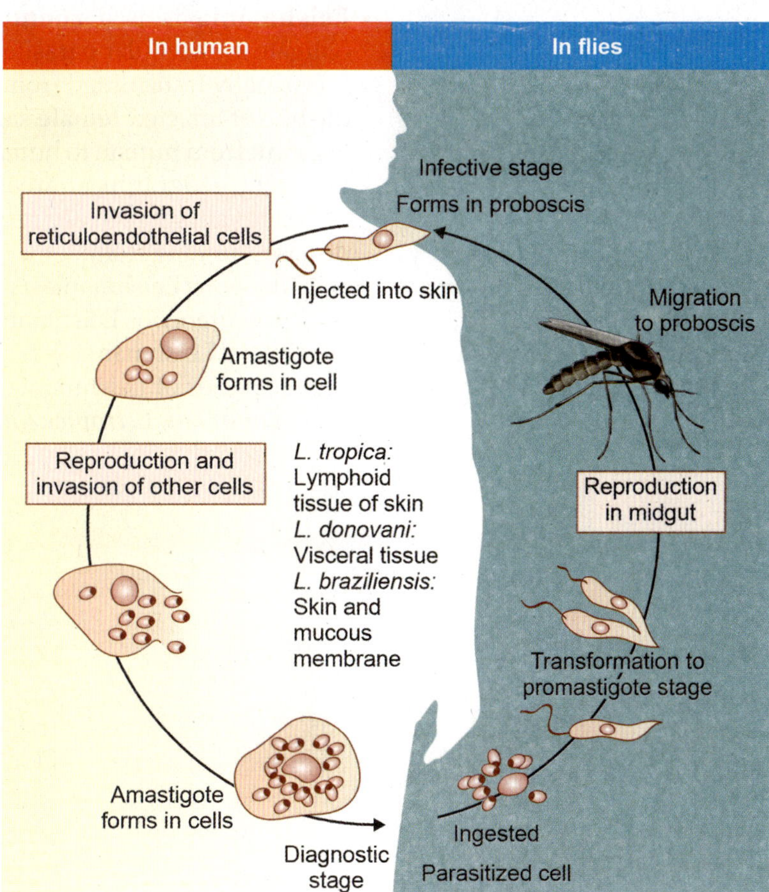

Fig. 46.4: Life cycle of *Leishmania* spp.

- *L. major and L. tropica* in Southern Europe, Asia, and Africa.
- *L. mexicana* and related species in Mexico and Central and South America.
- *L. braziliensis* and related species in Central and South America.

ii. **Visceral leishmaniasis** (kala-azar, Dumdum fever) is typically caused by *L. donovani* or *L. infantum* (previously called *L. chagasi* in Latin America) and occur in India, Africa (particularly the Sudan), Central Asia, the Mediterranean basin, South and Central America, and infrequently China. Most cases occur in northeastern India. Parasites disseminate from the site of the sandfly bite in the skin to regional lymph nodes, the spleen, the liver, and bone marrow and cause systemic symptoms. Subclinical infections are common; only a minority of infected patients develop progressive visceral disease. Symptomatic infection with *L. infantum* is more common among children than adults. Visceral leishmaniasis is an opportunistic infection in patients with AIDS or other immunocompromising conditions.

iii. **Mucosal leishmaniasis** (espundia) is caused mainly by *L. braziliensis* but occasionally by other *Leishmania* species. The parasites are thought to spread from the initial skin lesion through the lymphatics and blood to nasopharyngeal tissues. Symptoms and signs of mucosal leishmaniasis typically develop months to years after the appearance of the skin lesion.

Parasitic Pathogenesis

Given the wide diversity among human parasites, the pathogenesis is highly variable.

Although the human parasites exhibit direct pathogenic mechanisms, in most instances the organisms themselves are not highly virulent.

Visceral leishmaniasis is characterised by diversity and complexity of clinical manifestations ranging from asymptomatic infection to life-threatening illness. Experimental evidence and clinical studies indicate **multifaceted role of various factors leading to parasite survival and multiplication**.

Pathogenesis appears related to T cell cytotoxicity. Cutaneous leishmaniasis is caused by *L. tropica*; an animal reservoir for leishmaniasis caused by this organism has not been identified, although it has been found in some dogs in endemic areas. Morphologically, it is indistinguishable from *L. donovani*.

Prevention of Leishmaniasis

For prevention of leishmaniasis, the following may help:

- Treatment of leishmaniasis in a geographic area where humans are the reservoir.
- Reduction of the vector population by spraying residual insecticide (one that has prolonged duration of action) in sites of domestic transmission.
- Personal protective measures including insect repellents on exposed skin and protective clothing.
- Control of nonhuman reservoirs.

Travelers to endemic areas should use insect repellents containing DEET (diethyltoluamide) on exposed skin. Insect screens, bed nets, and clothing are more effective if treated with permethrin because the small sandflies can penetrate mechanical barriers.

Vaccines are not currently available.

Key Points

- Leishmaniasis is present in scattered areas worldwide and is transmitted by bites of sandflies.
- **Leishmaniasis** is a **zoonosis disease** caused by obligate intracellular parasites, i.e. ***Leishmania*** spp.
- It is usually transmitted from animal to humans or by the bite of infected **female sandflies** the parasites can transmit from human to human.
- Different geographical areas have different species of Leishmania which are responsible for a variety of diseases ranging from:
  - Cutaneous Leishmaniasis
  - Mucocutaneous Leishmaniasis
  - Visceral Leishmaniasis (kala-azar)
- Three species of Leishmania are extensively studied, i.e. ***L. donovani, L. tropica and L. braziliensis***.

Chapter 47

Entamoeba histolytica

(*Giardia lamblia*, Trichomonas)

Chapter Outline

- Protozoa
- Trichomonas
- *Trichomonas hominis*
- *Trichomonas vaginalis*

PROTOZOA

Amongst the protozoa, a medical lab has to mainly identify *Entamoeba histolytica* and *Giardia intestinalis*. In fresh stool, trophozoites are seen, whereas cysts should be identified in iodine preparations, preferably after concentration. The cyst may be presented in carriers. This is the infective form and carriers are public health hazards.

Entamoeba histolytica

Habitat: It lives in large intestine of man.

Morphology and life cycle

E. histolytica passes its life cycle only in one host, i.e. man.

E. histolytica is a natural parasite of man with worldwide distribution, but infection is more common in tropics. It passes its life cycle in one host only. The carrier stage is very common in this disease. Infection occurs from ingestion of contaminated food or drinks containing cysts, as vegetative (trophozoite) forms are destroyed by gastric juice. Excystation occurs in small intestine and young amoebae liberated penetrates the mucosa of intestine producing primary intestinal lesions and causing diarrhoea and dysentery. Secondary lesion (amoebic abscess) occurs when amoebae are carried via portal radicles to liver and in rare cases to lungs, brain or other organs. Trophozoites are found in tissues and in lumen of intestine in acute dysentery. Cysts are formed in intestine in acute dysentery. Cysts are formed in intestinal canal and are not found in tissues (Table 47.1 and Fig. 47.1).

Table 47.1: Morphology comparison of *E. histolytica*, *E. coli* and *E. nana*

Morphology	*E. histolytica*	*E. coli*	*E. nana*
1. Trophozoite			
(Fresh unstained) size	20–30 microns	20–40 microns	8 microns
Motility	Actively motile	Sluggish	Sluggish
Nucleus	Not visible	Visible	Visible
Cytoplasmic inclusions	Red cells, leucocytes tissue debris present, bacteria absent	Bacteria and other materials present	Red cells never found
Cytoplasm	Clearly defined into ectoplasm and endoplasm	No clear division	No clear division
(Iodine stained) nuclear character	Central karyosome, fine chromatin granules line nuclear membrance	Eccentric karyosome coarse, chromatin granules line nuclear membrane	Large, irregular and eccentric karyosome, no chromatin granules
2. Cyst (stained with iodine)			
1. Size	6–15 microns	15–20 microns	8–9 microns
2. Nucleus	1–4 central karyosome	1–8 eccentric karyosome	1–4 karyosome may be central or eccentric
3. Glycogen mass	Rounded bars Chromatoid bars	Filamentous with square or pointed ends	Not seen

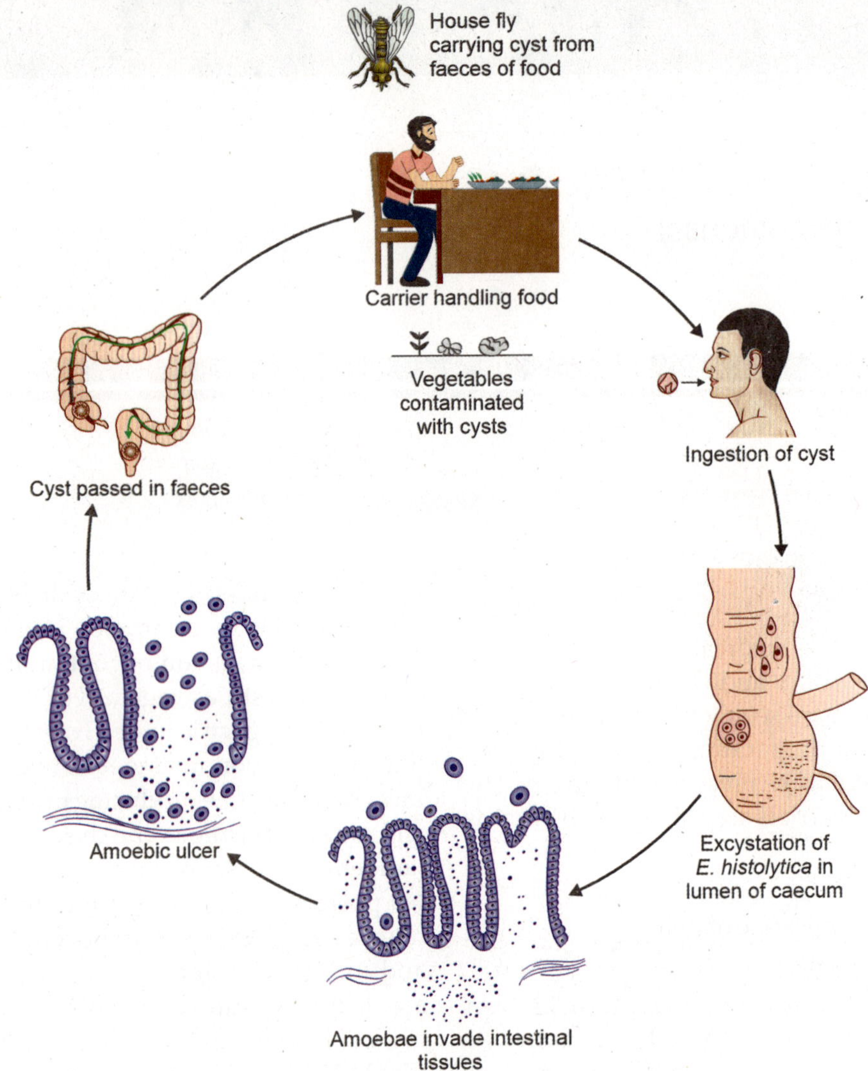

Fig. 47.1: Life cycle of *Entamoeba histolytica*

Trophozoite

It measures 10–60 µm (average 20–30 µm) in diameter. The cytoplasm of the trophozoite can be divided into a clear outer ectoplasm and an inner finely granular endoplasm in which red blood cells, leucocytes and tissue debris are found within the food vacuoles. Red blood cells may, however, be absent if infection is confined to the gut lumen. Trophozoites are motile. Movement results from long finger-like pseudopodial extensions of ectoplasm into which endoplasm flows. Trophozoite is the only form present in the tissues. It usually appears only in diarrhoeic faeces in active cases and survives only for a few hours. Nucleus is spherical in shape varying in size from 4–6 µm in diameter. In stained preparations it shows a central dot-like karyosome which is surrounded by a clear halo. The nuclear membrane is delicate and is lined by a single layer of fine chromatin granules. The space between the karyosome and the nuclear membrane is traversed by linin network (achromatic fibrils) having spoke-like radial arrangement (Fig. 47.2A and B).

Cyst

It is spherical. 10–15 µm in diameter. It is surrounded by a thick chitinous wall which makes it highly resistant to the gastric acid adverse environmental conditions and the chlorine concentration found in potable water. It starts as a uninucleate body, but later the nucleus divides to form two and then four nuclei. Uninucleate and bi-nucleate cysts in addition also possess a glycogen mass, which stains brown with iodine, and 1–4 chromidial or chromatoid bars (Fig. 47.3).

Comparison of *E. histolytica* and *E. coli* stages is shown in Fig. 47.3.

Entamoeba coli has no division in ecto- and endo-plasma, the pseudopodia consist of endoplasm, and it does not ingest red blood cells. The movement is sluggish and more like a flitting and quite different from the progressive directional movement of *Entamoeba histolytica*.

Macrophage does not send out pseudopodia and is not active moving, but often ingest red blood cells.

Amoebic cysts are usually absent in liquid stools, and the diagnosis depends upon the demonstration of

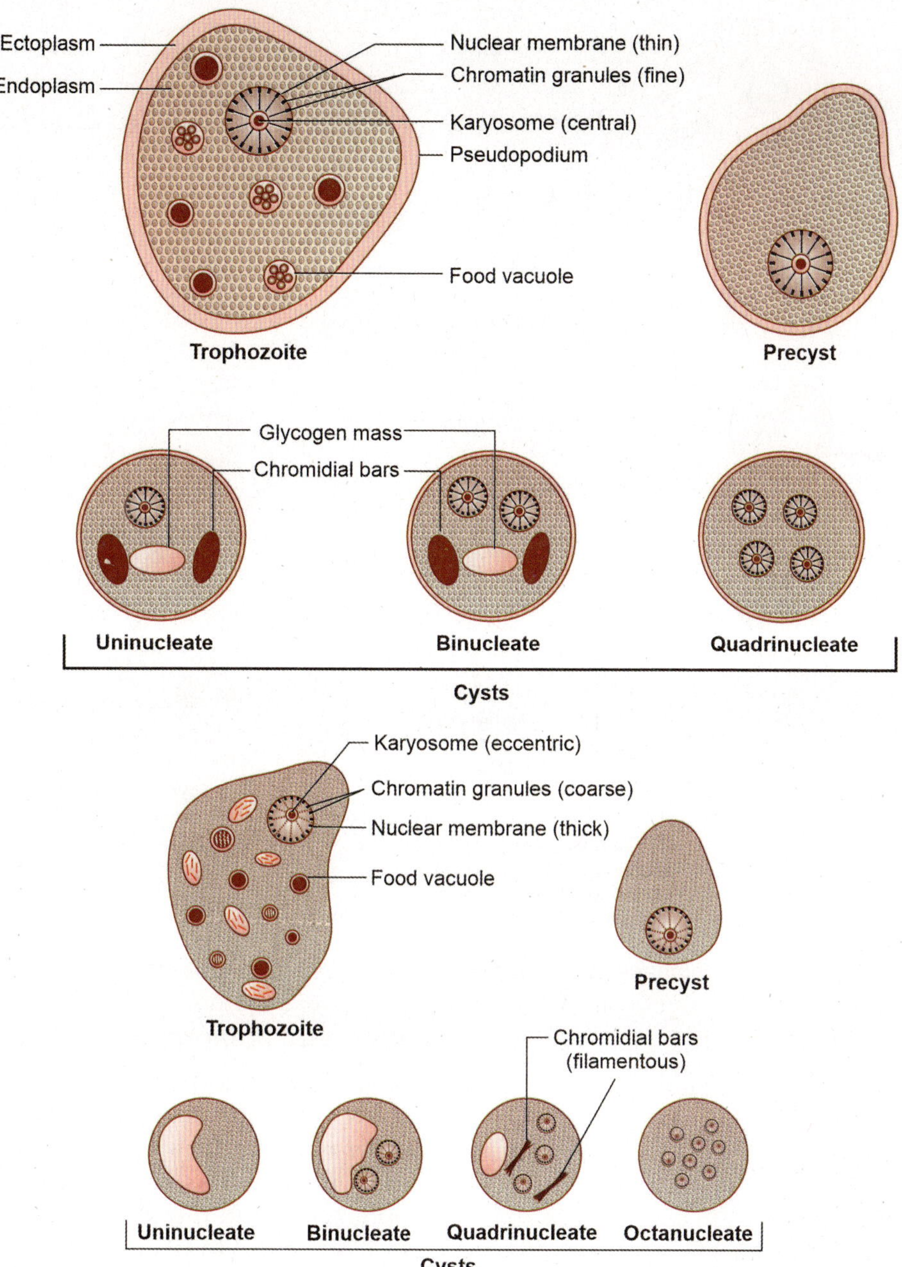

Fig. 47.2: *E. histolytica* showing morphological forms. (A) Well-labelled trophozoite, precyst and cystic stages; (B) Morphological forms of *Entamoeba coli*

moving trophozoites. The stool has to be fresh and protected against cooling. If the stool is left at room temperature for more than 1 hour, the trophozoites will lose their movement and start to degenerate or dye.

Various other morphological forms of *Endolimax nana, Iodaamoeba butschlii, Entamoeba hartmanni, Balantidium coli* to be differentiated from *E. histolytica* and *E. coli*.

Endolimax nana

Trophozoite

It is small, measuring 6–15 µm (average 10 µm) in diameter. The cytoplasm has an inner finely granular endoplasm and a clear outer ectoplasm. It exhibits sluggish motility by means of short, blunt, hyaline pseudopodia. Cytoplasmic inclusions contain bacteria, small vegetable cells, and crystals but never red blood cells. Nucleus is minute spherical with a large irregular karyosome lying eccentrically from which several achromatic strands extend to the nuclear membrane (Fig. 47.4).

Cyst

It is oval measuring 8–10 µm in diameter. The number of nuclei varies from 1 to 4 but mature cyst is quadrinucleate. Chromidial bars and glycogen vacuole are absent.

It is nonpathogenic and produces no symptoms.

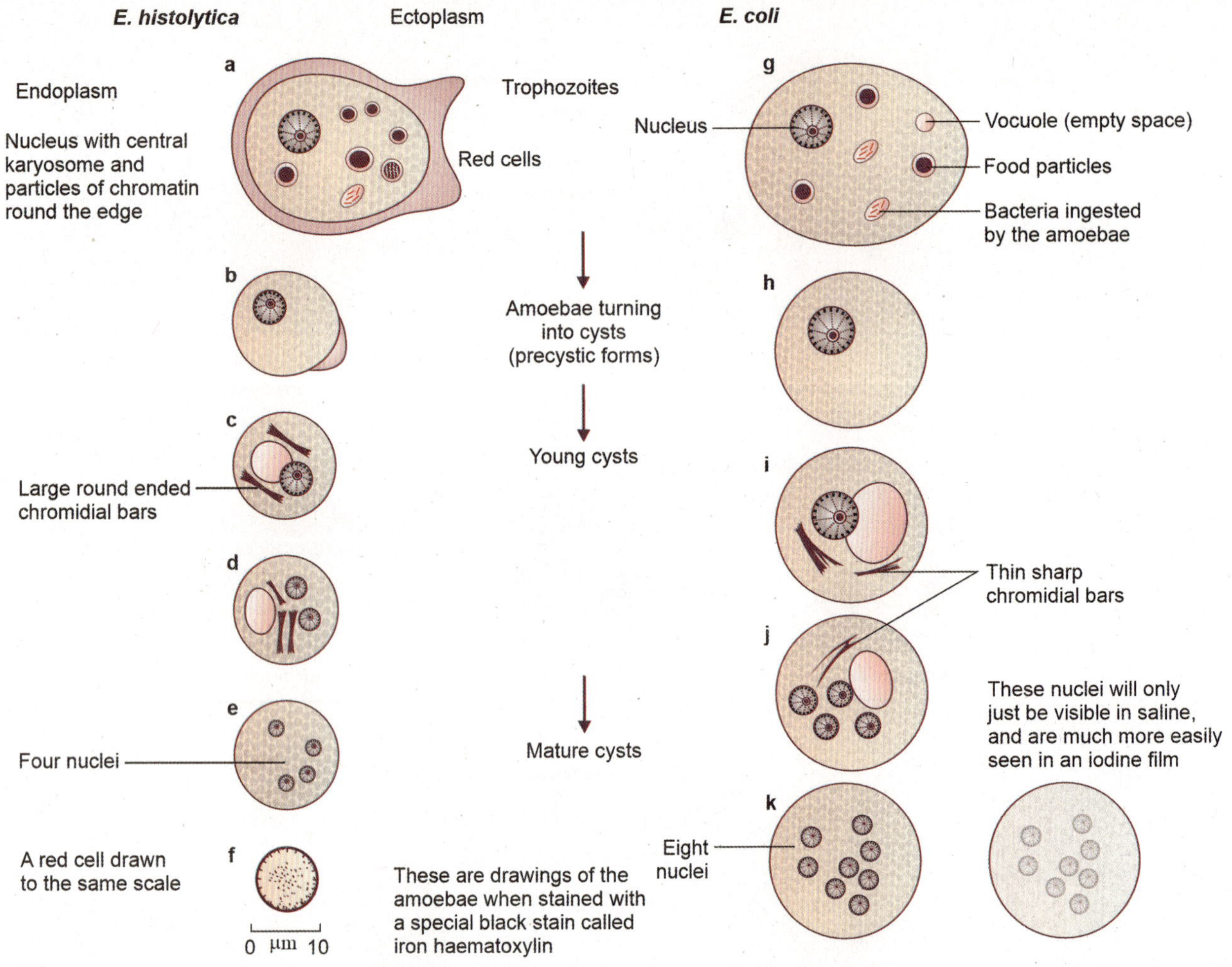

Fig. 47.3: Comparison of *E. histolytica* and *E. coli* (a to k)—well labelled

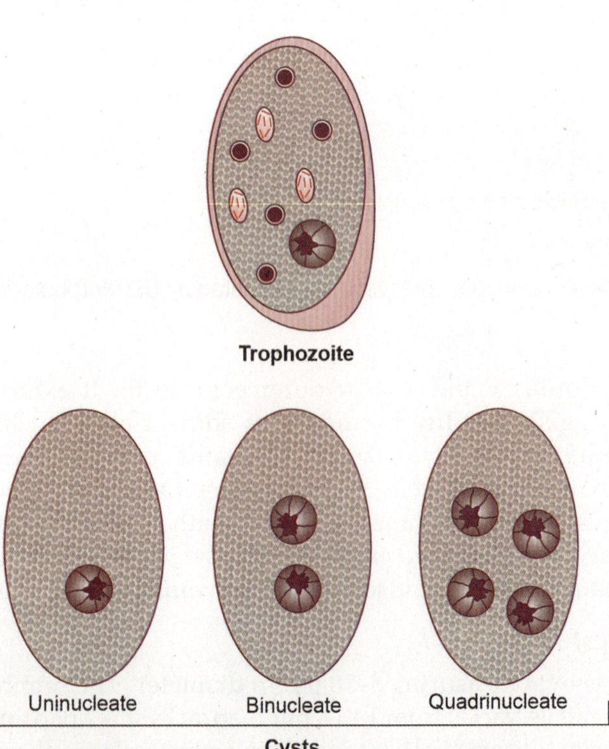

Fig. 47.4: Morphological forms of *Endolimax nana*

Entamoeba hartmanni

E. hartmanni is morphologically similar to *E. histolytica*, but both its trophozoites and cysts are smaller and the former never contain ingested red blood cells. Earlier it was regarded as small race of *E. histolytica*. The trophozoites and the cysts of *E. hartmanni* range from 4 to 12 μm and 5 to 10 μm in diameter respectively. It is nonpathogenic amoeba.

Iodamoeba butschlii

Trophozoite

Trophozoites vary in size from 6 to 20 μm in diameter and are fairly active in freshly evacuated unformed stools and show sluggish movement in older stools. The clear ectoplasm is not usually well differentiated from denser endoplasm that contains coarse and fine granules and has bacteria and yeast cells in food vacuoles. Occasionally, a discrete glycogen vacuole which stains golden brown with iodine may be demonstrated in the cytoplasm of the trophozoite (Fig. 47.5). The nucleus is relatively large measuring 2.0–3.5 μm in diameter. The karyosome is a large circular mass, central in position and surrounded by refractile globules. Peripheral chromatin lining is absent.

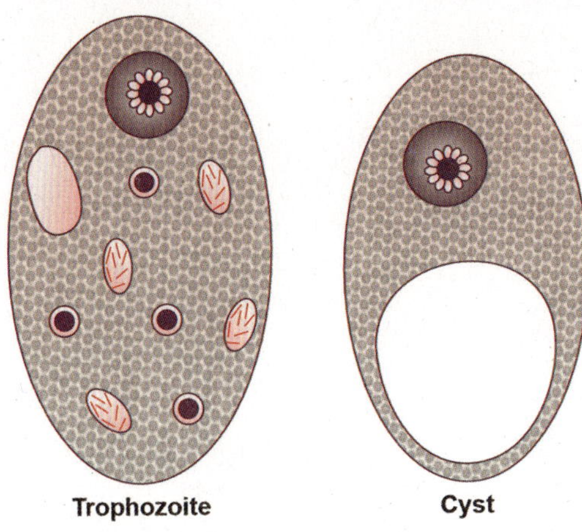

Fig. 47.5: Morphological forms of *Iodamoeba butschlii*

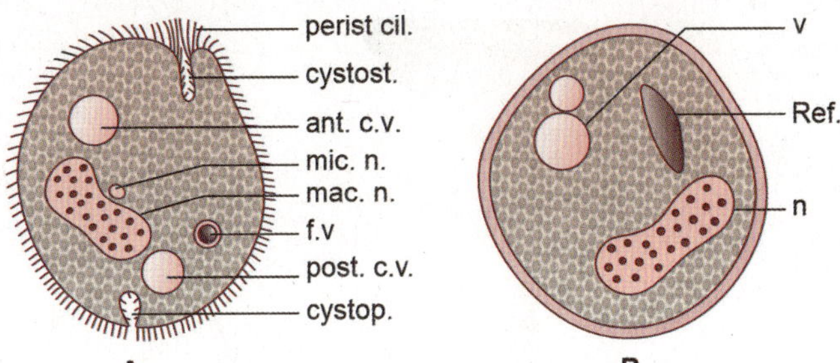

Fig. 47.6A and B: *Balantidium coli:* (A) *Trophozoite;* (B) *Cyst* (A) *c.v.*: Anterior contractile vacuole, *Cystost.*: Cystostome, *Cystop.* Cytophyge, *f.v.*: Food vacuoles, *mac. n.:* Macronucleus, *perist. cil.*: Peristonel cilia, post *c.v.*: Posterior contractile vacuoles, *mic. n.*: Micronucles (B) v: Contractile vacuole, Ref: Refractile vacuole, n: Vacuole

Cyst

The cyst of *I. butschlii* is ovoid or irregularly pyriform in shape, uninucleate and measure 8–15 µm in longest diameter. The cytoplasm contains a large glycogen vacuole chromidial bars are absent.

Balantidium coli

Trophozoite

Balantidium coli is the largest protozoal parasite inhabiting the large intestine of man. It is oval in shape and measures 60 × 45 mm or more. The anterior end is somewhat pointed and has a groove (*peristome*) leading to a mouth (*cytostome*) terminating in a short funnel-shaped gullet (*cytopharynx*) extending up to anterior one-third of the body. There is no intestine. The posterior end is broadly rounded and has an excretory opening known as *cytopyge* (Fig. 47.6A), through which the residual contents of food vacuoles empty periodically. The body is covered with a delicate pellicle showing longitudinal striations. Embedded in the pellicle are short cilia of relatively uniform length that, in the living organism, maintain a constant synchronized motion that vigorously propels the protozoan forward. The cilia that line the mouth part are longer and are called adoral cilia. These are used for propelling food into the cytopharynx. The cytoplasm of trophozoite has two nuclei (macronucleus and micronucleus), two contractile vacoules and numerous food vacuoles.

Cyst

The cyst of *B. coli* is spherical or oval measuring 40–60 µm in diameter. It is surrounded by a thick and transparent double-layered wall (Fig. 47.6B). Newly formed cyst shows movement, but as the cyst matures the cilia are absorbed and the movement ceases. The macronucleus, micronucleus and vacuoles are present in the cyst also.

Amoebiasis

Definition

Infection and manifestation of pathogenic *Entamoeba* species specifically *Entamoeba histolytica* giving intestinal and extraintestinal complication.

Introduction

Amoebiasis is an infection of the large intestine produced by *Entamoeba histolytica*. It is mostly asymptomatic but may cause chronic mild diarrhoea to fulminant dysentery. Among extraintestinal complications, the commonest is amoebic liver abscess (Fig. 47.7). In this section, apart from *Entamoeba histolytica*, we will also deal with certain other closely related pathogens.

Clinical Importance and Features

Amoebiasis is a disease of unhealthy sanitary conditions. Transmission is through faecal–oral route via contaminated water, vegetables, etc. Infected food handlers form a very important crosslink in transmission of disease.

Incubation period is usually 3–4 weeks. However, it may be much less with a massive infection with amoebic cysts. Trophozoites are the virulent forms of entamoebae. They invade the mucosa of large intestine producing amoebic ulcers which in turn are responsible for the intestinal manifestation of the disease. In 75–80% cases ulcers are confined to rectum and sigmoid colon.

Mild amoebic diarrhoea: There is intermittent diarrhoea consisting of 1–4 foul smelling loose or watery stools daily, sometimes containing blood and mucous.

Fulminant amoebic dysentery: Onset is abrupt with high fever, between 40° and 40.6°C, severe abdominal cramps and profuse bloody diarrhoea with tenesmus.

On examination, there is diffuse abdominal tenderness.

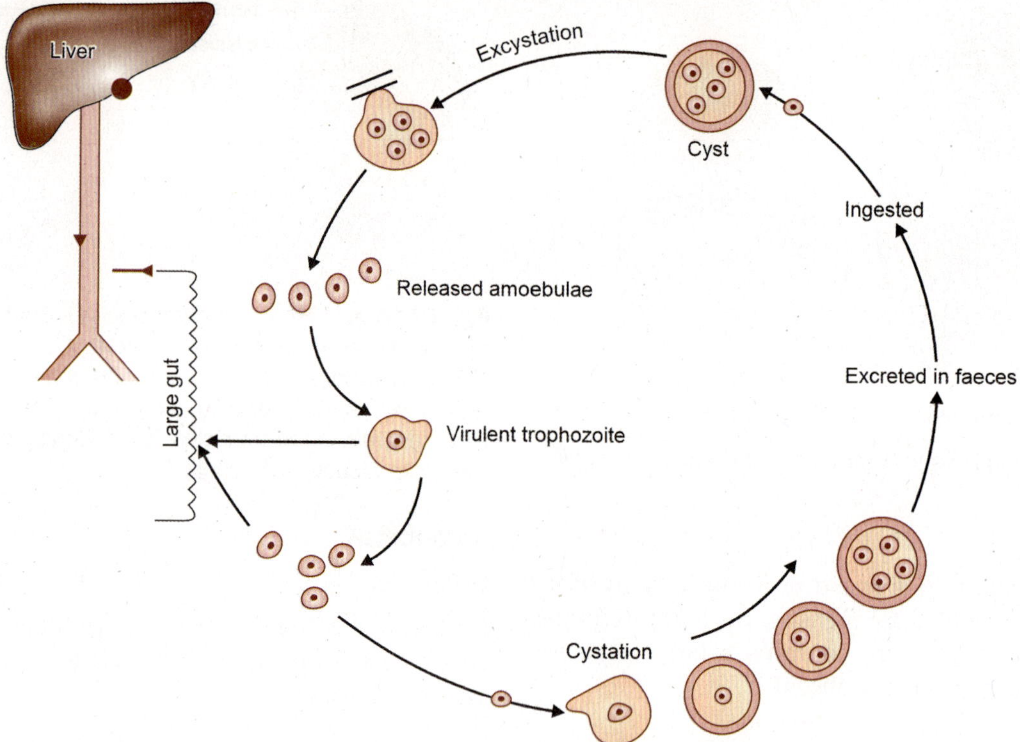

Fig. 47.7: Lifecycle of *E. histolytica* causing amoebiasis—intestinal and extraintestinal

Intestinal Complications

1. Amoebic typhlitis—amoebic infection of caecum is characterised by pain in right iliac fossa. On examination, there is tenderness over caecum. It has to be distinguished from appendicitis.
2. Amoebic appendicitis
3. Severe rectal haemorrhage
4. Amoeboma: A granulomatous lesion involving primarily caecum, although other parts of large intestine may also be involved.

Extraintestinal Complications

Commonest is amoebic liver abscess. It is characterised by:

1. Severe pain abdomen, localized to right hypochondrium
2. Vomiting
3. Fever may or may not be present.

These symptoms may or may not be accompanied by symptoms of amoebic diarrhoea. On examination, there is:

1. Tender hepatomegaly
2. Severe intercostal tenderness.

Laboratory Diagnosis of Amoebiasis

1. Examination of fresh stool acute dysentery for vegetative form.
2. Examination of specimen of stool for cysts.

Diagnosis of Intestinal Amoebiasis

Macroscopic examination of stool: An offensive (foul smelling) dark brown semifluid stool, acidic in reaction, mixed with blood, mucous and much faecal material which is representative of a case of amoebic dysentery.

Collection of Faeces

1. For the detection of trophozoites, collect fresh faecal sample and examine within 1 hour of collection.
2. For detection of cysts, stool is collected and placed in 10% formalin, and sent for examination.

Examination of Faeces

1. Place a drop of normal saline on one end of the slide and drop of iodine (2%) on the other end.
2. Pick up a very small portion of faeces with the help of a wooden applicator stick and emulsify in each solution separately.
3. Seal the preparation with a coverslip and examine.

Concentration Techniques

Used to increase the possibility of detection of the cysts in the stool sample. Various techniques used are basically of 2 types: (a) Floatation procedures, e.g. concentrated saline floatation and (b) sedimentation procedure, e.g. formalin-ether concentration.

A. Concentrated Saline Floatation

1. Take a vial 1″ diameter and 2–2½″ long of 20 ml capacity.
2. Fill up one-fourth with saline solution (saturated NaCl solution of specific gravity 1020).
3. Add faeces of size of a small marble and mix thoroughly. Fill up to brim with solution and

superimpose a grease-free 3″ × 2″ slide over it so that it under surface remains in contact with the suspension.

4. Invert the slide without allowing the drop to slide off and examine under microscope without a coverslip.

B. Formal-Ether Concentration

1. Take stool sample of the size of a marble in a mortar. Mix and suspend in about 10 cc of distilled water.
2. Strain the suspension through a funnel having gauze of 40 meshes inch and centrifuge at 2500 rpm for 2 minutes. Decant supernatant.
3. Add 7 ml of 10% formalin (buffered) to the sediment. Make a suspension by thorough mixing. Add 3 ml of ether, stopper the tube with a rubber stopper, shake vigorously in an inverted position for 30 seconds.
4. Remove stopper. Centrifuge at 2500 rpm for 1–2 minutes, when 4 layers are formed.
5. Carefully pour the 3 layers leaving the sediment undisturbed. Examine preparations of the sediment.

Amoebic and bacillary dysentery comparison is shown in Table 47.2.

Table 47.2: Amoebic and bacillary (bacterial) dysentery—a comparison

Macroscopic	*Amoebic dysentery*	*Bacillary dysentery*
1. Number of stools/day	6–8	10
2. Amount	Copious	Small
3. Odour	Offensive	Odourless
4. Colour	Dark red	Bright red
5. Nature	Blood and mucous with faeces	Only blood and water. Mucous may be present but faecal matter is absent
6. Reaction	Acidic	Alkaline
7. Consistency	Not adherent to container	Adherent to container
Microscopic		
1. RBCs	In clumps, red to yellow in colour	Discrete, bright red
2. Pus cells	Scanty	Numerous
3. Macro-phages	Scanty	Abundant
4. Eosinophils	Present	Scare
5. Pyknotic bodies	Present	Nil
6. Ghost cells	Nil	Numerous
7. Parasites	Trophozoites	Nil
8. Bacteria	Numerous (commensals)	Nil
9. Charcot-Leyden crystals	Present	Nil

Examination of blood: It shows leucocytosis.

- **Diagnosis of amoebic liver abscess:** Aspirated pus is examined for the trophozoite form of *Entamoeba histolytica*.
- **Liver biopsy:** In this case trophozoite form may be demonstrated in specimen of liver biopsy.
- **Stool examination:** Cysts of *E. histolytica* are present in less than 50% cases of amoebic liver abscess and gives the information of persistence of intestinal infection.
- **Blood examination:** It shows leucocytosis.

Morphological characteristics under microscope: It is very important to know that *Entamoeba histolytica* in the stool has to be distinguished from *Entamoeba coli* which is a normal commensal.

Microscopic examination of stool: The attention is given to:

a. **Character of the cellular exudate:** This is the scanty and consist of only the nuclear masses of a few pus cells, macrophages and epithelial cells. RBCs are clumped and reddish yellow or yellowish green in colour.
b. **Presence of Charcot-Leyden crystals:** These appear as a diamond-shaped and infact these are crystals of eosinophil.
c. **Demonstration of *Entamoeba histolytica*:** This is by examining an unstained preparation microscopically.

Cultural methods and complement fixation tests, may be of some value when causative organisms are not demonstrable by routine methods.

Other Serological Tests

Especially useful for extraintestinal complications of amoebiasis:

1. Indirect haemagglutination
2. Indirect immunofluorescence
3. CIEP
4. Agar gel diffusion

Giardia lamblia (Giardia intestinalis)

Giardia

Introduction: Giardia is an organism that is cosmopolitan in distribution, but is most common in warm climates. Children are particularly susceptible. *Giardia lamblia (intestinalis)* resides in the duodenum and upper jejunum. It may or may not cause, symptomatic infection.

Giardia diarrhoea occurs worldwide. *Giardia lamblia* is an intestinal flagellate. It lives in duodenum and upper part of jejunum of man.

Giardia lamblia

Morphology

- Trophozoite—14 µm × 7 µm size (Fig. 47.8A)
- Rounded at anterior end and narrow, pointed posterior end. Organism is dorsoventrally flattened with

dorsal surface convex. Ventral surface bears a bilobed adhesive disk. A pair of dark coloured median bodies behind the disks. There are 4 pairs of flagellae.

Cyst (Fig. 47.8B)

- 12 µm × 7 µm size
- Oval in shape, diagonal lie what are called false axostyles, four nuclei are distributed about these axostyles.

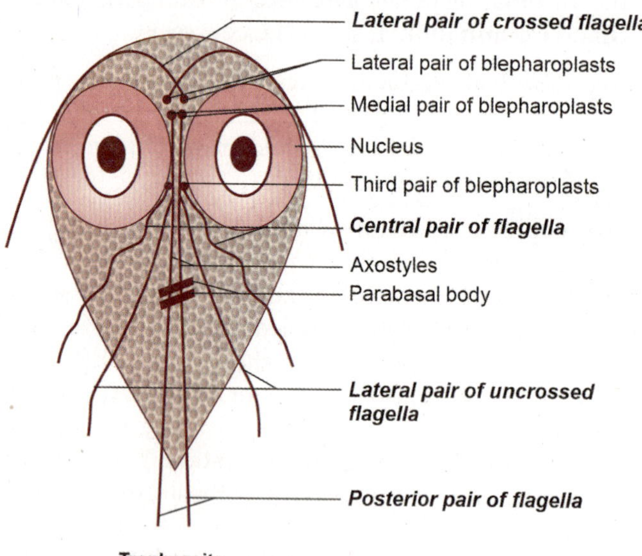

Fig. 47.8A: Trophozoite of *Giardia lamblia*

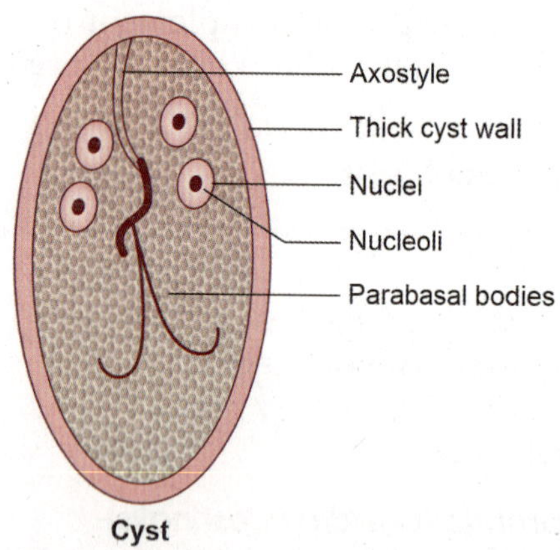

Fig. 47.8B: Cyst of *Giardia lamblia*

Life cycle (Fig. 47.9):

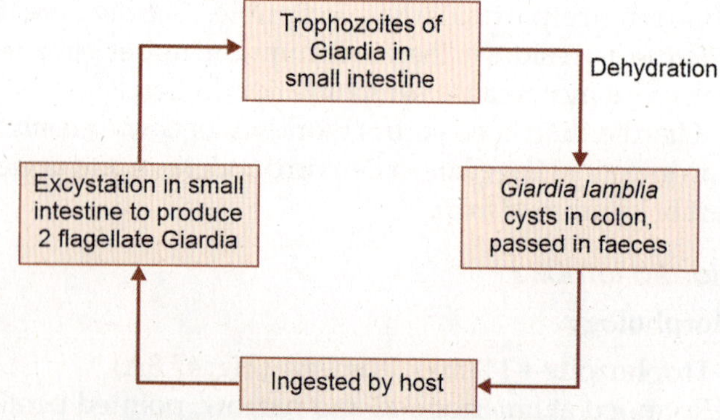

Fig. 47.9: Life cycle of *Giardia lamblia*

Clinical features and importance: Most of the persons who harbour Giardia remain asymptomatic. People who become symptomatic have varied symptoms as:

1. Vague abdominal pain
2. Diarrhoea
3. Flatulence
4. Weight loss
5. Anorexia

Diagnosis: Stool is examined as discussed earlier. Trophozoites are not usually seen in the stool. Usually only cysts are seen.

Giardia antibodies, in the patient serum, may be detected by ELISA and indirect fluorescent antibody tests. However, these may indicate present or past infection. Axenically cultured *G. lamblia* trophozoites are used as antigens in these tests.

Various conditions that have been associated with giardiasis in the compromised patient include hypogammaglobulinaemia, protein or calorie malnutrition, histocompatibility antigen or HLA YB-12. Gastric achlorhydria, blood group A, and reduced secretory IgA levels in the gut. Although patients with HIV infection have also been found to have giardiasis, the infection does not appear to be more severe among this group, regardless of the CD4+ cell count.

Pathogenicity: The presence of *G. lamblia* in the glandular crypts of duodenal–jejunal mucosa may not cause any pathology. These flagellates do not invade the tissues, but feed on mucus secretions. With the help of sucking disc the parasite attaches itself to the surface of the epithelial cells in the duodenum and jejunum and in an appreciable number of cases it may cause duodenal and jejunal irritation leading to duodenitis and jejunitis. Patient may complain of dull epigastric pain, flatulence and chronic diarrhoea of steatorrhoea type.

TRICHOMONAS

Introduction

There are 3 main species of Trichomonas

1. *Trichomonas vaginalis*
2. *Trichomonas tenax*
3. *Trichomonas hominis*

Trichomonas vaginalis is one of the normal flora of vagina and urethra in females and prostate, seminal vesicles and urethra in males.

Trichomonas tenax is a normal commensal of oral cavity and found primarily in tartar and pyrrhoeic sockets. It is transmitted by kissing, salivary droplets and fomites. Although *T. tenax* is considered to be harmless commensal in the mouth, there are reports of respiratory infections.

Trophozoites of Trichomonas morphology are shown in Fig. 47.10.

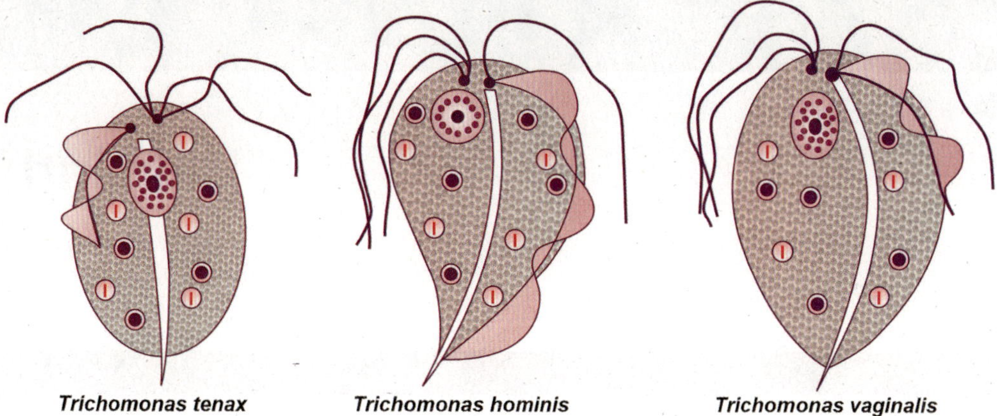

Fig. 47.10: Trophozoites of *Trichomonas* spp.

TRICHOMONAS HOMINIS

It is pyriform, measuring 5–14 µm in length and 7–10 µm in width (Fig. 47.10). It inhabits the caecum of man and several other primate species and feeds on enteric bacteria. It does not invade the intestinal mucosa. Though it has occasionally been found in the diarrhoeic stools, its pathogenicity is yet to be established.

TRICHOMONAS VAGINALIS

Morphology

1. **Trophozoite:** The size of trophozoite is 10–20 µm long and 5–15 µm broad. The shape of the trophozoites like tennis or badminton racket. Its end surface is convex and other surface is concave. There are two nuclei, two axostyles and four pairs of flagella. This moves with the help of flagella.
2. **Cyst:** The fully formed cyst is oval in shape and measures 11–14 µm long and 7–10 µm broad.

   Axostyle is situated in centre and there is 4 nuclei.

   Man is only host and cyst is infective stage.

Clinical features and importance

- It is the cause of vaginitis in females. It is transmitted during sexual intercourse and also by infected linen.
- It causes severe itching and a copious white discharge. (Acidity of vagina discourages infection but once established, it causes a shift towards alkalinity.)

Diagnosis: A drop of the vaginal secretion is placed on a 3″ × 1″ glass slide. 2 drops of methylene blue are added and examined under microscope. Highly motile organisms are seen.

Chapter 48

Helminthology I (Nematodes)

Chapter Outline

- Classification of Nematodes
- *Trichuris trichiura* (Whipworm)
- *Ascaris lumbricoides* (Roundworm)
- Life Cycle

CLASSIFICATION OF NEMATODES

1. Intestinal

1. **Caecum and appendix**
   a. *Enterobius vermicularis* (pinworm)
   b. *Trichuris trichiura* (whipworm)
2. **Small intestine**
   a. *Ascaris lumbricoides* (roundworm)
   b. *Ancylostoma duodenale* (hookworm)
   c. *Necator americanus*
   d. *Strongyloides stercoralis*
   e. *Trichinella spiralis*
   f. *Capillaria philippinensis*

2. Somatic or Tissue

1. **Lymphatic system**
   a. *Wuchereria bancrofti*
   b. *Brugia malayi* (filariasis)
2. **Subcutaneous tissue**
   a. *Loa loa*
   b. *Onchocerca volvulus*
   c. *Dracunculus medinensis* (guinea worm)
3. **Lungs**
   a. *Strongyloides stercoralis*
4. **Mesentery**
   a. *Dipetalonema perstans*
   b. *Mansonella ozzardi*
5. **Conjunctiva**
   a. *Loa loa*
6. **Skeletal muscle**
   a. *Trichinella spiralis*

Enterobius vermicularis

Geographical distribution: It has a cosmopolitan distribution with a special affinity for temperate zones, affecting at least 500 million people in the world.

Enterobius vermicularis is commonly called the **threadworm, pinworm** or **seat worm**. It causes an intestinal parasitic infection called enterobiasis (anal itching) that occurs commonly in children.

Habitat: Adult worm (gravid females) live in the caecum and vermiform appendix of human, where they remain until the eggs are developed. They generally remain on the surface of the mucosa and may occasionally encyst in the submucosa layer.

Morphology: These worms are 3–13 mm long and slender. Females are longer than the males. Both are white in colour. Life span is 2–3 weeks (Fig. 48.1).

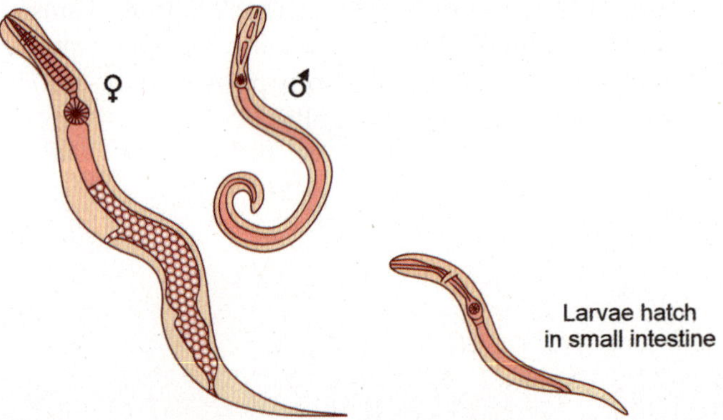

Fig. 48.1: *Enterobius vermicularis.* Females are longer than males and larvae hatch in small intestine

Male Worm

- An adult male measures 2–4 mm in length and 0.1–0.2 mm in breadth.
- The posterior third of the body is curved, sharply shortened and possess an exposed terminal copulatory spicule.
- The male worm dies immediately after fertilizing the females, therefore, are rarely seen.

Female Worm

- Adult female is longer, 8–12 mm in length and 0.3–0.5 mm in breadth.

- The posterior end is extremely straight and drawn out into a long, tapering and finely pointed tail, which is 1/3rd the length of the worm.
- The female reproductive organs are paired and T-shaped.

Life Cycle (Fig. 48.2)

Eggs

- The embryonated eggs are infective to human.
- The eggs are colourless, measuring 50–60 µm in length and 20–32 µm in breadth (Fig. 48.3).
- They are typically plane convex, with one flattened side and one convex side.
- The eggs are surrounded by a thin, hyaline, transparent shell composed of 2 layers of chitin.
- Egg contains a coiled tadpole-like larva.
- Egg can floats in saturated salt solution.
- The egg becomes infective after exposure to atmospheric oxygen for 6 hours and is more resistant to antiseptics.

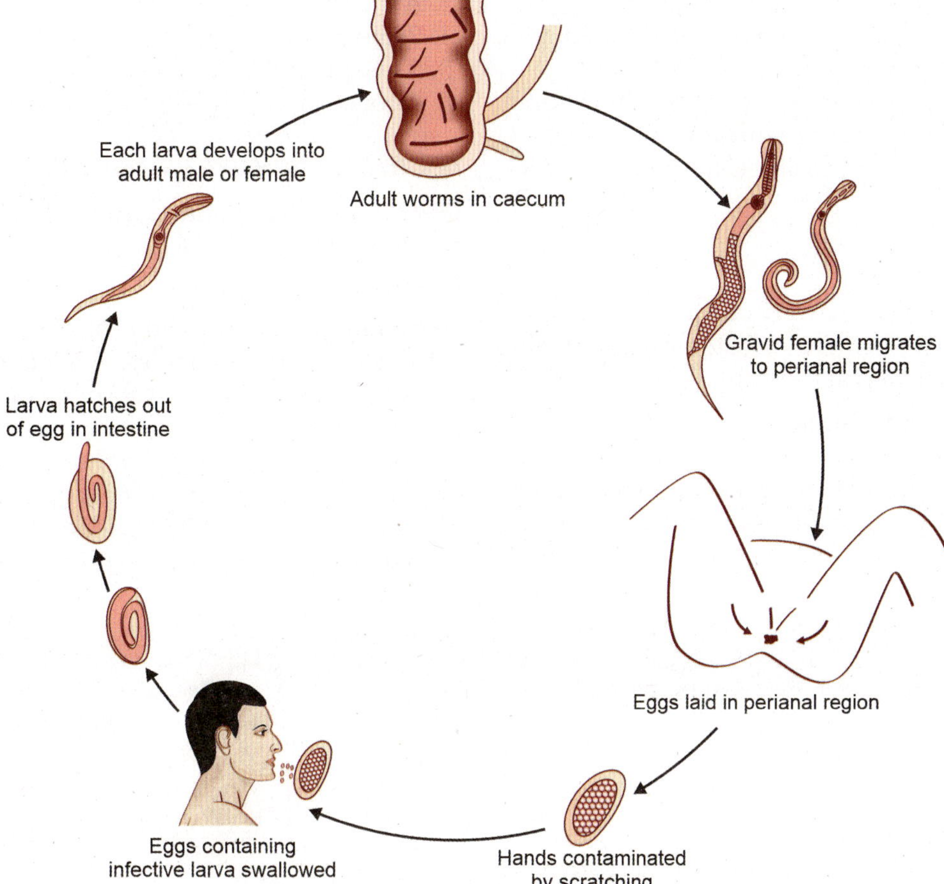

Fig. 48.2: Life cycle of *Enterobius vermicularis*

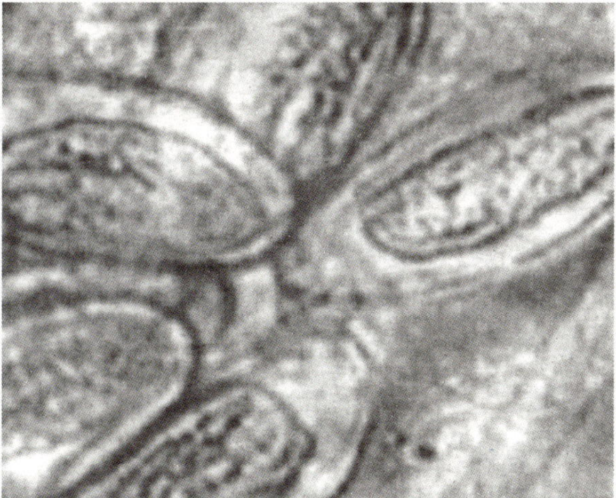

Fig. 48.3: A colourless plano convex egg *Enterobius vermicularis*

- A large number of eggs with an average of 11,105 eggs are present in the uterus of the gravid female that fill up the entire body of the female worm.
- The gravid female dies within 2–3 weeks after laying eggs.

Mode of Transmission

- Infected human beings are the only source of infection. No extra human reservoir is known.
- It is primarily a disease of children and intra-family transmission is very common.
- The different modes of transmission are:
  - Ingestion of eggs due to contaminated fingers, commonly seen in children.
  - Handling contaminated night clothes of the children.
  - Inhalation of air-borne eggs present in the dust.
  - Retro infection, occasionally seen mainly in adults.

Pathogenesis

Pathogenicity of eggs
- Significant pathological lesions are caused by the eggs.
- The eggs adhere well on surface of the skin and by thin natural perianal or perianal itching.

Pathogenicity of adult worms
- Adult worms attach to the mucosa and feed on intestinal content, bacteria and possibly epithelial cells, causing minute ulceration which may lead to mild catarrhal inflammation with diarrhoea, eosinophilia and bacterial infection.
- Infections are characterised by intense perianal itching.
- Patients vigorously scratch themselves.

Clinical Manifestation

Diseases
- Most patients are asymptomatic.
- In symptomatic patients, the most common complaint is perianal and perianal pruritus, usually nocturnal or in the early morning.
- Other complaints include abdominal pain, irritability and restlessness.
- Heavy infection in children may cause anorexia, behavioural changes such as sleep disturbance, nausea, nail bite, grinding teeth at night.

Complications: Urethritis, endometritis, appendicitis.

Diagnosis

a. **Detection of adult worms**
   1. Faecal examination (gross)
   2. Perianal examination early in the morning
   3. Discovery by patients in stool.
   4. Enema

b. **Detection of eggs (more commonly used)**
   1. Faecal examination
   2. Perianal swab

Perianal Swab

It is the surest method of diagnosing enterobius infection. Eggs are often left behind in the perianal folds.

Swab used consists of a cellophane tape held against a wooden applicator. Early in the morning before bathing, sticky side of the swab against anoperianal junction, reversed and stuck to a microslide. Add a drop of xylene which clears away the glue.

Diagnosis depends on identification of typical eggs.
1. Nonbile stained (white coloured).
2. Floats in saturated solution of saline
3. A transparent shell
4. Plano convex in shape
5. 50–60 µm × 30 µm
6. A coiled larva is present within the egg.

TRICHURIS TRICHIURA (WHIPWORM)

Distribution: It is worldwide in distribution, being more common in warm, moist climates.

Habitat: Ileocaecal region of human intestines.

Morphology: They are about 30–50 mm long with males being shorter than females. A whipworm is slender, thread-like throughout but abruptly becomes thick at the posterior end (reminiscent of a whip) (Fig. 48.4A).

The infection is very common. The adults measure 4 to 5 cm, and in general appearance resembles a whip. The worm has long thin cord-like anterior portion and a shout posterior portion. The female is a slightly larger

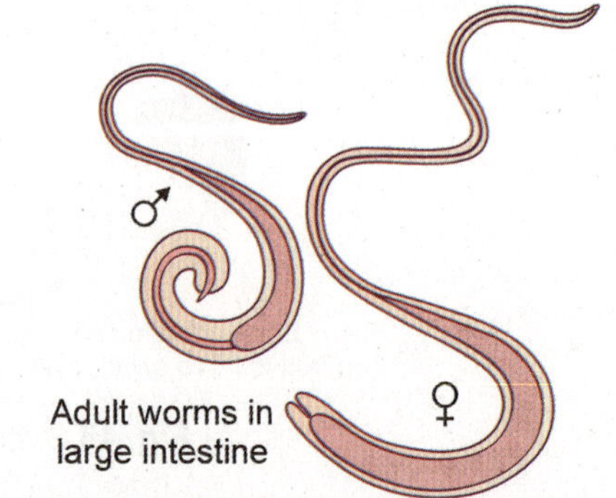

Fig. 48.4A: Adult worms in large intestine

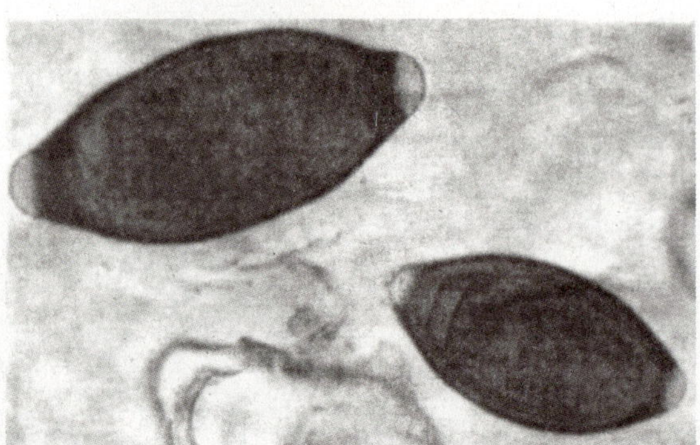

Fig. 48.4B: Eggs of *Trichuris trichiura* had a barrel-shaped, bile stained brown colour

worm. The posterior end of the female is rounded, whereas that of the male is curved and bear spicules. The adults are found in the caecum, ileum, appendix and colon—the anterior portion (which is really an oesophagus) is buried in the mucosa, the worm is oviparous, the eggs are passed in faeces. On moist ground, the larvae hatch within the eggs. Infection occurs by swallowing such eggs. The intestinal juice dissolves the egg-shell and the liberated larvae directly mature into adults.

Life Cycle (Whipworm) (Fig. 48.5)

- Eggs are passed in stool (1000–7000 per day) develop in moist and shady soil

↓

- Rhabditiform larva develops in eggs (infective)

↓

- Swallowed in contaminated food

↓

- Larva hatches in small intestine and migrates to ileocaecal area

↓

- Matures to adult worm

↓

- Females lay eggs

Clinical importance: Vast majority of infections are mild and cause no symptoms. In heavy infections, a patient may show:

1. Wasting
2. Diarrhoea with tenesmus
3. Blood streaked stools
4. Anaemia
5. Abdominal pain and flatulence

Hyperinfection is indicated by 30,000 eggs/g of faeces.

Diagnosis: Specific diagnosis depends on demonstrating characteristic eggs in the stool.

1. Bile stained.
2. Float in saturated soution of saline.
3. 50 µm × 25 µm in size.
4. Barrel-shaped with a mucus plug at each pole.
5. Contains an unsegmented ovum.

ASCARIS LUMBRICOIDES (ROUNDWORM)

Geographical distribution: It is most common in the tropics, though the distribution is worldwide, two populations of *Ascaris lumbricoides* exist, one in human and one in pigs, both show a strong host specificity.

Habitat: Jejunum of man.

Morphology: Adult worms are 15–45 cm long and 2–6 mm wide with females slightly longer and wider than males. Posterior ends are curved ventrally. Both sexes are brownish pink in colour.

The presence of adult *A. lumbricoides* in the intestine induces disordered changes in the jejunal mucosa and intestinal muscle layers. There is a coarsening of mucosal folds, shortening of the crypt depth, reduced mucus production and hypertrophy of the intestinal muscle layers.

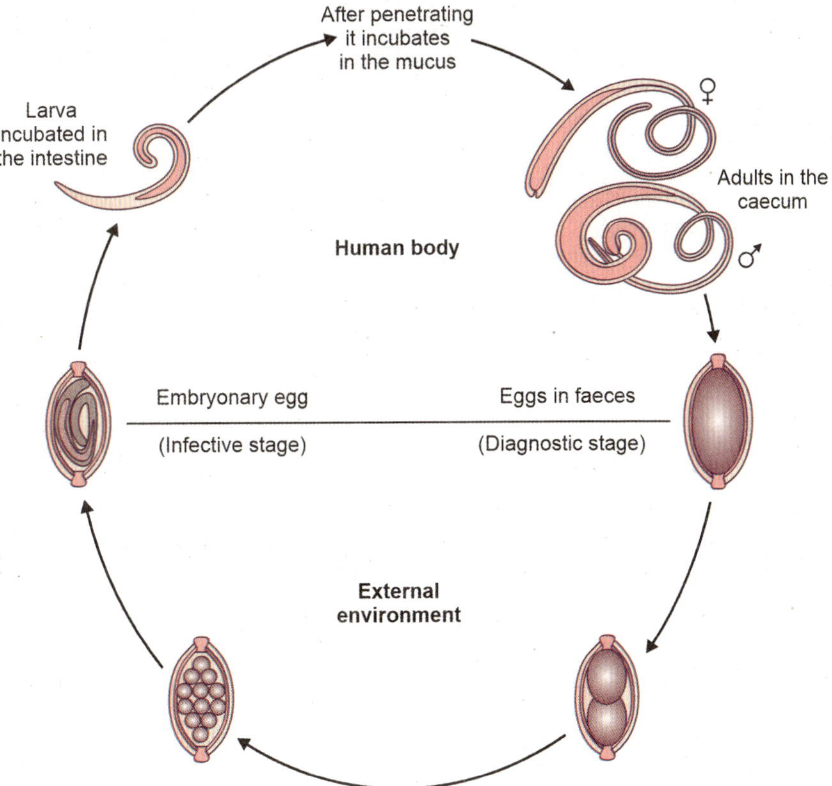

Fig. 48.5: Life cycle of *Trichuris trichiura* (whipworm)

Structure of eggs: Eggs are rounded or oval in shape (Fig. 48.6).

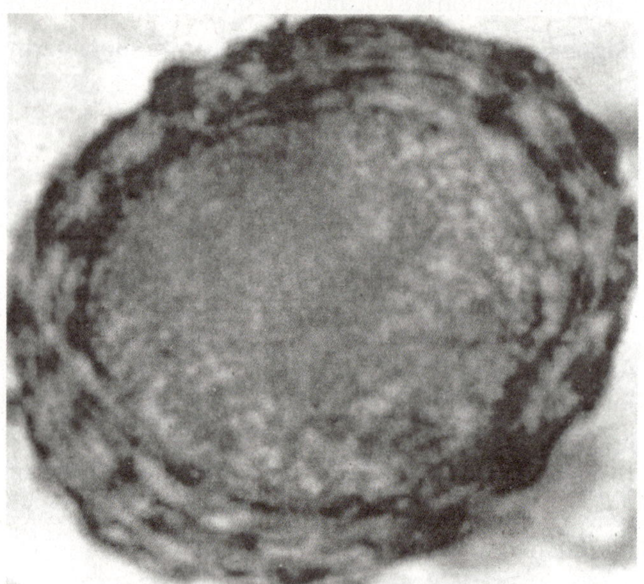

Fig. 48.6: Fertilised egg *Ascaris lumbricoides*

The eggs are brown in colour and their outer shell is thick and there is albuminous coat on outer shell.

Structure of unfertilised egg: This is elongated and narrow (Fig. 48.7). Egg shell is thin and brown in colour. Its ovum is degenerated and disorganised. This ova does not float in saturated salt solution.

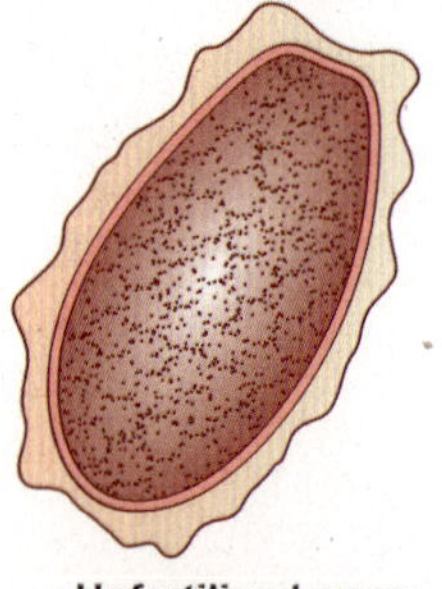

Size: 60–70 × 30–50 mm
Shape: Broad ovoid
Colour: Outer layer yellow-brown
Shell: 3 layers
Ovum: Unembryonated

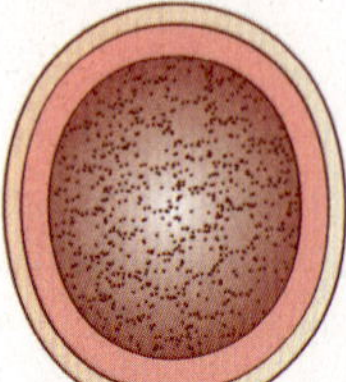

Fig. 48.7: Unfertilised and decorticated egg *A. lumbricoides*

Fertilised egg: Bile stained, brown, thick albuminous coat.

- Size: 88–94 × 40–44 mm.
- Shape: Narrow elongate
- Colour: Outer layer yellow-brown
- Shell: Thick, 3 layers
- Outer layer irregular and coarse mamillated.
- Ovum: Refractile granules

Life Cycle (Fig. 48.8)

The adult worm: Eggs and larine cycle.

i. Adults are found in the small intestine of man, pig, sheep and cattle.
ii. Eggs are passed in human faeces and are non-infective to man till the larvae are developed inside.
iii. Infective larvae are found either in egg on soil or vegetable, contaminated with water containing the larvae.

Man is infected by ingest ion of eggs containing infective larvae which escapes into the intestine. The rhabditiform larvae penetrate the intestinal wall, passess to the blood stream.

Clinical manifestations: The clinical manifestations are very variable, may be presented as nausea, vomiting or lobar pneumonia may be encountered. Sometimes the worms are passed through nose or in stools.

Pathogenesis: The pathogenesis of ascariasis is generally related to organ damage and host reactions to larval migration as well as the number and location of adult worm in the body. Ascaris larvae migrating through the intestinal mucosa, liver and lungs provoke hypersensitivity reaction in the human host. Some of the larvae may be immobilised and covered with eosinophils, resulting in the formation of granulomas. In the lungs, movement of the larvae from the blood vessels into the air spaces results in haemorrhage. There is oedema of the alveoli. Alveolar sacs are filled with a serous exudate, the peribronchial tissues becoming infiltrated with eosinophils and neutrophils, and mucus production in the bronchi is increased. Known as Loeffler's syndrome, it gives rise to dry cough, high fever and bronchial asthma. The effect is severe when the number of larvae is large or when transmission is seasonal.

Although persons infected with Ascaris worms often are asymptomatic, heavy infestation can cause severe complications, particularly in children, who may experience malnutrition, growth stunting, or intestinal obstruction.

Clinical importance

1. **Of larvae:** On reaching lung, when larvae break into the alveolar space and cause minute haemorrhages, larvae may cause:
   1. Mild chest pain
   2. Dry cough
   3. Mild rusting of sputum
   4. Breathlessness on exertion

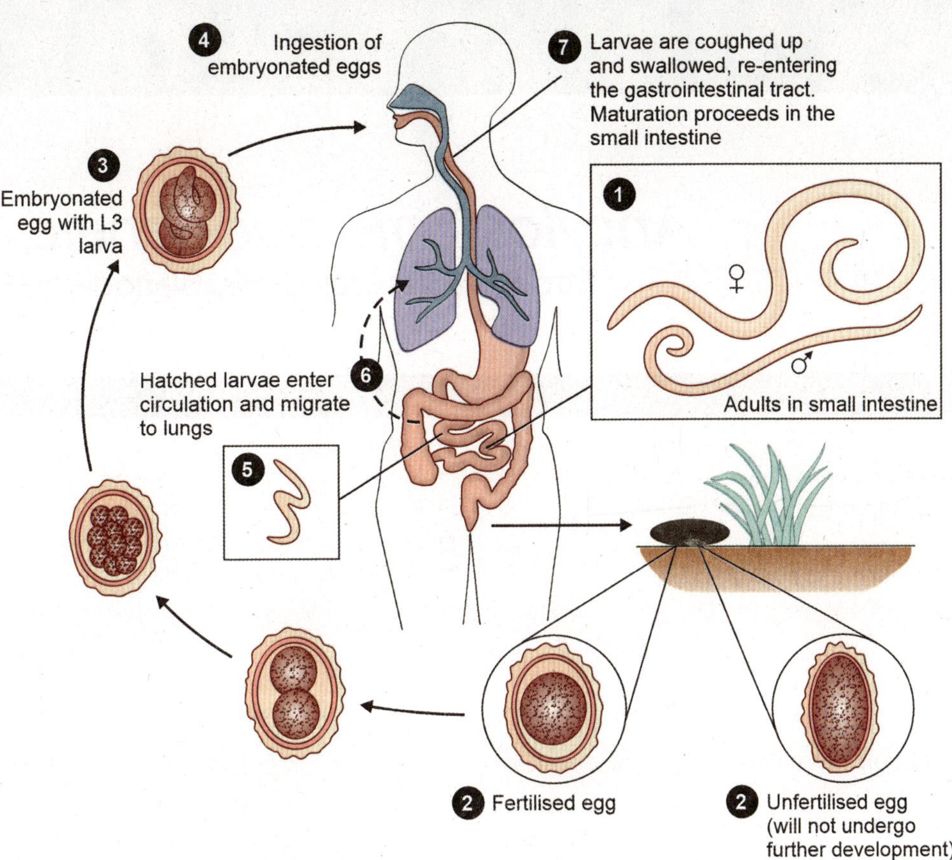

Fig. 48.8: Life cycle of *Ascaris lumbricoides*

Superimposed bacterial infection may occur. Investigation may reveal eosinophilia.

2. **Of adult worms:** May cause a variety of symptom complexes in small intestine.
   a. Malnutrition and under-development in children
   b. Abdominal pain which may be colicky
   c. Sensitisation phenomena including:
      1. Skin rashes
      2. Eye pain
      3. Breathlessness
      4. Insomnia and restlessness
   d. Fatal intestinal obstruction.

   Wandering worms may lead to:
   1. Clogging of appendix, leading to appendicitis.
   2. Anal irritation.
   3. Obstructive jaundice by blockage of bile ducts.
   4. Nausea and vomiting on entering stomach where gastric acidity irritates them.
   5. Sudden consternation as a result of exit through nose and mouth.
   6. Extensive damage of eustachian tubes and middle ear.

Diagnosis

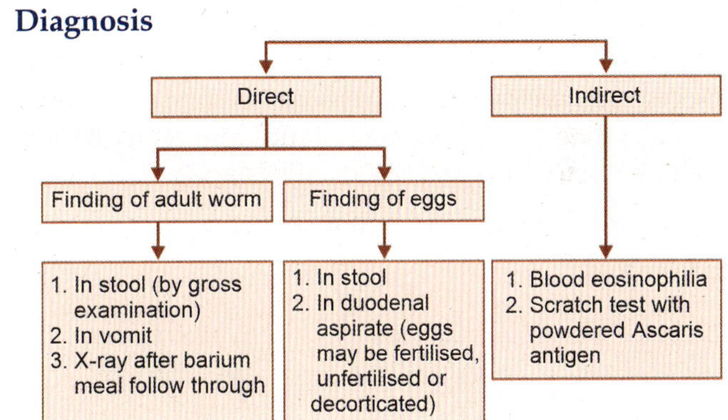

Characteristics of ova:

1. Bile stained
2. Floats in saturated saline
3. 70 μm × 45 μm mammillations.
4. Thick outer shell surrounded by an albuminous coat thrown into mammillations.
5. A large unsegmented ovum containing yolk granules.
6. A clear crescentic space at each end.

Unfertilised egg is narrower, longer with an inconspicuous ovum and it settles down in saturated saline.

Chapter 49

Ancylostoma duodenale (Hookworms)

Strongyloides stercoralis, Filariodeae (Filaria Worms)

Chapter Outline

HOOKWORM

Two main species of hookworm known to cause infection are:

1. *Ancylostoma duodenale*
2. *Necator americanus*

Geographical distribution: *Ancylostoma duodenale* is abundant in Southern Europe, North Africa, India, China and SE Asia and in small scattered areas of United States, Caribbean Islands and South America. *Necator americanus* is more abundant than *A. duodenale*. It was first discovered in Brazil, then Texas. Now, it is indigenous in Africa, India, SE Asia, China and SW Pacific Islands.

Habitat: Small intestine of human being.

Morphology

Characteristic	*A. duodenale*	*N. americanus*
1. Size	8–13 mm long thicker (stouter)	7–11 mm long slender
2. Anterior end	Bends in direction of body curvature	Bends opposite to the body curvature
3. Buccal capsule	6 teeth, 4 hook-like on ventral surface and 2 knob-like on dorsal surface	4 chitinous plates, 2 ventral and 2 dorsal. A pair of subventral and subdorsal teeth
4. Posterior end of female	A spine is present	No spine is present

Ancylostoma duodenale is a species of the roundworm genus *Ancylostoma*. It is a parasitic nematode worm and commonly known as the Old World hookworm. It lives in the small intestine of hosts such as humans, cats and dogs, where it is able to mate and mature (Fig. 49.1). *Ancylostoma duodenale* and *Necator americanus* are the two human hookworm species that are normally discussed together as the cause of hookworm infection.

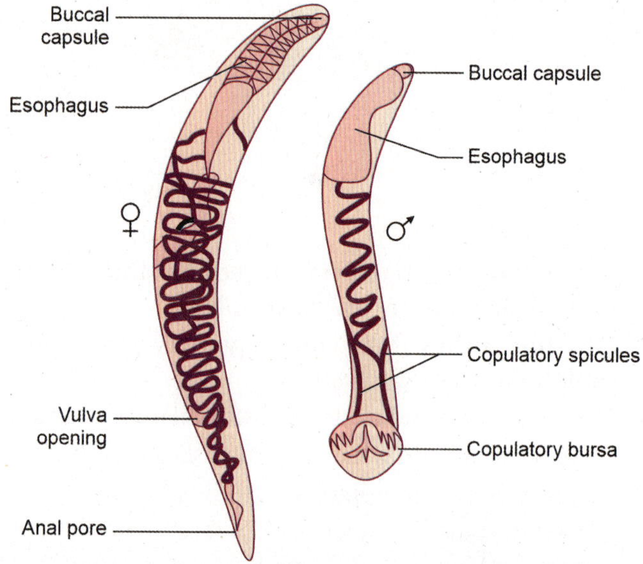

Fig. 49.1: Structure of hookworm: Male and female

They are dioecious. *Ancylostoma duodenale* is abundant throughout the world, including Southern Europe, North Africa, India, China, southeast Asia, some areas in the United States, the Caribbean, and South America.

Morphology: Occur as parasites in the small intestine of their hosts.

These worms are very small; only 2 mm in length.

Recognised by their elongate oesophagus and single row of eggs within the uterus.

Both males and females are found in part of the life cycle as free-living soil organisms.

The adult attach themselves firmly to the mucosa of the small intestine and feed on blood. Eggs, when passed, are in various stages of development, further development takes place on soil—rhabditiform larvae hatch, come out of eggs and moult to form filariform larvae (Fig. 49.2A and B). The latter are infective and penetrate the skin entering the venous stream they are earned to the right side of the heart and through the pulmonary artery to the capillaries, of two lungs. Here they break out of the blood vessels into the alveolar lumina. Migrating up the respiratory tract and epiglottis they come to the oesophagus, to pass down to the small intestine and to develop into adults (Fig. 49.3).

This parasite has two dorsal and two ventral cutting plates around the anterior margin of the buccal capsule. It also has a pair of subdorsal and a pair of subventral teeth located close to the rear. Males are usually 7–9 mm long, whereas females are about 9–11 mm long. The typical lifespan of these parasites is 3–5 years. They can produce between 5,000 and 10,000 eggs per day (Fig. 49.4).

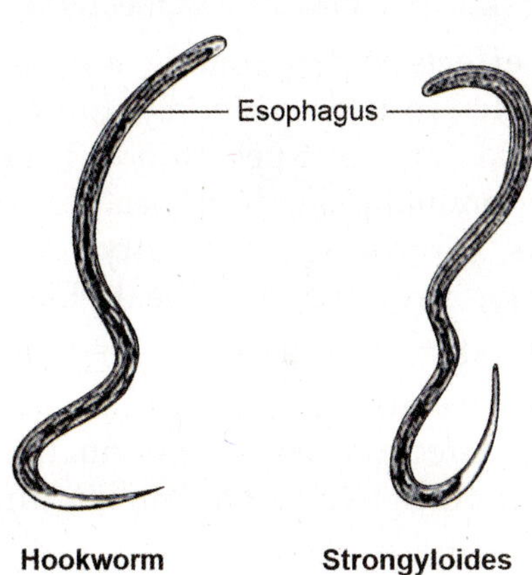

Fig. 49.2A: Filariform stage with comparison of strongyloides larvae

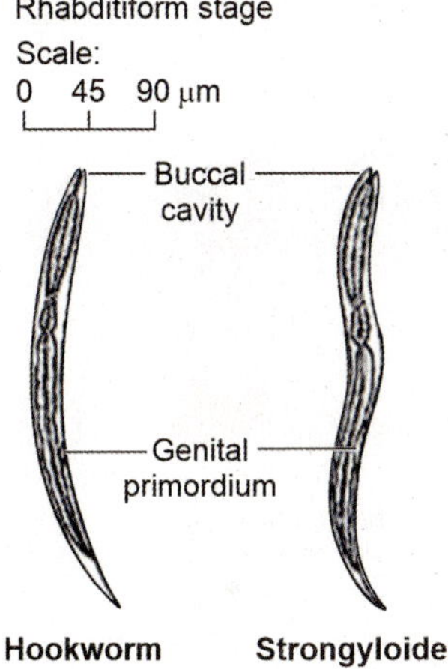

Fig. 49.2B: Rhabditiform stage with hookworm and comparison of Strongyloides

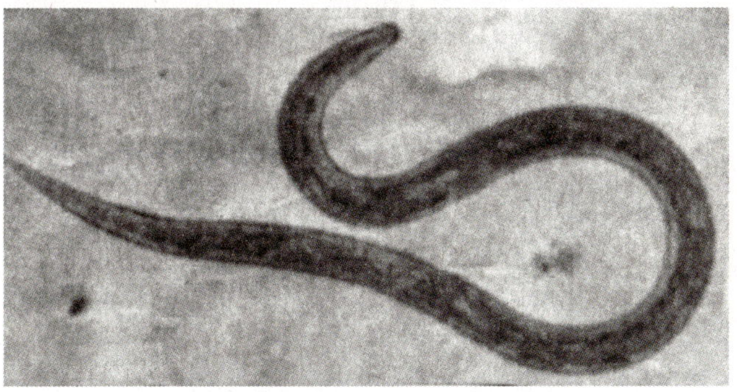

Fig. 49.3: Adult hookworm

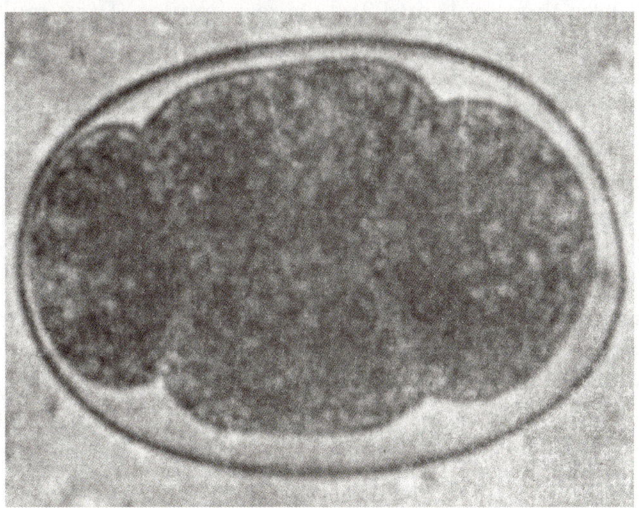

Fig. 49.4: Hookworm egg, showing 4 blastomeres

Necator americanus is a species of hookworm (a type of helminth) commonly known as the New World hookworm. Like other hookworms, it is a member of the phylum nematode. It is an obligatory parasitic (Fig. 49.5) nematode that lives in the small intestine of human hosts. Necatoriasis—a type of helminthiasis—is the term for the condition of being host to an infestation of a species of Necator. Since *N. americanus* and *Ancylostoma duodenale* (also known as Old World hookworm) are the two species of hookworms that most commonly infest humans, they are usually dealt with under the collective heading of "hookworm infection". They differ most obviously in geographical distribution, structure of mouthparts, and relative size.

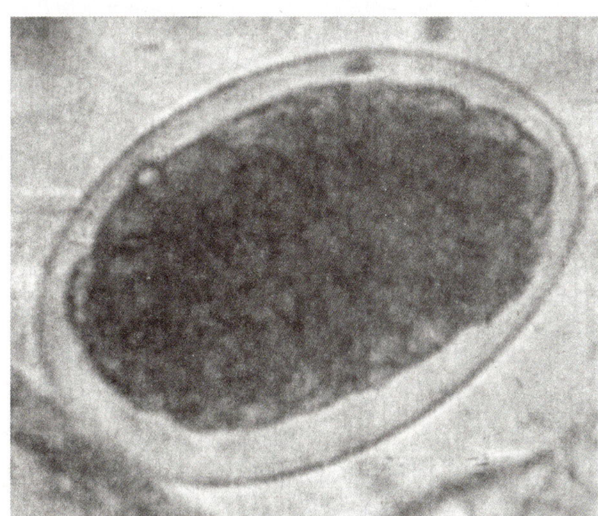

Fig. 49.5: Ova of hookworm (*Necator americanus*) showing early mitosis 2–16 cells

Life cycle (Fig. 49.6): Life cycle and reproduction—eggs are passed in the faeces and hatch into rhabditiform larvae in about 48 hours in the faeces or in the soil *A. duodenale* and *N. americanus*. Eggs are generally 57–76 µm by 35–47 µm and are oval-shaped with a thin shell.

Life cycle continued juveniles feed or faeces for about 3 days then molt into 2nd stage juveniles. They molt again 5–10 days later into filariform larvae. Can survive 3–4 weeks outside host.

Life cycle infect humans by penetrating skin and then travel to the heart and lungs where they penetrate the pharynx and are swallowed. When they reach the small intestine, they attach to the intestinal wall and feed on blood. Cutting plates in *N. americanus*. Cutting teeth in *A. duodenale*.

Life cycle worms molt again two more times to reach maturity. *A. duodenale* adult males measure 8–11 mm with females being 10–13 mm. *N. americanus* adult males measure 7–9 mm and females measure 9–11 mm. Adult worms copulate and eggs appear in the faeces in about 6 weeks (females can produce several thousand eggs in one day). Cycle starts over again and adults live 1–2 years.

Adults, penetrates blood vessels, and sucks blood. The incubation process of the larvae begins once entered into the small intestine; therefore, symptoms may not arise for up to 40 days, but this is variable from person to person. Blood loss from sites of intestinal attachment may cause iron deficiency anaemia and protein loss.

Pathology and pathogenesis: The pathology of *N. americanus* is divided into two stages—larvae and adults. The larvae penetrate the uninfected skin and travel through various organs, including the respiratory tract and lymph nodes. Once in the lymph nodes, the larvae start entering the blood, lungs, and intestines. Some larvae cannot readily enter the dermis and remain trapped in the skin, causing skin irritation and cutaneous larva migrans.

Pathogenic effects: Asymptomatic until worms have already started multiplying. Symptoms include: Irritation of skin at site of penetration, iron deficiency anaemia, abdominal pain, diarrhoea, loss of appetite, weight loss, tiredness, difficulty in breathing, cardiomegaly, irregular heartbeat. Extreme cases include stunted growth and mental retardation.

Clinical manifestations: The clinical manifestations of hookworm infection consist of dermatitis at the site of entry (ground itch) and pneumonia during larval

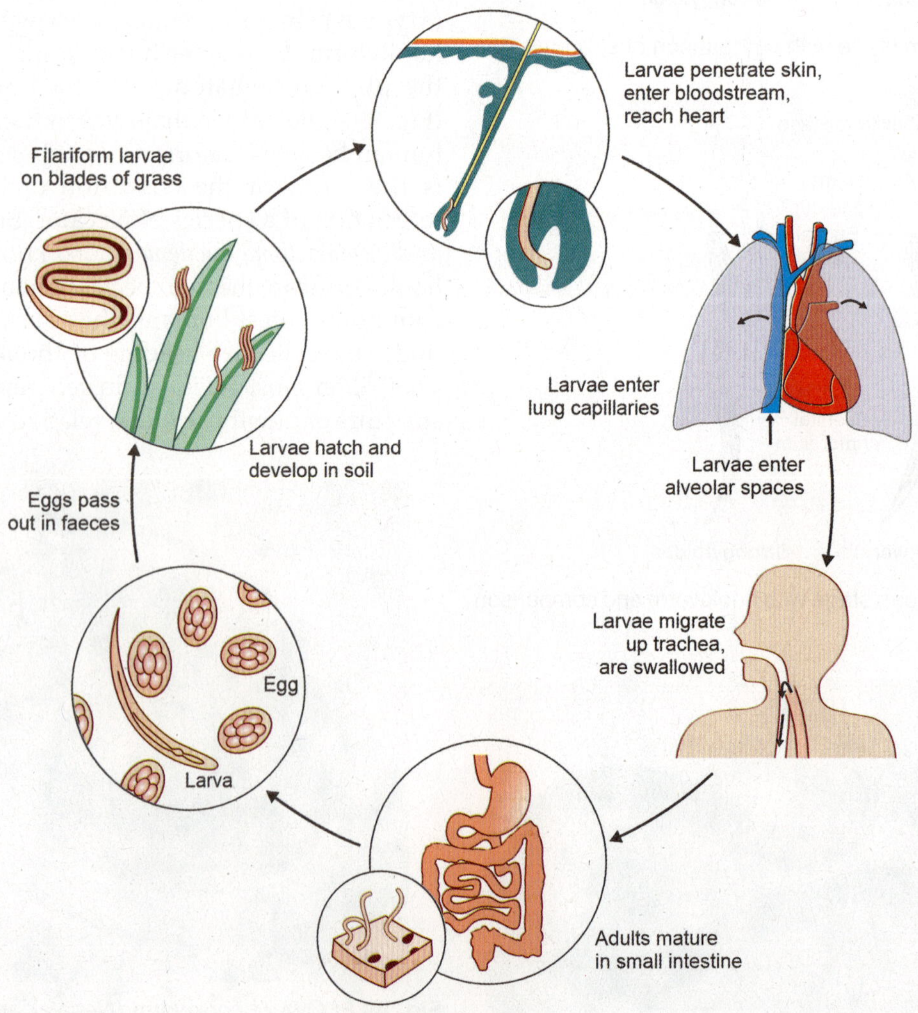

Fig. 49.6: Life cycle: Hookworm

migration through the lungs, the adults produce severe anaemia, usually of microcytic hypochromic type.

Clinical importance: Whether hookworm infestation, manifests as hookworm disease, depends on 3 factors.

No. of worms present:	*A. duodenale*	*N. americanus*
5	Asymptomatic	
25	Mild symptoms	Asymptomatic
25–100	Moderate symptoms	Mild symptoms
100–500		Moderate symptoms
100–1000	Severe symptoms	Severe symptoms
1000	Fatal	Fatal

Thus, *A. duodenale* infection is in general more severe in comparison to *N. americanus* infection. This is because while one *N. americanus* sucks 0.03 ml blood/day; one *A. duodenale* sucks 0.15 ml blood/day, i.e. 5 times more.

A. Symptoms during Cutaneous Phase

This phase is symptomatic only if there is secondary *bacterial infection*; when urticarial rash results in ground itch. One thing that must be discussed here is:

Cutaneous larva migrans or creeping eruption: It is caused when animal invading strains or species of hookworm invade human beings (caused by *A. braziliense* and *A. connum*). After penetrating the superficial layers, they are incapable of penetrating stratum germinativum. So, they begin an aimless wondering leaving a red, itchy, scaly wound that usually gets infected.

B. Symptoms during Pulmonary Phase

It is usually asymptomatic, though there may be some amount of dry cough and sore throat.

C. Intestinal Phase

It is the most important clinical phase because juvenile after attaching themselves to intestinal mucosa, begin to feed on blood up to 200 ml of blood may be lost daily in severe infections.

Additional symptoms of heavy infection are

1. Dry skin and hair
2. Oedema and potbelly in children (due to protein deficiency).
3. Mental dullness
4. Even heart failure

Hookworm anaemia is usually a microcytic hypochromic anaemia, severity depending on worm load and dietary iron intake.

I. A moderate infection manifests as

1. Iron deficiency anaemia
2. Slight, intermittent abdominal pain
3. Loss of normal appetite
4. Desire to eat soil.

Diagnostics

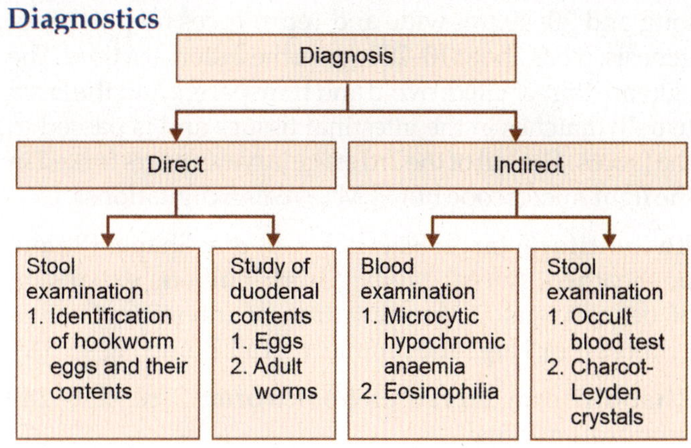

Laboratory Diagnosis

- **Direct methods**
  - *Stool examination:* To find the adult worm or characteristic hookworm eggs.
  - *Stool concentration:* Required to detect light infections.
  - *Larva:* Seen if stool is kept at room temperature after 24 hours (not preserved).

Diagnosis: Identify the eggs in the faeces

- All hookworm eggs look the same so cannot ID species
- Eggs are ovoid with thin, smooth eggshell.
- Internally, eggs are always early in mitosis—contain 2–16 cells.
- Size: 55–75 µm × 35–40 µm (Fig. 49.7)

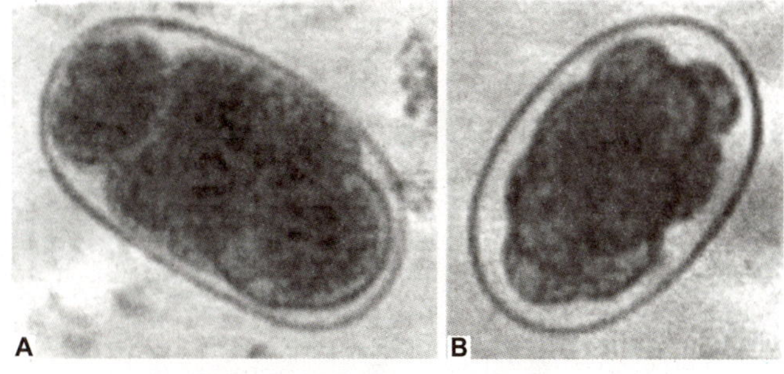

Fig. 49.7: (A) Eggs of *A. duodenale*; (B) Egg of *N. americanus* (*see also* Figs 49.4 and 49.5)

Strongyloides stercoralis (Threadworm)

It is a curious organism capable of free living as well as living as a parasite. It has a worldwide distribution in the tropics and temperate climates. Free living forms exist mostly in the moist tropics. They are not common in India.

Geographical distribution: This is widely distributed in the tropical areas of Asia, Africa and South America. Recent reports from Poland indicate that infection can also spread in temperate regions.

S. stercoralis can persist for many years in man by autoinfection. Some Australians are still carrying infections from World War II.

Morphology: The adult parasitic female resides in the mucosa of the small intestine and is about 2.7 mm long and 30–40 µm wide and reproduces by parthenogenesis. It has about 10–20 eggs in the 2 uteri at a time. The eggs are thin-shelled, ovoid and transparent and the larva usually hatches in the intestinal tissues and is passed in the faeces. The tail of the 3rd stage larva appears forked in the light microscope but SEM reveals 6 digitations.

Rhabditiform larva: Size: 225 × 18 µm; Shape: Plump, unsheathed; Buccal cavity: Short; Bulbous expansion of oesophagus at the transition of intestine; Genital primordium: Large and prominent; Tail: Blunt (Fig. 49.8A).

Rhabditiform larvae of hookworm: Size: 250–280 primordium: Small.

Filariform larva: Size: 550 × 20 µm: Shape: Long, slender, gracile, unsheathed; Oesophagus: 1/2 of body length with no bulbous expansion; Tail: Forked or blunt (Fig. 49.8B).

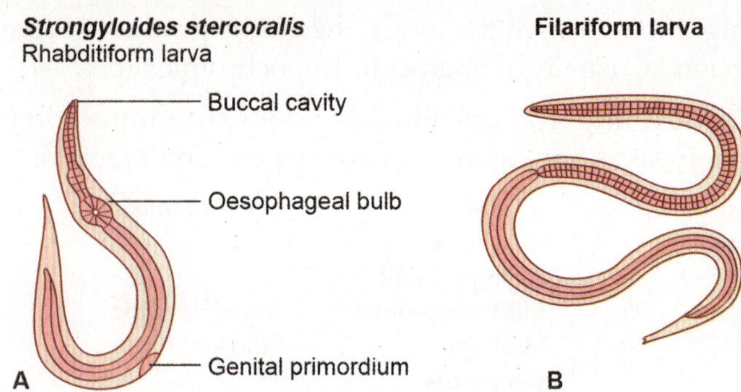

Fig. 49.8: (A) *Strongyloides stercoralis*—rhabditiform larvae; (B) *Strongyloides stercoralis*—filariform larvae

Life cycle of *Strongyloides stercoralis* (Fig. 49.9A and B)

Life cycle: The parasite shows 3 different modes of development: Indirect development, direct development

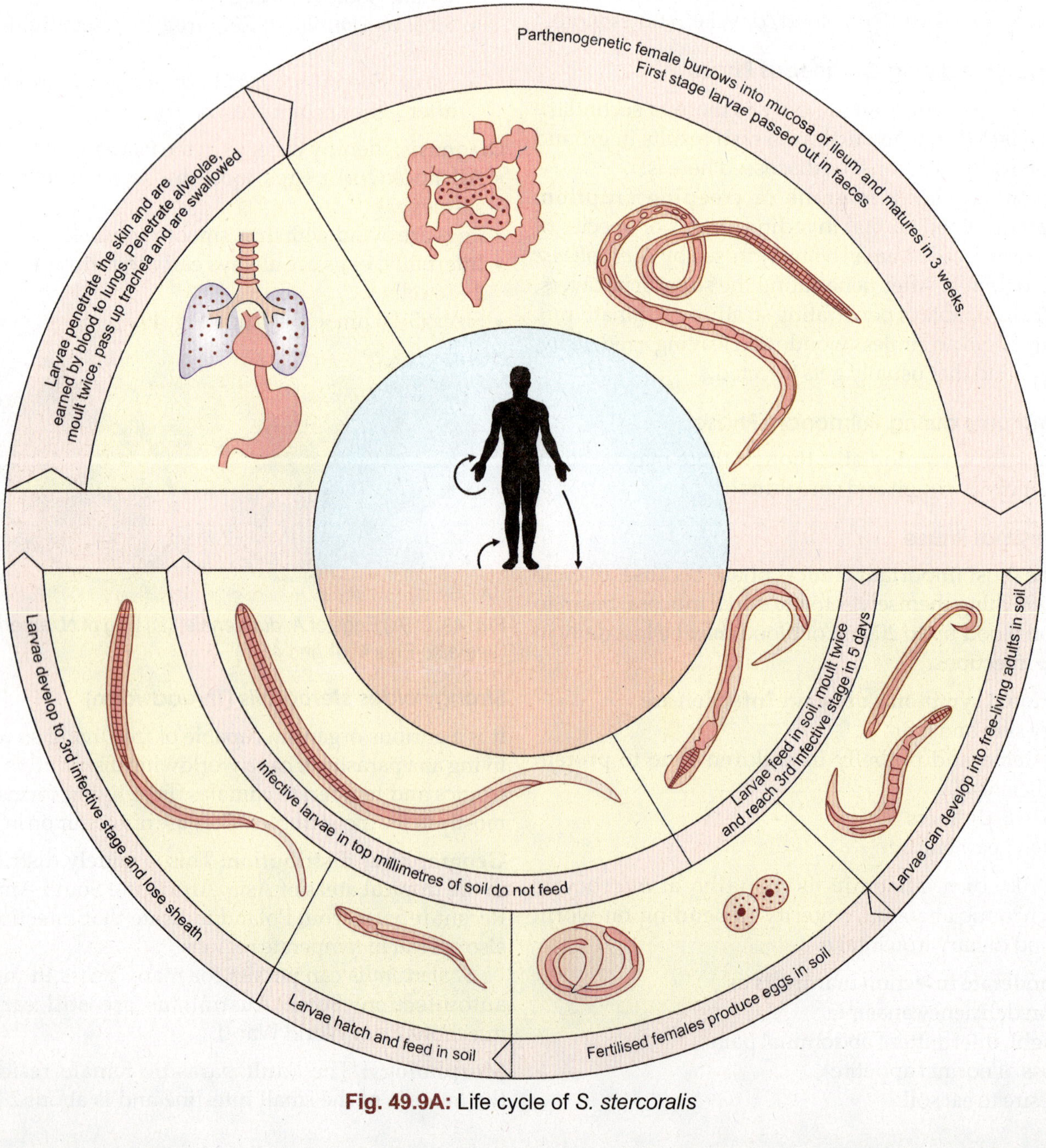

Fig. 49.9A: Life cycle of *S. stercoralis*

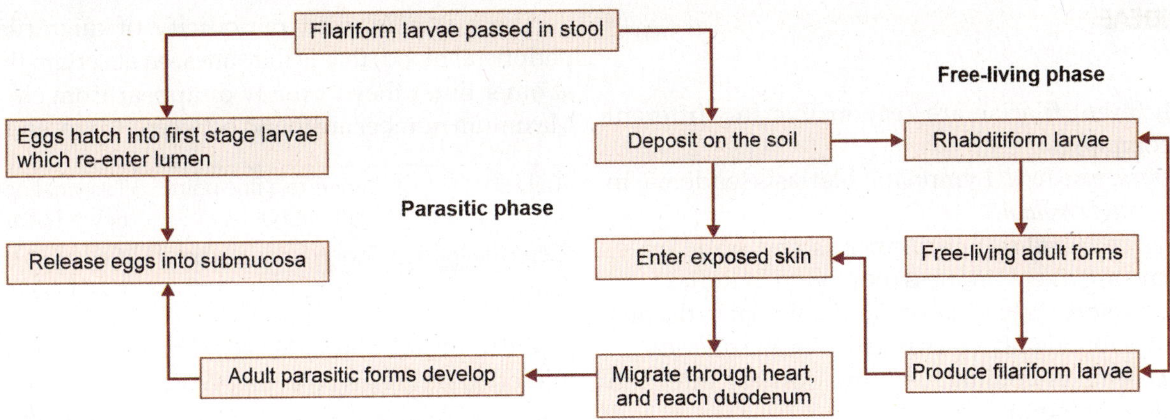

Fig. 49.9B: Life cycle of *S. stercoralis*

and autoinfection (Fig. 49.9). Indirect development occurs in the external environment where the free-living adults produce eggs, rhabditiform larvae and filariform larvae. The filariform larvae can penetrate the skin, enter the circulation, pass through the lungs and can be swallowed to become adult females in the intestinal tissues. The rhabditiform larvae passed in the faeces can undergo direct development to become filariform larvae without developing into adults. Autoinfection occurs when rhabditiform larvae become filariform larvae in the host tissues and penetrate the intestine or perianal skin to undergo the same cycle of development. Autoinfection leads to a continuous build-up of the worm burden.

Clinical aspects: Skin reactions, often seen at the site of entry of larvae, which occur as rash and pruritus. There may be pneumonitis during larval migration and intestinal symptoms on maturation. The intestinal symptoms consist of epigastric pain, diarrhoea, flatulence and vomiting. The gluteal region may show dermatitis indicating that autoinfection is taking place.

Diagnosis: Best means of diagnosis is demonstration of filariform larvae in fresh stools. Larvae are 490–630 μm long and 9 μm in breadth and possess a cylindrical oesophagus (Fig. 49.10).

Duodenal intubation and examination of aspirates, or a string test (enterotest) and examination of intestinal mucus, is recommended in suspected cases, even when serial stool examinations are negative. A number of reliable serology tests are also available to aid in the diagnosis of strongyloidiasis.

Larval stages of *S. stercoralis* must be distinguished from hookworm larvae. The rhabditiform larvae resemble those of hookworms but can be distinguished by the shorter buccal capsule and larger genital primordium. The filariform larvae also resemble those of hookworms, but the tail is notched and the esophagus is about one-half the length of the body (*see* Fig. 49.2A and B).

Clinical importance: Clinical manifestations of strongyloidiasis are:

1. Watery mucous diarrhoea (occasionally alternating with constipation)
2. Fat malabsorption cause steatorrhoea
3. Vitamin B_{12} deficiency
4. Eosinophilia with cough and dyspnoea
5. Skin rashes, etc.

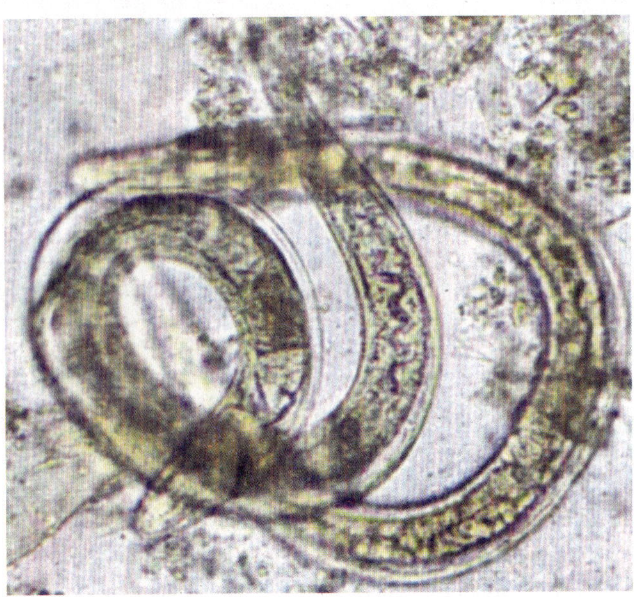

Fig. 49.10: Filariform larvae passed in the stool

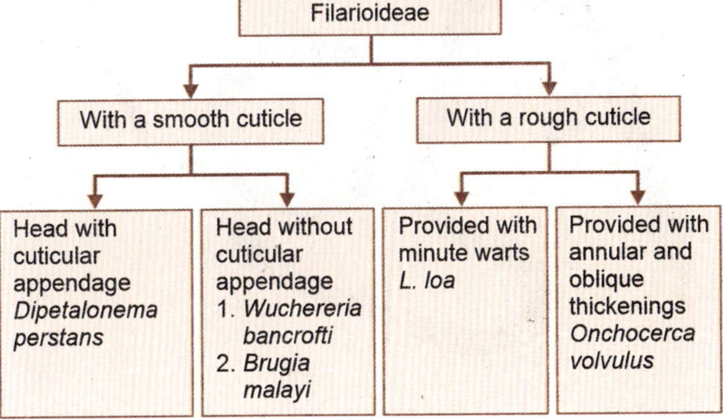

FILARIOIDEAE

Filaria

These different filariae are responsible for different disease complexes.

- *Wuchereria bancrofti:* Lymphatic filariasis (endemic in India), *Brugia malayi*.
- *Onchocerca volvulus:* Subcutaneous and optic infections causing river blindness (not found in India) .
- *Dipetalonema perstans*—causes illness similar to the first two but is found only in Africa and South America.
- *Loa loa*—causes conjunctival and corneal infection (not found in India).

Therefore, we will limit our discussion to *Wuchereria bancrofti* and *Brugia malayi*.

1. Bancroftian filariasis is widespread in the world, particularly in Asia, Africa, and parts of south America. In India, it is endemic along sea coasts and the big river systems.
2. *Brugia malayi* is indigenous primarily in Asia. In India, it has been seen in Kerala, Odisha, Madhya Pradesh and Assam.

Habitat

- Adult worm—lymphatic system
- Microfilariae—in blood

Morphology: Here we will discuss the morphology of adult worms. That of microfilaria will be discussed under the diagnosis of filariasis.

Feature	*W. bancrofti*	*B. malayi*
1. Size	Female 60–100 mm long Male 40 mm long (about 250–300 µm wide) (both the species are cuticular)	Half the size of *W. bancrofti*
2. Papillae	2 circles of well-defined post-anal papillae	3–4 pairs of post-anal papillae

The tail of both worms is finger-like and curved ventrally. Differences are more pronounced in the microfilaria (Fig. 49.11).

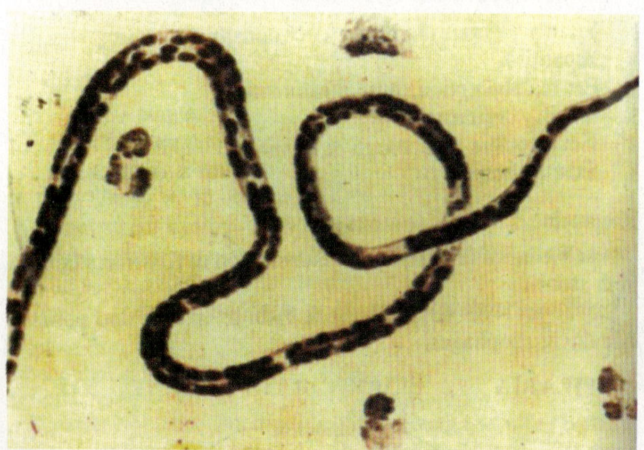

Fig. 49.11: Microfilaria in peripheral blood smear

There is a marked periodicity of microfilariae in peripheral blood, that is they are seen at certain times and at other times they virtually disappear from circulation. Maximum number are found between 10 p.m. and 2 a.m.

Tail	Tapers to a fine point contains nuclei	Terminal portion devoid of nuclei
Cephalic space	Twice as long as broad	As long as broad
Sheath	Well stained	Hardly visible

Differential characteristics of various species in microfilariae are given in Fig. 49.12.

Life cycle: (Fig. 49.13).

Pathogenesis and stages of filarial infection (Fig. 49.14).

Filariasis

Filariasis is an infectious disease that spreads through mosquito bites. Some people have no symptoms. Others may have inflammation, swelling or fever. Filariasis can lead to lymphoedema (fluid retention) or hydrocoele (swelling in the scrotum).

Clinical Importance

1. **Incubation phase:** Period between infection and appearance of microfilariae (mf) in the blood. It is largely asymptomatic but there may be:
   1. Mild fever
   2. Malaise
2. **Acute phase:** This starts when females reach maturity and start releasing microfilaria. There is intense inflammation, usually in the lower half of the body, symptoms include:
   a. Chills especially at midnight
   b. Fever with midnight rise
   c. Tender, inflamed inguinal lymph nodes
   d. There may be orchitis (testicular inflammation)
   e. Epididymitis.
   Acute febrile episode of elephantoid fever recur frequently
   a. Sudden onset of rigors
   b. Fever (up to 104°F)
   c. Sweating and lysis of fever
   It recurs periodically after a few days.
   - Serous cavity filariasis is caused by the worms *Mansonella perstans* and *Mansonella ozzardi*, which occupy the serous cavity of the abdomen.
   - The adult worms, which usually stay in one tissue, release early larval forms known as microfilariae into the person's blood. These circulating microfilariae can be taken up during a blood meal by an insect vector; in the vector, they develop into infective larvae that can be spread to another person.
3. **Obstructive phase:** It is caused by obstruction of lymphatics by adult worms and are marked by chronic inflammatory reaction. It is characterised by:

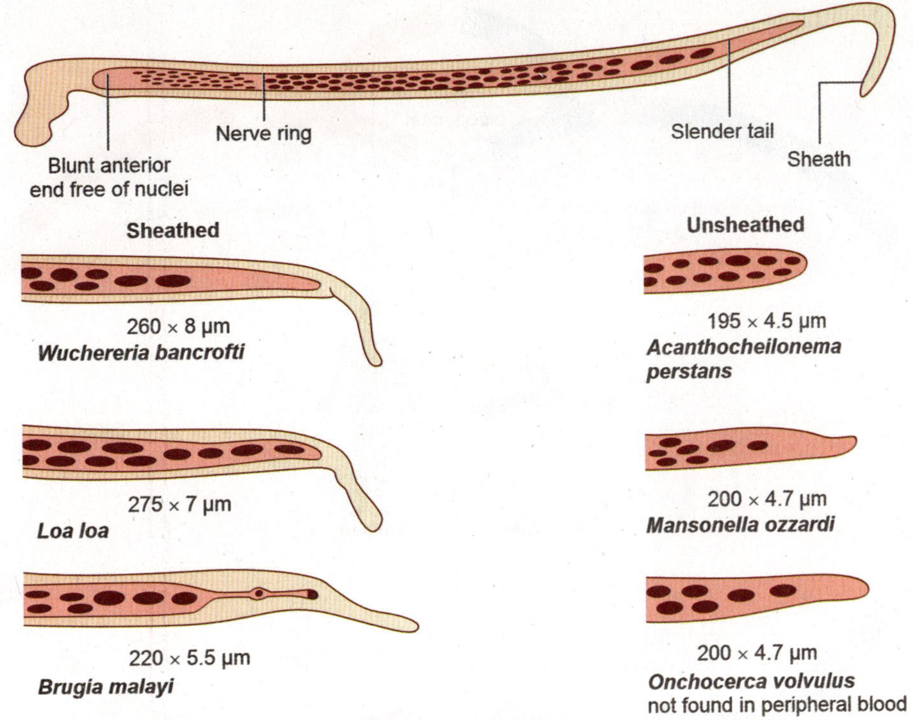

Fig. 49.12: Differential characteristics of microfilariae

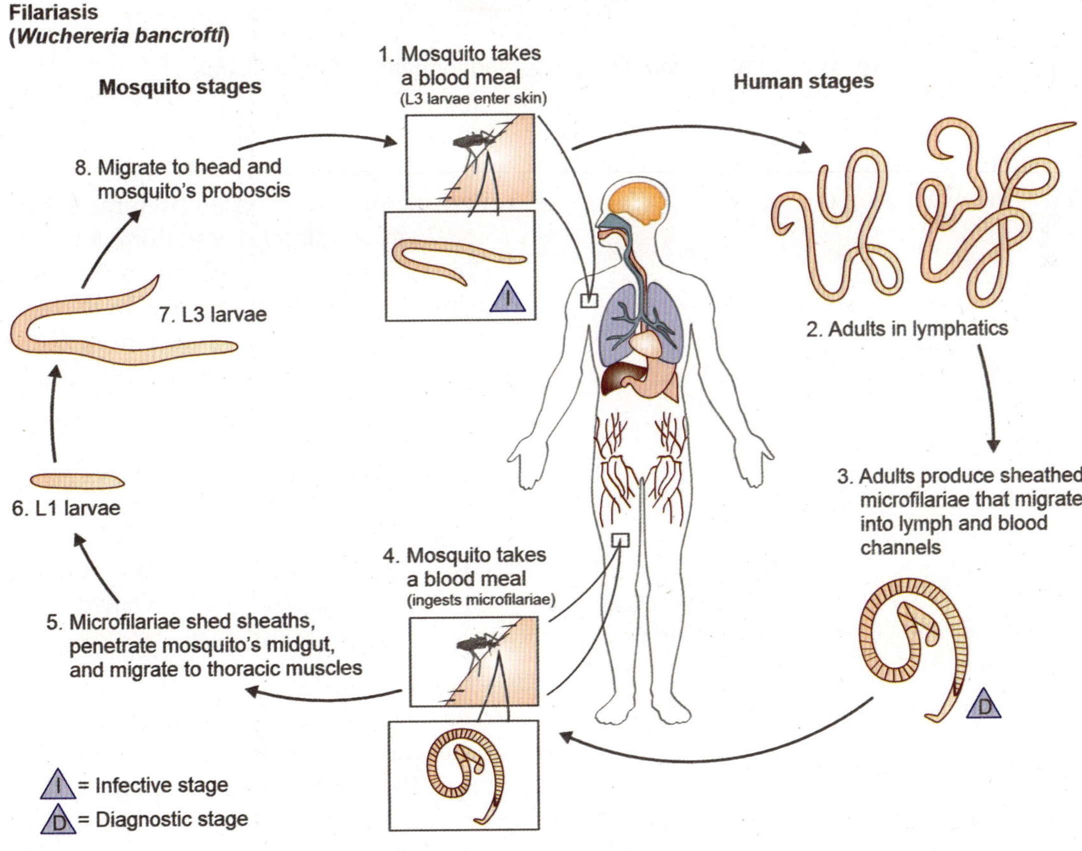

Fig. 49.13: Life cycle

a. Lymph varices
b. Chyluria
c. Hydrocele

4. **Elephantiasis**
   - Swelling of limbs and genitalia
   - *Male:* Enlargement of scrotum, penis retracted under skin, spermatic cords thickened.

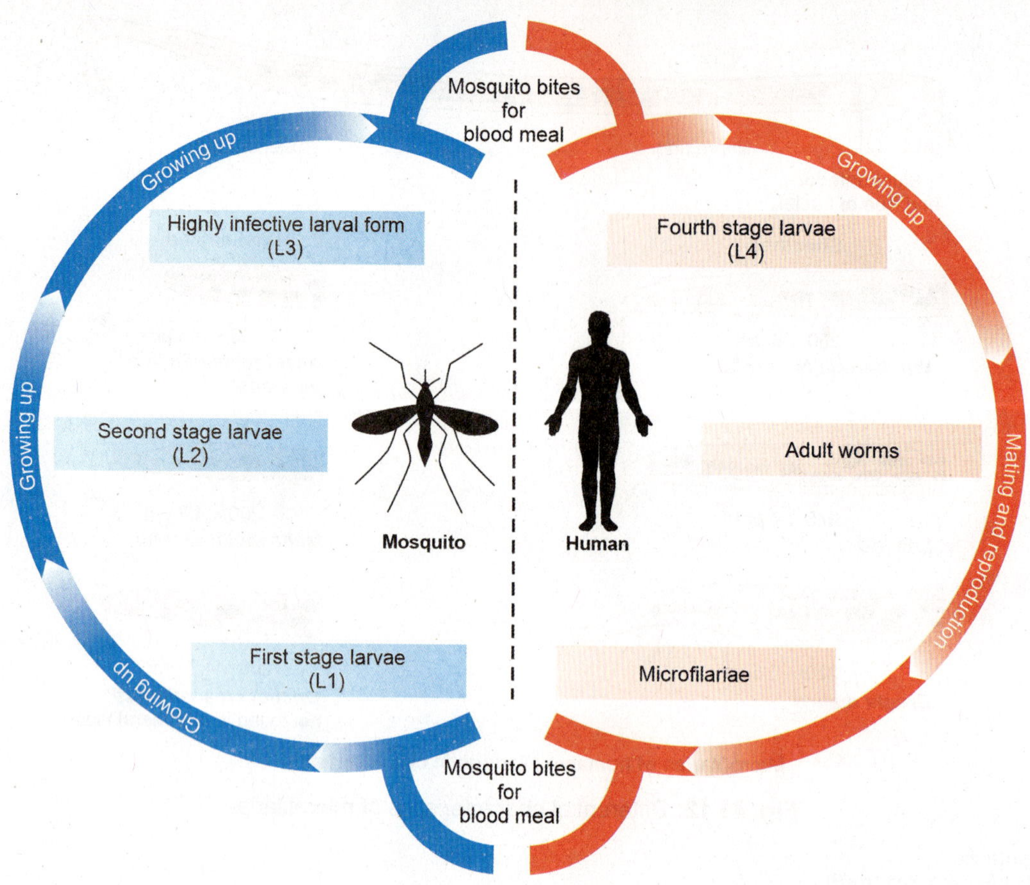

Fig. 49.14: Various stages L_1 to L_4 and formation of microfilariae

- *Female:* Long tumorous mass covered by thickened ulcerated skin develops on the vulva.

Diagnosis

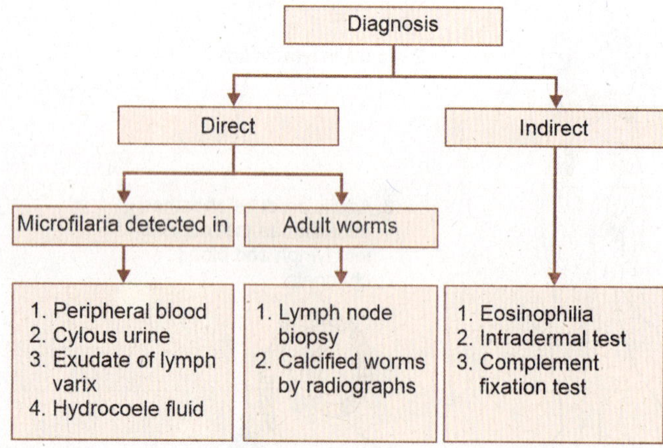

Detecting Microfilaria in Blood

Diethylcarbamazine provocative test: Nocturnally periodic microfilariae may be demonstrated in the blood at any time of the day by giving 100 mg diethylcarbamazine and taking blood 45 minutes later. (Administration of 4–6 mg/kg with examination at 30–60 minutes for *W. bancrofti*, 90 minutes for *B. malayi*. It is of no use in subperiodic filariasis.)

Can be detected by many techniques:

1. Peripheral smears taken preferably between 10 pm and 2 am and stained with Romanowsky stains.
2. Put 0.25 ml of fresh blood in 0.5 ml of 3% acetic acid. Then smears are made. In these preparations, microfilaria appears as transparent fibrils.

Characteristics as seen by Romanowsky stains

	Microfilaria malayi	Mf. bancrofti
General	Minor angulations besides 4–5 major curves	Shows 3–4 major curves with a graceful appearance
Nucleus	Blurred and intermingled	Well-defined and spaced. Quite discrete

Individuals infected by filarial worms may be described as either "microfilaraemic" or "amicrofilaraemic", depending on whether microfilariae can be found in their peripheral blood. Filariasis is diagnosed in microfilaraemic cases primarily through direct observation of microfilariae in the peripheral blood. Occult filariasis is diagnosed in amicrofilaraemic cases based on clinical observations and, in some cases, by finding a circulating antigen in the blood.

A diagrammatic sketch of *W. bancrofti* is shown in Fig. 49.15, also *see* Fig. 49.11, microfilariae in peripheral blood.

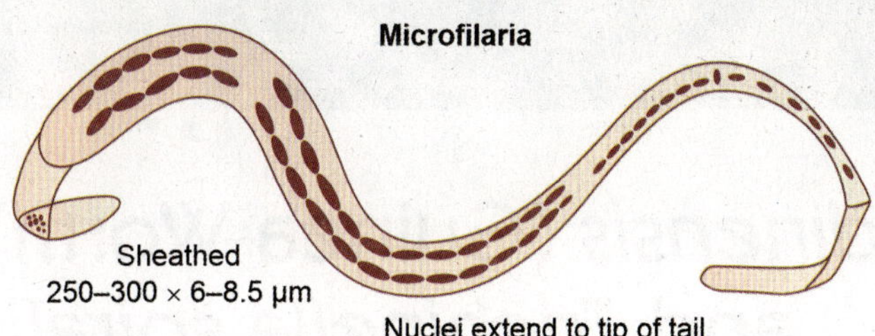

Fig. 49.15: Sketch diagram of microfilariae (labelled)

Prevention and Control

The best way to prevent filariasis is to avoid mosquito bites, particularly in tropical areas.

- Sleep under a mosquito net.
- Use insect repellent on exposed skin, especially at night.
- Wear long pants and long sleeves.
- Using bed nets while sleeping.
- Applying repellent creams on skin.

Chapter 50

Dracunculus medinensis (Guinea Worm) and *Trichinella spiralis*

Chapter Outline

- *Dracunculus medinensis*: Guinea Worm Disease (GWD)
- Habitat
- Classification
- Morphology
- Life Cycle of *Dracunculus medinensis*
- Clinical Manifestation
- *Trichinella spiralis*
- Habit and Habitat

DRACUNCULUS MEDINENSIS: GUINEA WORM DISEASE (GWD)

Introduction

Dracunculiasis, also known as guinea worm disease (GWD), is an infection caused by the parasite *Dracunculus medinensis*. A parasite is an organism that feeds off another organism to survive. GWD is spread by drinking water containing guinea worm larvae.

Guinea worm is on target to be the second infectious disease of humans to be eradicated, after smallpox. It was formerly endemic to a wide swath of Africa and Eurasia; as of 2021, it remains endemic in five countries: Chad, Ethiopia, Mali, South Sudan and Angola, with most cases in Chad and Ethiopia. Guinea worm spreads to Angola in 2018, and it is now considered endemic there. Infection of domestic dogs is a serious complication in Chad.

The common name "guinea worm" is derived from the guinea region of Western Africa.

Dracunculus medinensis is among the longest nematodes affecting humans. It is also known as guinea worm, Medina worm, serpent worm or dragon worm.

It causes dracunculiasis or dracontiasis, a nodular dermatosis produced by the development of Dracunculus parasite in the subcutaneous tissue.

Habitat

The adult females inhabit the subcutaneous tissue usually of the foot or lower limbs.

Less frequently they also inhabit other parts of the body including the head and neck.

The guinea worm is found predominantly in Africa from Senegal (west) to Ethiopia (east).

Also found in India, Pakistan, Saudi Arabia, and Yemen.

Inhabits freshwater lakes and rivers.

Classification

Phylum: Nematoda
Class: Chromadorea
Chromadoria
Rhabditida
Spirurina
Dracunculoidea
Family: Dracunculidae

Morphology

Adult Worms

Male: Male worms are difficult to demonstrate as they are immediately after fertilizing the females. Hence, it has not yet been recovered from man.

The male measures 12–30 mm in length and 0.4 mm in breadth.

Female: It is slender long worm and is one of the longest nematodes known to cause infection in man.

It measures 60 cm to 1 mm or more in length and 1.5 to 1.7 mm in diameter, resembling a piece of long twine thread.

The body is cylindrical, smooth and milk white in colour.

The posterior end is extremely tapering and is bent to form a hook.

A minute triangular mouth is present in an anterior end.

An inner layer of 4–6 papillae and outer layer of 4 pairs of papillae surrounded the mouth.

Female worm is of the thickness of a knitting needle. Body is cylindrical, white and smooth. Tail is pointed, forming a blunt hook. Head is rounded, terminating in a thickened cuticle cap or cephalic shield mouth is triangular, small and surrounded by 6 papillae and an outer circle of 4 double papillae. Whole worms occupied by a double uterus filled with empryos.

A pair of uteri, oviducts and tubules and a single unpaired vagina constitutes the female genital tract.

The worm is ovoviviparous and discharge embryos in successive batches for a period of about 3 weeks until the gravid female completely implies its uterine contents.

The body fluid is toxic and causes a bluster if female escapes into the tissue. The life span of female is about 1 year and that of the male is not more than 6 months.

After 100 days of infection the adult female fertilized sexually, then male die, then female migrates to subcutaneous tissue.

After a year of infection, females cause blister in skin, mostly in lower limbs, where they produce thousands of larvae when host contact water (Fig. 50.1).

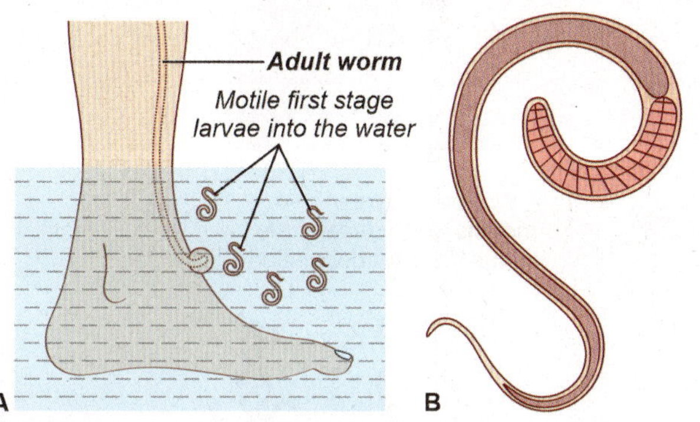

Fig. 50.1: (A) Adult worm liberating first stage larvae into water; (B) First stage larvae, hook structure

Life Cycle of *Dracunculus medinensis*

Life cycle is completed in two hosts:

- *Definitive host:* Human
- *Intermediate host:* Cyclops and other twelve species.

Entrance into man and development into adult worms:

- Man acquires infections by drinking unfiltered water containing infected cyclops.
- On reaching the stomach, the cyclopses are digested by the gastric juices and L_3 larvae are liberated.

Life cycle (Fig. 50.2):

Entrance into man and development into adult worms

- Man acquires infections by drinking unfiltered water containing infected cyclops.
- On reaching the stomach, the cyclopses are digested by the gastric juices and L_3 larvae are liberated.
- The larvae penetrated the gut wall and enter the retroperitoneal connective tissue where they grow and become sexually mature.
- The males die after fertilizing the females and disappear within 6 months of infection.
- The gravid female migrates and selects those parts of the skin labile to come in contact with water such as the backs of water carriers, anus and legs of washerman and legs of those who fill water in containers in 'step wells' and ponds.

First Stage Larva

- It is unsheathed and coiled with a round anterior end and a long slender filariform tail.
- It is large, measuring 650–750 mm in length and 17–20 mm in breadth.
- The cuticle is conspicuously striated.
- It moves about with a shift motion, briskly coiling and uncoiling body.
- It shows a tad-pole like movement in water.
- These larvae are set-free only at the time of partition when the affected part is submerged in water.
- Further development proceeds in the body of a minute fresh water crustacean of the genus Cylops.
- On reaching the skin surface, it secretes a toxin, producing a blister which later ruptures and forms an ulcer, contact with water stimulates the worm to protrude its head through the center of the ulcer and causes a reflex discharge of a milky fluid containing a large number of first stage rhabditiform larva.

Development of Larva in Cyclops

- The larva discharged in water swims vigorously in water with tad-pole like movement.
- These larvae further develop when ingested by suitable *Cyclops* species.
- In the body cavity of Cyclops, the first stage larva moults twice to develop into third stage larva, the infection from the parasite.
- These infected Cyclops have short life span than normal non-infected ones.

Third Stage Larva

- It is the infective stage of the parasite.
- It is found in the body cavity of Cyclops.
- The larvae are ingested by the copepod crustacea, Cyclops, which actively chase them. Once ingested, the larvae mature into their infective stage in approximately 14 days and can then reinfect humans.
- After mating inside the definitive (human) host, the female burrows through the skin, creating an ulcerated area, usually in a lower part of the host's anatomy.
- When the ulcerated area is exposed to water (as in a river or lake), the female's uterus ruptures, releasing many juveniles into the water (Fig. 50.3).

Feeding

Dracunculus medinensis is parasitic, feeding on the blood of its vertebrate host.

The male worm dies shortly after mating, and the female matures over the subsequent 10–14 months, slowly migrates to the surface of the body and emerges through the skin. When affected body parts are submerged in water, the female worm releases larvae, which are ingested by copepods, thus completing the life cycle.

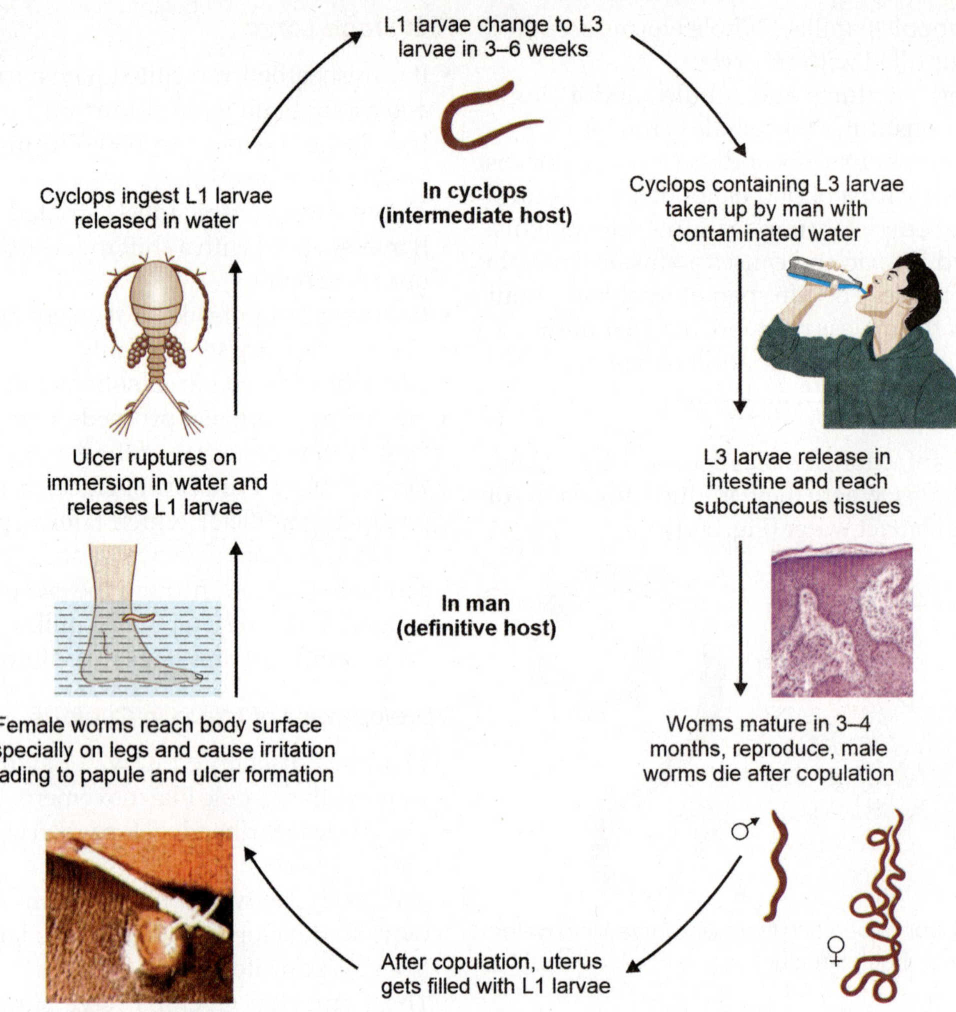

Fig. 50.2: Life cycle of *Dracunculus medinensis*. L_1 larvae change to L_3

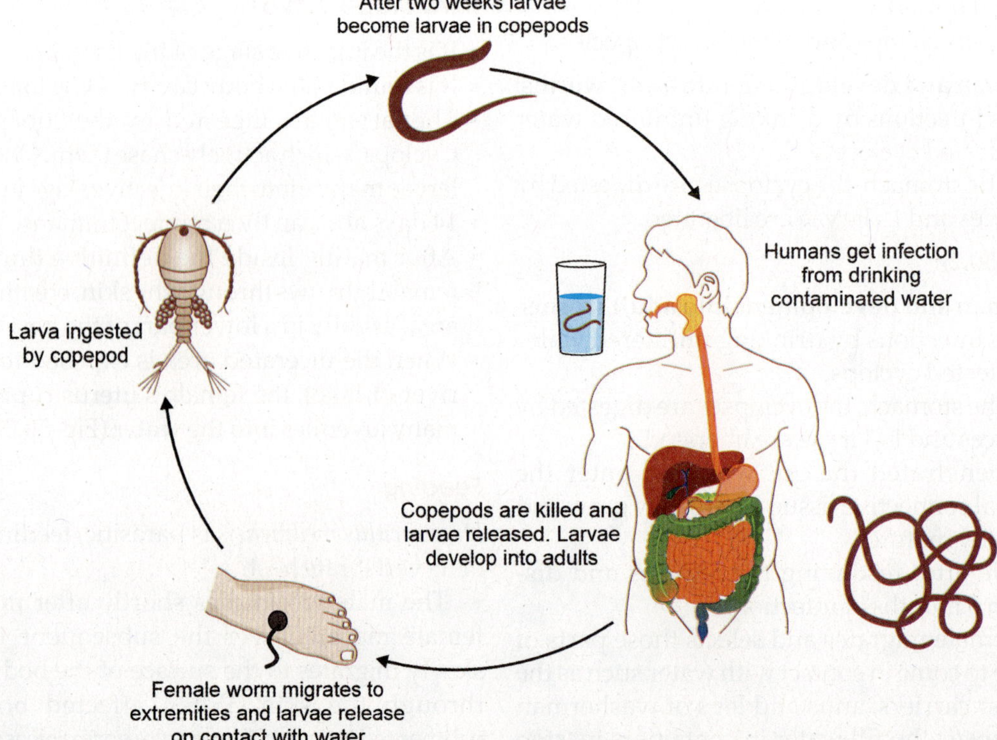

Fig. 50.3: Life cycle of *D. medinensis*, larvae release on contact with water, larvae develop in copepod and develops

Pathogenesis and Pathology

- The third stage larva is not pathogenesis and does not produce any pathological lesions.
- Only female adult worm is pathogenic.
- It produces a toxin, forming blister which is formed at the site at which the female worm comes out of the surface of the skin on coming contact with water.
- The blister is filled with the fluid which is bacteriologically sterile and contains numerous larvae and leucocytes.
- Diffusible toxins produced by the parasite are believed to cause urticaria, dyspnoea, vomiting, mild fever and occasional fainting.
- Blister formation is accompanied by intense burning pain, fiery serpent.
- This may be accompanied by generalised reactions such as urticaria, nausea, vomiting, diarrhoea and giddiness and marked burning sensation over the next few days, the lesion vesiculates and blister ruptures producing a painful ulcer.
- The worm is often visible in the opening of ulcer.
- If the female worms break during the attempts of extractions the larva remains trapped in the subcutaneous tissue and may give rise to cellulitis and abscesses.
- If the female worms break during the attempts of extractions the larva remain trapped in the subcutaneous tissue and may give rise to cellulitis and abscesses.
- In uncomplicated cases, lesions may only last for several weeks until the worm is completely expelled.
- However, many cases infection of the worm track with persistence of the lesions, chronic ulceration and possible sequelae, involving disseminated infection, phlegma of limbs, contractures of tendons, fibrous ankylosis or arthritis in the joints, die prematurely and calcify. The calcified worms can be triggered arthritis, locked joints or permanent clipping and deformations.

Clinical Manifestations

- The pre-patent period is 10–14 months.
- The symptoms are manifested during parturition of the female and are due to the liberation of a toxic substance causing allergic manifestation and blister formation.
- Septic infection can occur as a result of contamination by secondary organisms drawn in by the worm at the time of retraction.
- Blister formation appears wherever the female worms make an attempt to come to the surface of the body where it can readily discharge its larva.
- The blister is usually found on the lower extremities of the body especially between the metatarsal bones, sole of the feet or on the ankle and less frequently in arms, buttock, scrotum.
- The death of the worm causes the formation of an abscess which, when secondarily infected, results in cellulitis and local blistering of the skin.
- Aseptic abscesses and cystic swelling can also occur when worms rupture before emerging, causing an acute inflammatory response from the host's immune system.
- Also, chills, fever and local painful swellings commonly precede the emergence of the worm. *D. medinensis* has also been found coiled in the hernial sac and in the placenta, causing bleeding in pregnancy.

Clinical Importance

At onset of migration to subcut tissue and skin of limbs, there may be an allergic reaction, Characterised by:

1. A rash
2. Nausea and vomiting
3. Dizziness
4. Localized oedema

Worms remain under skin for a month before a reddish papule develops. This rapidly becomes a blister. Feet and legs are the commonest site of blisters. On rupture of blister the allergic reactions subside. A tiny hole remains through which the worm protrudes; when expelled, complete healing occurs. Secondary bacterial infection may ensue and lead to a host of complications including tetanus, abscesses, etc.

Laboratory diagnosis: It depends on:

1. **Detection** of adult worm on the skin.
2. **Detection of embryos**: Bathe the affected part in water. Now, mount the water on a side and observe under microscope.

Detection of adult worms: This is possible when the female worm appears at the surface of the skin.

Detection of first stage larva

- Specific diagnosis is made by the microscopic demonstration of the first stage larva in the discharge fluid.
- Dracunculiasis is usually diagnosed simply by seeing the worm exit the body through the blister on the skin. Once the worm is completely removed from the skin, the worm and its larvae can be examined under a microscope to ensure it is a *D. medinensis* worm.

TRICHINELLA SPIRALIS

Introduction

Trichinella spiralis which causes trichinosis was first observed in 1821 in the muscles of a patient at autopsy by James Paget. Richard Owen in 1835 described the encysted larval form in muscles and named it Trichina spiralis. Virchow discovered its life cycle in 1859. Name *Trichinella spiralis* was given by Raillet in 1895. (*Trichos*—hair, *ella*—dimunitive, spiralis refers to the spirally coiled appearance of larvae in muscles.) It occurs in humans both as an adult in the intestine and as a larva in the tissues (usually muscles).

Trichinellosis, also called trichinosis, results from roundworms (nematodes) from the genus Trichinella. It is a parasitic infection. It is caused by consuming undercooked or raw meat (usually pork). *Trichinella spiralis* is the common cause of human disease by eating raw or undercooked pork. Other mammals like wild carnivores and horses can be reservoirs of infection.

Habit and Habitat

Habitat

Human skeletal muscle

Nematode parasite, occurring in rodents, pigs, bears, hyenas and humans, and is responsible for the disease trichinosis. It is sometimes referred to as the "pork worm" due to it being typically encountered in undercooked pork products. It should not be confused with the distantly related pork tapeworm.

It is the widespread organism in the world. It is less common in tropical regions but is well known in Mexico, South America, Southern Asia and Middle East.

Morphology

- **Adult worms:** Males are 1.4–1.6 mm long and are more slender anteriorly than at posterior end. Anus terminal and has a large papilla on each side.
- **Females** are 2.6–3.4 mm long. They also taper anteriorly. Anus is nearly terminal. Vulva is located about the middle.
- **Larvae:** Measure 100 µm × 6 µm. They remain encysted in adult worms remain buried in the duodenal or jejunal mucosa of pig, rat and human. The encysted larvae are present in the striated muscles of these hosts (Fig. 50.4A) due to the fertilised females discharging embryos into the circulating blood and reaching the muscles where they ultimately remain encysted (Fig. 50.4B). Inside the cysts, larvae continue to grow and become 1 mm, which is the infective stage. However, when encysted in human skeletal muscle, they reach a dead end and are calcified.

Female Trichinella worms live for about six weeks, and in that time can produce up to 1,500 larvae; when a spent female dies, she passes out of the host. The larvae

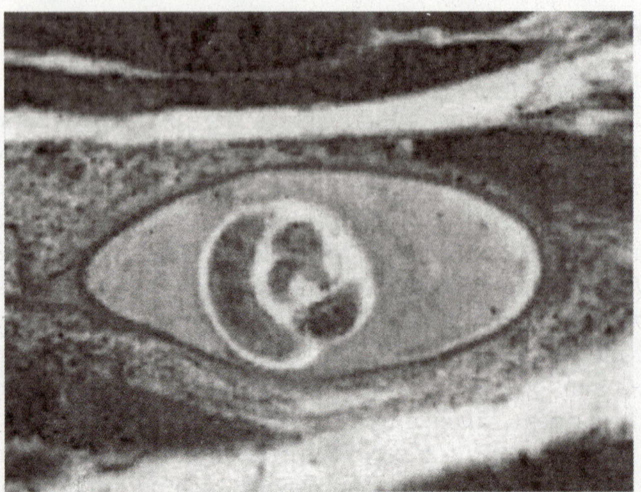

Fig. 50.4A: Encysted larvae in muscle tissue

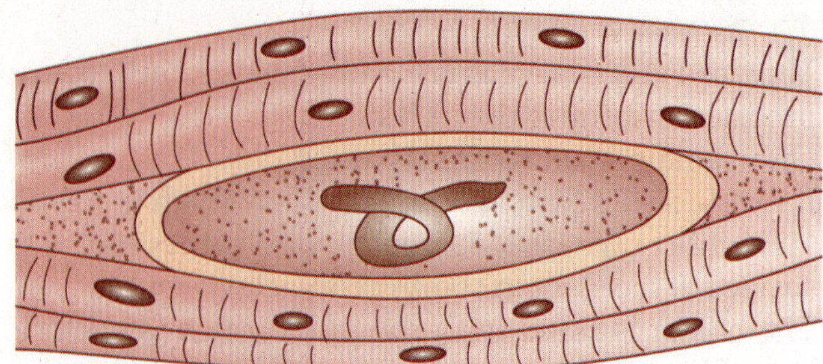

Fig. 50.4B: Diagrammatic representation of striated muscle showing encysted larvae

gain access to the circulation and migrate around the body of the host, in search of a muscle cell in which to encyst. The migration and encystment of larvae can cause fever and pain, brought on by the host inflammatory response. In some cases, accidental migration to specific organ tissues can cause myocarditis and encephalitis that can result in death.

Trichinella spiralis is the smallest known nematode parasite of humans. The males measure about 1.4 to 1.6 mm in length and the females are twice the size of the males. The body of the worm is more slender at the anterior then at the posterior end (Fig. 50.5).

Pathophysiology: Ingestion of undercooked or raw meat from domestic or sylvatic animals containing encysted larvae of *Trichinella* species can lead to Trichinellosis. *T. spiralis* results from the consumption of inadequately cooked or raw pork from domestic pigs.

Clinical importance: Symptoms are diverse and may include generalized fever, abdominal pain, diarrhoea, nausea, vomiting, or myalgias.

Can be studied under three headings:

1. **Penetration of adult females into mucosa:** It results in:
   1. Intestinal pain
   2. Nausea and vomiting
   3. Diarrhoea
   4. Red blotches on skin
2. **Migration of larvae:** Migration of larvae usually damage small blood vessels with resultant localised oedema, particularly in face and hands. Wandering larvae may rarely cause any of the following:
   1. Pneumonitis
   2. Encephalitis
   3. Nephritis
   4. Eye damage (subconjunctival haemorrhage)
   5. Myocarditis
   6. Sublingual haemorrhage.
3. **Penetration and encystment in skeletal muscle:** It may cause:
   1. Intense muscular pain
   2. Swelling of masseters
   3. Nervous symptoms such as hallucinations

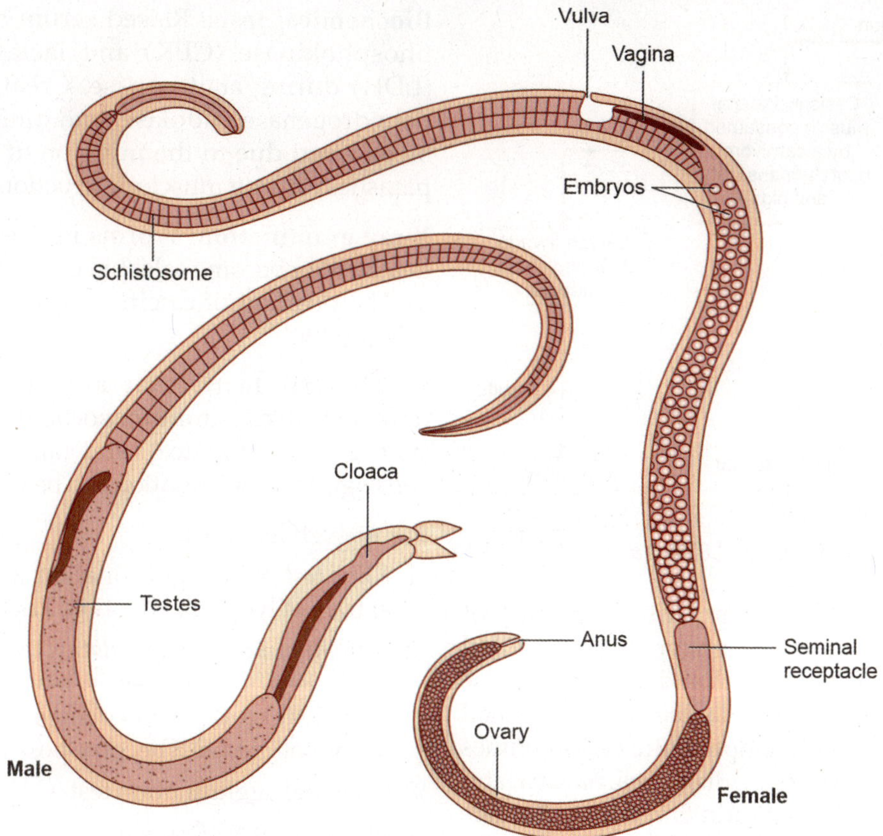

Fig. 50.5: *Trichinella spiralis:* Parasite of male and female

4. Difficulty in breathing and/or swallowing.
5. Extreme eosinophilia

Complications

- Myocarditis
- Pneumonitis
- Secondary bacterial pneumonia
- Nephritis
- Chronic diarrhoea
- Neurotrichinellosis

Life cycle: The life cycle (Fig. 50.6A and B) of trichinellosis divides into two stages: (1) Domestic cycle and (2) sylvatic cycle.

1. **Domestic cycle:** Affects domestic animals, particularly swine, rodents, and horses.
2. **Sylvatic cycle:** Affects wildlife like bear, wild boar, and moose.

The life cycle of *Trichinella spiralis* (**causing trichinosis or trichinellosis in human**)

Systemic (parenteral) phase: Larvae enter the lymphatic circulation and then into the blood, reaching skeletal muscles, myocardium, and brain which are high in oxygen content. This phase leads to systemic symptoms like fevers, myositis, myalgias, periorbital oedema and can even cause myocarditis and encephalitis.

The larvae provoke significant eosinophilia, especially in patients who develop cardiac and CNS dysfunction.

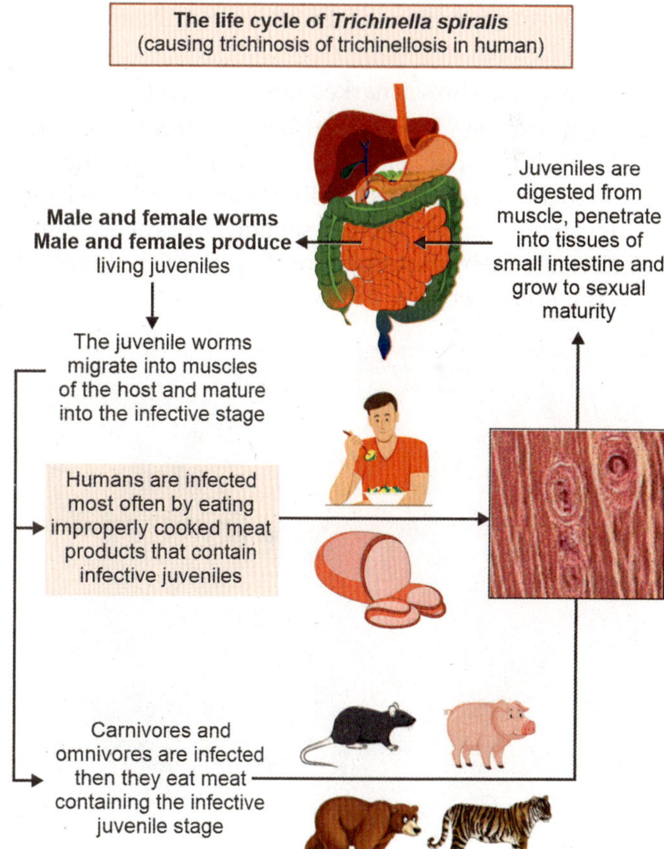

Fig. 50.6A: Life cycle of *Trichinella spiralis:* Cause and effects

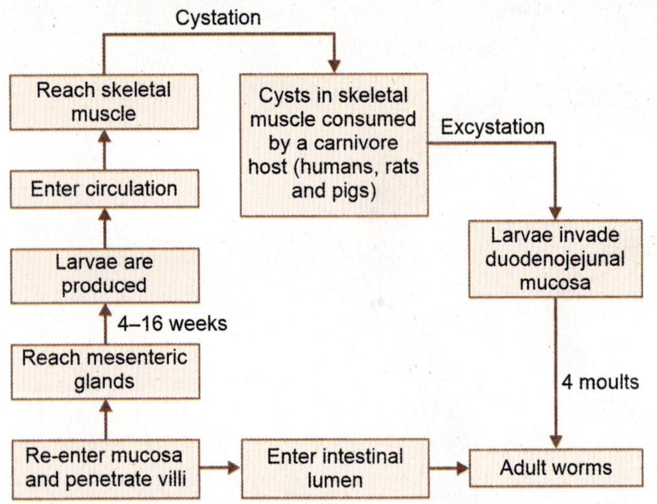

Fig. 50.6B: Life cycle of *T. spiralis*

Enteric or gastrointestinal phase: After ingestion of infected meat by humans, the enzymes pepsin and hydrochloric acid act in the stomach and cause the release of the 1st stage of the larvae. These larvae invade the small intestine. Invasion can be asymptomatic or sometimes associated with abdominal pain, diarrhoea, nausea, and vomiting. Larvae then turn into adults and mate. Female Trichinella worms produce larvae, which complete the gastrointestinal or enteric phase.

Diagnosis

1. Routine examinations of stool, blood, milk, etc. rarely detect larvae.
2. Haemogram shows marked eosinophilia (20–60%).
3. Trichinoscopy: Larvae can be detected in skeletal muscle by biopsy. Small samples of deltoid, biceps, gastrocnemius and pectoralis major are obtained and digested by gastric juice for several hours at 37°C and concentrated by centrifugation. Larvae can be detected in this specimen (Fig. 50.7).

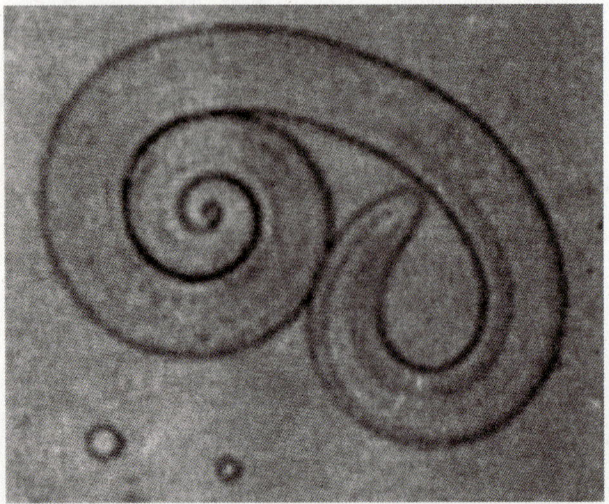

Fig. 50.7: *Trichinella spiralis* under microscope

Biochemical tests: Raised serum creatinine, creatine phosphokinase (CPK) and lactate dehydrogenase (LDH) during acute phase. Creatine kinase, lactate dehydrogenase, aldolase, and aminotransferases can be elevated due to the invasion of skeletal muscle by parasites causing muscle destruction.

X-ray examination: Worms in deeper tissue after the death either become calcified or absorbed.

The position of calcified worm may be located by skiagraphy.

Serological tests, that are available, are ELISA (enzyme-linked immunosorbent assay), indirect IF (immunofluorescence), and latex agglutination test. Serologic test confirmation can be via Western blot.

Serology: It includes:

1. *Kline test:* Slide agglutination test using an alkaline extract of lyophilized whole Trichinella.
2. *Bentonite and latex flocculation test (BFT and LFT):* Test of choice for diagnosis in man. Bentonite and latex particles are added to Trichinella extract and glycerin saline solution test become positive on the 15th day.
3. Charcoal agglutination test (CAT)
4. Fluorescent antibody test
5. Complement fixation test
6. Intradermal test (Bachman)

Sometimes serology is not reliable mainly during the early course of the disease (during the first 3 weeks or more). Infection with other organisms like nematodes or other helminths and autoimmune diseases can cause a false positive serologic reaction.

Evaluation: Diagnosis is initially made usually based on clinical signs and symptoms. Diagnostic confirmation is by serology; or occasionally muscle biopsy may be needed.

The definitive diagnosis method is a muscle biopsy.

Sensitivity is high if the biopsy is performed 4 weeks after infection. If performed early in the disease course, it may be negative.

Prevention and control: The disease can be transmitted only by drinking contaminated water and can be completely prevented through to relatively simple measures.

- Preventing people from drinking cyclops contaminated water:
- Avoid drinking contaminated water
- Filtering water
- Boiling
- Treatment of water with larvicides to kill cyclops
- Preventing people infected with the worm from entering water sources used for drinking.

Chapter 51

Helminthology II
(Cestodes)

Chapter Outline

- Helminthology
- Cestodes
- *Taenia saginata* and *T. solium* (Taeniasis)
- Cysticercosis

HELMINTHOLOGY

Classification of Helminths

The helminths are tripoblastic (having 3 germ layers) metazoa.

The helminths of medical importance are classified as follows:

Helminths
Phylum: Platyhelminthes
Classes: Cestoidea and Trematoda
Phylum: Nemathelminthes
Class: Nematoda

Features of Platyhelminthes
(*Classess:* Cestoidea and Trematoda).
- Body flattened, leaf-like or tape-like and segmented.
- Body cavity absent.
- Alimentary canal incomplete, or entirely absent.
- Mostly hermaphrodites.

Features of Nemathelminthes
(*Class:* Nematoda)
- Body elongated, cylindrical, unsegmented.
- Body cavity present.
- Nemathelminthes

CESTODES

The following tapeworms—all infecting men are to be studied in this class (1) *Taenia saginata* (beef tapeworm): (2) *Taenia solium* (pork tapeworm); (3) *Diphyllobothrium latum* (fish tapeworm); (4) *Hymenolepis nana* (dwarf tapeworm; and (5) *Echinococcus granulosus* (hydatid worm).

TAENIA SAGINATA AND *T. SOLIUM* (TAENIASIS)

Taenia saginata

This is the largest infective tapeworm of human being. This is commonly found in beaf eaters. Adult worm lives in small intestine. This worm is hermaphrodite (both sexes in single worm). Length of adult worm is 5–10 metres but it can be 24 metres. It has three parts, i.e. head or scolex, neck and body. Body is made up of many segments (proglottides). There are 1000–2000 proglottides.

Mode of infection: Man acquires infection by eating raw or undercooked beef containing viable cysticerci. Infection in humans is related to the habit of eating food preparations, which contains insufficiently cooked or raw meat.

Various factors are responsible for transmission of infection in a community. These are high prevalence of *T. saginata* eggs in the field contaminated by indiscriminate defecation by man, dispersal of egg by flies and increased travel and tourism. The poor personal hygiene and low socioeconomic condition are the other important factors.

Morphology (*T. saginata* and *T. solium*): They are usually on an average 5–20 feet in length (exceptionally long species up to 30–75 feet have been on record). They are white and transparent. *T. solium* is much smaller than *T. saginata* (6–10 feet). They have two basic parts, head and body consisting of proglottides, 1500 or more in *T. saginata*, 1000 in *T. solium*. Tapeworms are hermaphrodites.

Head or scolex is different in the two species.

1. *T. solium* has a typical, nonretractable rostellum one with 2 circles of 22–32 hooks. It has 4 circular suckers. It is spheroid in shape.
2. *T. saginata* has no rostellum, but has 4 powerful suckers. Proglottides or segments of *T. solium* are smaller than those of *T. saginata* and contain half the number of testes ($\leq$200). Eggs of both species are similar in morphology and will be discussed in detail under the diagnosis of taeniasis. Usually gravid proglottides are discharged in stool and these liberate ova. However, occasionally eggs may also be found in stool.

Life cycle of *Taenia saginata* (Fig. 51.1): This passes its life cycle in two hosts. Man is primary host and cattles (cow) are secondary host.

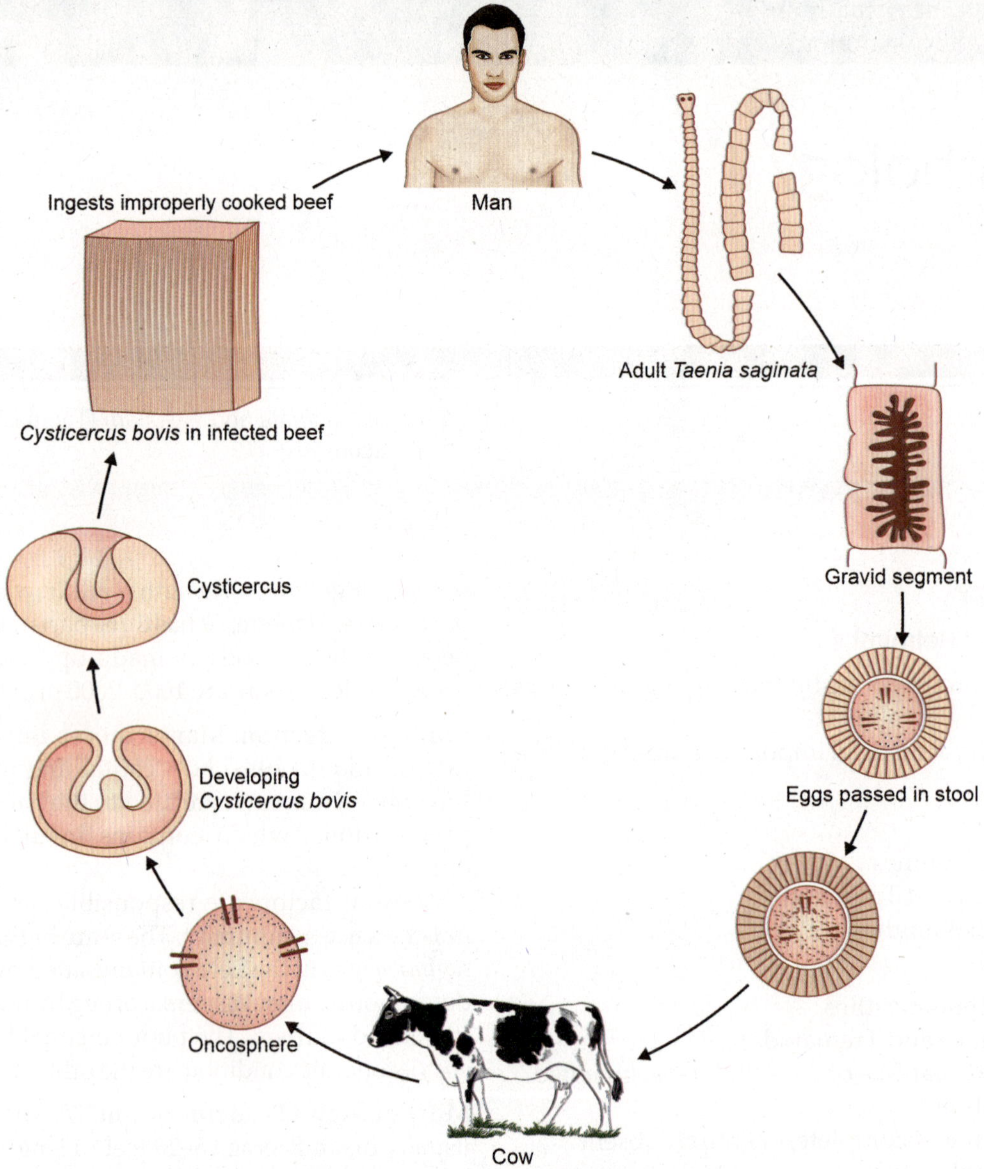

Fig. 51.1: Life cycle of *Taenia saginata*

Taenia solium

It is commonly found in pork eaters. Adult worm lives in small intestine. This worm is hermaphrodite. This is 2–3 metres long. There is armed rostellum and four suckers in head. The number of proglottides is less than 1000.

Primary host is man and secondary host is pig. The larval stage of *Taenia solium* is known as cysticercus cellulosae (Fig. 51.2).

Scatch diagrams of all cystodes are shown in Fig. 51.4.

CYSTICERCOSIS

Cysticercosis is infection by the larval stage of *Taenia solium*, the pork tapeworm. The adult tapeworm resides in the human intestines. The eggs are passed in human faeces which are ingested by pigs or they infect vegetables. These eggs then develop into larval stages in the host, spread by blood to any site in the body and form cystic larvae termed *cysticercosis cellulosae* (Fig. 51.5).

Morphology of Cysticerci

Cysticercus has a small unvaginated scolex and neck resembling an adult taenia. The external tissue consists of hair-like processes, a peripheral collagenous fibrous layer, two muscle layers, peripheral cells, calcareous corpuscles.

Human beings may acquire infection by the larval stage by eating undercooked pork (measly pork), by ingesting uncooked contaminated vegetables, and sometimes, by autoinfection.

Pathologic Changes

The cysticercosis may be single or there may be multiple cysticerci in the different tissues of the body.

The cysts may occur virtually anywhere in the body and accordingly produce symptoms. The cysticercus consists of a round to oval white cyst, about 1 cm in diameter, contains milky fluid and invaginated scolex with birefringent hooklets. The cysticercus may remain viable for a long time and incite no inflammation. But when the embryo dies, it produces granulomatous reaction with eosinophils. Later, the lesion may become scarred and calcified.

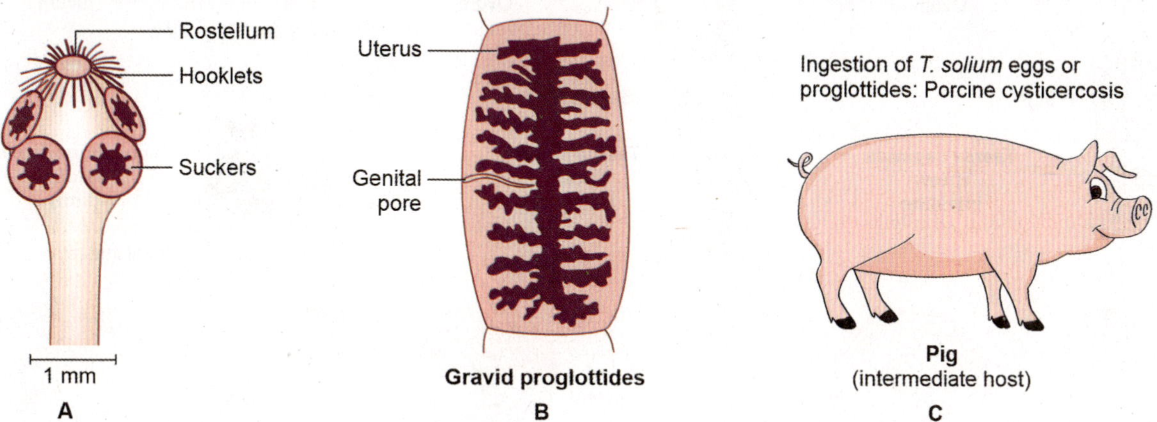

Fig. 51.2: (A) Rostellum, hooklets, suckers; (B) Gravid proglottides; (C) Intermediate host—pig

Life Cycle of *Taenia solium* (Fig. 51.3)

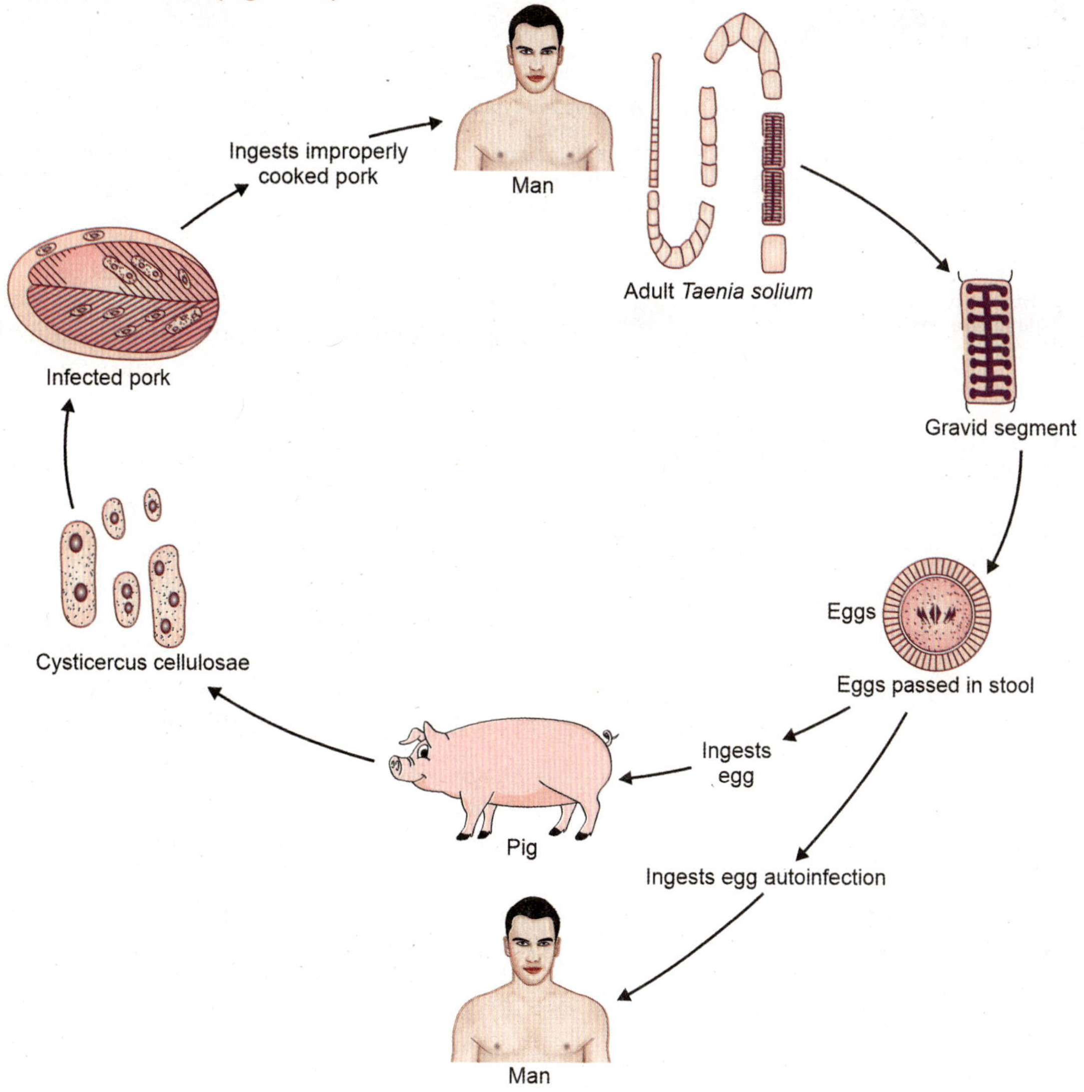

Fig. 51.3: Life cycle of *Taenia solium*

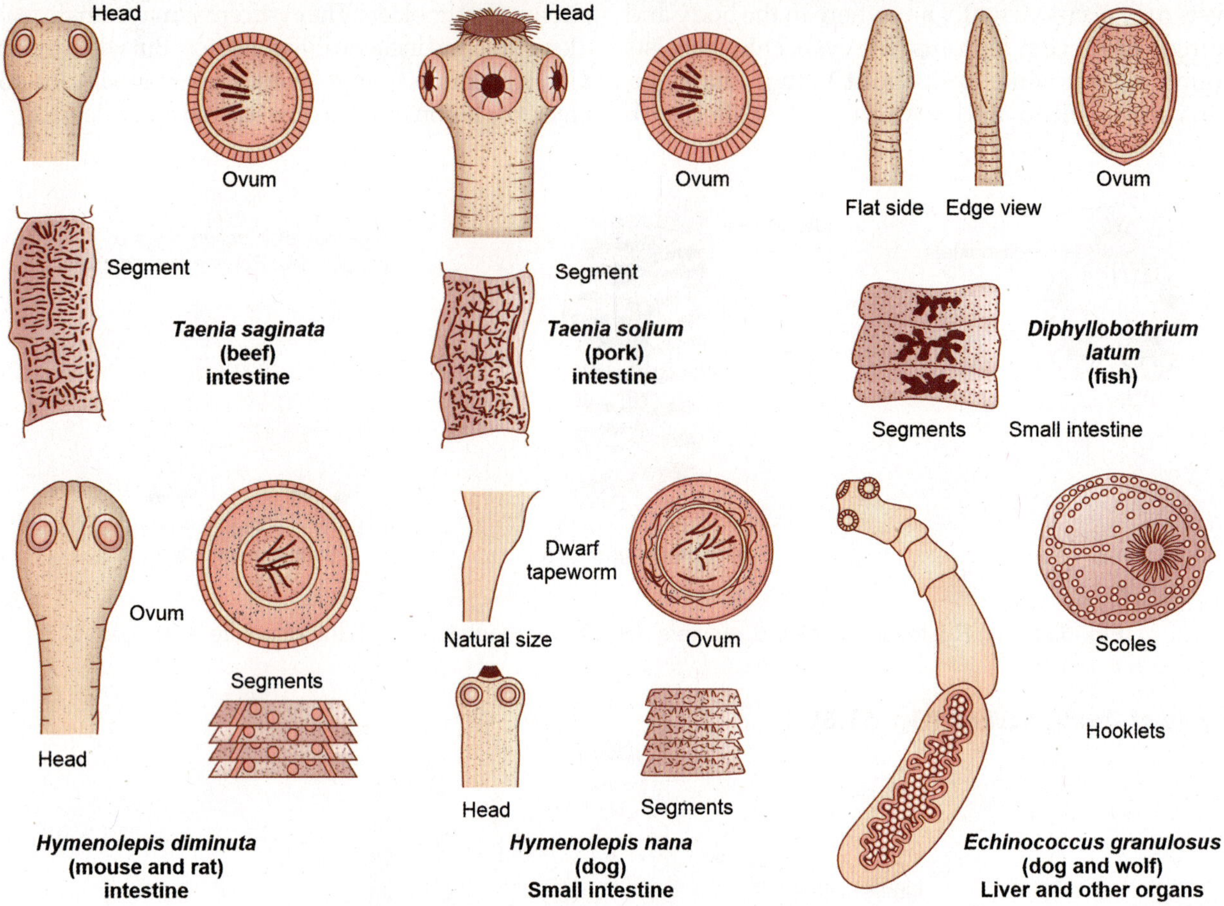

Head
Ovum
Segment
Taenia saginata
(beef)
intestine
Head
Ovum
Segment
Taenia solium
(pork)
intestine
Flat side
Edge view
Ovum
Diphyllobothrium latum
(fish)
Segments
Small intestine
Ovum
Head
Segments
Hymenolepis diminuta
(mouse and rat)
intestine
Dwarf tapeworm
Natural size
Ovum
Head
Segments
Hymenolepis nana
(dog)
Small intestine
Scoles
Hooklets
Echinococcus granulosus
(dog and wolf)
Liver and other organs

Fig. 51.4: Cystodes—tapeworms

Human being
(definitive host)
Ingestion of infected pork, poorly cooked:
Taeniasis
Ingestion of *T. solium* eggs by faecal contamination:
Human cysticercosis

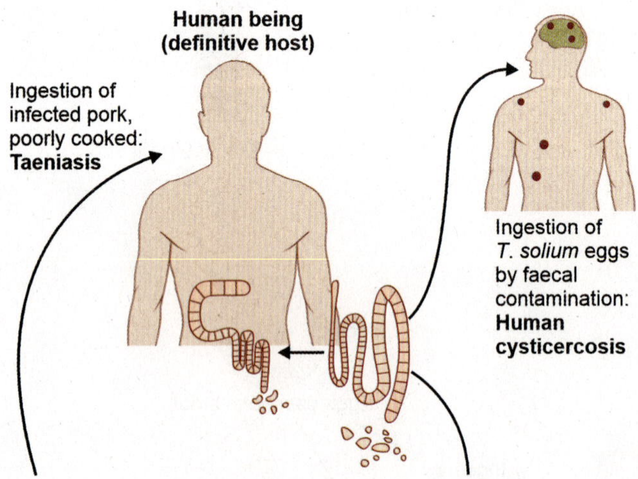

Fig. 51.5: Human cysticercosis

Pathogenicity of *T. saginata* and *T. solium*

Generally patient has no problem. But in case of heavy infestation, there could be abdominal pain, diarrhoea, anaemia, constipation, etc.

Clinical Symptoms

Due to adult worm: Anaemia, abdominal symptoms like dyspepsia (increased acidity in stomach), abdominal pain and discomfort. Other symptoms like hypoproteinemia, oedema, growth reduction, mental retardation, deficiency of iron, pale skin, etc.

Laboratory Diagnosis

Stool examination: It includes:

i. Macroscopic examination of stool for adult worm.
ii. Microscopic examination of stool for demonstration of ova of hookworm either by direct smear method or salt floatation method.
iii. Test for occult blood: Usually positive. (Caution: Positive due to bleeding from peptic ulcer, or due to a meat diet may mislead the diagnosis.)

Diagnosis of cysticercosis may really be quite difficult and in fact impossible. Various methods include:

i. Biopsy of subcutaneous nodule containing cysticerci.
ii. Roentgenograms of skull and soft tissues may reveal calcified cysticerci.
iii. Haemogram may reveal eosinophilia.
iv. CT scan may reveal multiple small, opaque masses in the brain.
v. A positive indirect haemagglutination test using antigen from swine cysticerci.

Ova of Taeniae (Fig. 51.6)

- Spherical in shape.
- 31–32 mm in diameter.
- Bile stained
- Does not float in saturated saline solution.
- Consists of a thick embryospore which is brown in colour and striated.
- Contains an encosphere (14–20 mm) with 3 pairs of hooklets.

Blood examination: Hb, RBC count, PCV, MCV, MCHC, MCH are decreased; DLC shows eosinophilia; PBF shows microcytic hypochromic anaemia.

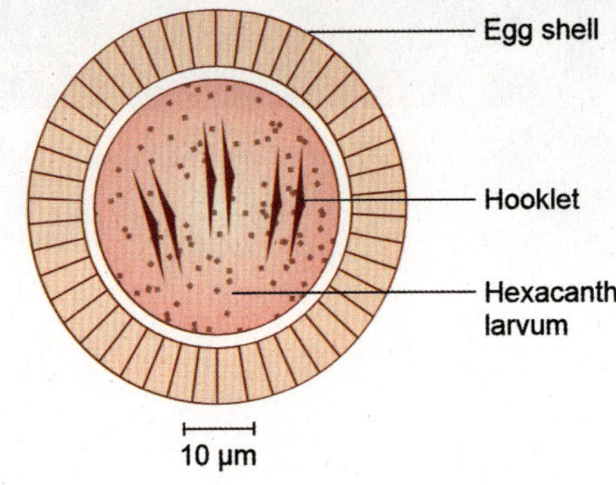

Fig. 51.6: Ova of tapeworm showing 3 pairs of hooklet

Chapter 52

Echinococcus granulosus

(Hydatid Cyst)

Chapter Outline

ECHINOCOCCUS GRANULOSUS (HYDATID CYST DISEASE)

Introduction

Echinococcus spp.

Cestodes of the genus Echinococcus are distributed in many parts of the world. At present, 4 species are regarded as valid. These are: *Echinococcus granulosus*, *E. multilocularis*, *E. oligarthrus* and *E. vogeli*.

Geographical distribution: Cosmopolitan. It is common in areas where there is a close relationship between man, sheep and dog. It is more common in temperate climates.

E. granulosus is found worldwide with main endemic areas in Argentina, Brazil, Chile, Uruguay, Peru, Sardinia, Cyprus, the Middle East, Northern India, Pakistan, some East European countries and Kenya. It is maintained mainly in a domestic transmission cycle consisting of dog as final host and livestock as intermediate hosts. It produces the so-called 'unilocular' type of echinococcosis in man.

Habitat: Man harbours only the larvae, adult worms reside in intestines of canine animals.

Morphology of hydatid cyst: Commonest sites for cysts are liver (50%) and lung (40%). Other uncommon sites include omentum, mesentery, peritoneum, pleura, skin, subcutaneous tissues, muscles, spleen, brain, kidney, etc. Hydatid cysts may vary in size from being microscopic to very large containing up to 40 litres of fluid.

Contents of cyst consist of hydatid sand and clear, watery fluid of specific gravity 1007–1015 containing albumin, and a protein allied to casein, sodium chloride (0.5%), phosphates and sulphates of sodium and calcium, succinates, traces of sugar and a toxin allied to albumin.

Life Cycle and Morphology of *E. granulosus*

The adults are located in the small intestine of the dog and other carnivores and are 3–6 mm long with 3 to 4 proglottides. The spherical scolex has 2 rows of 28 to 40 hooks and 4 suckers. The worms are firmly attached to the wall of the small intestine by their scolex and suckers. The terminal segment is gravid and contains about 5000 eggs. The eggs are similar in morphology to those of their *Taenia* spp.

The gravid proglottides disintegrate in the dog intestine and the eggs are then discharged in the faeces. If they are deposited on pasture, they are ingested by various grazing animals or other suitable intermediate hosts. The oncosphere hatches in the duodenum and penetrates the intestinal wall. It then reaches various organs of the body via the blood stream. The liver is principally involved because of capillary filtering. The hooks then disappear and the parasite begins to grow into a hydatid cyst. The structure and the development of the parasite within the cyst are shown in Fig. 52.1. Hydatid fluid fills the cyst cavity. The fluid is secreted by the parasite and is bacteriologically sterile in living cysts. It is clear or slightly yellowish in colour with a specific gravity of about 1.012. The development of the cyst is slow and protoscolices are formed only after 1 to 2 years.

The carnivores which act as the definitive host become infected by eating hydatid cysts from the viscera of the infected intermediate hosts. The scolices are then liberated from the cyst and attach themselves to the intestinal tissues where they develop into adults.

Man becomes accidentally involved in the life cycle of the parasite by ingesting the eggs. This may happen by swallowing the eggs that contaminate the hands after petting dogs.

Illustration of life cycle of *E. granulosus* is given in Fig. 52.2.

Clinical features and importance: Hydatid cyst is usually asymptomatic because of its insidious growth. Once, it is very large it becomes symptomatic depending on the site of involvement.

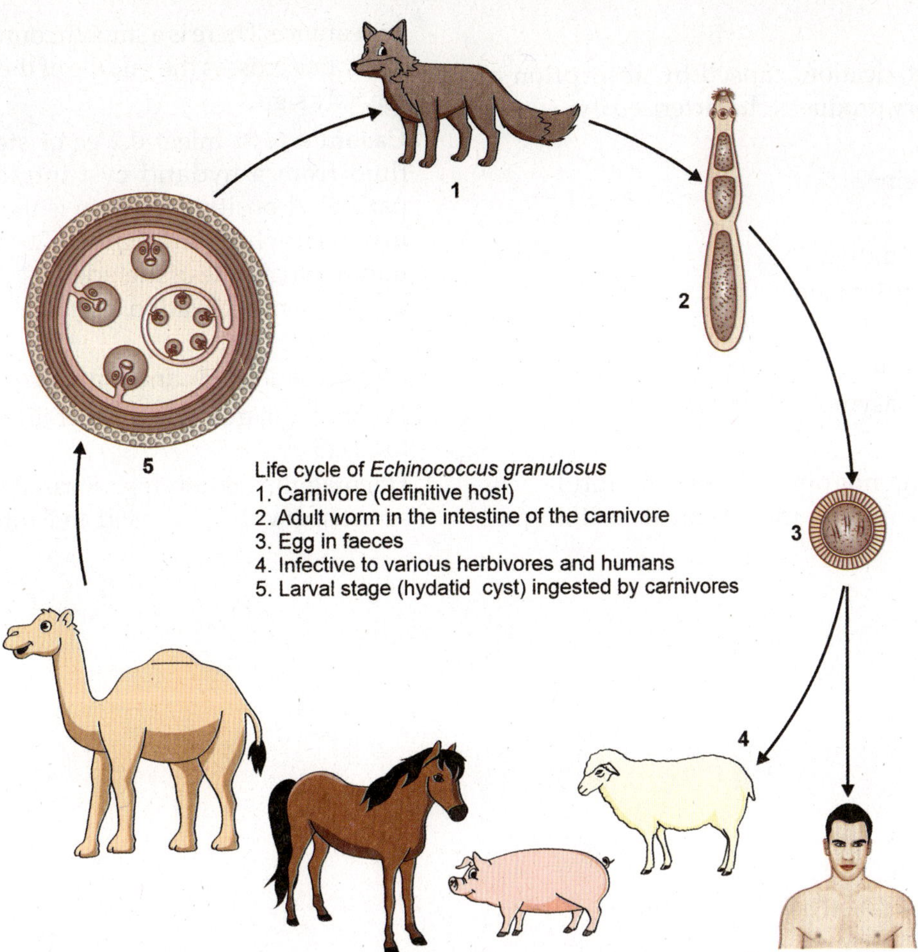

Fig. 52.1: Life cycle of *E. granulosus*

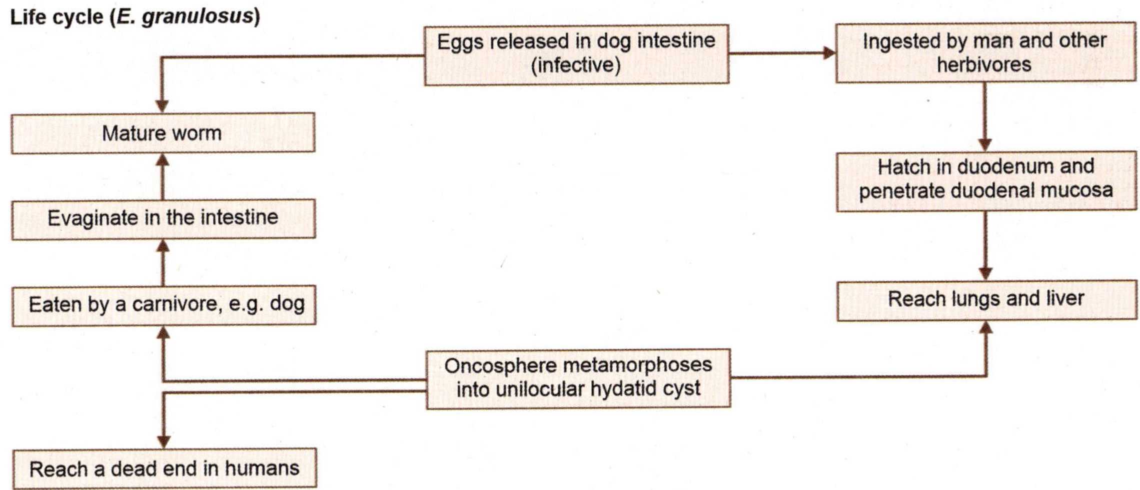

Fig. 52.2: Life cycle of *E. granulosus*

1. **Liver:** It may appear as an insidiously increasing tumour of the liver. It can cause portal hypertension but jaundice is usually absent.
2. **Lung:** Lung lesions are usually detected accidentally on routine X-rays, although occasionally they may cause pressure on adjoining structures.
3. **Kidney:** Presentation resembles that of hypernephroma.
4. **Brain:** Presentation of a cerebral tumour.

If a hydatid cyst ruptures, it is a serious complication characterised by:

i. Immediate pyrexia
ii. Urticaria
iii. Multiple cutaneous eruptions
iv. Anaphylactic shock
v. Peritonitis if cyst is on liver surface.

Importance

1. Verminous intoxication, caused by absorption of worm's excretory products, characterised by:
   - Dizziness
   - Abdominal pain
   - Headache
   - Nausea and vomiting
   - Diarrhoea/constipation
   - Anorexia
2. Anaemia may occur
3. Infection may be asymptomatic

Diagnosis

1. **Routine roentgenograms:** Detect hydatid cysts quite often because of their typical radiological appearance. There is a smooth round outline. In lung a wavy line crosses the middle of the cyst, representing the holy sign.
2. **Casoni's test:** Inject 0.2 cc of sterile unpreserved fluid from a hydatid cyst intradermally into the patient. A positive reaction is the appearance of an urticarial wheel and flare in 20–20 minutes. Other immunological tests include:
   a. Complement fixation test
   b. Precipitin test
   c. Latex slide agglutination test.
3. Haemogram may show generalized eosinophilia (up to 20–25%)
4. Haemagglutination test: Formalinised sheep RBCs sensitised with tannic acid and antigen are used.

Chapter 53

Hymenolepis nana

Chapter Outline

HYMENOLEPIS NANA (H. nana—Dwarf Tapeworm)

Geographical distribution: *H. nana* is cosmopolitan and is a common parasite in children in the Middle East, Central Asia, North India, Pakistan, Mediterranean regions, North Africa and some parts of South and Central America.

Habitat: Human small intestine.

Morphology: This is the smallest tapeworm that infects man. Its length varies from 25 to 40 µm, and has about 200 segments. The eggs are ovoid, measuring 20 to 47 µm in diameter, with 2 membranous shells. The inner shell has 2 poles; from each pole 4 to 8 filaments arise. Inside the egg is the oncosphere or the hexacanth embryo which bears 6 hooks (Fig. 53.1).

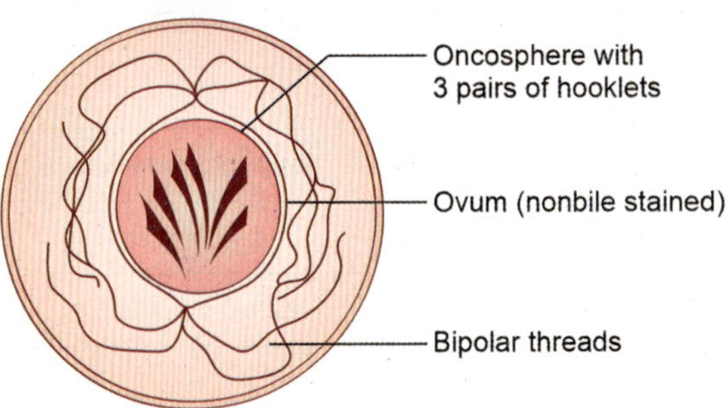

Fig. 53.1: *Hymenolepis nana*

Life cycle: Infection occurs by swallowing the eggs as a result of faecal contamination of water and food. After ingestion the oncosphere hatches and penetrates the villus of the small intestine where the cysticercoid develops (Fig. 53.2). Later the cysticercoid emerges from the villus and develops into an adult worm. Gravid proglottides disintegrate in the lumen of the intestine and eggs are discharged in the faeces.

Illustration of *H. nana* (Fig. 53.3)

Summary of life cycle, pathogenesis, pathology is given in Fig. 53.4.

Clinical importance: It is rarely symptomatic. When present, symptoms represent those of simple taeniasis. Light infection with *H. nana* generally does not produce any symptoms. In heavy infections gastrointestinal disturbances such as anorexia, vomiting and diarrhoea.

Diagnosis: Depends on identification of eggs in stool

1. 30–47 µm in diameter
2. Floats in common salt solution (saturated)
3. Nonbile stained
4. Oncosphere is covered with a thin, hyaline membrane
5. There is also an outer vitelline membrane.

DIPHYLLOBOTHRIUM LATUM

This tapeworm is capable of infecting many fish-eating mammals such as seals, seal-lions, bears, cats, dogs, foxes, and also man.

Geographical distribution: Mainly in temperate and sub-arctic areas of Europe and Asia and including Finland, parts of Russia, Alaska and Siberia. It is also known to occur around lakes in North and South America, Switzerland, Ireland, Italy, Japan, France and Romania.

Habitat: Human small intestine.

Morphology: Adult worm is 40 mm in length and 1 mm in width. Scolex bear 4 suckers and a retractable rostellum, armed with a single circle of 20–30 hooks. Proglottides are wider than long.

Proglottid contains both female and male reproductive organs and a uterine pore through which the eggs are discharged. The uterine pore is on the ventral surface; adjoining it is a coiled uterus containing eggs. A large number of testes and vitellaria are scattered laterally in each proglottid. The eggs are operculated and measure 60 to 80 × 40 to 60 mm. The operculum is loosely attached and can be lifted by pressing the coverglass when examining the eggs under the microscope. Operculum is one end of the egg, apical knob is the other end of the egg (Fig. 53.5).

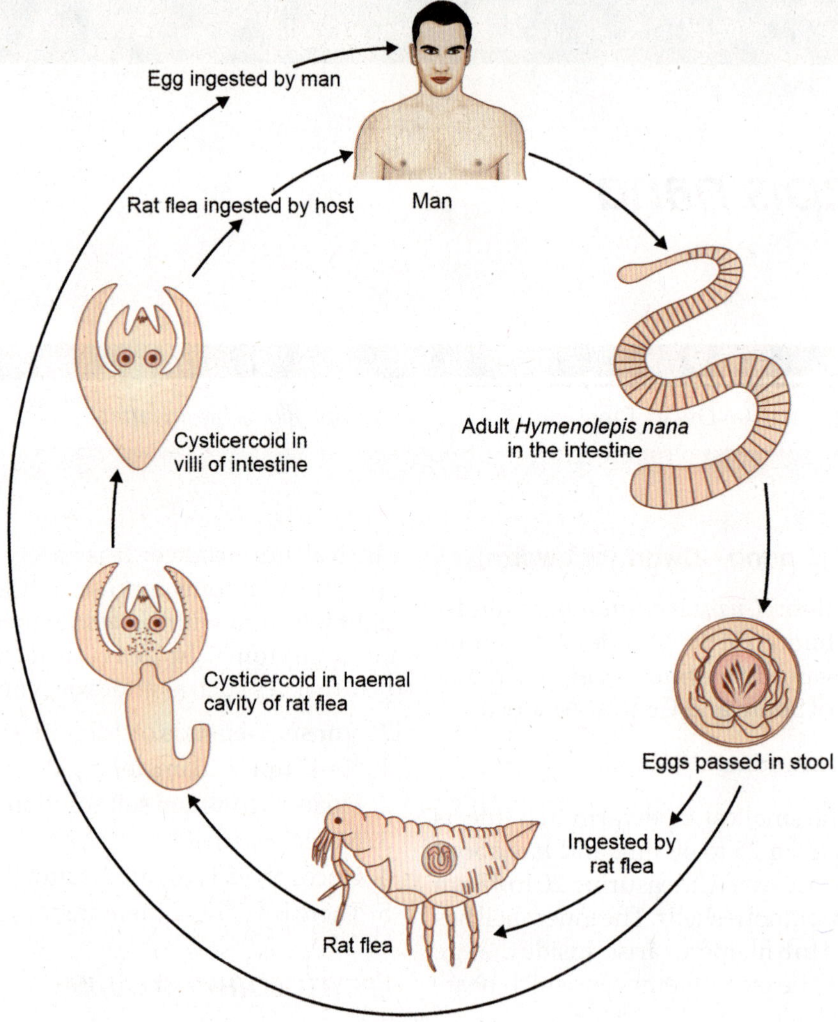

Fig. 53.2: Life cycle of *H. nana*

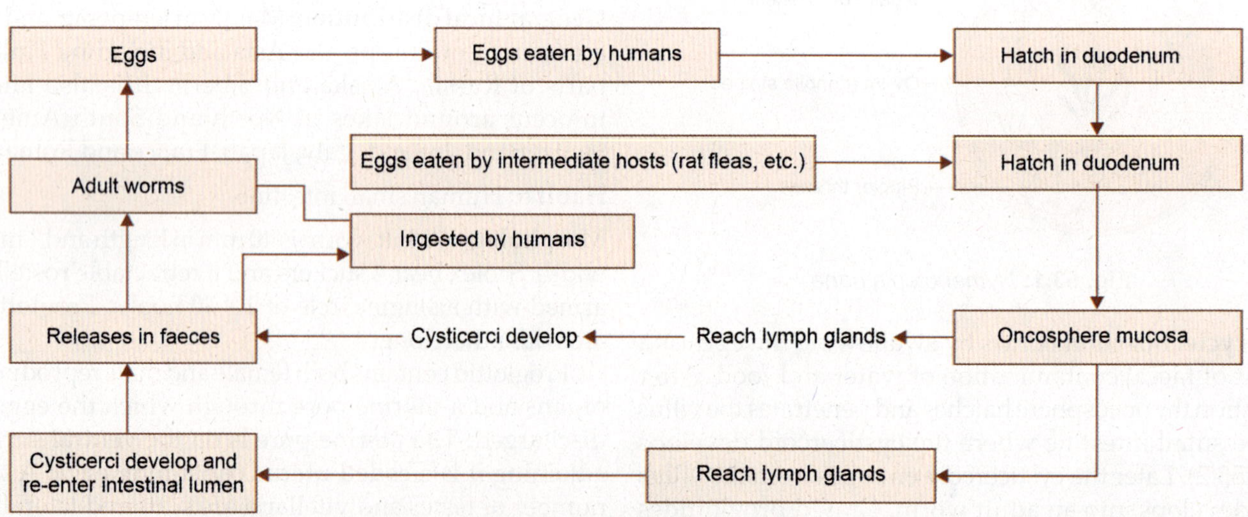

Fig. 53.3: Life cycle of *H. nana*

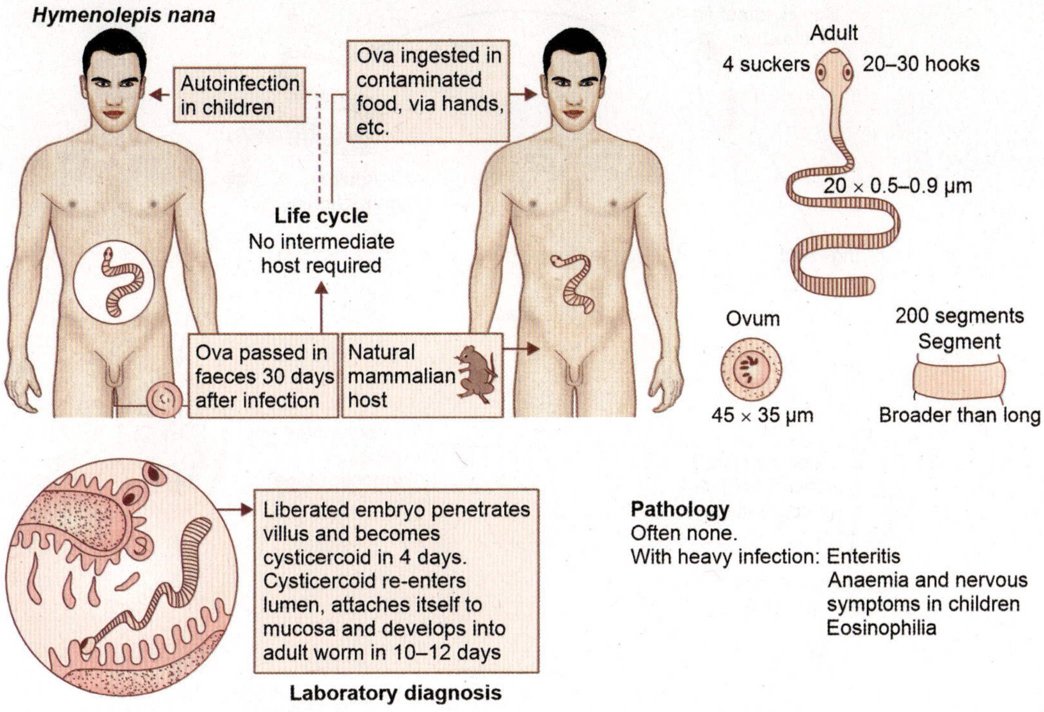

Fig. 53.4: Summary of life cycle, morphology and pathophysiology of *H. nana*

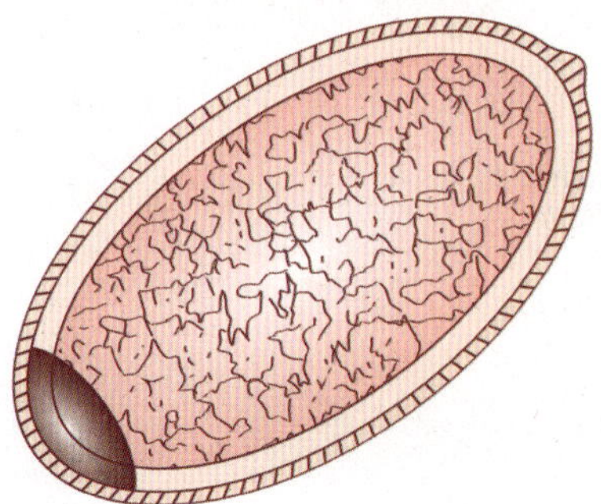

Fig. 53.5: Diphyllobothrium

Pathogenicity: The infection of fish tapeworm in man is known as diphyllobothriasis. The symptoms are gastrointestinal disturbances and anaemia.

Life cycle (Fig. 53.6): Eggs are unembryonated at the time of evacuation.

A ciliated embryo develops in 11–15 days and is known as a coracidium. The coracidium emerges from the egg by pushing out the operculum and it swims freely in water. It can survive for 1–2 days but for further development it must be ingested by a crustacean. If ingested by a suitable crustacean it transformed into a procercoid larva. If the infected crustacean is eaten by a fish, the procercoid larva changes into a plerocercoid larva. Humans become infected by eating raw or semi-cooked infected fish. The released larva then enters the small intestine and develops into an adult worm. The parasite has a long life span and is known to survive in man for up to 25 years.

Clinical aspects: The patient may remain asymptomatic or have mild gastrointestinal symptoms. Patients sometimes complain of fatigue and numbness of the extremities. In some cases, a megaloblastic anaemia develops. This may lead to neurological symptoms as seen in pernicious anaemia. The anaemia is apparently due to competitive uptake of vitamin B_{12} by the parasite.

Laboratory diagnosis: Microscopical examination of sample of faeces.

This is made by finding operculated eggs in the faeces. Proglottides are rarely passed.

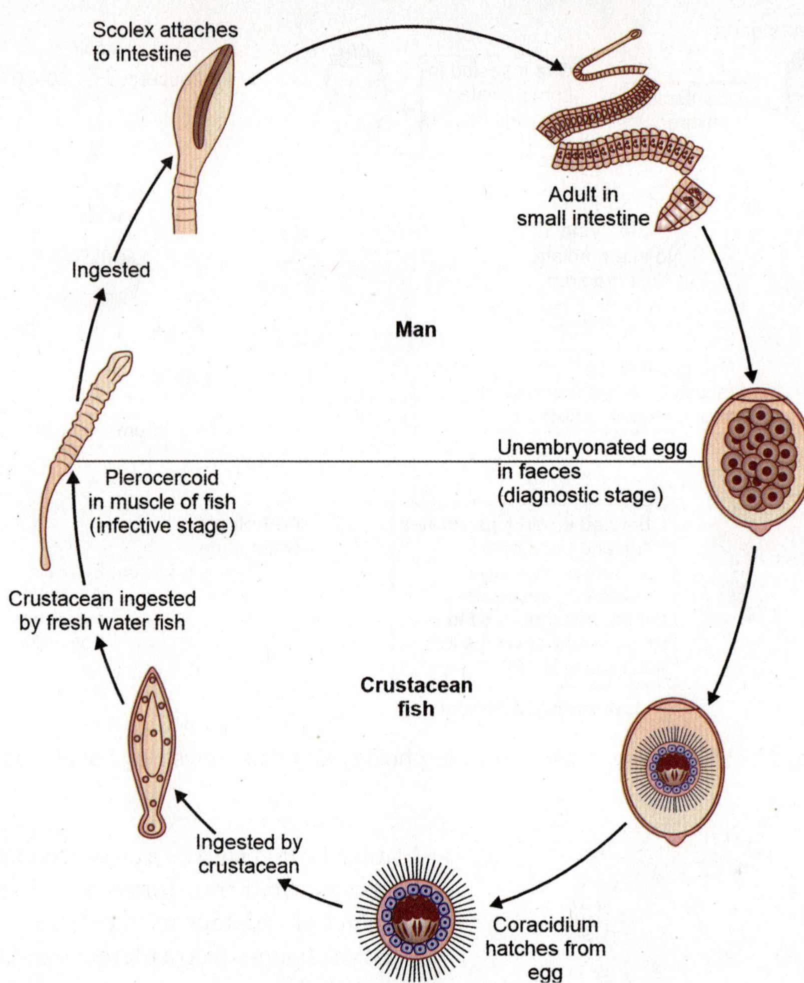

Fig. 53.6: Life cycle of *Diphyllobothrium latum*

Trematodes
(Schistosomes)

Chapter Outline

TREMATODES (FLUKES): CLASSIFICATION

Classification

Phylum	Platyhelminthes
Class	Trematoda
Subclass	Digenea
Order	Protostomata
Suborder	Strigeata
	Amphistomata
	Distomata

Out of the above trematodes, family Schistosomatidae is considered in this chapter.

According to the habitat of trematodes (flukes)

1. Intestinal trematodes (intestinal flukes)
   a. Small intestine: *F. buski, H. heterophyes, M. yokogawai, W. watsoni*
   b. Large intestine: *G. hominis*
2. Hepatic trematodes (liver flukes): *C. sinensis, O. felineus. F. hepatica*
3. Lung trematodes (lung flukes): *P. westermani*
4. Blood trematodes (blood flukes)
   a. In the vesical venous plexus: *S. haematobium*
   b. In the rectal venous plexus and portal venous system: *S. mansoni, S. japonicum*

Modes of infection

A. Ingestion of encysted cercariae:
   a. Vegetables, e.g. *E. aepatica, F. buski*
   b. Fish, e.g. *C. sinensis, H. heterophyes*
   c. Crab, crayfish, e.g. *P. westermani*
B. Skin penetration by free cercariae: *Schistosoma* species

Blood Flukes

Schistosoma spp. causative organism	*Disease*
Schistosoma japonicum	Intestinal schistosomiasis
Schistosoma mansoni	Intestinal schistosomiasis
Schistosoma haematobium	Urinary schistosomiasis
Schistosoma intercalation	Intestinal schistosomiasis

S. japonicum (Table 54.1)

S. japonicum discharges more eggs per worm than *S. mansoni*. Therefore, the pathology produced by *S. japonicum* is greater. The eggs travel in 2 directions. Some eggs find their way into the lumen of the bowel and appear in the faeces. Others flow with the blood in the portal circulation and enter the liver. Most of these are trapped in the liver and give rise to pathology in that organ. Some eggs find their way through the liver tissue and enter the systemic circulation. These may circulate with the blood and settle down in any other organ of the body. Fibrosis of the liver may produce portal hypertension leading to splenic enlargement, oesophageal varices, haemorrhoids and ascites.

S. japonicum is located mainly in the superior mesenteric vein and its branches. *S. mansoni* is located mainly in the inferior mesenteric vein and its branches.

Schistosoma haematobium

Habitat: Adult worm lives in the vesical and pelvis plexus of veins.

Morphology and life cycle: The male is 10–15 mm long by 1 mm thick and covered by a finally tuberculated cuticle. The adult female is long and slender. 20 mm by 0.25 mm, with the cuticular tubercles confined to the two ends. The gravid worm contains 20–200 eggs in its uterus at one time and may pass up to 300 eggs a day. The eggs are ovoid, about 110–170 µm × 40–70 µm with a brownish yellow transparent shell carrying a terminal spine at one pole (Fig. 54.1).

Pathogenicity: The terminal spined eggs of *S. haematobium* may erode blood vessels and cause haemorrhages.

Table 54.1: Eggs of *Schistosoma* species

Feature	*Schistosoma haematobium*	*Schistosoma mansoni*	*Schistosoma japonicum*
No. of eggs in uterus	10–50	1–2	50–200
Shape of eggs	Terminal spined	Lateral spined	Round with small knob
Dimensions (μm)	150 × 52	140 × 61	85 × 60
Mode of avoiding eggs Eggs produced/day	Urine	Faeces	Faeces
Female	20–300	100–300	3500
Reaction to Zlehl-Neelsen staining	Negative	Positive	Positive
Cercariae (cephalic glands) Oxyphilic	2 pairs	2 pairs	5 pairs
Basophilic	3 pairs	4 pairs	None
Intermediate snail host	Spp. of Bulinus	Spp. of Biomphalaria and Australorbis	Spp. of Oncomelania
Definitive host	Man	Man	Man and domestic animals
Geographical distribution	Africa to Iran	Africa and South America	Far East
Habitat	Vesical, prostatic or uterine venous plexus	Mesenteric plexus of sigmoido-rectal area (inferior mesenteric vein and its radicles)	Mesenteric plexus of ileocaecal region (superior mesenteric vein and its radicles)

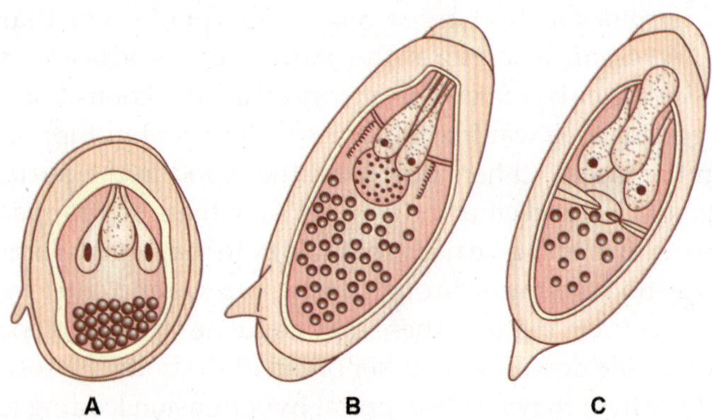

Fig. 54.1: Eggs of *Schistosoma* species. (A) *S. japonicum*, (B) *S. mansoni;* (C) *S. haematobium*

Laboratory diagnosis: Eggs can be demonstrated by microscopic examination of centrifuged deposits of urine. They may occasionally be found in faeces.

Schistosoma mansoni

Habitat: Adult worm lives in the mesenteric veins of the sigmoidorectal area, also in the branches of the portal vein in the liver.

- Definitive host: Man
- Intermediate host: Fresh-water snail

Pathogenicity: The disease caused by *S. mansoni* is designated as *Schistosoma mansoni;* also known as intestinal bilharziasis, schistosomal dysentery. Patient develops abdominal pain and bloody diarrhoea which may continue for many years.

Laboratory diagnosis: Eggs are demonstrated by microscopic examination of stool.

Schistosoma spp. life cycle (Fig. 54.2)

1. Infected human host
2. Adults in human tissues
3. Eggs shed in water via urine and faeces (diagnostic stage)
4. Miracidia hatches out
5. Invades snail
6. Sporocyst in snail
7. Cercaria (infective stage)

General features of schistosomes

1. The schistosomes are diocious trematodes (sexes are separate).
2. They measure 10–20 mm in length with shorter and stouter males. The males have a deep ventral groove known as the gynaecophoric canal.
3. There is no muscular pharynx.
4. A single canal is formed behind the ventral sucker by the union of bifurcated caeca to form the intestinal caecum.
5. Laurer's canal is absent in female, males have 4–8 testes.
6. Non-operculated eggs are produced and there is no redia stage or metacercariae stage.
7. Cercariae are fork tailed and enter definitive host by penetration.
8. Eggs have long sharp spines, all the eggs do not develop and mature together but instead, gradually.
9. Adult worms reside in the lumen of portal vein, venules of intestine and urinary tract.

Morphology of schistosome development stages is shown in Fig. 54.3 and differentiation of all three species given in Table 54.2.

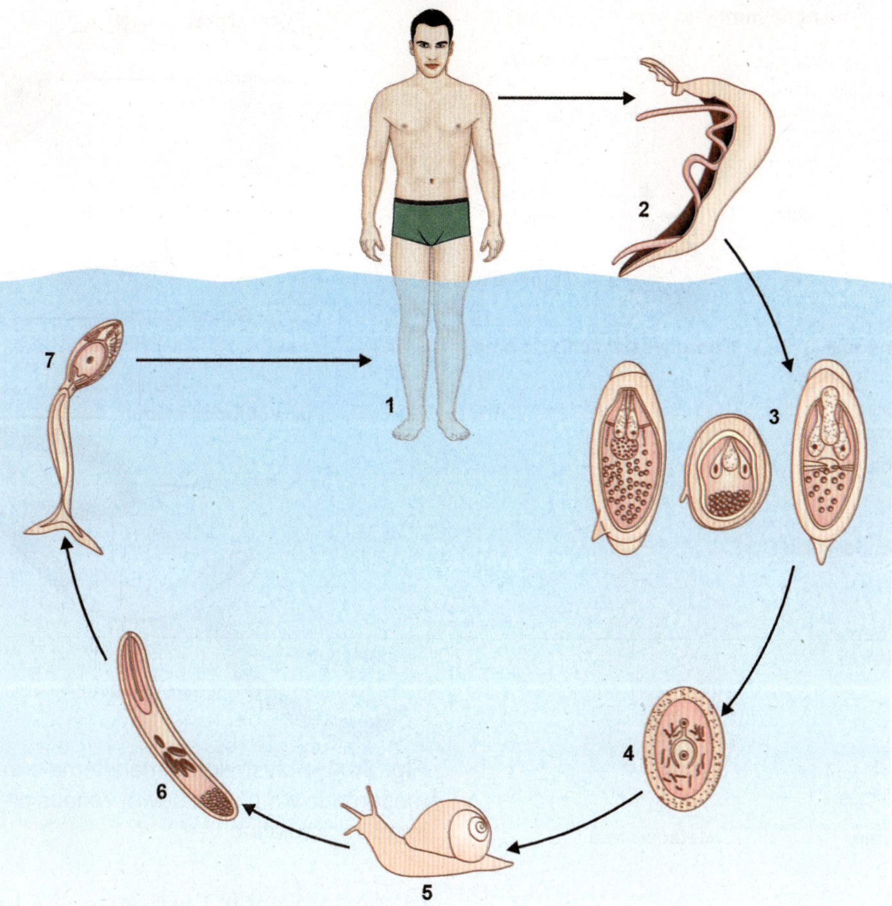

Fig. 54.2: Life cycle of *Schistosoma* spp.

Clinical Aspects

1. **Invasive stage:** Cercarial dermatitis, which is also known as 'swimmer's itch' is a pruritic papular rash and may appear on parts of the body which have come in contact with water containing cercariae. The dermatitis often develops 24 hours after exposure and may last for 2–3 days and then spontaneously disappears. Dermatitis is not often seen in inhabitants of the endemic areas, probably because they have been desensitised to cercarial antigens.
2. **Acute stage (Katayama fever):** This occurs 5–10 weeks after infection and symptoms are due to pulmonary involvement and migration of the worms through the circulation. The patient may have a cough, fever and asthma-like symptoms. Lymphadenopathy, hepatic and splenic enlargement may be present (Fig. 54.4).
3. **Chronic stage:** During this stage adult worms mature in their respective sites and egg production generally starts 10–12 weeks after infection. For many years patient may remain asymptomatic. In *S. japonicum* and *S. mansoni* infections, symptoms pointing to gastrointestinal involvement appear first. These may consist of diarrhoea, abdominal pain and headache. As more and more eggs enter the portal circulation, symptoms resulting from portal hypertension gradually develop. These consist of enlargement of liver and spleen, anaemia, haematemesis and ascites. Central nervous system involvement, due to the present of eggs and ectopic worms, is sometimes seen with *S. japonicum*. This can have serious consequences and the patient may present as a space-occupying lesion, encephalitis or focal epilepsy. Renal involvement has been reported with *S. mansoni* in the form of immune complex disease. In *S. haematobium* infection, the most common, symptom is haematuria. In addition, there may be polyuria and dysuria. Papilloma formation in the bladder is common. Urethritis, structure of the ureter and obstruction due to papillomas may lead to hydronephrosis, kidney failure and uraemia. There is a general belief that chronic infection predisposes the patient to cancer of the bladder.

Pathology: The adults do not multiply and the egg is the main cause of pathology in schistosomiasis. The eggs penetrate the blood vessels and the host tissues by secreting proteolytic enzymes through ultramicroscopic pores in their shell. However, many eggs become standed in the tissues or are carried by the blood stream to other organs of the body. The host reaction to the eggs may vary from small granulomas to extensive fibrosis. The extent of damage is generally related to the number

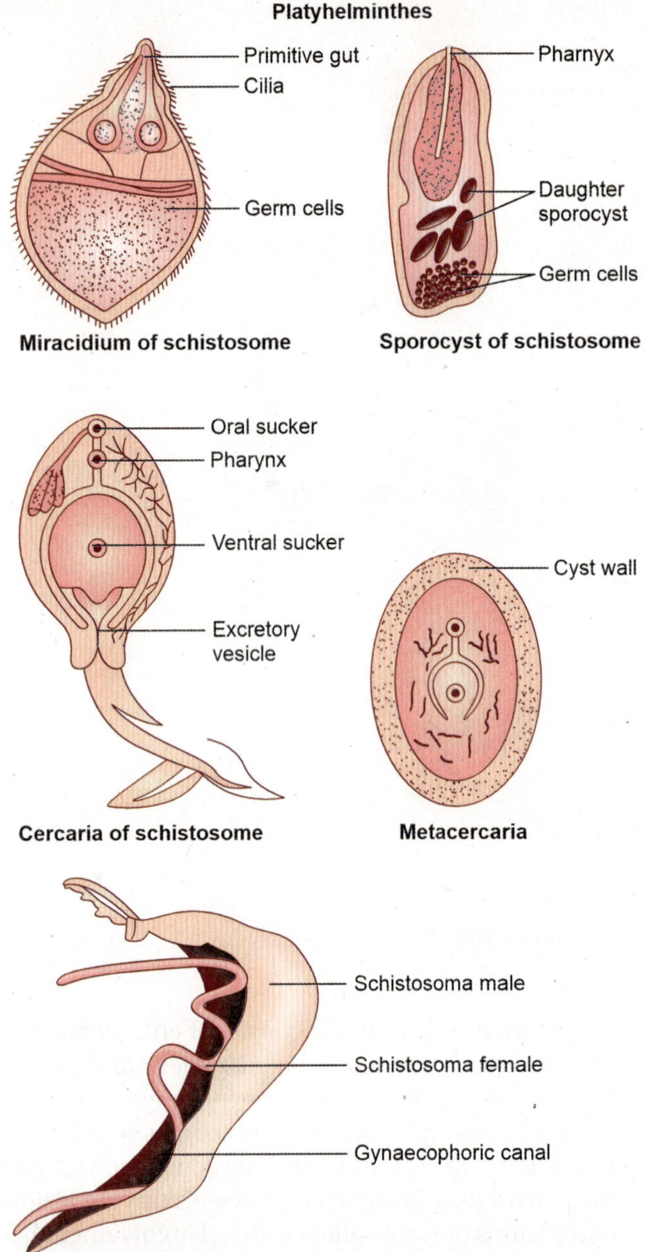

Fig. 54.3: Morphology of development of schistosome stages

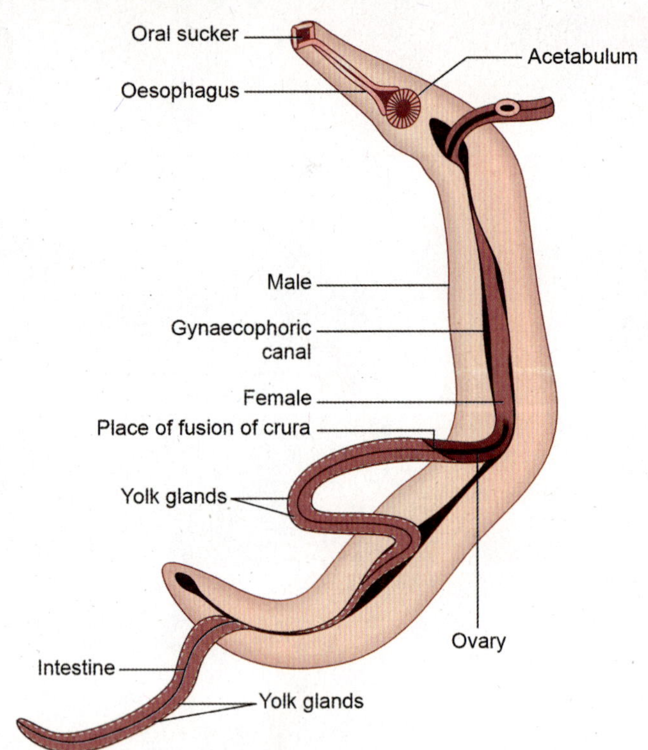

Fig. 54.4: Schistosome male/female in copulation migrate to mesenteric venules of bowel venous plexus of bladder. Laying eggs in circulation

of eggs present in the tissues. Complete immunity does not occur with initial infection and repeated infections are common in endemic areas adding to the pathological damage.

Diagnosis: Detection of eggs in the faeces (*S. japonicum* and *S. mansoni*) and urine (*S. haematobium*) is the definitive method of diagnosis. Kato thick smear is useful for the detection and quantitation of eggs in the faeces and micropore filtration for detection of eggs in the urine. In light infection, rectal biopsy is useful for *S. japonicum* and *S. mansoni*. *Cystoscopy* is similarly of value in *S. haematobium* infection. Various immunodiagnostic tests are available including intradermal,

Table 54.2: Differentiating features of *Schistosoma* species

Feature	*Schistosoma haematobium*	*Schistosoma mansoni*	*Schistosoma japonicum*
Location in human body			
Veins in which located	Vesical	Mesenteric	Mesenteric
Length of male (mm)	10–14	6–12	10–20
Length of female (mm)	16–20	10–20	20–30
Male			
Size	1–1.5 cm × 1 mm	1 cm × 1 mm	2 cm × 0.25 mm
Cuticle	Finely tuberculated	Coarsely tuberculated	Not tuberculated
Testes	4–5, in aggregates	8–9, arranged in a zigzag fashion	6–8 in single row

Contd.

Table 54.2: Differentiating features of *Schistosoma* species (Contd.)

Feature	*Schistosoma haematoblum*	*Schivosome mansoni*	*Schistosome Japonicum*
Female			
Size	2 cm × 0.25 mm	1.4 cm × 0.25 mm	2.6 cm × 0.3 mm
Ovary	Behind the middle of the body	Anterior to the middle of the body	In the middle portion
Uterus contains	20–30 eggs	1–3 eggs (often only one)	50 or more eggs
Reunited intestine	Long, reunion occurs at roughly the middle of the body	Longest of all three species, reunion occurs in the anterior half	Shortest, reunion occurs in the posterior fourth of the body

cercarian Hullen reaction (CHR), the fluorescent antibody test using cercariae (FAT), the circumoval precipitin (COP) reaction and ELISA test. The egg morphology is shown in Fig. 54.1 and Table 54.1.

Section 4

Immunology

55. Immunity
56. Immunopathology (Immune Responses and Immunoglobulins)
57. Major Histocompatibility: HLA Complex, Transplantation and Complement System
58. Antigen–Antibody Reactions
59. Hypersensitivity (Allergy), Tolerance and Autoimmune Disease and Tumour Immunity

Chapter 55

Immunity

Chapter Outline

- Introduction to immunology
- Immunological apparatus
- Humoral Immunity
- B Cells and T Cells

INTRODUCTION TO IMMUNOLOGY

Immunology is a young branch of medicine. The first effective immunization was performed by Edward Jenner (1749–1823), who introduced vaccination with cowpox in 1796 as a means of protection against smallpox.

Before going further, certain terms used in immunology must be clarified as follows:

1. **Antigen:** A substance that can induce a detectable immune response.
2. **Antibody:** A protein produced as a result of introduction of an antigen which has the ability to combine with that antigen.
3. **Anaphylaxis:** A reaction of immediate hypersensitivity which results from sensitization of tissue fixed mast cells by cytotropic antibodies following exposure to antigen.
4. **Allergy:** An altered state of immune reactivity, usually denoting hypersensitivity.
5. **Allergen:** Antigens that give rise to allergic reaction by IgE antigens.
6. **Anergy:** The inability to react to a battery of common skin test antigens.
7. **Antitoxin:** Protective antibodies that inactivate soluble toxic protein product of bacteria.
8. **Capping:** The movement of cell surface antigen toward one pole of a cell after antigens are cross-linked by specific antibody.
9. **Chemotaxis:** A process whereby phagocytic cells are attracted to the vicinity of invading pathogen.
10. **Complement:** A system of serum proteins that is primary humoral mediator of antigen–antibody reactions.
11. **Hapten:** A substance that is not immunogenic but can react with an antibody of appropriate specificity.
12. **Immunogen:** A substance that, when introduced into an animal provokes the immune response.
13. **Opsonin:** Substance capable of enhancing phagocytosis, e.g. antibody and complement.
14. **Serology:** Determination of antibodies to infectious agents in serum, important in clinical medicine.
15. **Tolerance:** Condition in which responsive cell clones have been eliminated or inactivated by prior contact with antigen, with the result, that no immune response occurs on administration of antigen.
16. **Toxoid:** Antigenic but nontoxic derivative of toxins.

IMMUNOLOGICAL APPARATUS

The immunological apparatus is a highly developed system belonging to reticuloendothelial system which is diffusely scattered throughout the body. The two principal cells constituting this organ are macrophages and lymphocytes which are widely distributed through all the organs and tissues.

The principal cellular component in both types of reactions is the lymphocyte bursa dependent lymphocytes (B cells) and thymus dependent lymphocytes (T cells).

T Lymphocytes

These are present in the peripheral lymphoid tissues as well as in blood. In blood, they constitute 70–80% of all lymphocytes.

Functions

1. **Cellular immune reactions:** Delayed hypersensitivity reactions.
   - Resistance against infections by certain bacteria and viruses.
   - Rejection of solid organ transplant.
   - Resistance against tumours.
2. **Regulatory functions:** Modulation of immune response mediated by other T cells and B cells.

Function: B cells secrete immunoglobulins after they are transformed into plasma cells. Immunoglobulins, as will be discussed later, play the most important part in antigen–antibody reaction.

Macrophages

They are widely distributed in lymphoid tissues, blood and monocytes. They process and present the antigen to immune competent cells. They also act as powerful effect on cells in cell-mediated immune reactions. They also produce a number of soluble factors that influence the growth and functions of lymphocytes.

K Cells

They are characterised by the presence of Fc receptor but they lack Ig and surface markers of T cells and are non-phagocytic. Functionally, they are responsible for antibody-dependent cellular cytotoxicity (ADCC).

Natural Killer (NK) Cells

These are capable of lysing a variety of antigens, tumour cells and virus infected cells.

Immunity is of two types:

1. **Cellular immunity:** The concept was introduced by Metchnikoff (1887). Infective organisms are engulfed in the body by two types of circulating cells, i.e. polymorphonuclear leucocytes and macrophages, the phenomenon known as phagocytosis.
2. **Humoral immunity:** Introduced by Fodor in 1886, who observed a direct action of an immune serum on microbes during the course of his studies on anthrax bacilli.

Types of Immune Response

The functional anatomy of the lymphoid system can be appreciated only against the background of the two component concept of immunity. The immune response to an antigen, whatever its nature, can be of two broad types:

1. **Humoral or antibody-mediated immunity (HMI or AMI):** Humoral immunity is mediated by antibodies produced by plasma cells and present in blood and other body fluids (hence the name 'humoral' from 'humor', the old term for body fluids).
2. **Cellular or cell-mediated immunity (CMI):** Cellular immunity is mediated directly by sensitised lymphocytes. Cells for each of these components develop through separate channels and remain independent.

Antibody-Mediated Immunity (AMI)

Antibody synthesis typically involves the cooperation of 3 cells: Macrophages, helper T cells, and B cells. After processing by a macrophage, fragments of antigen appear on the surface of the macrophage in association with class II MHC proteins. These molecules bind to specific receptors on the surface of a helper T cells, which then produces lymphokines such as interleukin-2, B cell growth factor, and B cell differentiation factor. These factors activate the antigen-specific B cell. The activated B cell proliferates and differentiates to form many plasma cells that secrete large amounts of immunoglobulins (antibodies). Although antibody formation usually involves helper T cells, certain antigens, e.g. bacterial polysaccharides, can activate B cells directly, without the help of T cells, and are called T cell-independent antigens.

Overall AMI

1. Provides primary defense against most extracellular bacterial pathogens
2. Helps in defense against viruses that infect through the respiratory or intestinal tracts
3. Prevents recurrence of virus infections
4. It also participates in the pathogenesis of immediate (types 1, 2 and 3) hypersensitivity and certain autoimmune diseases.

Cell-Mediated Immunity (CMI)

Antibody-mediated immunity is directed primarily against (1) toxin-induced diseases, (2) infections in which virulence is related to polysaccharide capsules (e.g. pneumococcus, meningococcus, *Haemophilus influenzae*), and (3) certain viral infections. However, in many microbial infections, especially intracellular ones such as tuberculosis, cell-mediated immunity imparts resistance and aids in recovery. Furthermore, cell-mediated immunity is important in defense against parasites and tumours and in the rejection of organ transplants. The strongest evidence for the importance of cell-mediated immunity comes from clinical situations in which its suppression (by immunosuppressive drugs or disease, e.g. AIDS) results in overwhelming infections or tumours.

The constituents of the cell-mediated immune system include several cell types: (1) Macrophages, which present the antigen to T cells; (2) helper T cells, which participate in antigen recognition and in regulation (helper and suppressor) functions; (3) natural killer (NK) cells, which can inactivate pathogens; and (4) K (killer) and cytotoxic T cells, which can kill with or without antibody. Macrophages and helper T cells produce cytokines that activate helper and cytotoxic T cells leading to the killing of the pathogen or tumour cell.

Although the complexity of cell and lymphokine interactions is enormous, the result is relatively simple: In the person with competent cellular immunity, opportunistic pathogens rarely or never cause disease, and the spread of other agents, for example, certain viruses (e.g. herpes viruses) or tumours (e.g. Kaposi's sarcoma) is limited. The assessment of the competence of cell-mediated immunity is therefore important.

The main function of the immune system is to prevent or limit infections by microorganisms such as bacteria, viruses, fungi, and parasites. Protection is provided primarily by the cell-mediated and antibody-mediated (humoral) arms of the immune system. (Complement and phagocytes are essential also.)

The cell-mediated arm consists primarily of T lymphocytes (e.g. helper T cells and cytotoxic T cells), whereas the antibody-mediated arm consists of B lymphocytes (and plasma cells). Some of the major functions of T cells and B cells are shown in Table 55.2. The main functions of antibodies are (1) to neutralize toxins and viruses and (2) to opsonize bacteria, making them easier to phagocytize. Cell-mediated immunity, on the other hand, is directed primarily against organisms such as fungi, parasites, and certain intracellular bacteria, it is also involved in the killing of virus-infected cells and tumour cells. Cell-mediated immunity and antibody are both highly specific for the invading organism. How do these specific protective mechanisms originate? The following examples briefly describe how immunity to microorganisms occurs.

Overall CMI

- Protects against fungi, viruses and facultative intracellular bacterial pathogens like *Mycobacterium tuberculosis*, *Mycobacterium leprae*, Brucella and Salmonella, and parasites like Leishmania and trypanosomes.
- It also participates in the rejection of homografts and graft-versus-host reaction.
- It mediates the pathogenesis of delayed (type 4) hypersensitivity and certain autoimmune diseases.
- It provides immunological surveillance and immunity against cancer.

HUMORAL IMMUNITY

Synthesis of Antibody

On exposure to antigen, antibody production follows a characteristic pattern (Fig. 55.1). The production of antibodies consists of three steps.

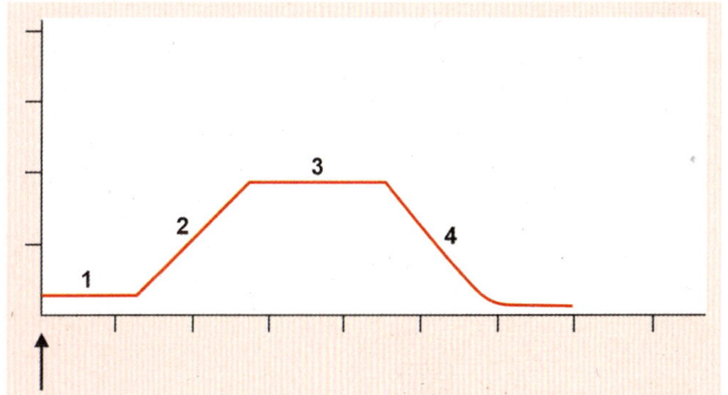

Fig. 55.1: Primary immune response. An antigenic stimulus: 1. Latent period: 2 Log phase (rise in titer of serum antibody): 3. Steady state of antibody titer, 4. Decline of antibody titer

1. **Lag phase:** A lag phase, the immediate stage following antigenic stimulus during which no antibody titer in circulation. This is the time taken for the interactions described above to take place and antibody to reach a level that can be measured.
2. **Log phase:** A log phase in which there is steady rise in the titer of antibodies. There is an exponential rise in the antibody level or titer.
3. **A plateau or steady state:** This log phase is followed by a plateau with a constant level of antibody when there is equilibrium between antibody synthesis and catabolism.
4. **Decline phase:** Decline of antibody titer.

The Primary Response

When an antigen is first encountered, a rise of antibody detectable in the serum occurs within days or weeks (typically 7–10 days), depending on the nature and dose of the antigen and the route of administration (e.g. parenteral or oral). The serum antibody concentration continues to rise for several weeks, then declines and may drop to very low levels. The first antibodies to appear are IgM followed by IgG or IgA. IgM levels decline earlier than IgG levels.

The Secondary Response

When there is a second encounter with the same antigen or a closely related (or cross-reacting) one, months or years after the primary response, there is a rapid antibody response (typically 3–5 days) to higher levels than the primary response. This is attributed to the persistence of antigen-sensitive "memory cells" after the first contact.

During the secondary response, the amount of IgM produced is similar to that after the first contact with antigen. However, a much larger amount of IgG antibody is produced and the levels tend to persist much longer than in the primary response. Also, such antibodies tend to bind antigen more firmly (i.e. have higher avidity) and thus dissociate less easily.

Active and Passive Immunity

Active immunity is resistance induced after contact with foreign antigens, e.g. microorganisms or transplanted cells. This contact may consist of clinical or subclinical infection, immunization with live or killed infectious agents or their antigens, exposure to microbial products (e.g. toxins and toxoids), or transplantation of foreign cells. In all these instances, the host actively produces antibodies and lymphoid cells acquire the ability to respond to the antigens.

The main advantage of active immunity is that resistance is long-term. Its major disadvantage is its slow onset, especially the primary response.

Passive immunity is resistance based on antibodies preformed in another host. Administration of antibody against diphtheria, tetanus, botulism, etc. makes large amounts of antitoxin immediately available to neutralize the toxins. Likewise, preformed antibodies to certain viruses (e.g. rabies and hepatitis A and B viruses) can be injected during the incubation period to limit viral multiplication.

The main advantage of passive immunization is the prompt availability of large amounts of antibody; disadvantages are the short life-span of these antibodies and possible hypersensitivity reactions if globulins from another species are used.

Natural and Acquired Immunity

Immunity may be natural (innate) or acquired (adaptive).

a. **Natural immunity** is resistance not acquired through contact with an antigen. It is nonspecific and includes host defenses such as barriers to infectious agents (e.g. skin and mucous membranes), certain cells (e.g. natural killer cells), certain proteins (e.g. the complement cascade and interferons), and other processes such as phagocytosis and inflammation (Table 55.1).
b. **Acquired immunity** occurs after exposure to an agent, is specific, and is mediated by antibody and by lymphoid cells. It can be active or passive.

Table 55.1: Natural immunity

Mechanism	*Factor*
Entry of micro-organisms limited	× Keratin layer of intact skin (mechanical barrier) × Lysozyme in tears and other secretions (degrades peptidoglycan in bacterial cell wall) × Fatty acids of the skin (inhibit growth of microorganisms) × Respiratory cilia (elevate mucus containing trapped organisms) × Normal flora of throat, colon, and vagina (inhibits colonization by pathogens) × Low pH of vagina and stomach × Surface phagocytes, e.g. alveolar macrophages
Growth of micro-organism in body limited	× Natural killer cells × Phagocytes, e.g. neutrophils × Interferons (inhibit virus replication) × Transferrin and lactoferrin (sequester iron required for bacterial growth) × Complement × Elevated body temperature × Inflammatory response

B CELLS AND T CELLS (Fig. 55.2)

Origin and features: T cells are subdivided into 2 major categories on the basis of whether they have CD4 or CD8 proteins on their surface. Mature T cells have either CD4 or CD8 proteins but not both.

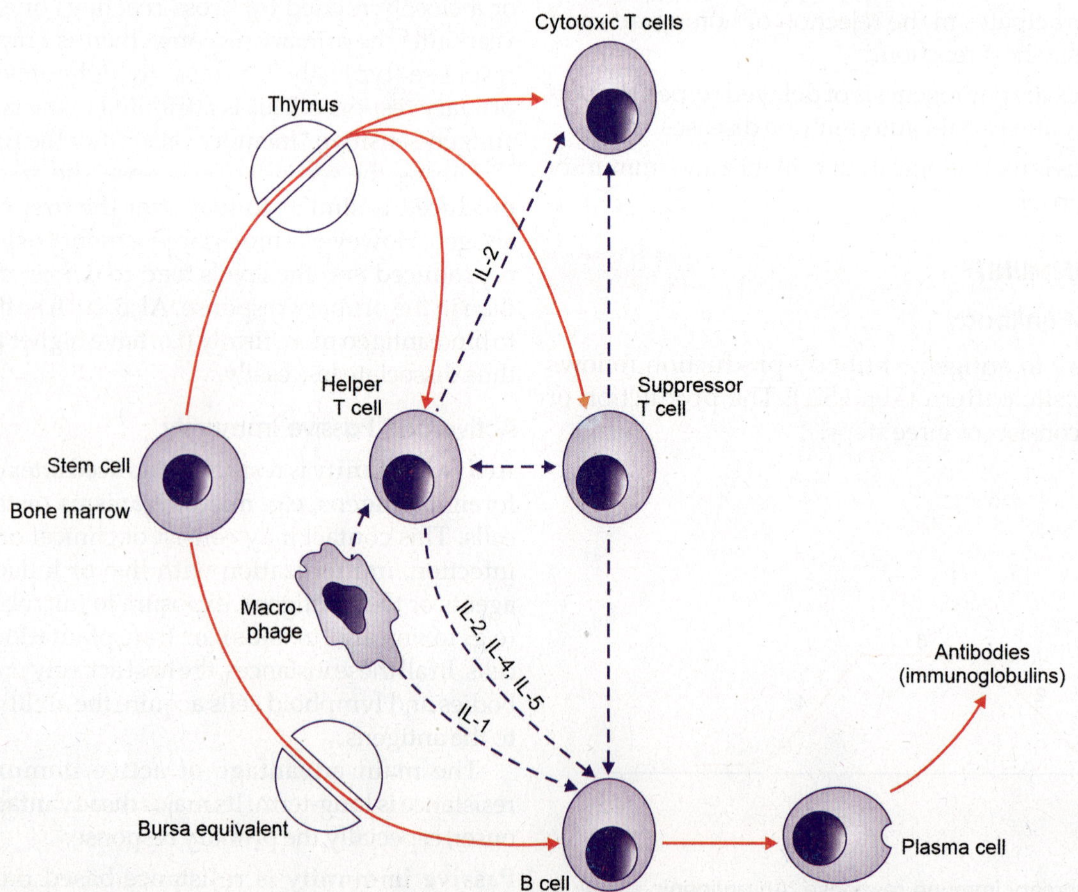

Fig. 55.2: Origin of T and B cells. Dotted lines indicate interactions mediated by interleukins, mediators of suppressor T cell activity have not been characterised

CD4 lymphocytes perform the following helper and effector functions: (1) They help B cells develop into antibody-producing plasma cells; (2) they help CD8 T cells to become activated cytotoxic T cells; and (3) they effect delayed hypersensitivity. CD4 cells make up about 65% of peripheral T cells and predominate in the thymic medulla, tonsils, and blood.

CD8 lymphocytes perform both cytotoxic and suppressor functions: (1) They are cytotoxic for virus-infected, tumour, and allograft cells; (2) they suppress immunoglobulin production by B cells; and (3) they suppress delayed hypersensitivity reactions and cellular immunity. CD8 cells predominate in human bone marrow and gut lymphoid tissue and constitute about 35% of peripheral T cells.

Features of T Cells

T cells constitute 65–80% of the recirculating pool of small lymphocytes. Within lymph nodes, they are located in the inner, subcortical region, not in the germinal centers. Their life span is long: Months or years. They can be stimulated to divide when exposed to certain mitogens, e.g. phytohemagglutinin or concanavalin A (endotoxin, a lipopolysaccharide found on the surface of Gram-negative bacteria, is a mitogen for B cells but not T cells). Most human T cells have receptors for sheep erythrocytes on their surface and can form "rosettes" with them; this finding serves as a means of identifying T cells in a mixed population of cells.

B CELLS

Origin: During embryogenesis, B cell precursors are recognised first in the foetal liver. From there they migrate to the bone marrow, which is their main location during adult life. Unlike T cells, they do not require the thymus for maturation. Pre-B cells lack surface immunoglobulins and light chains but do have μ heavy chains in the cytoplasm. The maturation of B cells has two phases: The antigen-independent phase consists of stem cells, pre-B cells, and B cells, whereas the antigen-dependent phase consists of the cells that arise subsequent to the interaction of antigen with the B cells, e.g. activated B cells and plasma cells. Comparison of T cells and B cells is given in Table 55.2.

Table 55.2: Comparison of T cells and B cells

Feature	*T Cells*	*B Cells*
Antigen receptors on surface	Yes	Yes
IgM on surface	No	Yes
CD3 proteins on surface	Yes	No
Clonal expansion after contact with specific antigen	Yes	Yes
Immunoglobulin synthesis	No	Yes
Helper/suppressor regulator of antibody synthesis	Yes	No
Mediator of cellular immunity and delayed hypersensitivity	Yes	No
Maturation in thymus	Yes	No
Maturation in bursa or its equivalent	No	Yes

B cells constitute about 30% of the recirculating pool of small lymphocytes, and their life span is short, i.e. days or weeks. Approximately over a billion new B-cells are produced each day. Within lymph nodes, they are located in germinal centers; within the spleen, they are found in the white pulp. They are also found in the gut associated lymphoid tissue, e.g. Peyer's patches.

Major functions of T cells and B cells are shown in Table 55.3.

Table 55.3: Major functions of T cells and B cells

Antibody-mediated immunity (B cells)	*Cell-mediated immunity (T cells)*
1. Host defense against infection (opsonize bacteria, neutralize toxins and viruses) 2. Allergy, e.g. hay fever 3. Autoimmunity	1. Host defense against infection (especially *M. tuberculosis*, viruses, and fungi) 2. Allergy, e.g. poison oak 3. Graft and tumour rejection 4. Regulation of antibody response (help and suppression)

Immunopathology

(Immune Responses and Immunoglobulins)

Chapter Outline

- Immunopathology
- Auto Immunity
- Immune Response
- Important Cytokines
- Macrophages
- Natural Killer Cells
- Antibodies
- Immunoglobulins
- Immunoglobulin Structure
- Isotypes, Allotypes, and Idiotypes

IMMUNOPATHOLOGY

Immunopathology is a study of diseases caused by immune reactions. Immunity (Immune—exempt) is a specific protective response to an agent or micro-organisms.

Terminology

Antigen: The genesis of an immune response requires contact of cells/molecules of immune system with a molecule, which can be recognised as being of the non-self or foreign type. Those substances which can induce a specific response from the components of the immune system are called "antigens".

Antigens are usually protein, polysaccharide or carbohydrate in nature and mostly have a molecular weight in excess of 10,000. A molecular weight below 2,500 seems to be the lower limit below which a substance cannot be antigenic. Sometimes molecules which are very small cannot by themselves act as antigens but with the help of a carrier molecule can act as complete antigen. Antigens which are on the surface areas, elicit specific recognition from the immune system. These are called determinants or epitopes. Antigens can be exogenous or endogenous.

Endogenous antigens can be
1. Heterologous
2. Autologous
3. Homologous or iso-antigens

Antibodies: They constitute the globulin fraction of the serum. They are also called immunoglobulins. Those molar studied by action of proteolytic enzymes consist of a basic molecule—a monomer. This is made up of four polypeptide chains held together by disulphide bonds. The immunoglobulins are divided into 5 types—IgG, IgA, IgD, IgE, IgM depending on the composition of the heavy chains.

Functions of antibodies
1. Neutralization of bacterial toxins
2. Preventing viral and bacterial entry
3. Opsonization
4. Complement mediated cell lysis
5. ADCC—Antibody dependent cell mediated cytotoxicity.

Immune response: It has 2 main components
A. Central system—which includes thymus, GIT and lymphoid organs
B. Peripheral—spleen and lymph nodes.

Thymus: Produces thymic lymphocytes, only 1% of which leave the thymus and 99% are destroyed. Thymus is responsible for maturation of paracortical areas of lymph node and development of 'T'mediated, cellular immune response.

GI lymphoid tissue is considered necessary for development of secretory antibody forming mucosa, lymphoid aggregates. It plays an important role in immunity to infectious agents entering the body through the mouth.

Functional population of lymphoid cells
1. T lymphocytes 'T' cells ("Thymus derived")
2. B lymphocytes or B cells (Bursa derived or "Bone-marrow derived")
3. Macrophages

Complement system: It is made up of at least 9 proteins and is involved in the process of inflammation, phagocytosis and clotting. There are two pathways by which the complement system can act
1. Classical pathway
2. Alternate pathway

Functions of complement: Complement can act by

1. Opsonization—through adhesion of C3b to bacterial surface and to neutrophil and macrophage
2. Lysis of bacterial cells through action of C8 and C9
3. Increasing the speed and magnitude of the acute inflammatory reaction.

Disorders of Immune Reactions

- **Immune deficiency:** Where the host cannot innovate an adequate response against the antigen
- **Hypersensitivity:** Where immune response is abnormal and inappropriate so that there is a resultant tissue damage
- **Autoimmunity:** Where there is tissue damage because immune system cannot distinguish between self and non-self.
- **Neoplastic proliferations** of elements of immune system—plasma cell myeloma, Waldenstorm's macroglobulinaemia.

Immune deficiency can be classified as:

i. Primary immune deficiency.
ii. Secondary immune deficiency.

- **Primary deficiency**
  - T cell defect, e.g. DiGeorge syndrome, Nezelof syndrome.
  - B cell defect, e.g. Bruton-type agammaglobulinaemia.
  - B and T cells defect: Reticular dysgenesis, Swiss agammaglobulinaemia.
- **Secondary deficiency**
  - AIDS
  - Malnutrition
  - Iatrogenic (immunosuppressant/cytotoxic drugs)
  - Age

Hypersensitivity Reactions

- Type I: Immediate or anaphylactic sensitivity.
- Type II: Cytotoxic hypersensitivity.
- Type III: Immune complex-mediated
  i. Localised, e.g. Arthus reactions
  ii. Generalised, e.g. serum sickness
- Type IV: Cell mediated immunity.
- Type V: Stimulatory reactions.

Transplantation and Immune Response

Types

- **Allograft:** Same species but genetically different
- **Autograft:** One part of body to another.
- **Synograft:** Between two genetically identical individuals such as twins.
- **Xenograft:** Between 2 different species.

Mechanism of transplant rejection

1. T cell-mediated reaction.
2. Antibody-mediated reaction.

Rejection reactions can be of the following types:

1. Acute rejection
2. Hyperacute rejection
3. Chronic rejection.

AUTOIMMUNITY

Autoimmunity, also called auto-allergy, auto-sensitivity, auto-antigen production and immunopathy, is an immune response against an animal's own antigens. It indicates a failure of immunological tolerance to the body's own antigens. Macromolecular substances of animal cells, tissues, organs and body-fluids are antigenic. Sometimes these tissue antigens become antigenic to their own hosts and cause autoimmune disease; then they are described as "auto-antigens".

Immunologic tolerance is defined as the absence of a specific immune response resulting from a previous exposure to the inducing antigen. This non-reactivity is specific to the particular antigen, immune reactivity to other antigens being unaffected. The most no example is immunologic tolerance to self. Any antigen that comes into contact with the immunological system during embryonic life would be recognised as a self antigen and would not induce any immune response.

I. **Alteration in antigenicity of tissue proteins:** This may be due to:
   1. Degenerative lesions, e.g. lens protein in cataracts and skin burns.
   2. Attachment of hapten, e.g. allergic contact dermatitis.

II. **Release of an antigen which has always been "isolated":** From the cells or tissue which have become "sequestrated" during development, e.g. lens protein. Such a protein will be labeled "non-self" and the immune system will mount a specific response (B cell/T cell mediated), against it.

III. **Loss of tolerance:** Tolerance of self proteins might be expected to be lost in a variety of ways, e.g. lymphoma—"forbidden clones" might be formed as a result of some disease of the lymphoreticular system; the defect might be a failure to eliminate a forbidden clone (recognising self), during embryogenesis due to disorder of the regulatory mechanism—this forbidden clone might persist in the thymus.

Types of Antibody

It may be postulated that the autoantibodies will either be immunoglobulins or cell-bound. The immunoglobulins might be of any class and of one of two types.

1. Organ specific immunoglobulins, whose specificity is directed against a determinant present in one organ, e.g. haemolysins and antithyroid antibodies.
2. Non-organ specific antibodies directed against DNA, mitochondria, smooth mu chain in immunoglobullin (IgM) determinants (rheumatoid factor) fall into this group.

Mackay and Burnet have listed five "markers" of autoimmune disease.

1. Hypergammaglobulinemia.
2. Circulating autoantibodies.
3. Deposition of globulin or its derivatives at sites of action.
4. Accumulation of lymphocytes and plasma cell in specific lesions.
5. Significant temporary or lasting benefit from corticosteroid therapy. Autoimmune diseases occur in human beings are as follows.

Probable Autoimmune Diseases

1. Autoimmune haemolytic anaemias.
2. Hashimoto's chronic thyroiditis.
3. Systemic lupus erythematosus.
4. Rheumatic fever
5. Lupoid hepatitis.
6. Myasthenia gravis.
7. Glomerulonephritis (nephrotoxic).
8. Sjögren's disease.
9. Autoimmune encephalomyelitis.
10. Autoimmune thrombocytopenic purpura.

Possible Autoimmune Diseases

1. Polyarteritis nodosa.
2. Systemic sclerosis (scleroderma).
3. Polymyositis (dermatomyositis).
4. Autoimmune adrenalitis.
5. Autoimmune orchitis.
6. Pernicious anaemia.
7. Rheumatoid arthritis.

IMMUNE RESPONSE

Definition: The immune response is the specific reactivity induced in a host by an antigenic stimulus. For the generation of immune response, antigen must interact with and activate a number of different cells. In addition, these cells must interact with each other. It is generally equated with protection against invading microorganisms in infectious disease. But the immune response has a much wider scope and includes reactions against any antigen, living or nonliving. It may lead to consequences that are beneficial, indifferent or injurious to the host. The state of specific non-reactivity (tolerance) induced by certain types of antigenic stimuli is also included in it.

Type: Immune Response

The immune response can be divided into two types: The humoral (antibody mediated) and the cellular (cell mediated) types. The generation and control of immune responses are a consequence of a complex series of antigen-mediated interactions between various cell types. The two are usually developed together, though at times one or the other may be predominant or exclusive. They usually act in conjunction but may sometimes act in opposition.

Mediators of Immunological Reactions

The Complement System

The complement system is the primary humoral mediator of antigen–antibody reactions. It consists of at least 20 chemically and immunologically distinct plasma proteins capable of interacting with each other. The various functions they carry-out are increased vascular permeability, chemotaxis, opsonization prior to phagocytosis and lysis of target organisms.

Pathways: Activation occurs via two pathways:

i. **Classic pathway:** Initiated by antigen–antibody complexes.
ii. **Alternate pathway:** Initiated by a variety of largely non-immunologic stimuli.

The Kinin System

This system results in the ultimate release of the vasoactive non-apeptide bradykinin, a potent agent that increases vascular permeability; contraction of smooth muscle, dilatation of blood vessels and pain when injected into the skin.

The Lymphokines

When antigen is injected intradermally into an appropriate sensitised host, a delayed skin reaction may develop over the course of 24–48 hours, characterised by mononuclear cell infiltrate. The initial reaction of antigen with a few specifically sensitised lymphocyte results in the production of soluble mediators called lymphokines.

The functions of lymphokines are:

1. Recruit host inflammatory cells
2. Activate the inflammatory cells
3. Keep them at site of inflammation
4. Amplify the cell-mediated hypersensitivity reaction (type IV).

While these substances exert marked biological effects on the cells, they are produced in only minute quantities by activated lymphocytes.

A variety of lymphokines, detected usually by diverse functional assays, has been described. It is not yet clear, how many chemically distinct molecules are involved, nor how many of the lymphokine activities detected *in vitro* are relevant *in vivo*.

IMPORTANT CYTOKINES

Mediators Affecting Lymphocytes

1. IL-1 is a protein produced mainly by macrophages. It activates a wide variety of target cells, e.g. T and B lymphocytes, neutrophils, epithelial cells, and

fibroblasts, to grow, differentiate, or synthesize specific products. For example, it stimulates T lymphocytes to differentiate and produce IL-2 (*see* below). In addition, it is "endogenous pyrogen," which acts on the hypothalamus to cause the fever associated with infections and other inflammatory reactions.

2. IL-2 is a protein produced mainly by helper T cells that stimulates both helper and cytotoxic T cells to grow. Resting T cells are stimulated by antigen (or other stimulators) both to produce IL-2 and to form IL-2 receptors on their surface, thereby acquiring the capacity to respond to IL-2. Interaction of IL-2 with its receptor stimulates DNA synthesis. IL-2 acts synergistically with IL-4 (*see* below) to stimulate the growth of B cells.
3. IL-4 and IL-5 are proteins produced by helper T cells, they promote the growth and differentiation of B cells, respectively. IL-4 also enhances the synthesis of IgE and hence may predispose to type I (anaphylactic) hypersensitivity. IL-5 enhances the synthesis of IgA and stimulates the production and activation of eosinophils. Eosinophils are an important host defense against many helminths (worms), e.g. Strongyloides).
4. Other lymphokines (IL-6 through IL-10) have also been reported but are of lesser importance than those described above.
5. Transfer factor is a dialyzable extract of lymphocytes (MW 2000) that can transfer specific delayed hypersensitivity to a nonreactive recipient and may temporarily restore competent cellular immunity to immunocompromised individuals.

Mediators Affecting Macrophages and Monocytes

1. Chemotactic factor attracts monocytes, which then become macrophages.
2. Migration-inhibitory factor inhibits the migration of normal macrophages *in vitro* and may act to retain macrophages at the site of a delayed hypersensitivity reaction *in vivo*.
3. Macrophage-activating factors, like migration-inhibitory factor, are produced by lymphocytes and can activate macrophages to phagocytize certain organisms, e.g. *M. tuberculosis*. Gamma interferon (*see* below) is one of the most important macrophage-activating factors.

Mediators Affecting Polymorphonuclear Leukocytes

1. Leukocyte-inhibitory factor inhibits migration of neutrophils, analogous to migration inhibitory factor (above).
2. Chemotactic factors for neutrophils, basophils, and eosinophils selectively attract each cell type.

Mediators Affecting Stem Cells

IL-3 is made by activated helper T cells and supports the growth and differentiation of bone marrow stem cells. Granulocyte-macrophage colony-stimulating factor (GM-CSF) is made by various cells including T lymphocytes. It stimulates bone marrow cells to produce granulocytes and macrophages, GM-CSF is used to reduce the risk of infection in patients whose neutrophil numbers are reduced as a result of cancer chemotherapy.

Mediators with Other Effects

1. **Interferons** are glycoproteins that block virus replication and exert many immunomodulating functions. Alpha interferon (from leukocytes) and beta interferon (from fibroblasts) are induced by viruses (or double-stranded RNA) and have antiviral activity. Gamma interferon is a lymphokine produced by activated CD4 and CD8 T lymphocytes. It is one of the most potent activators of the phagocytic activity of macrophages, NK cells, and neutrophils, thereby enhancing their ability to kill microorganisms and tumour cells. It also increases the synthesis of class II MHC proteins in a variety of cell types. This enhances antigen presentation by these cells, gamma interferon also increases antibody production by enhancing the production of B cell-stimulating lymphokines.
2. **Tumour necrosis factor (TNF-α)** is an inflammatory mediator released primarily by macrophages. It has many important immunologic effects, e.g. it increases lymphokine and IL-2 receptor synthesis by helper T cells, increases proliferation of B cells, and attracts and activates neutrophils. TNF-α has other striking biologic effects as well. It is an important mediator of endotoxin-induced septic shock; antibody to TNF-α prevents the action of endotoxin. TNF-α is also known as cachectin because it inhibits lipoprotein lipase in adipose tissue, thereby reducing the utilization of fatty acids. This results in cachexia. TNF, as its name implies, can cause the death and necrosis of certain tumours in experimental animals. It may do this by promoting intravascular coagulation that causes infarction of the tumour tissue. The role of TNF in the death of human tumour cells is unclear.
3. **Lymphotoxin** (also known as TNF-β) is made by activated T lymphocytes and causes effects similar to those of TNF-α. It binds to the same receptor as TNF-α, hence has the same effects as TNF-α.

MACROPHAGES

Macrophages have 3 main functions: Phagocytosis, antigen presentation, and cytokine production.

a. **Phagocytosis:** Macrophages ingest bacteria and other particles. They have surface Fc receptors that interact with the Fc portion of immunoglobulins, thereby enhancing the uptake of opsonized organisms.
b. **Antigen presentation:** Foreign material is ingested and degraded, and fragments of antigen are presented

on the macrophage cell surface (in conjunction with MHC molecules) for interaction with the T cell receptor.

c. **Cytokine production:** They produce several cytokines (macrokines, monokines), the most important of which are IL-1 and tumour necrosis factor (TNF). IL-1 plays an essential role in the activation of helper T cells and TNF is an important inflammatory mediator (*see* below).

Macrophages are derived from bone marrow histiocytes and exist both free, e.g. monocytes, and fixed in tissues, e.g. Kupffer cells of the liver. Macrophages migrate to the site of inflammation, attracted by certain mediators, especially C5a, an anaphylatoxin released in the complement cascade.

NATURAL KILLER CELLS

Natural killer (NK) cells play an important role in the innate host defenses. They specialize in killing virus-infected cells and tumour cells by secreting cytotoxins (perforins) similar to those of cytotoxic T lymphocytes. They are called "natural" killer cells because they are active without prior exposure to the virus, are not enhanced by exposure, and are not specific for any virus. They can kill without antibody, but antibody enhances their effectiveness, a process called antibody-dependent cellular cytotoxicity (ADCC). From 5 to 10% of peripheral lymphocytes are NK cells.

NK cells are lymphocytes with some T cell markers, but they do not have to pass through the thymus in order to mature. They have no immunologic memory, and, unlike cytotoxic T cells, have no T cell receptor, also, killing does not require recognition of MHC proteins. IL-2-activated NK cells (LAK cells) are being used for the treatment of certain cancers.

ANTIBODIES

Antibodies are immunoglobulins that react specifically with the antigen that stimulated their production. They make up about 20% of the protein in blood plasma.

Antibodies that arise in an animal in response to typical antigens are heterogeneous, because they are formed by several different clones of cells; i.e. they are polyclonal. Antibodies that arise from a single clone of cells, e.g. in a plasma cell tumour (myeloma), are homogeneous; i.e. they are monoclonal. Monoclonal antibodies also can be made in the laboratory by fusing a myeloma cell with an antibody-producing cell. Such hybridomas produce virtually unlimited quantities of monoclonal antibodies that are useful in diagnostic tests and in research (*see* below).

Hybridomas and Monoclonal Antibodies

One of the most important scientific advances of this century is the hybridoma cell, which has the remarkable ability to produce large quantities of a single molecular species of immunoglobulin. These immunoglobulins, which are known as monoclonal antibodies, are called "monoclonal" because they are made by a clone of cells that arose from a single cell. Note, however, that this single cell is, in fact, formed by the fusion of 2 different cells, i.e. it is a hybrid, hence the term "hybridoma."

Hybridoma cells are made in the following manner:

1. An animal, e.g. a mouse, is immunized with the antigen of interest.
2. Spleen cells from this animal are grown in a culture dish in the presence of mouse myeloma cells. The strain of myeloma cells chosen has 2 important attributes: It grows indefinitely in culture, and it does not produce immunoglobulins.
3. Fusion of the cells is encouraged by adding certain chemicals, e.g. polyethylene glycol.
4. The cells are grown in a special culture medium (HAT medium) that supports the growth of the fused, hybrid cells but not of the "parental" cells.
5. The resulting clones of cells are screened for the production of antibody to the antigen of interest.

Monoclonal Antibodies

When a clone of lymphocytes or plasma cells undergoes selective proliferation, as in multiple myeloma, antibodies with a single antigenic specificity accumulate. Such antibodies produced by a single clone and directed against a single antigenic determinant are called monoclonal antibodies, e.g. plasma cell tumour (myeloma). In myeloma, antibodies are produced by a single clone of plasma cells directed against a single antigenic determinant and hence the antibodies are homogeneous and monoclonal.

Polyclonal Antibodies

Antibodies that are produced ordinarily by infection or immunization in an animal in response to a single antigen are heterogeneous as they are synthesised by several different clones of B cells against different epitopes of the same antigen, i.e. they are polyclonal. Such antisera contain immunoglobulins of different classes with specificities against different epitopes of the antigen.

Function of Antibodies

The primary function of antibodies is to protect against infectious agents or their products. Antibodies provide resistance because they can

1. Neutralize toxins and viruses
2. Opsonize microorganisms.

Opsonization is the process by which antibodies make microorganisms more easily ingested by phagocytic cells. This occurs by either of 2 reactions:

1. The Fc portion of the immunoglobulin interacts with its receptors on the phagocyte surface to facilitate ingestion; or
2. IgG or IgM activates complement to yield C3b, which interacts with its receptors on the surface of the phagocyte.

Antibodies can be induced actively in the host or acquired passively and are thus immediately available for defense. In medicine, passive immunity is used in the neutralization of the toxins of diphtheria, tetanus, and botulism by antitoxins and in the inhibition of such viruses as rabies and hepatitis A and B viruses early in the incubation period.

IMMUNOGLOBULINS

The immunoglobulins are the protein molecules that carry antibody activity.

Classes of Immunoglobulins: There are 5 classes of immunoglobulins IgG, IgA, IgM, IgD and IgE.

Biological Activities of Different Classes of Immunoglobulins

- **IgG:** In normal human adults, IgG constitutes approximately 75% of the total serum immunoglobulins. There are 4 subclasses of IgG, IgG1, IgG2, IgG3 and IgG4. IgG is the only immunoglobulin that can cross the placenta, IgG is also capable of fixing serum complement.
- **IgA:** IgA is the predominant immunoglobulin class in body secretions comprising 15% of the total immunoglobulins. Secretory IgA provides the primary defence mechanism against some local infections owing to its abundance in salvia, tears, bronchial secretions and mucous secretions of small intestine.
- **IgM:** It is prominent in early immune responses to most antigens and predominates in certain antibody responses like natural blood group antibodies. IgM is the most efficient complement fixing immunoglobulin.
- **IgD:** The main function of IgD has not been determined, though there are isolated cases reported of IgD activity against certain antigens like insulin, penicillin, milk proteins, diphtheria oxoid and thyroid antigens.
- **IgE:** Its main function lies in allergic reactions.

IMMUNOGLOBULIN STRUCTURE

Immunoglobulins are glycoproteins made up of light (L) and heavy (H) polypeptide chains. The terms "light" and "heavy" refer to molecular weight; light chains have a molecular weight of about 25,000, whereas heavy chains have a molecular weight of 50,000–70,000. The simplest antibody molecule has a Y shape (Fig. 56.1).

L chains belong to one of 2 types, κ (kappa) or λ (lambda), on the basis of amino acid differences in their constant regions. Both types occur in all classes of immunoglobulins (IgG, IgM, etc.), but any one immunoglobulin molecule contains only one type of L chain. The amino-terminal portion of each L chain participates in the antigen-binding site. H chains are distinct for each of the 5 immunoglobulin classes and are designated γ, α, μ, ε, and δ (Table 56.1). The amino-terminal portion of each H chain participates in the antigen-binding site; the carboxy terminal forms the Fe fragment, which has the biologic activities.

If an antibody molecule is treated with a proteolytic enzyme such as papain, peptide bonds in the "hinge" region are broken, producing 2 identical Fab fragments, which carry the antigen-binding sites, and one Fe fragment, which is involved in placental transfer, complement fixation, attachment for various cells, and other biologic activities.

L and H chains are subdivided into variable and constant regions. The regions are composed of 3-dimensionally folded, repeating segments called domains. An L chain consists of one variable (VL) and one constant (CL) domain. Most H chains consist of one variable (VH) and 3 constant (CH) domains. (IgG and IgA have 3 CH domains, whereas IgM and IgE have 4.) Each domain, is approximately 110 amino acids long. The variable regions are responsible for antigen binding, whereas the constant regions are responsible for various biologic functions, e.g. complement activation and binding to cell surface receptors.

Table 56.1: Properties of human immunoglobulins.

Property	*IgG*	*IgA*	*IgM*	*IgD*	*IgE*
Percentage of total immunoglobulin in serum (approx)	75	15	9	0.2	0.004
Serum concentration (mg/dl) (approx)	1000	200	120	3	0.05
Sedimentation coefficient	7S	7S or 11S[1]	19S	7S	8S
Molecular weight (× 1000)	150	170 or 400[1]	900	180	190
Structure	Monomer	Monomer or dimer	Pentamer	Monomer	Monomer
H-chain symbol	γ	α	μ	δ	ε
Complement fixation	+	-	+	-	-
Transplacental passage	+	-	-	?	-
Mediation of allergic responses	-	-	-	-	+
Found in secretions	-	+	-	-	-
Opsonization	+	-	-	-	-

[1]The 11S form is found in secretions (e.g. saliva, milk, and tears) and fluids of the respiratory, intestinal and genital tracts.
[2]IgM opsonizes indirectly by activating complement. This produces C3b, which is an opsonin.

Properties of Human Immunoglobulins (Fig. 56.1)

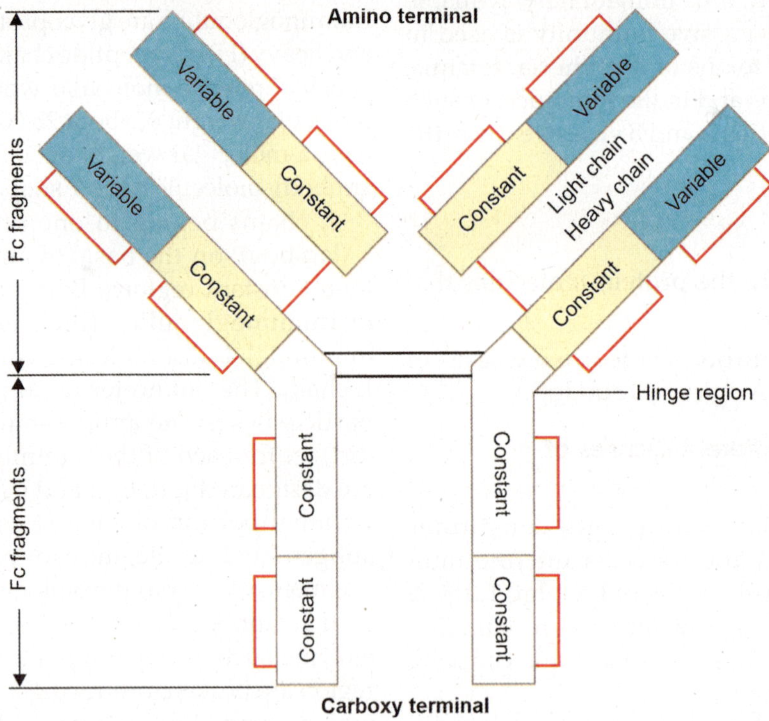

Fig. 56.1: Structure of IgG

Major functions of immunoglobulin are given in Table 56.2.

Table 56 2. Important functions of immunoglobulins

Immuno-globulin	*Major functions*
IgG	Opsonizes bacteria, making them easier to phagocytize. Fixes complement, which enhances bacterial killing. Neutralizes bacterial toxins and viruses, crosses the placenta.
IgA	Secretory IgA prevents attachment of bacteria and viruses to mucous membranes. Does not fix complement.
IgM	Produced in the primary response to an antigen. Fixes complement but does not cross the placenta. Found on the surface of B cells as well as in serum.
IgD	Uncertain. Found on the surface of many B cells as well as in serum.
IgE	Mediates immediate hypersensitivity by causing release of mediators from mast cells and basophils upon exposure to allergen.

ISOTYPES, ALLOTYPES, AND IDIOTYPES

Because immunoglobulins are proteins, they are antigenic, and that property allows them to be subdivided into various isotypes, allotypes, and idiotypes.

1. **Isotypes** are immunoglobulins that can be distinguished antigenically yet are found in all normal humans. For example, IgG and IgM are different isotypes; the constant region of their H chains. (γ and μ) is different antigenically (the 5 immunoglobulin classes—IgG, IgM, IgA, IgD, and IgE— are different isotypes, their heavy chains are antigenically different). Similarly, IgA1 and IgA2 are different isotypes (the antigenicity of the constant region of their H chains is different), and κ and λ chains are different isotypes (their constant regions also differ antigenically).
2. **Allotypes,** on the other hand, are additional antigenic features of immunoglobulins that vary among individuals. They vary because the genes that code for the L and H chains are polymorphic, and individuals can have different alleles. For example, the γ H chain contains an allotype called Gm, which is due to a 1- or 2-amino acid difference that provides a different antigenicity to the molecule. Each individual inherits different allelic genes that code for one or another amino acid at the Gm site.
3. **Idiotypes** are the antigenic determinants of the hypervariable region. Each idiotype is unique for the V domain of the immunoglobulin produced by a specific clone of antibody-producing cells. Anti-idiotype antibody reacts only with the V domain of the specific immunoglobulin molecule that induced it. The network theory of immune regulation employs anti-idiotype antibody as both a positive and a negative regulator. Because the antibody could interact with the antigen-binding site, it could mimic antigen and induce B cell differentiation. Alternatively, it could suppress it.

Chapter 57

Major Histocompatibility: HLA Complex, Transplantation and Complement System

Chapter Outline

HISTOCOMPATIBILITY ANTIGENS (HLA)

Definition: The term HLA refers to human leucocyte antigen displayed on the various cell surfaces, that evoke the rejection of transplanted organs. This is brought about by the recognition of histocopatibility antigens displayed on the cell surfaces of the donor organ through the recipient's immune system. It is called human leucocyte antigen because MHC encoded antigens were initially detected on white cells.

MAJOR HISTOCOMPATIBILITY COMPLEX

HLA Complex

The name histocompatibility complex arose because its discovery was based on transplantation experiments, and only later were the other two components of the complex identified. The major antigens determining histocompatibility in human beings are alloantigens, characteristically found on the surface of leucocytes. Human MHC antigens are therefore synonymous with human leucocyte antigens (HLA), and the MHC complex of genes with the HLA complex.

The HLA complex of genes is located on the short arm of chromosome 6 (Fig. 57.1). It consists of three separate clusters of genes:

Structure and genetic constitution: The structure and organization of HLA and corresponding HLA genes is complex and still incompletely understood

Several genes code for histocompatibility antigens, but those that code for the most important transplantation antigens are clustered on a small segment of chromosome 6. This cluster of genes constitutes the human major histocompatibility complex (MHC) or HLA complex.

The HLA complex is composed of four closely linked loci called HLA complex on chromosome 6.

HLA—HLA loci show high degree of polymorphism, i.e. the existence of multiple allelic forms in a population. Each of the several allelic determinants at these loci is identified by a number, e.g. HLA-B5, etc.

Already, more than 40 antigens have been recognised at HLA-B locus. These antigens are designated by a W, e.g. HLA-BW 21. Antigens coded by HLA—A, B and C loci are called class I antigens and those coded by HLA-D/DR loci are called class II antigens. These are ME-MT and SB antigens.

MHC Antigens

Class I MHC Antigens

These are glycoproteins found on the surface of virtually all nucleated cells. There are approximately 20 different

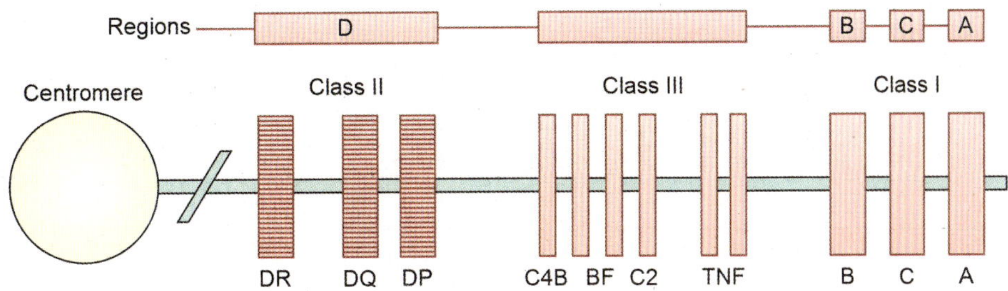

Fig. 57.1: HLA complex loci on chromosome

proteins encoded by the allelic genes at the A locus, 40 at the B locus, and 8 at the C locus. The complete class I antigen is composed of a 45,000-molecular-weight heavy chain noncovalently bound to a beta-2 microglobulin. The heavy chain is highly polymorphic and is similar to an immunoglobulin molecule; it has hypervariable regions in its N-terminal region. The polymorphism of these molecules is important in the recognition of self and nonself. Stated another way, if these molecules were very similar, our ability to reject foreign grafts would be correspondingly lower.

Class I antigens are detected in the laboratory by reacting lymphocytes (as antigen) with a battery of specific antibodies plus complement. If lymphocyte and antibody match, the cell is lysed. This test, along with the test for class II antigens (*see* below), is used to identify the haplotypes of donors being considered for transplant surgery.

Class II MHC Antigens

These occur on the surface of certain cells, including macrophages, B cells, dendritic cells of the spleen, and Langerhans cells of the skin. They are highly polymorphic glycoproteins composed of 2 polypeptides (MW 33,000 and 28,000) that are noncovalently bound. Like class I antigens, they have hypervariable regions that provide much of the polymorphism. Unlike class I antigens, which have only one chain encoded by the MHC locus (beta-2 microglobulin is encoded on chromosome 15), both chains of the class II antigens are encoded by the MHC locus.

Class II antigens were first demonstrated by the "mixed-leukocyte reaction." In this test, "stimulator" lymphocytes from a potential donor are first killed by irradiation and then mixed with live "responder" lymphocytes from the recipient, the mixture is incubated in cell culture to permit DNA synthesis, which is measured by incorporation of tritiated thymidine. The greater the amount of DNA synthesis in the responder cells, the class II MHC antigens of the donor cells are more foreign. A large amount of DNA synthesis indicates an unsatisfactory "match", i.e. donor and recipient class II (HLA-D) MHC antigens are not similar, and the graft is likely to be rejected. Currently, clinical laboratories can determine the important class II antigens (DR loci) by using serologic tests analogous to those used for the class I antigens.

Distribution: Class I antigens are present on virtually all the nucleated cells. They evoke the formation of humoral antibody in genetically non-identical recipients.

Class II antigens: These are present on mainly B lymphocytes, monocytes/macrophages, dendritic/Langerhans' cells and some endothelial cells. Class II antigens are products of Ir (immune response) genes, which determine individual pattern of responses to foreign antigens.

Between the class I and class II gene loci is a third locus (Fig. 57.2). This locus contains several immunologically important genes, namely 2 cytokines (tumour necrosis factor and lymphotoxin) and two complement components (C2 and C4).

Inheritance of HLA haplotype: A set of closely linked genes on one chromosome constitutes a haplotype and these tend to be inherited en bloc including one gene each from HLA—A, B, C, D and DR loci. Parents share one haplotype with all children and differ in the other. However, if both parents had shared one haplotype, there would be a 1 in 2 chance of parents and offspring being identical. This degree of haplotype sharing is of fundamental importance in predicting graft survival.

Biologic Importance of MHC

The ability of T cells to recognize antigen is dependent on association of the antigen with either class I or class II proteins. For example, cytotoxic T cells respond to antigen in association with class I MHC proteins. Thus, a cytotoxic T cell that kills a virus-infected cell will not kill a cell infected with the same virus if the cell does not also express the same class I proteins. This finding

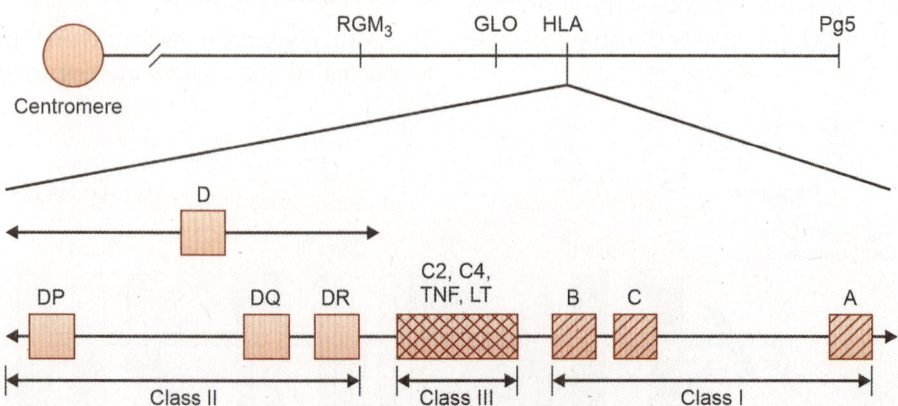

Fig. 57.2: The human leukocyte antigen (HLA) gene complex: A, B, and C are the class I loci. DP, DQ, and DR are class II loci. C2 and C4 are complement loci. TNF is tumour necrosis factor. LT is lymphotoxin. PGM_3, GLO, and Pg 5 are adjacent, unrelated genes

was determined, using inbred animals, by mixing virus-infected cells and cytotoxic T cells bearing different class I proteins and observing that no killing of the virus infected cells occurred. Helper T cells recognize class II proteins. Helper-cell activity depends in general on both the recognition of the antigen on antigen-presenting cells and the presence on these cells of "self" class II MHC proteins. This requirement to recognize antigen in association with a "self" MHC protein is called MHC restriction. Note that T cells recognize only antigens bound to the surface of cells, whereas B cells can recognize soluble antigens that interact with immunoglobulin receptors.

Significance of HLA Complex

1. **Organ transplantation:** In organ transplantation, HLA antigens of the graft evoke both humoral and cell mediated response, which leads to graft destruction, if there is a disparity between donor and recipient. Hence, HLA typing is very important in the selection of donor–recipient combinations.
2. **Regulation of immune responses:** Class II antigens having a Ir gene control, regulate the immune response of an individual.
3. **Cell to cell interaction in immune response:** The ultimate expression of immune response both humoral and cellular results from interaction of various immunologically active cells. These interactions are critically dependent on the recognition of class II FILA antigens.
4. **Role in host defence:** The T cell-mediated lysis of the virus and tumour cells by cytotoxic T cells are brought about in the presence of class I antigen as follows (Fig. 57.3):

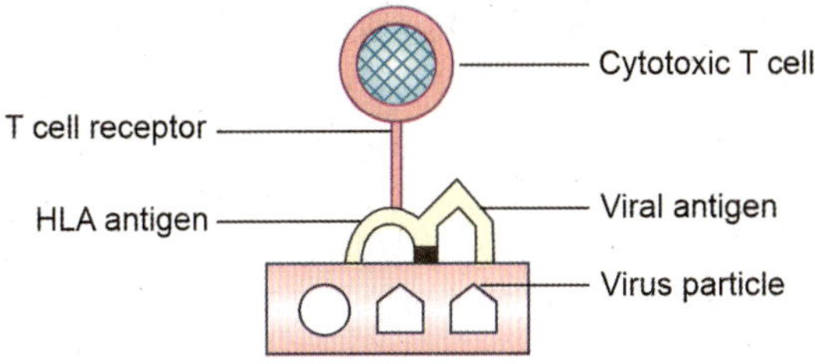

Fig. 57.3: Diagrammatic representation of role in host defence

As we can see, it is the HLA antigen present on the surface of virus infected cell which is recognised by the cytoxic T cell via, its surface receptor for the same, that the Olysis is brought about cytotoxic T cell cannot recognize viral antigens independent of HLA antigen (HLA restriction).

5. **HLA and disease association:** A variety of diseases have been found in association with certain HLA types. Selected examples of HLA and disease association is given in Table 57.1.

Table 57.1: Diseases and HLA with estimated relative risk

Disease	*HLA*	*Estimated relative risk*
Ankylosing spondylitis	B 27	90
Reiter's disease	B 27	48
Acute anterior uveitis	B 27	16.9
Rheumatoid arthritis	DW4/DR4	4.2
Hashimoto's disease	DR3	2.6
Addison's disease	B-8, DW3	4.0
Hemochromatosis	BW A3	6.3
21-Hydroxylase deficiency	A3, BW 47	4, 15
Dermatitis herpetiformis	B8, DW3	8, 7, 13.5

The best known is the association of ankylosing spondylitis and HLA-B 27.

In view of physiologic role of HLA complex in regulation of immune response, the following two mechanisms are postulated in their association with immunologically mediated diseases.

i. Involvement of immunoresponse genes which regulate the levels of autoantibody responses. Hence, association with autoimmune diseases.
ii. Direct participitation of HLA macromolecule in disease in which pathogens may share cross-reacting antigens with HLA or molecule may provide receptors for viruses and this may facilitate virus cell interaction leading to disease process.

Transplantation

An autograft (transfer of an individual's own tissue) is always accepted. A syngeneic graft is a transfer of tissue hetween genetically identical individuals, i.e. identical twins, and usually "takes" permanently: A xenograft, a transfer of tissue between different species, is always rejected by an immunocompetent recipient.

An allograft is a graft between genetically different members of the same species, e.g. from one human to another. Unless specific measures are taken, it is rejected by the "allograft reaction." Initially, vascularization of the graft is normal, but in 11–14 days, marked reduction in circulation and mononuclear cell infiltration occurs, with eventual necrosis. A T cell-mediated reaction is the main cause of rejection of many types of grafts, e.g. skin, but antibodies contribute to the rejection of certain transplants, especially bone marrow. In experimental animals, rejection of most types of grafts can be transferred by cells, not serum. Also, T cell-deficient animals do not reject grafts but B cell-deficient animals do. The role of cytotoxic T cells in allograft rejection is described earlier.

If a second allograft from the same donor is applied to a sensitised recipient, it is rejected in 5–6 days. This accelerated ("second-set") rejection is caused primarily by presensitised cytotoxic T cells.

The acceptance or rejection of a transplant is determined, in large part, by the class I and class II MHC proteins, with class II playing the major role. The proteins encoded by the DR locus are especially important. Prior to transplantation surgery, laboratory tests are performed to determine the closest match of MHC antigens in the donor and recipient. Class I antigens and certain class II antigens, especially DR, are detected by using a panel of known antibodies plus complement to lyse donor lymphocytes. Additional information regarding the compatibility of the class II antigens is determined by the mixed leukocyte reaction with cultured cells. In addition to the tests used for matching, preformed cytotoxic antibodies in the recipient's serum reactive against the graft are detected by observing the lysis of donor lymphocytes by the recipient's serum plus complement. This is called "crossmatching" and is done to prevent hyperacute rejections from occurring. (ABO blood group tests are also done on the donor and recipient.)

Among siblings in a single family, there is a 25% chance for both haplotypes to be shared and a 50% chance for one haplotype to be shared. For example, if the father is haplotype AB, the mother is CD, and the recipient child is AC, there is a 25% chance for a sibling to be AC, i.e. a 2-haplotype match, and a 50% chance for a sibling to be either BC or AD, i.e. a one-haplotype match.

The success of tissue and organ transplants depends on the donor's and recipient's human leukocyte antigens (HLA) encoded by the HLA genes. These proteins are alloantigens; i.e. they differ among members of the same species. If the HLA proteins on the donor's cells differ from those on the recipient's cells, an immune response occurs in the recipient. The genes for the HLA proteins are clustered in the major histocompatibility complex (MHC), located on the short arm of chromosome 6. Three of these genes (HLA-A, HLA-B, and HLA-C) code for the class I MHC antigens. Several HLA-D loci determine the class II MHC antigens, i.e. DP, DQ, and DR. Each person has 2 haplotypes, i.e. 2 sets of these genes, one on the paternal and the other on the maternal chromosome 6. These genes are very diverse (polymorphic) (i.e. there are many alleles of the class I and class II genes), but any individual inherits only a single allele at cach locus from each parent and thus can make no more than 2 class I and II proteins at each gene locus. Expression of these genes is codominant; i.e. the proteins encoded by both the paternal and maternal genes are produced. Each person can make as many as 12 HLA proteins: 3 at class I loci and 3 at class II loci, from both chromosomes.

Graft-versus-Host Reaction

Well-matched transplants of bone marrow may establish themselves initially in 85% of recipients, but subsequently a graft-versus-host (GVH) reaction develops in about two-thirds of them. This reaction occurs because grafted immunocompetent T cells proliferate in the irradiated, immunocompromised host and reject cells with class II antigens, resulting in severe organ dysfunction especially in the skin, liver, and gastrointestinal tract. The GVH reaction can be reduced by administering antithymocyte globulin or monoclonal antibodies before grafting; this eliminates mature T cells from the donor marrow. Immunotoxins, e.g. ricin, linked to monoclonal anti-T cell antibody can also be used to reduce this reaction.

Effect of Immunosuppression on Graft Rejection

To reduce the chance of rejection of transplanted tissue, immunosuppressive measures, e.g. cyclosporin A, corticosteroids, azathioprine, and radiation, are used. Cyclosporin A prevents the activation of T lymphocytes by inhibiting signal transduction within the cytoplasm of T cells. This drug is well-tolerated and is remarkably successful in preventing the rejection of transplants. Unfortunately, immunosuppression enhances the recipient's susceptibility to opportunistic infections and neoplasms. Immunosuppressive drugs, e.g. cyclosporine, also reduce GVH reactions.

Complement

The complement system consists of approximately 20 proteins that are present in normal human (and other animal) serum. The term "complement" refers to the ability of these proteins to complement, i.e. augment, the effects of other components of the immune system, e.g. antibody. There are 3 main effects of complement:

1. Lysis of cells such as bacteria, allografts, and tumour cells;
2. Generation of mediators that participate in inflammation and attract phagocytes; and
3. Opsonization, i.e. enhancement of phagocytosis.

Complement proteins are synthesized mainly by the liver. Complement is heat-labile, i.e. it is inactivated by heating serum at 56°C for 30 minutes. Immunoglobulins are not inactivated at this temperature.

Activation

Several complement components are proenzymes, which must be cleaved to form active enzymes.

Activation of the complement system can be initiated either by antigen–antibody complexes or by a variety of nonimmunologic molecules, e.g. endotoxin.

Sequential activation of complement components occurs via one of 2 pathways. Both pathways lead to the production of C3b, the central molecule of the complement cascade. Of the two pathways, the alternative one is more important the first time we are infected by a microorganism, since the antibody required to trigger the classic pathway is not present.

1. In the classic pathway, antigen–antibody complexes activate C1 to form an esterase, which cleaves C2 and C4 to form a C4b2b complex. The latter is C3 convertase, which cleaves C3 molecules into 2 fragments, C3a and C3b. C3s, an anaphylatoxin, is discussed below. C3b forms a complex with C462b, producing a new enzyme, C5 convertase (C4b2b3b), which cleaves C5 to form C5a and C5b. C5a is an anaphylatoxin and a chemotactic factor (*see* below). C5b binds to C6 and C7 to form a complex that interacts with C8 and C9 to produce the "membrane attack" complex (MC 5b, 6, 7, 8, 9), which causes cytolysis (Fig. 57.4).
2. In the alternative pathway, many unrelated cell surface substances, e.g. bacterial lipopolysaccharides (endotoxin), fungal cell walls, and viral envelopes, activate a different C3 convertase (C3bBb), which generates more C3b. The additional C3b binds to form C3bBbC3b, a C5 convertase that generates C5b, leading to the production of the membrane attack complex described above.

Regulation of the Complement System

Several serum proteins regulate the complement system at different stages.

1. C1 inhibitor binds to and inactivates the esterase. Complement activation proceeds past this point by generating sufficient C1 to overwhelm the inhibitor.
2. Factor I cleaves C3b, thereby reducing the amount of C5 convertase available.
3. Factor H enhances the effect of factor I on C3b. C3b deposited on certain membranes or activators is protected from factors H and I.
4. Factor P (properdin) protects C3b and stabilizes the convertases of the alternative pathway.
5. Factors B and D interact with C3b to form C3bBb (C3 convertase) in the alternative pathway.
6. Decay-accelerating factor (DAF) is a protein on the surface of human cells that inactivates C3bBb, thereby protecting these cells from damage by membrane attack complexes generated by the alternative pathway.

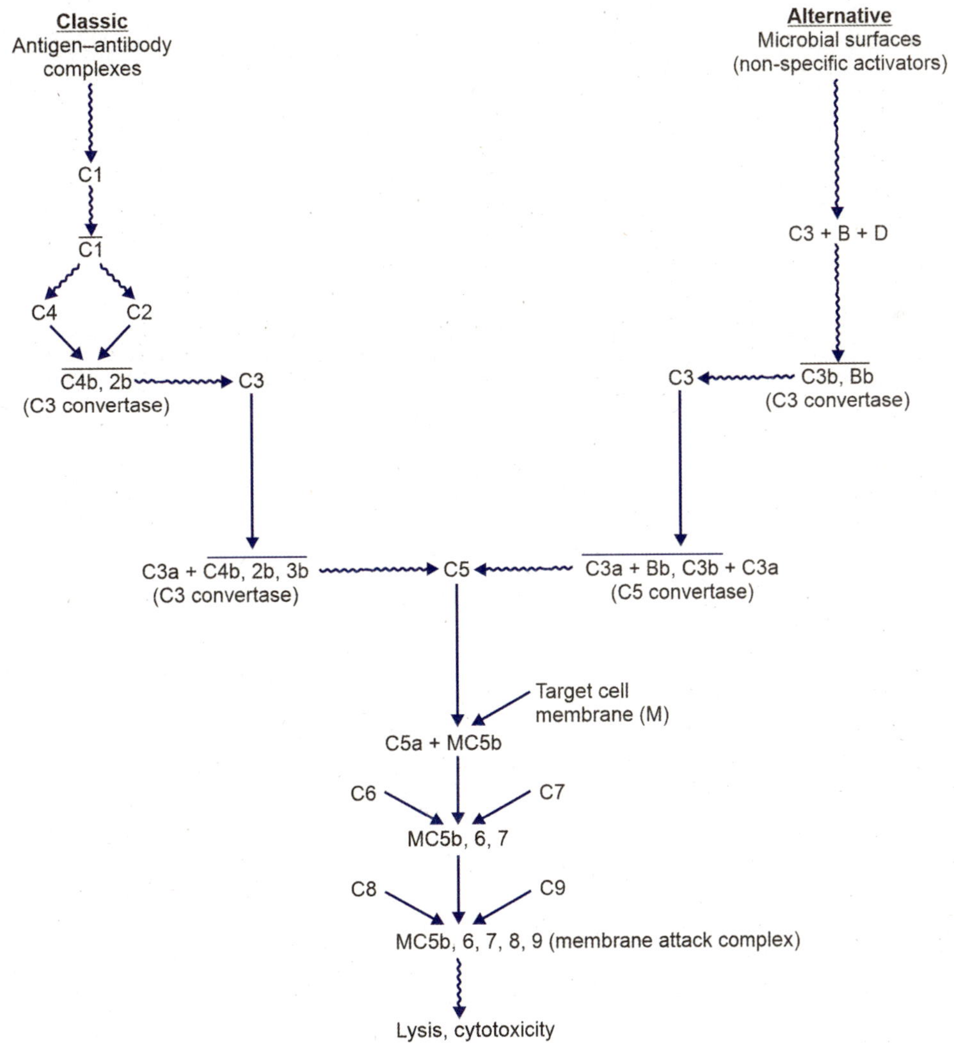

Fig. 57.4: The classic and alternative pathways of the complement system → indicates that proteolytic cleavage of the molecule at the tip of the arrow has occurred, → points toward the products of a reaction; a line over a complex indicates that it is enzymatically active

Cytolysis

Insertion of the C5b6789 complex into the cell membrane leads to killing or lysis of many types of cells including erythrocytes, bacteria, and tumour cells. Cytolysis is not an enzymatic process; rather, it appears that insertion of the complex results in disruption of the membrane and the entry of water and electrolytes into the cell (Fig. 57.4).

Clinical Aspects

1. Inherited (or acquired) deficiency of some complement components, especially C5–C8, greatly enhances susceptibility to Neisseria bacteraemia and other infections.
2. Inherited deficiency of C1 esterase inhibitor results in angioedema. When the inhibitor is reduced, an overproduction of esterase occurs. This leads to an increase in anaphylatoxins, which cause capillary permeability and oedema.
3. Immune complexes bind complement, and thus complement levels are low in immune complex diseases, e.g. acute glomerulonephritis. Binding (activating) complement attracts polymorphonuclear leukocytes, which release enzymes that damage tissue.

BIOLOGIC EFFECTS

Opsonization: Cells, antigen–antibody complexes, and viruses are phagocytized much better in the presence of C3b. This is due to the presence of C3b receptors on the surface of many phagocytes.

Chemotaxis: C5a and the C567 complex attract leukocytes. They migrate especially well toward C5a.

Anaphylatoxin: C3, C4a, and C5a cause degranulation of mast cells with release of mediators, e.g. histamine, leading to increased vascular permeability and smooth muscle contraction.

Chapter 58

Antigen–Antibody Reactions

Chapter Outline

INTRODUCTION

Reactions of antigens and antibodies are highly specific. An antigen will react only with antibodies elicited by itself or by a closely related antigen. Because of the great specificity, reactions between antigens and antibodies are suitable for identifying one by using the other. This is the basis of serologic reactions. However, cross-reactions between related antigens can occur, and these can limit the usefulness of the test. The results of many immunologic tests are expressed as a titer which is defined as the highest dilution of the specimen, e.g. serum, that gives a positive reaction in the test. Microorganisms and other cells possess a variety of antigens and thus induce antisera containing many different antibodies, i.e. the antisera are polyclonal. Monoclonal antibodies excel in the identification of antigens because cross-reacting antibodies are absent, i.e. monoclonal antibodies are highly specific.

Types of Reactions

1. Immunodiffusion
2. Electrophoresis
3. Immunoelectrophoresis
4. Radioimmunoassay
5. Immunochemical and physicochemical methods.
6. Immunofluorescence
7. Agglutination
8. Complement fixation

The important, and commonly used techniques will be described.

IMMUNODIFFUSION

Principle: The antigen and antibody are detected by their reaction to form a precipitate line. It is the most common technique. It may be single or double. In single immunodiffusion, the antigen or antibody remains fixed and the other one is allowed to move in agar-filled tube and form precipitate complex with it. Double immunodiffusion: Both reactants are free to move towards each other and precipitate.

Movement in either form may be radial or linear.

Clinical application: Most important application is in estimation of serum immunoglobulins or serum proteins.

Technique: Quantitative determination of the immunoglobulins IgG, IgA and IgM by tri-partigen-plates.

Composition of tri-partigen plates: Tri-partigen immunodiffusion plates contain a prepared agar gel in which H-chain specific antiserum to the respective immunoglobulins is incorporated. (The antiserum is produced by immunization of sheep and goats.) Preservative sodium azide: 1 mg/ml.

Sodium P—ethyl

Mercury mercaptobenzene sulfonates ≤0.1 mg per ml.

Method

1. Open the plate and leave the opened plate to stand for about 5 minutes, at room temperature to allow any condensation water that may have accumulated in the walls to evaporate.
2. IgA and IgM are determined with undiluted serum. Only when IgG is to be determined, sera to be tested and control serum used must be diluted 1: 10 with normal saline.

Procedure

1. Well 1 is filled with 5 µl of control serum. Wells 2–12: Each filled with 5 µl of sera under tests.

2. Close the plate tightly and leave it to stand at room temperature.
3. Diffusion time of 50 hours. (IgG and IgA) and 80 hours (IgM).
4. At the end of the given diffusion time, the diameter D of the precipitin rings should be measured accurately to 0.1 mm using a suitable calibrated instrument.
5. The immunoglobulin concentrations related to the measured diameters are read directly from the tables of reference values.
   The results are reliable only when the value found for the control sera applied to well 1 lies within the confidence range taken from the table of values enclosed with each pack of control sera.
   Confidence range with Hoechst packing: 15% of immunoglobulin concentration with each pack. When determining IgG, value found must be multiplied by the dilution factor 10.
6. If the protein concentration of the sera samples diverge considerably from normal value, this means that resultant ppt rings will fall outside the assay range of the plate. In this case examination is repeated using high dilution (tripartigen IgM is not suited for IgM determination in seminal fluid).

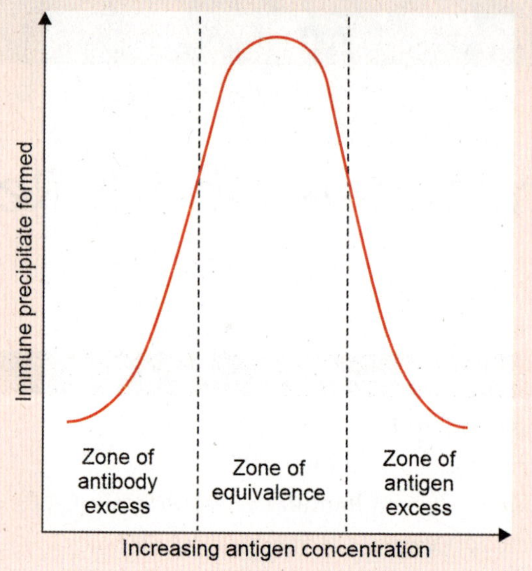

Fig. 58.1: Precipitin curve. In the presence of a constant amount of antibody, the amount of immune precipitate formed is plotted as a function of increasing amounts of antigen

Precipitation

In this reaction, the antigen is in solution (soluble antigen). The antibody cross-links antigen molecules in variable proportions, and aggregates (precipitates) form. In the zone of equivalence, optimal proportions of antigen and antibody combine; the maximal amount of precipitates forms, and the supernatant contains neither an excess of antibody nor an excess of antigen (Fig. 58.1). In the zone of antibody excess, there is too much antibody for efficient lattice formation, and precipitation is less than maximal.† In the zone of antigen excess, all antibody has combined but precipitation is reduced because many antigen–antibody complexes are too small to precipitate, i.e. they are "soluble." Procipitin reactions can be done in solution or in semisolid medium (agar).

A. **Precipitation in solution:** This reaction can be made quantitative; i.e. antigen or antibody can be measured in terms of micrograms of nitrogen present. It is used primarily in research.

B. **Precipitation in agar:** This is done as either single or double diffusion. It can also be done in the presence of an electric field.

   1. *Single diffusion:* In single diffusion, antibody is incorporated into agar and antigen is measured into a well. As the antigen diffuses with time, precipitation rings form depending on the antigen concentration. By calibrating the method, such radial immunodiffusion is used to measure IgG IgM, complement components, and other substances in serum (IgE cannot be measured because its concentration is too low.)
   2. *Double dillusion:* In double diffusion, antigen and antibody are placed in different wells in agar and allowed to diffuse and form concentration gradients. Where optimal proportions (*see* zone of equivalence, above) occur, lines of precipitate form. This method (Ouchterlony) indicates whether antigens are identical, related but not identical, or not related (Fig. 58.2).

C. **Precipitation in agar with an electric field:**

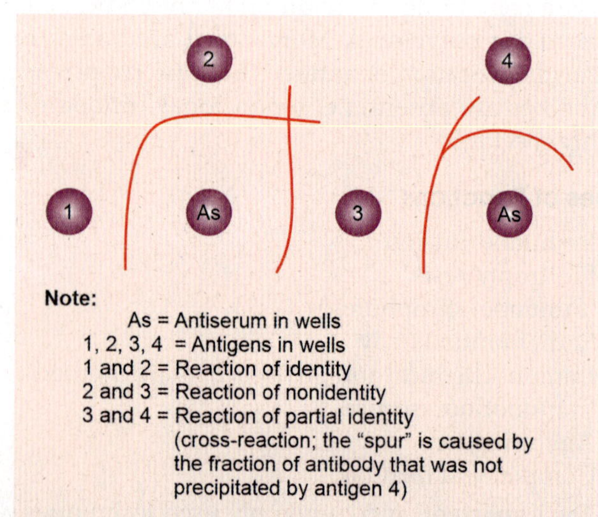

Fig. 58.2: Double-diffusion (Ouchterlony) precipitin reactions

†"The term "prizone" refers to the failure of a precipitate or flocculate to form because too much antibody is present. For example, a false-negative serologic test for syphilis (VDRL) is occasionally reported because the antibody titer is too high. Dilution of the serum yields a positive result.

Immunoelectrophoresis (IEP)

Principle: Immunoelectrophoresis combines electrophoretic separation diffusion in the electric field and immune precipitation of proteins simultaneously. Hence both identification and approximate quantities can thereby be accomplished for individual proteins present in serum, urine or other biologic fluid.

Immunoelectrophoresis as described by Graber and Williams (1953) added the immunological discrimination of double diffusion to zone electrophoretic separation of protein solutions. The original method was rather cumbersome and demanded large volumes of antiserum. Scheidegger (1955) modified the method by scaling the whole technique down to the 76 × 26 mm microscope slide. This allowed the initial electrophoretic separation to be conducted in 45 min instead of 6 hour and the diffusion phase to be completed in 24 hours instead of 10 days. The restricted space available on 76 × 26 mm glass slide did, however, make for difficulties in comparison between separation pattern and was restrictive when non-specific antisera were used to identify individual precipitin arcs.

Materials

1. Electrophoresis apparatus: Any low voltage power pack is suitable provided it can produce a maximum of 50 MA or 50 V current or voltage stabilised (Shandon Southern VOKAM).
2. Universal electrophoresis tank (Shandon Southern). Electrophoresis wicks: Filter paper or lint laid over the electrophoresis bridge supports of the electrophoresis tank.
3. Gel Punch and suction device and suitable template. Glass plates 80 × 80 mm. The plates should be precoated with 2–5% agar and dried. This skinning process makes the gel adhere to the plate so that it does not become detached during subsequent washing procedures.
4. Wooden blocks 10 × 2 × 2 cm metal rule double bladed knife for through cutting. A double bladed knife can be made by blotting two surgical scalpel blades on either side of a 1 mm metal spacer bar. Water bath horizontal table micropipette.
5. Agar: Various commercial agar preparations are suitable including Difco special agar noble and Behringwerke purified agar noble in barbiturate buffer is dispensed in 6 ml aliquots. Difco special agar noble, 3.6 g barbitone buffer pH 8.6, 150 ml and distilled water 150 ml.
6. Barbitone buffer (Venoral) pH 8.6 (dilute stock solution 1 in 2). Stock solution: Sodium barbitone 154 g. Barbitone 27.6 g distilled water to 10 litre. Add sodium azide, 10 G as an antimicrobial preservative. Stain solution: ponceau S 2 g. Trichloracetic acid 30 g distilled water to 1 litre. Dissolve and leave overnight before use. Staining time: 10 min. Destain solution: 5% acetic acid solution.
7. Anti-serum in appropriate quantity.

Method

1. **Preparation of the gel:** 6 ml of predispensed agar is melted in the water bath and pour into the "Preskinned" glass plate on a horizontal table. The gel is left to set and then allowed to handen at 4°C in a moist chamber.
2. **Origin wells:** Place the gel over the template and cut origin wells 1–2 mm diameter according to template. The wells should be evacuated by suction.
3. **Samples loading:** The origin wells are filled to the brim with the test samples. One well should be reserved for a control sample stained with Bromophenol blue to provide a marker of electrophoretic migration
4. **Electrophoresis:** the gel is inverted and placed in the electrophoresis tank so that the agar is in direct contact with the wicks or the support bridges. A constant current of 1.5 mA/cm gel (12 mA per 30 mm plate) is applied and or until the Bromophenol blue mark has migrated to within 1 cm of anode wick.
5. On completion of the electrophoretic separation the gel is removed from the tank and placed over the templates. The wooden blocks are placed on either side of the gel and the metal rule supported over the gel. With the rule as a guide out the antiserum troughs with the double bladed knife. Gently lift out the and remove the agar from the troughs.
6. Fill the troughs with antiserum (approx 100 µl).
7. Place the gel in a moist chamber to diffuse for 18–24 hours at ambient temperature. The gel should be maintained horizontal during this diffusion phase. On completion of diffusion, the precipitin lines can be examined by incident light illumination against a dark background.
8. To prepare permanent preparations, unreacted protein must be washed from the gel. This is achieved by washing in saline for 24 hours. and in distilled water for 1 hr. The gel is covered either with filter paper and dried in a warm air oven or with three layers of Whatman 3 mm paper and press dried. The plate can be now stained, excess stain being removed by washing in 5% acetic acid.

Possible Sources of Error

1. Electrophoretic separation must be adequate. Too long or too short separation will lead to difficulties in interpretation.
2. Too short an antiserum trough or irregularities in cutting it, will distort the precipitin pattern.
3. Bacterial contamination or proteolytic degradation of the serum sample will distort the pattern and alter the electrophoretic mobility of many proteins.
4. Diffusion will occur more rapidly at a high temperature. With a high ambient temperature precipitin pattern should be examined sooner than the usual 18–20 hours.

5. When testing for small molecular weight proteins, such as Bence Jones protein, the precipitin pattern should be examined at 30 min intervals to avoid loss of the preciptin lines due to rapid diffusion of the antigen towards the antiserum trough.

Identification of Precipitin Lines

The analysis of a precipitin pattern requires a certain degree of practice and familiarity. Albumin, transferrin and the major immunoglobulin lines are readily identified, but other lines often need other techniques to aid their identification.

Specific antisera: The use of two antisera in troughs on either side of an electrophoretic separation allows the direct comparison of the precipitin lines produced by a polyspecific antiserum and the corresponding line produced with a monospecific antiserum. The advantage of the 80 × 80 mm plate over the 76 × 26 mm slide can be seen where direct comparison can be made between different test samples developed against monospecific and polyspecific antisera.

Specific stains: Certain plasma proteins can be stained with specific stains. Liporoteins can be stained with oil red or Sudan black. Haptoglobin and haemopexin can be stained with benzidine which identifies the haemoglobin or haem-components. Ceruloplasmin can be stained with Litatic P-phenylenediamine

Purified proteins: In certain instances where purified proteins are available these can be used to identify precipitin arcs in an immunoelectrophoretic pattern. Method utilising purified proteins have been described by Clausen and Hermens (1960). A serum sample is placed in a well in agar on a glass slide (Fig. 58.3).

A current is passed through the agar, and the proteins move in the electric field according to their charge and size. Then a trough is cut into the agar and filled with antibody. As the antigen and antibody diffuse toward each other, they form a series of arcs of precipitate. This permits the serum proteins to be characterised in terms of their presence, absence, or unusual pattern (e.g. human myeloma protein).

Counter Current Immunoelectrophoresis (CIEP)

Principle: The basic principles of the method involve electrophoresis in a gel medium of antigen and antibody in opposite directions simultaneously from separate wells. With resultant precipitation line at a point intermediate between their origins.

Clinical applications: In detection of the following:

- HBs Ag (Australia antigen)
- Cord IgM in intrauterine infection
- α (Alpha) fetoprotein
- Fungal precipitins

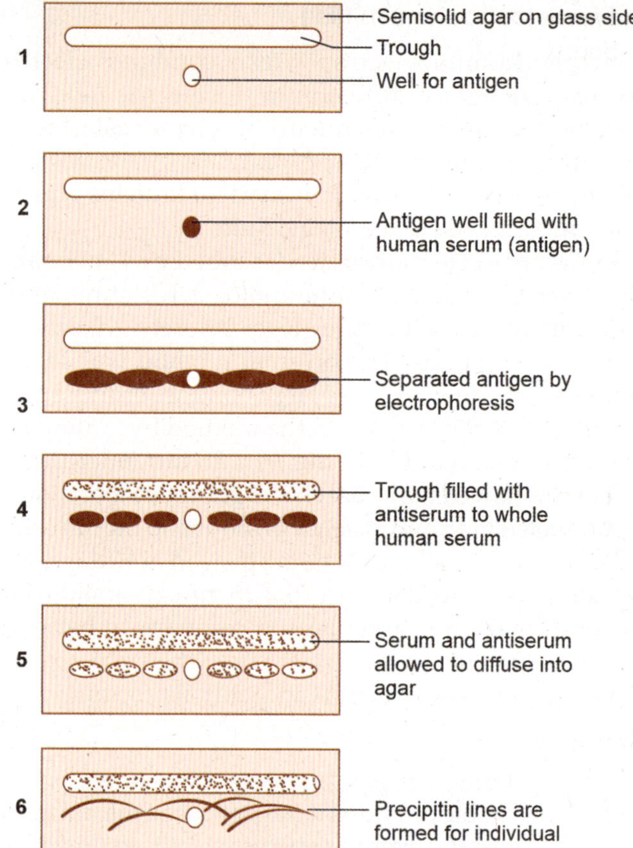

Fig. 58.3: Immunoelectrophoresis (IEP) human serum (1–6)

Prozone phenomenon: It refers to suboptimal precipitation which occur in the region of antibody excess. Thus dilution of antisera need to be reacted with fixed amounts of antigen in order to obtain maximum precipitation line. This is a common to phenomenon seen in paraproteinemias.

Electrophoresis

Electrophoresis is the separation of proteins in an electric field on the basis of the surface charge. It was perfected in 1937 by Tiselius. Generally paper, agarose or cellulose acetate strips are employed as supporting media which do not interfere in the flow of molecules in the electric field.

Electrophoresis of Serum Proteins

Principle: Various charged fractions of serum proteins are separated by subjecting serum to an electric field.

Paper Electrophoresis

Reagents

1. Venoral buffer (ionic strength 0.05, pH 8.6). Diethyl barbituric acid 1.84 g. Sodium diethylbarbiturate 10.3 g in water. Add water to 1 litre.
2. *Staining solution:* 0.01% bromphenol blue, 5 g of $ZnSO_4$, $7H_2O$ added and dissolved in 5% acetic acid. Made to 100 ml with 5% acetic acid.
3. *Wash solution:* 5% acetic acid.

4. *Fixative solution:* 5% acetic acid containing 0.3% Sodium acetate.

Execution: Buffer is poured into two tanks of electrophoresis apparatus (vertical type, horizontal type, vertical type discussed here). Whatman 1 mm. Filter paper strips (4 cm × 32 cm) are moistened with buffer, removing the excess buffer with a blotting paper. 20 µl of serum are applied exactly on the line drawn previously on the middle of the paper. The paper is mounted on the apparatus.

The apparatus is closed tightly and the electrophoretic run is started.

Voltage applied: 150 volts.

Current strength 1 to 1.5 milliamps for a 4 cm strip.

Time of run: 6 hours.

At the end of the run, the strips are removed and dried at 110°C for 20 minutes. They are then washed for 6 minutes, each time in two changes of wash solution. Subsequently the strips are washed with the fixative solution for 6 minutes and dried at room temperature or at 100°C for about 15 minutes.

Scanning/Elution: The stained bands on the strips can be scanned directly in a densitometer.

Cellulose Acetate Membrane Electrophoresis

Requisites:

1. Cellulose acetate membrane
2. Filter paper strips
3. Venoral buffer (pH 6.6, 0.07 M)
   - Barbituric acid 0.38 g.
   - Add distilled water to 500 ml.
   - Add thiomersal 0.01% for preservative purposes.
4. Staining solution: 0.8% Poneau 3R in 6% trichloro-acetic acid.
5. Decolourization solution: 1% Acetic acid.
6. Alkaline solution for elution: 0.01 N-NaOH solution.

Execution

1. Pretreatment of cellulose acetate membrane (6 cm × 3.4 cm) with buffer.
2. Preparation of electrophoretic bath, set the apparatus and connect with electricity. Pour buffer solution in the tanks and mount the membrane on the supporter bridge of the apparatus and wet by buffer solution
3. *Sampling:* Apply 0.0006–0012 ml per 1 cm of membrane.
4. Pass a constant current at 0.4–0.8 mA per 1 cm, of membrane for 45–60 minutes.
5. *Staining:* After time-up, separate the membrane from bath and put in the staining solution for 3 minutes.
6. Decolourise the background of the membrane with 1% acetic acid using several changes of acetic acid.
7. Scanning by densitometry or elution with 0.01 N NaOH, as described previously.

Agglutination

In this reaction, the antigen is particulate (e.g. bacteria and red blood cells) or is an inert particle (latex heads) coated with an antigen. Antibody, because it is divalent or multivalent, cross-links the antigenically multivalent particles and forms a latticework, and clumping (agglutination) can be seen. This reaction can be done in a small cup or tube or with a drop on a slide.

Agglutination Techniques

Agglutination and precipitation reactions are the basis of most commonly used, techniques in laboratories.

The agglutination of insoluble native antigens or antigen coated particles can be simply assessed with or without the aid of a microscope. Requirements in agglutination tests are three:

1. Stable cell or particle suspension.
2. Antigen close to the surface.
3. The knowledge that incomplete or non-agglutinating antibodies are not detectable without modifications.

Types of Agglutination Reactions

1. **Direct agglutination test:** In this, red blood cells, bacteria, fungi, etc. can be agglutinated by serum antibody. The clumping can be seen directly or under microscope after incubating for some time.
2. **Indirect (passive) agglutination test:** In this, the soluble antigen is passively absorbed or chemically coupled to red blood cells or other inert particles and thereby form stable reagents for antibody detection. Agglutination tests may be performed in tubes or microtitre plates.

Clinical Applications

In detection of rheumatoid factor, antistreptolysin-O (ASL-O); C-reactive protein (CRP), Coombs' test. Detection of HBs Ag. Factor VIII antigen in haemophilia and related clotted disorder, HCG detection in urine.

Latex agglutination inhibition test: In this test, instead of red blood cells, latex particles are used as the agent for coating the antigen. The most important clinical application of this test is the *Pregnancy test* or the detection of human chorionic gonadotrophin (HCG) in the urine of pregnant female. The test employs antiserum (anti-HCG produced in female rabbits) and antigen which consists of latex particles coated with HCG.

Neutralization tests: These use the ability of antibodies to block the effect of toxins or the infectivity of viruses. They can be used in cell culture (e.g. inhibition of cytopathic effect and plaque-reduction assays) or in host animals (e.g. mouse protection tests).

Neutralization reactions: In neutralization reactions, the harmful effects of a bacterial exotoxin or virus are eliminated by a specific antibody.

Opsonization is immune opsonization or nonimmune opsonization.

Immune complexes: Immune complexes in tissue can be stained with fluorescent complement. Immune complexes in serum can be detected by binding to Clq or by attachment to certain (e.g. Raji lymphoblastoid) cells in culture.

Hemagglutination tests: Many viruses clump red blood cells from one species or another (active hemagglutination). This can be inhibited by antibody specifically directed against the virus (hemagglutination inhibition) and can be used to measure the presence and concentration of such antibody. Red blood cells also can absorb many antigens and, when mixed with matching antibodies, will clump (this is known as passive hemagglutination).

Antiglobulin (Coombs) test: In many haemolytic anaemias, e.g. haemolytic disease of the newborn (Rh incompatibility) and drug- related haemolytic anaemias, antibodies are bound to the red cell surface. These immunoglobulins can be detected by the direct antiglobulin (Coombs) test, in which antiserum against human immunoglobulin is used to agglutinate the patient's red cells. In some cases, the amount of antibody bound is too small to be detected in the direct Coombs test and the indirect antiglobulin test for antibodies in the patient's serum should be performed. In this test, the patient's serum is mixed with normal red cells and antiserum to human immunoglobulins is added. If antibodies are present in the patient's serum, agglutination occurs.

Enzyme-Linked Immunosorbent Assay (ELISA)

There are many variations of this method that depend on the conjugation of an enzyme to either an antigen or an antibody. The enzyme is detected by assaying for enzyme activity with its substrate. The method is nearly as sensitive as RIA yet requires no special equipment or radioactive labels. For measurement of antibody, known antigens are fixed to a solid phase (e.g. plastic microplate), incubated with test serum dilutions, washed, and then reincubated with an anti-immunoglobulin labeled with an enzyme, e.g. horseradish peroxidase. Enzyme activity is measured by adding the substrate for the enzyme and estimating the colour reaction in a spectrophotometer. The amount of antibody bound is proportional to the enzyme activity.

Various types of enzyme-linked immunosorbent assay (ELISA) depends on an enzyme-substrate reaction and are direct ELISA, indirect ELISA, sandwich ELISA and competitive ELISA.

The ELISA test (enzyme-linked immunosorbant assay) is one of the most widely employed variants of enzyme immunoassay. Enzyme immunoassays have emerged as quantitative techniques for detection of antigens, haptens and antibodies. They all employ various enzymes linked to either antigen or antibody as a label which can easily be detected by measurement of enzyme activity.

Principle: The ELISA assay can be used to measure either antigen or antibody. To measure antigen, the antibody is bound to solid phase, incubated with test serum and then a second enzyme labelled antibody is added, substrate is then added and enzyme activity is related to antigen concentration.

Clinical applications: In detection of HBs Ag, HCG levels in urine or blood, CEA levels, steroid hormones, immunoglobulins, antibodies to bacteria, viruses, DNA and allergens.

Procedure

Material and Methods

1. Test sample: Serum sample stored at 4°C till the time test is performed.
2. Enzyme conjugate: Antibody to the specific antigen is conjugated to enzyme. The commonly used enzyme being horse-radish peroxidase. Others are alkaline phosphatase, lysozyme and glucose-6-phosphate dehydrogenase. The enzyme is coupled to antigen or antibody by various cross-linking agents, e.g. glutaraldehyde and dimaleimide.
3. Substrate: Orthophenylenediamine. (OPD) or 5-amino salicylic acid.
4. Antibody microtest plate: Precoating of antibody carried out in flat bottomed, 96 well microtest plates with specific dilution.
5. Diluent: Phosphate buffer saline (PBS) pH 7.2, 0.1 M or carbonate buffer pH 9.5 or normal saline with 0.1% sodium azide.

Method

1. The antibody is diluted to 1:500 in PHS at pH 7.2 and 75 µm is added to the bottom of each well.
2. Incubate the plates at 4°C in a moist chamber overnight for 18–20 hours.
3. Wash the plate three time with PBS supplemented with 0.05% tween 20 (BS-T) for 5 minutes each.
4. Add 200 µ of 1% bovine serum albumin in each well and incubate overnight at 4°C in a moist chamber.
5. Add 25 µl of the test samples positive and negative control into the test plates coated with antibody.
6. Incubate the plate for 2 hours at room temperature.
7. Wash three times with PBS-T and add 50 µl of peroxidase conjugated antibody to each well.
8. Incubate the plates at room temperature for 2 hours and wash five times with PBS-T.
9. Add 100 ml of freshly prepared substrate, i.e. orthophenyldiamine in citrate buffer pH 5.0 and hydrogen peroxide.
10. After 30 minutes incubation at room temperature in a dark box, add 75 µl of 2 M sulfuric acid to stop the reaction.
11. Add 75 µl of PBS to make final volume of reaction mixture as 250 µl.
12. A positive test is indicated by the production of yellow colour as a result of the product of enzyme

reaction. This is read by the naked eye against a white background or by measuring the optical density at 492 nm in a spectrophotometer using a microcuvette ora micro ELISA reader.

Calculations

$$\frac{\text{OD Test} - \text{OD Blank II}}{\text{OD Blank I} - \text{OD Blank II}} = \text{OD of sample} > \text{OD Mean}$$

Interpretation of Results

A sample is labelled positive if the yellow colour is stronger than that of the negative control and if the optical density, measured as the ratio of test to negative control is more than 2:1 (OD of Blank I is the average optical density of 5–7 negative controls and OD of Blank II is the optical density of 100 µl substrate, 75 µl of 2 M sulphuric acid and 75 µl of PBS). A test sample with a ratio between 1.5 and 2.1 is repeated and if the ratio is still less than 2.1, the test should be considered negative.

Advantages of ELISA Technique

1. Simple and easy to perform
2. Sensitivity at low cost
3. Stability of reagents
4. Lack of radiation hazards
5. Potential for automation
6. Relatively inexpensive equipment.

EIA Assays Currently Available

1. Hepatitis	HBs Ag, anti-HBs Ag, anti-HBc Ag, IgM anti-HBc Ag HBe/anti-HBe, anti-HA V anti-delta
2. Cancer	CEA, AFP, beta-HCG, estrogen receptor, TdT, PAP
3. STD	*N. gonorrhoeae* *Chlamydia trachomatis*
4. Infections	Rubella, rotavirus cytomegalovirus, IgE, Toxo-G
5. Metabolic	Ferritin, prealbumin
6. Thyroid	TSH
7. AIDS	HTLV-III

Immunofluorescence

Fluorescent dyes, e.g. fluorescein and auramine, can be covalently attached to antibody molecules and made visible by ultraviolet (UV) light in the fluorescence microscope. Such "labeled" antibody can be used to identify antigens, e.g. on the surface of bacteria (such as streptococci and treponemes), in cells in histologic section, or in other specimens. The immunofluorescence reaction is called direct when known labeled antibody interacts directly with unknown antigen and indirect when a 2-stage process is used (e.g. known antigen is attached to a slide, unknown serum is added, and the preparation is washed; if the unknown serurn antibody matches the antigen, it will remain fixed to it on the slide and can be detected on addition of a fluorescent dye-labeled antiglobulin antibody and examination by UV microscopy). The indirect test is often more sensitive than direct immunofluorescence, because more labeled antibody adheres per antigenic site. Furthermore, the labeled anti-globulin becomes a "universal reagent", i.e. independent of the nature of the antigen used, the antiglobulin is reactive with all IgG of that species.

Radioimmunoassay (RIA) is a highly sensitive and quantitative procedure that utilizes radioactively labeled antigen or antibody.

Radioimmunoassay (RIA)

This method is used for the quantitation of antigens or haptens that can be radioactively labeled. It is based on the competition for specific antibody between the labeled (known) and the unlabeled (unknown) concentration of material. The complexes that form between the antigen and antibody can then be separated and the amount of radioactivity measured. The more unlabeled antigen present, the less radioactivity there is in the complex. The concentration of the unknown (unlabeled) antigen or hapten is determined by comparison with the effect of standards. RIA is a highly sensitive method and is commonly used to assay hormones or drugs in serum. The radioallergosorbent test (RAST) is a specialized RIA that is used to measure the amount of serum IgE antibody that reacts with a known allergen (antigen).

Complement-fixation reactions are serological tests based on the depletion of a fixed amount of complement in the presence of an antigen–antibody reaction and are: (i) Complement fixation test; (ii) Immune adherence test; (ii) Immobilization test; (iv) Cytolytic or cytocidal reactions.

Complement Fixation

The complement system consists of 20 or more plasma proteins that interact with one another and with cell membranes. Each protein component must be activated sequentially under appropriate conditions for the reaction to progress. Antigen–antibody complexes are among the activators, and the complement fixation test can be used to identify one of them if the other is known.

The reaction consists of the following 2 steps (Fig. 58.4): (1) Antigen and antibody (one known and the other unknown) are mixed, and a measured amount of complement (usually from guinea pig) is added. If the antigen and antibody match, they will combine and take up ("fix") the complement. (2) An indicator system, consisting of "sensitised" red blood cells (i.e. red blood cells plus anti-red blood cell antibody), is added. If the antibody matched the antigen in the first step, complement was fixed and less is available to attach to the sensitised red blood cells. The red blood cells remain unhaemolyzed, i.e. the test is positive. If the antibody did not match the antigen in the first step, complement is free to attach to the sensitised red blood cells and they are lysed; i.e. the test is negative.

Complement must be carefully standardized, and the patient's serum must be heated to 56°C for 30 minutes to inactivate any human complement activity. The antigen must be quantitated. The result is expressed as the highest dilution of serum that gives positive results. Controls to determine whether antigen or antibody alone fixes complement are needed to make the test results valid. If antigen or antibody alone fixes complement, it is said to be anticomplementary.

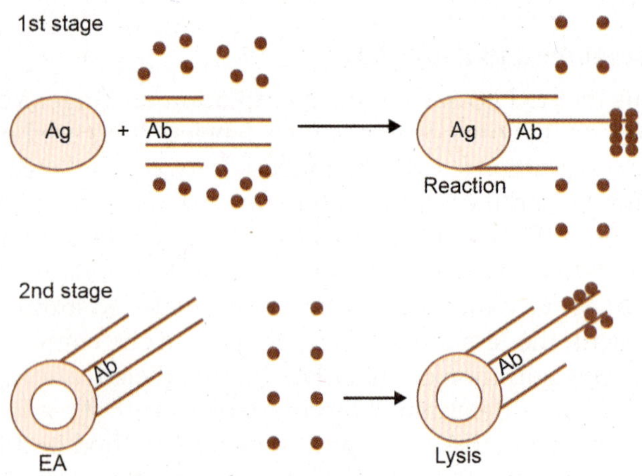

Fig. 58.4: Complement fixation. In the first stage, if the antigen and antibody are homologous, complement (black circles) is fixed. In the second stage, sensitised red cells (EA) are added. If complement was fixed in the first stage, loss complement remains free. Therefore, lysis of EA is reduced.

USEFUL STOCK SOLUTIONS

1. **Ficoll Hypaque**
   - 11.40 g of Ficoll is dissolved in 160 ml of distilled water. Add 40 ml of Conray 280
   - 22 ml of Conray 420
2. **Phosphate Buffers:** (Table 58.1)
   - 0.2 M
     - Solution A—Na_2HPO_4—14.32 g/200 ml.
     - Solution B—KH_2PO_4—5.44 g/200 ml.
   - 0.15 M
     - Solution A—Na_2HPO_4, $12H_2O$—53.70 g/L
     - 30 Solution B—KH_2PO_4—20.41 g/L.

Table 58.1: Phosphate buffer stock solution preparation

S. No.	Solution (A) Ml	Solution (B) Ml	Ph
1.	0.25	9.75	5.29
2.	0.50	9.50	5.59
3.	1.0	9.0	5.91
4.	2.0	8.0	6.24
5.	3.0	7.0	6.47
6.	4.0	6.0	6.64
7.	5.0	5.0	6.81
8.	6.0	4.0	6.98
9.	7.0	3.0	7.17
10.	8.0	2.0	7.38
11.	9.0	1.0	7.73
12.	9.5	0.5	8.04

Contd.

3. **Phosphate buffered saline (PBS) pH 7.2**
   - 18 ml of 0.2 M Solution A
   - 7 ml of 0.2 M Solution B 4.38 g NaCl.
   - Add distilled water to make up to 500 ml. Store in refrigerator. Make a fresh every third day.
4. **Hank's solution:**
   1. 775 ml distilled water in a flask.
   2. Dissolve by shaking after each addition A
      80 g NaCl
      4 g KCl
      2 g Na_2HPO_4, $12H_2O$
      1 g KH_2PO_4
      (Slight heating may be used to dissolve the last two)
   3. To 100 ml distilled water, add 2 g $CaCl_2$, without heating. Add to A—gives B.
   4. To 100 ml distilled water, add 2 g $MgSO_4$, without heating. Add to B—gives C.
   5. Add 20 g glucose to C—gives D (dissolve without heat)
   6. To 25 ml distilled water add 200 mg phenol red. Dissolve by stirring and pulverising. Add to D and make volume to 1000 ml. Filter using a millipore filter. Store in refrigerator. Make a fresh after 2–3 weeks, unless sterile.

      For use dilute 1: 10 in distilled water and adjust pH with $NaHCO_3$ (2.8 g/100 ml).
5. **Alsever's solution:**
   - For storing sheep red cells
   - 24.6 g glucose
   - 9.6 g trisodium citrate (dihydrate)
   - 5.04 g NaCl.
   - Dissolve in 1200 ml distilled water
   - Adjust pH to 6.1 with 10% citric acid.
   - Use 50 ml of Alsever's solution for 50 ml of whole blood.

Chapter 59

Hypersensitivity (Allergy), Tolerance and Autoimmune Disease and Tumour Immunity

Chapter Outline

HYPERSENSITIVITY (ALLERGY)

Introduction

When an immune response results in exaggerated or inappropriate reactions harmful to the host, the term hypersensitivity or allergy is used. These reactions are typical in a given individual and occur upon a second contact with a specific antigen. The first contact sensitizes, i.e. induces the antibody, and then the subsequent contacts elicit the allergic response. Hypersensitivity reactions can be subdivided into 4 main types. Types I, II, and III are antibody mediated, whereas type IV is cell-mediated (Table 59.1).

Table 59.1: Classification hypersensitivity reactions

Mediator	*Type*	*Reaction*
Antibody	I (immediate, anaphylactic)	IgE antibody is induced by allergen and binds via its Fc receptor to mast cells and basophils. After encountering the antigen again, the fixed IgE becomes cross-linked, inducing degranulation and release of mediators, e.g. histamine
Antibody	II (cytotoxic)	Antigens on a cell surface combine with antibody, this leads to complement-mediated lysis, e.g. transfusion or Rh reactions, or autoimmune haemolytic anaemia
Antibody	III (immune complex)	Antigen–antibody immune complexes are deposited in tissues, complement is activated, and polymorphonuclear cells are attracted to the site, causing tissue damage
Cell	IV (delayed)	Helper T lymphocytes sensitised by an antigen release lymphokines upon second contact with the same antigen. The lymphokines induce inflammation and activate macrophages, which, in turn, release various mediators

MECHANISMS OF IMMUNOLOGIC TISSUE INJURY (HYPERSENSITIVITY REACTIONS)

Classification: The immune disorders are classified by the source of antigen are as follows:

Immune disorders classified by source of antigen

Exogenous: Atopic disease (e.g. poison ivy contact dermatitis; reactions to plant pollens, sera and drugs).

Homologous: Reactions to isoantigens (e.g. transfusion reaction, erythroblastosis foetalis, transplant rejection).

Autologous: Autoimmune diseases (e.g. systemic lupus erythematosus, rheumatoid arthritis, Sjögren's syndrome).

The second classification is based on the mechanisms of immunologically mediated disorders as follows:

It occurs as a systemic disorder or a local reaction.

Systemic reaction: It usually follows an intravenous injection of an antigen to which host has already become sensitised. This often leads to a state of shock, which is sometimes fatal.

Local reaction: It depends on the portal of entry of the allergen and takes the form of localized cutaneous reaction, conjunctival discharge, nasal discharge or bronchial asthma or food allergy.

TYPE I: IMMEDIATE (ANAPHYLACTIC) HYPERSENSITIVITY

An antigen induces the formation of IgE antibody, which binds firmly by its Fc portion to basophils and mast cells. Re-exposure to the same antigen results in cross-linking of the cell-bound IgE, and release of pharmacologically active mediators within minutes ("immediate reaction"). Cyclic nucleotides and calcium play essential roles in release of the mediators*. The reactivity can be transmitted by serum but not by cells. No single mediator accounts for all the manifestations of anaphylaxis. Some important mediators and their effects are as follows:

Mediators of Type I Reaction: Type I reactions are mediated by IgE antibodies produced by lymphocytes and plasma cells in response to an allergen. Once released, IgE antibodies attach to mast cells and basophils through cell surface receptors. Once attached, these cells release a variety of powerful vasoactive mediators after a series of reactions which are shown as follows:

Primary mediators released	*Secondary mediators*
1. Histamine	1. Arachidonic acid metabolites
2. Eosinophil chemotactic factor of anaphylaxis (ECE-A)	2. Leukotrienes
3. Neutrophilic chemotactic factor	3. Platelet activating factors (PAF)
4. Neutral proteases	

1. Histamine occurs in platelets and in granules of tissue mast cells and basophils in a preformed state. Its release causes vasodilatation, increased capillary permeability, and smooth-muscle contraction. Clinically, disorders such as allergic rhinitis (hay fever), urticaria, and angioedema can occur. The bronchospasm so prominent in acute anaphylaxis is due, in part, to histamine release. Anti-histamine drugs can block histamine receptor sites and can be relatively effective in allergic rhinitis but not in asthma (*see* below).
2. Slow-reacting substance of anaphylaxis (SRS-A) consists of several leukotrienes, which do not exist in a preformed state but are produced during anaphylactic reactions. This accounts for the slow onset of the effect of SRS-A. Leukotrienes are formed from arachidonic acid by the lipoxygenase pathway and cause increased vascular permeability and smooth-muscle contraction. They are the principal mediators in the bronchoconstriction of asthma and are not influenced by anti-histamines.
3. Eosinophil chemotactic factor of anaphylaxis (ECF-A) is a tetrapeptide that exists preformed in mast cell granules. When released during anaphylaxis, it attracts eosinophils that are prominent in immediate allergic reactions.
4. Serotonin (hydroxytryptamine) is preformed in mast cells and blood platelets. When released during anaphylaxis, it causes capillary dilation, increased vascular permeability, and smooth-muscle contraction but is of minor importance in human anaphylaxis.
5. Prostaglandins and thromboxanes are related to leukotrienes. They are derived from arachidonic acid via the cyclooxygenase pathway. Prostaglandins cause dilation and increased permeability of capillaries and bronchoconstriction. Thromboxanes aggregate platelets.

The above-mentioned mediators are active only for some minutes after release; they are enzymatically inactivated and resynthesized slowly. Manifestations of anaphylaxis vary among species.

Because mediators are released at different rates in different amounts and tissues vary in their sensitivity to them. For example, the respiratory tract (bronchospasm, laryngeal edema) is a principal shock organ in humans but the liver (hepatic veins) plays that role in dogs.

Reactions of systemic anaphylaxis: After administration of heterologous proteins, e.g. antisera, penicillin, enzymes, within minutes there is itching, hives, skin erythema followed shortly by contraction of respiratory bronchioles leading to respiratory distress. There is vomiting, diarrhoea, laryngeal obstruction leading to shock and death.

Reactions to local anaphylaxis: These are exemplified by atopic reaction which is defined as a genetically controlled predisposition to the production of specific IgE antibodies upon inhalation or ingestion of minute amounts of antigen like pollen, dust, animal dander, etc. Specific diseases like urticaria, allergic rhinitis, angio-oedema and bronchial asthma.

Atopy

Atopic disorders are immediate-hypersensitivity reactions that exhibit a strong familial predisposition and are associated with elevated IgE levels. The predisposition to atopy is genetic, and symptoms are induced by exposure to the specific allergens. These antigens are typically found in the environment (e.g. pollens and house dust) or in foods (e.g. shellfish and nuts). Exposure of nonatopic individuals to these substances does not elicit an allergic reaction. Common clinical manifestations include hay fever, asthma, eczema, and urticaria. Many sufferers give immediate-type reactions to skin tests (injection, patch, or scratch) containing the offending antigen.

Atopic hypersensitivity is transferable by serum, not by lymphoid cells. In the past, this observation was used for diagnosis in the passive cutaneous anaphylaxis (Prausnitz-Küstner) reaction, which consists of taking serum from the patient and injecting it into the skin of a normal person. Some hours later the test antigen, injected into the "sensitised" site, will yield an immediate wheal-and-flare reaction. This test is now impractical because of the danger of transmitting certain viral infections. Radioallergosorbent tests (RAST) permit the identification

(*An increase in cyclic GMP within these cells increases mediator release, whereas an increase in cyclic AMP decreases release. Therefore, drugs that increase intracellular cyclic AMP, such as epinephrine, are used to treat type I reactions. Epinephrine also has sympathomimetic activity, which is useful in treating type I reactions.)

of specific IgE against potentially offending allergens if suitable specific antigens for *in vitro* tests are available.

The cause of atopy is speculative. Reduced number of suppressor T cells and abnormal "mediator feedback" have been proposed, as well as a predisposition to an abnormally high IgE response.

Drug Hypersensitivity

Drugs, particularly antimicrobial agents, are now among the most common causes of hypersensitivity reactions. Usually it is not the intact drug that induces antibody formation. Rather, a metabolic product of the drug, which acts as a hapten and binds to a body protein, does so. The resulting antibody can react with the hapten or the intact drug to give rise to type I hypersensitivity. When re-exposed to the drug, the person may exhibit rashes, fevers, or local or systemic anaphylaxis of varying severity. Reactions to very small amounts of the drug can occur, e.g. in a skin test with the hapten. A clinically useful example is the skin test using penicilloyl-polylysine to reveal an allergy to penicillin.

Desensitization

Major manifestations of anaphylaxis occur when large amounts of mediators are suddenly released as a result of a massive dose of antigen abruptly combining with IgE on many mast cells. This is systemic anaphylaxis, which is potentially fatal. Desensitization can prevent systemic anaphylaxis.

Acute desensitization involves the administration of very small amounts of antigen at 15 minutes intervals. This causes small-scale formation of complexes and not enough mediator release to produce a major reaction. This permits the administration of a drug or foreign protein to a hypersensitive person, but hypersensitivity is restored days or weeks later.

Chronic desensitization involves the long-term administration at weekly intervals of the antigen to which the person is hypersensitive. This stimulates the production of IgG-blocking antibodies in the serum, which can prevent subsequent antigen from reaching IgE on mast cells, thus preventing a reaction.

TYPE II: CYTOTOXIC HYPERSENSITIVITY

This type is mediated by antibodies directed toward antigens present on the surface of cells or other tissue components. The antigenic determinants may be intrinsic to the cell membrane or extrinsic adsorbed on the cell surface. In either case the reaction takes place by the binding of antibody to normal or altered cell surface antigens. There are two antibody dependent mechanisms as follows:

1. **Complement mediated cytotoxicity:** In this reaction, antibody (IgM or IgG) reacts with an antigen present on the surface of the cell, causing activation of complement system and resulting in direct membrane damage and lysis. At the same time, the antibody coated cells become susceptible to phagocytosis example of such reaction is seen in Goodpasture disease, autoimmune haemolytic anaemia and erythroblastosis foetalis.
2. **Antibody dependent cell mediated cytotoxicity (ADCC):** In this, the target cells coated with IgG antibody can be killed by a variety of non-sensitised cells that have Fc receptors. This is carried out by K cells, eosinophils, neutrophils and monocytes which bind to the target cell by the receptor for Fc fragment of IgG and carry out lysis without phagocytosis.
   This mechanism has been studied *in vitro* and whether it plays role *in vivo* is not known.
3. **Chemotactic factors:** These are for neutrophils, eosinophils, basophils, monocytes and other lymphocytes.
4. **Interleukin-2:** This substance also called T cells growth factor is produced by antigen of mitogen activated T cells. It, in turn, causes proliferation of the T cells involved in mediating cellular immunity.
5. **Transfer factor:** This is an ill-defined substance present only in humans, which has the ability to transfer delayed hypersensitivity and enables to prepare the non-sensitised lymphocytes to respond to specific antigen without preparing the host to make antibody against the same antigen. The exact mechanism is not known, but it is postulated to be a single-stranded polynucleotide which either is informational or may provide some part of a receptor for antigen.

Antibody directed at antigens of the cell membrane activates complement and damages those cells. The antibody (IgG or IgM) attaches to the antigen via the Fab region and acts as a bridge to complement via the Fc region. As a result, there may be complement-mediated lysis as in haemolytic anaemias, ABO transfusion reactions, or Rh haemolytic disease. In addition to causing lysis, complement activation can attract phagocytes to the site, with consequent release of enzymes that damage cell membranes.

Drugs (e.g. penicillins, phenacetin, quinidine) can attach to surface proteins on red blood cells and initiate antibody formation. Such autoimmune antibodies (IgG) then may combine with the cell surface and result in haemolysis.

TYPE III: IMMUNE-COMPLEX HYPERSENSITIVITY

This type of hypersensitivity reaction is induced by antigen–antibody complexes that produce tissue damage as a result of their capacity to activate a variety of serum mediators, principally complement system and biologically active fragments, e.g. kinins. The toxic reaction is initiated when antigen combines with antibody, either within the circulation (circulating immune complexes) or at extravascular sites (*in situ* immune complexes).

There are two types of antigens that cause such reaction.

Exogenous antigen, e.g. foreign protein, bacteria, viruses.

Edogenous antigen: In which the individual can produce antibody against its own body component.

When antibody and antigen coexist, immune complexes are formed. Normally, they are promptly removed by the reticuloendothelial system, but occasionally they persist and are deposited in tissues, resulting in several disorders. In persistent microbial or viral infections, immune complexes may be deposited in organs, e.g. the kidneys, resulting in dysfunction. In autoimmune disorders, "self" antigens may elicit antibodies that bind to organ antigens or deposit in organs as complexes, especially in joints (arthritis), kidneys (nephritis), or blood vessels (vasculitis). Wherever immune complexes are deposited, they activate the complement system. Polymorphonuclear cells are attracted to the site, and inflammation and tissue injury occur. Two typical type III hypersensitivity reactions are the arthus reaction and serum sickness.

Arthus Reaction

If animals are given an antigen repeatedly until they have high levels of precipitating IgG antibody and that antigen is then injected subcutaneously or intradermally, intense oedema and haemorrhage develop, reaching a peak in 3–6 hours. Antigen, antibody, and complement are deposited in vessel walls; polymorphonuclear cell infiltration and intravascular clumping of platelets then occur. These reactions can lead to vascular occlusion and necrosis. A likely clinical counterpart of the Arthus reaction is hypersensitivity pneumonitis (allergic alveolitis) associated with the inhalation of thermophilic actinomycetes ("farmer's lung").

Serum Sickness

Following the injection of foreign serum (or certain drugs), the antigen is excreted slowly. During this time, antibody production starts. The simultaneous presence of antigen and antibody leads to the formation of immune complexes, which may circulate or be deposited at various sites. Typical serum sickness results in fever, urticaria, arthralgia, lymphadenopathy, and splenomegaly a few days to 2 weeks after injection of the foreign serum. Although it takes several days for symptoms to appear, serum sickness is classed as an immediate reaction because symptoms occur promptly after immune complexes form. Symptoms improve as the immune elimination of the antigen continues and subside when it is complete. Nowadays, serum sickness is caused more commonly by drugs, e.g. penicillin. than by foreign serum because foreign serum is used so infrequently.

IMMUNE-COMPLEX DISEASES

Many clinical disorders associated with immune complexes have been described, although the antigen is often in doubt. Several representative examples are described below.

A. **Glomerulonephritis:** Acute post-streptococcal glomerulonephritis is a well-accepted immune complex disease. Its onset follows several weeks after a group A beta-haemolytic streptococcal infection, particularly of the skin, and often with nephritogenic serotypes of *Streptococcus pyogenes*. Typically, the complement level is low, suggesting an antigen–antibody reaction. Lumpy deposits of immunoglobulin and C3 are seen along glomerular basement membranes by immunofluorescence, suggesting the presence of antigen–antibody complexes, although streptococcal antigens have rarely been demonstrated. It is assumed that streptococcal antigen–antibody complexes, after being filtered out by glomeruli, fix complement, attract polymorphs, and start the inflammatory process. Similar lesions with "lumpy" deposits containing immunoglobulin and C3 occur in infective endocarditis, serum sickness, and certain viral infections, e.g. hepatitis B and dengue haemorrhagic fever. Lesions containing immune complexes also occur in the nephritis of systemic lupus erythematosus, where the "lumpy" deposits contain DNA as the antigen.

B. **Arthritis:** Rheumatoid arthritis is a chronic inflammatory joint disease, especially of young women. Serum and synovial fluid of patients contain "rheumatoid factor," i.e. IgM and IgG antibodies that bind to the Fc fragment of normal human IgG. It is assumed that there are deposits of immune complexes (containing the normal lgG and rheumatoid factor) on synovial membranes and in blood vessels that activate complement and attract polymorphonuclear cells, causing inflammation. Patients have high titers of rheumatoid factor and low titers of complement in serum during active rheumatoid disease.

C. **Autoimmune disease:** In many autoimmune diseases, antigen–antibody complexes related to the organ site of activity (e.g. thyroid hormone receptors and acetylcholine receptors) have been demonstrated.

TYPE IV: DELAYED (CELL-MEDIATED) HYPERSENSITIVITY

Delayed hypersensitivity is a function of helper (CD_4) T lymphocytes, not antibody. It can be transferred by immunologically committed (sensitised) T cells, not by serum. The response is "delayed"; i.e. it starts hours (or days) after contact with the antigen and often lasts for days. It consists mainly of mononuclear cell infiltration (macrophages and helper (CD_4 T cells) and tissue induration, as typified by the tuberculin skin test.

This type of hypersensitivity is initiated by specifically sensitised T lymphocytes. It induces the classic delayed hypersensitivity reactions and cell mediated cytotoxic reactions.

i. **Delayed hypersensitivity:** The type of reaction is initiated by specifically sensitised T lymphocytes generated during the initial contact with antigen, some of the memory cells remain in the circulation for a long time. When the individual is re-exposed to the specific antigen, e.g. tuberculin, T lymophocytes are stimulated to divide and release a variety of biologically active molecules K/a lymphokines. The lymphokines amplify the inflammatory response by recruiting inflammatory cells, activating them and keeping them it site. The most important result is stimulation and activation of macrophages within the lesion which further cause tissue damage and inflammatory reactions. Example of this type of reaction is tuberculin reaction, mantoux test (MX-test).

ii. **T cell-mediated cytotoxicity:** The process of CTLs is complex and ill understood. They however, once sensitised, kill the antigen bearing target cells. This group of T cells are characterised by the presence of OK T5/T8 antigens on their surface. The CTL after causing lysis of the target cell, survives the encounter and is then recycled to kill other target cells.

This CTL mediated lysis is highly specific and the cells are not affected. It is now clear that this specificity is due to the presence of cell surface HLA antigens by which CTLs recognize their target cells. It is suggested that the infection of the cell with the antigen, e.g. virus, changes the cell surface HLA antigen, which is different from the normal self HLA antigen, so as to evoke the CTIS, capable of recognizing altered self and thereby kill the virus infected target cell, e.g. transplant rejection reaction.

Clinically Important Delayed Hypersensitivity Reactions

A. **Contact hypersensitivity:** This manifestation of cell-mediated hypersensitivity occurs after sensitization with simple chemicals (e.g. nickel, formaldehyde), plant materials (e.g. poison ivy, poison oak), topically, applied drugs (e.g. sulfonamides, neomycin), some cosmetics, soaps, and other substances. In all cases, the small molecules acting us haptens, enter the skin, attach to body proteins, and become complete antigens. Cell-mediated hypersensitivity is induced, particularly in the skin. Upon a later skin contact with the offending agent, the sensitised person develops erythema itching, vesication, eczema, or necrosis of skin within 12–48 hours. Patch testing on a small area of skin can sometimes identify the offending antigen. Subsequent avoidance of the material will prevent recurrences.

B. **Tuberculin-type hypersensitivity:** Delayed-type hypersensitivity to antigens of micro-organisms occurs in many infectious diseases and has been used as an aid in diagnosis. It is typified by the tuberculin reaction. When a patient previously exposed to *Mycobacterium tuberculosis* is injected with a small amount of tuberculin in the epidermis, there is a little reaction in the first few hours. Gradually, however, induration and redness develop and reach a peak in 48–72 hours. A positive skin test indicates that the person has been infected with the agent, but it does not confirm the presence of current disease. However, if the skin test converts from negative to positive, it suggests recent infection and possible current activity. Infected persons do not always have a positive skin test, because overwhelming infection, disorders that suppress cell-mediated immunity (e.g. uraemia, measles, sarcoidosis, lymphoma, and AIDS), or the administration of immunosuppressive drugs (e.g. corticosteroids, antineoplastics) may cause anergy.

A positive skin test response assists in diagnosis and provides support for chemoprophylaxis or chemotherapy. In leprosy, a positive lepromin test indicates the presence of tuberculoid leprosy with competent cell-mediated immunity, whereas a negative lepromin test suggests the presence of lepromatous leprosy with impaired cell-mediated immunity. In systemic mycotic infections (e.g. coccidioidomycosis and histoplasmosis), a positive delayed-type skin test with the specific antigen indicates exposure to the organism. Cell-mediated hypersensitivity develops in many viral infections, however, serologic tests are more specific than skin tests both for diagnosis and for assessment of immunity. In protozoan and helminthic infections, skin tests may be positive but they are generally not as useful as specific serologic tests.

Clinical Laboratory Methods for Detection of Cellular Immune Function

The immune system in humans can be divided into 2 major parts, one involving humoral immunity (antibody and complement) and the other immuno-competent cells, i.e cellular immunity. The present chapter reviews the tests that have medical application in the detection of cellular immune function. This is studied through the following tests:

1. Delayed hypersensitivity skin tests.
2. Lymphocyte transformation test.
3. Assays for T and B lymphocytes.
4. Neutrophil function.

1. Delayed Hypersensitivity Skin Tests (PPD-MX test)

Principle: The tests is based on recall of T lymphocyte immunologic memory and thus overall T lymphocyte function is assessed. The postulated sequence of events leading to the appearance of the delayed hypersensitivity type skin test is that circulating T lymophocytes come into contact with antigen (mainly held by skin macrophages) and presensitised cells present are stimulated to lymphokine production and blast cell transformation. The lymphokines encourage the trapping of circulating mononuclear cells at the site of antigen and the activation of nonsensitised by stander cells into the reaction. A cascade effect is produced with increasing localization of mononuclear cells which is clinically manifest as induration. Local persistence of antigen favours the production of a more vigorous response and vica versa. Thus, subcutaneous (instead of intradermal) injection of antigen result in its rapid removal before a local response is apparent. The presence of oedema of the skin will result in false negative results due to increased lymphatic clearance of antigen.

Method: The volar aspect of the forearm is the most convenient site for testing.

1. Prepare the arm by shaving and cleaning with isopropyl alcohol, finally drying thoroughly with a sterile swab.
2. Mark out the area to be tested with the code numbers of the antigens to be tested with a skin pencil or suitable non-washable marker (e.g. ball-point pen).
3. Inject the appropriate antigen solution using a disposable syringe. The skin is stretched taut with the free hand and then, with the needle of the syringe at a very shallow angel with the bevel uppermost, the needle is introduced, intradermally. Care should be taken not to inject subcutaneously causing bleeding, or not to penetrate enough resulting in an exit puncture and leakage of antigen solution over the skin. Once the needle is in place the solution is gently injected and the skin should blanch and a small bleb is rainsed. Some of the antigen solution are painful on injection and the subject should be warned in advance to obviate inadvertent movements of the arm. When the needle is withdrawn, ideally there should be no bleeding at the site of injection indicating that dermal vessels have not been punctured. There may occasionally be very slight blood leakage with good technique but persistent oozing suggests that the injection has been subcutaneous and not intradermal; a false negative result may thus be obtained.
4. The test sites are examined 48 hours later. If problems are expected in distinguishing Arthus reactions, the tests can be read at 6 and 24 hours.
5. Both erythema and induration are measured in mm. The response is not always symmetrical and irregular induration can be measured in two directions at right angles and the result averaged. A positive response is conventionally assessed as one giving 7.5 mm induration. Response can be graded with 3–4 mm = ±, 5–8 mm = +, 9–11 mm = ++, 12 mm or more = + + + +.

Comments

There are no normal values as such available for skin test responses and there is very little information as to the percentage of normal population responding to the various antigens. It is for this reason that a battery of antigens is used with the expectation that, at least one positive result indicates normal cell mediated immunity. It is conventional to mesure a positive response as one with 5 mm or more of induration, although again information is lacking as to the normal range of induration in those giving a positive response.

Tests for Evaluation of Cell-mediated Immunity

Evaluation of the immunocompetence of persons depends either on the demonstration of delayed-type hypersensitivity to universally present antigens (equating the ability to respond with the competence of cell-mediated immunity) or on laboratory assessments of T cells.

Skin tests for the presence of delayed-type hypersensitivity: Most normal persons respond with delayed-type reactions to skin test antigens of *Candida*, streptokinase streptodornase, or mumps because of past exposure to these antigens. Absence of reactions to several of these skin tests suggests impairrnent of cell-mediated immunity.

Skin tests for the ability to develop delayed-type hypersensitivity: Most normal persons with competent cell-mediated reactions can readily develop reactivity to simple chemicals (e.g. dinitrochlorobenzene; DNCB) applied to their skin in lipid solvents. When the same chemical is applied to the same area 7–14 days later, they respond with a delayed-type skin reaction. Immunocompromised persons with incompetent cell-mediated immunity fail to develop such delayed-type hypersensitivity.

In Vitro Tests for Lymphoid Cell Competence

A. **Lymphocyte blast transformation:** When sensitised T lymphocytes are exposed to the specific antigen, they transform into large blast cells with greatly increased DNA synthesis, as measured by incorporation of tritiated thymidine. This specific effect involves relatively few cells. A larger number of T cells undergo nonspecific blast transformation when exposed to certain mitogens. The mitogens phytohemagglutinin and concanavalin A are plant extracts that stimulate T cells specifically. (Bacterial endotoxin, a lipopolysaccharide, stimulates B cells specifically.)

B. **Macrophage migration inhibitory factor:** Macrophage migration inhibitory factor is elaborated by cultured T cells when exposed to the antigen to which they are sensitised. Its effect can be measured by observing the reduced migration of macrophages in the presence of the factor compared with the level in controls.

TOLERANCE

Tolerance is specific immunologic unresponsiveness, i.e. an immune response to a certain antigen (or epitope) does not occur, although the immune system is otherwise functioning normally. In general, antigens that are present during embryonic life are considered "self" and do not stimulate an immunologic response. The lack of an immune response is the result of the deletion of self-reactive T cell precursors in the thymus. On the other hand, antigens that are not present during the process of maturation, i.e. that are encountered first when the body is immunologically mature, are considered "nonself" and usually elicit an immunologic response.

The main process by which T lymphocytes acquire the ability to distinguish self from nonself occurs in the foetal thymus. This process, called clonal deletion, involves the removal of T cells that react against antigens present in the fetus at that time. (Note that exogenous substances injected into the fetus early in development are treated as self.) The mechanism of this "negative selection" is unknown. A second process which also plays a role is clonal inactivation (clonal anergy). This process, which can occur outside the thymus, involves functional inactivation of certain T cells. The mechanism of clonal anergy is also unknown but may involve suppressor cells or inappropriate presentation of antigen, leading to a failure of interleukin-2 production. Whether an antigen will induce tolerance rather than an immunologic response is largely determined by the following:

1. The immunologic maturity of the host; e.g. neonatal animals are immunologically immature and will accept allografts that would be rejected by mature animals.
2. The structure and dose of the antigen, e.g. a very simple molecule induces tolerance more readily than a complex one, and very high or very low doses of antigen may result in tolerance instead of an immune response. Purified polysaccharides or amino acid copolymers injected in very large doses result in "immune paralysis"—a lack of response.

Other aspects of the induction or maintenance of tolerance are as follows:

1. T cells become tolerant more readily and remain tolerant longer than B cells.
2. Administration of a cross-reacting antigen tends to terminate tolerance.
3. Administration of immunosuppressive drugs enhances tolerance, e.g. in transplants.
4. Tolerance is maintained best if the antigen continues to be present.

Autoimmune Diseases

The adult host usually exhibits tolerance to tissue antigens present during foetal life that are recognised as "self." However, in certain circumstances tolerance may be lost and immune reactions may develop to host antigens, resulting in autoimmune diseases. Either humoral or cell-mediated reactions can be involved, but most are antibody-mediated. Many autoimmune diseases exhibit a marked familial incidence, which suggests a genetic predisposition to these disorders. There is a strong association of some diseases with certain human leukocyte antigen (HLA) specificities, especially the class II genes. For example, rheumatoid arthritis occurs predominantly in individuals carrying the HLA-DR4 gene.

Diseases: Some examples of diseases that involve autoimmune reactions are described below.

A. **Allergic encephalitis:** This is due to a cell-mediated response to the basic protein of brain myelin. For example, when animal brain substance, mixed with adjuvant, is injected into an animal of the same species, a demyelinating encephalitis develops. It resembles postvaccinal encephalitis seen in persons injected with older rabies vaccines made in rabbit brains. Rarely, it occurs following certain viral infections, e.g. measles or influenza, or following immunizations against these viral infections.

B. **Chronic thyroiditis:** When animals are injected with thyroid gland material, they develop humoral and cell-mediated immunity against thyroid antigens and a chronic thyroiditis. Humans with Hashimoto's chronic thyroiditis have antibodies to thyroglobulin, suggesting that these antibodies may provoke an inflammatory process that leads to fibrosis of the gland.

C. **Rheumatic fever:** Group A streptococcal infections regularly precede the development of rheumatic fever. Cross-reactions occur between cell membrane antigens of streptococci and human heart muscle sarcolemma, which may play a causative role in disease.

D. **Haemolytic anaemias, thrombocytopenias, and granulocytopenias:** Various forms of these disorders have been attributed to the attachment of autoantibodies to cell surfaces and subsequent cell destruction. Pernicious anaemia is caused by an autoimmune reaction to intrinsic factor, a protein secreted by parietal cells of the stomach that facilitates the absorption of vitamin B_{12} idiopathic thrombocytopenic purpura is due to antibody directed against platelets.

E. **Diabetes, myasthenia gravis, and hyperthyroidism (Graves' disease):** In these diseases, antibodies to receptors play a pathogenic role. In extreme insulin resistance in diabetes, antibodies to insulin receptors have been demonstrated that interfere with insulin binding. In my asthenia gravis (a nervous system disease), antibodies to acetylcholine receptors of neuromuscular junctions occur in the serum. Some patients with Graves' disease have circulating antibodies to thyrotropin receptors, which, when they bind to the receptors, resemble thyrotropin in activity and stimulate the thyroid to produce more thyroxine.

F. **Systemic lupus erythematosus (SLE), rheumatoid arthritis, and other collagen vascular diseases:** These disorders feature vasculitis and collagen degeneration plus a variety of focal inflammatory lesions and the presence of autoantibodies against many different "self" antigens. For example, antibodies to DNA are found in SLE and antibodies to IgG (rheumatoid factor) occur in rheumatoid arthritis. Complement levels are low, and the nephritis associated with these disorders appears to be an immune-complex disease. Although the causes of these disorders are unknown, typical cases have followed sensitization by drugs, foreign proteins, and other immune stimuli.

Mechanisms: The following mechanisms for autoimmunity have been proposed.

A. **Release of sequestered antigens:** Certain tissues, e.g. sperm, central nervous system, and the lens and uveal tract of the eye, are sequestered so that their antigens are not exposed to the immune system. When such antigens enter the circulation accidentally, e.g. after damage, they elicit both humoral and cellular responses, producing aspermatogenesis, encephalitis, or endophthalmitis, respectively.

B. **Escape of tolerance at the T cell level:** Unresponsiveness to a "self" antigen may be maintained by tolerance at the T cell level. Such tolerance may be terminated by cross-reactions, i.e. when the host responds to antigens that cross-react with tolerated "self" antigens. For example, in rheumatic fever, antibodies against streptococcal antigens cross-react with heart tissue antigens.

C. **Diminished suppressor T cell function:** In normal immune regulation, suppressor T cells may limit an immune response to "self" antigens. If suppressor T cell functions decrease, antibodies to "self" antigens, e.g. an antibody to normal IgG, may be formed. Such antibody (IgM or IgG) occurs in rheumatoid arthritis, in which antigen–antibody complexes form in joints.

Tumour Immunity

Tumour-associated Antigens

Animals carrying a chemically or virally induced malignant tumour can develop resistance to that tumour and cause its regression. In the course of neoplastic transformation, **new antigens**, called tumour-associated antigens (TAA), develop at the cell surface and the host recognizes such cells as "nonself." In chemically induced tumours in experimental animals, TAAs are highly specific, i.e. cells of one tumour will have different TAAS from those on cells of another tumour even when they arise within the same animal. In contrast, virally induced tumours possess TAAs that cross-react with one another if induced by the same virus. TAAS on tumour cells induced by different viruses do not cross-react.

Mechanism of Tumour Immunity

Cell-mediated reactions attack these "nonself" tumour cells and limit their proliferation. Such immune responses probably act as a surveillance system to detect and eliminate newly arising clones of neoplastic cells. In general, the immune response against tumour cells is weak and can be overcome experimentally by a large dose of tumour cells. Some tumour cells can escape surveillance by "modulation," i.e. internalizing the surface antigen so that it no longer presents a target for immune attack. The cell-mediated immune responses that affect tumour cells *in vitro* include natural killer (NK) cells, which act without antibody, killer (K) cells, which mediate antibody-dependent cytolysis (antibody-dependent cellular cytotoxicity), cytotoxic T cells; and activated macrophages. Whether these immune responses function to prevent or control tumours *in vivo* is unknown.

Tumour antigens can stimulate the development of specific antibodies as well. Some of these antibodies are cytotoxic, but others enhance tumour growth, perhaps by blocking recognition of tumour antigens by the host. Spontaneously arising human tumours may have new cell surface antigens against which the host develops both cytotoxic antibodies and cell-mediated immune responses. Enhancement of these responses at times permits containment of some tumours. For example, the administration of BCG vaccine (bacillus Calmette-Guérin, a bovine mycobacterium) into surface melanomas can lead to their partial regression. Immunomodulators, such as interleukins and interferons, are also being tested in such settings. One interleukin, tumour necrosis factor (cachectin), is experimentally effective against a variety of solid tumours. In addition, lymphocytes activated by interleukin-2 (lymphokine-activated killer (LAK) cells) may be useful in cancer immunotherapy.

Carcinoembryonic Antigen and Alpha-Fetoprotein

Some human tumours contain antigens that normally occur in foetal but not in adult human cells.

a. Carcinoembryonic antigen circulates at elevated levels in the serum of many patients with carcinoma of the colon, pancreas, breast, or liver. It is found in foetal gut, liver, and pancreas and in very small amounts in normal sera. Detection of this antigen (by radioimmunoassay) is not helpful in diagnosis but may be helpful in management of such tumours. If the level declines after surgery, it suggests that the tumour is not spreading. Conversely, a rise in the level of carcinoembryonic antigen in patients with resected carcinoma of the colon suggests recurrence or spread of the tumour.

b. Alpha-fetoprotein is present at elevated levels in the sera of hepatoma patients and is used as a marker for this disease. It is produced by foetal liver and is found in small amounts in some normal sera. It is, however, nonspecific; it occurs in several other malignant and nonmalignant diseases.

Monoclonal antibodies directed against new surface antigens on malignant cells (e.g. B cell lymphomas) can be useful in diagnosis. Some day, such antibodies might carry toxic chemicals specifically to such cells and be useful for therapy.

Index

I

K

L

M

U

V

Y

Z